Textbook of Pharmacotherapy for Child and Adolescent Psychiatric Disorders

Textbook of Pharmacotherapy for Child and Adolescent Psychiatric Disorders

David R. Rosenberg, M.D.
John Holttum, M.D.
Samuel Gershon, M.D.

University of Pittsburgh Medical Center

Brunner/Mazel *Publishers* • New York

Note: With dramatic advances continually being made in the clinical sciences, it is a challenge for physicians to keep abreast of both modifications in treatment that such advances require and of new drugs being introduced each year. The authors and publisher of this volume have taken care to make certain that the doses of drugs, schedules of treatment, and routes of administration are correct and compatible with the standards generally accepted at the time of publication. However, it is essential for the reader to become fully cognizant of the information on the instruction inserts provided with each drug or therapeutic agent prior to administration or prescription.

Library of Congress Cataloging-in-Publication Data

Rosenberg, David R.
    Textbook of pharmacotherapy for child and adolescent psychiatric
disorders / David R. Rosenberg, John Holttum, Samuel Gershon.
        p.   cm.
    Includes bibliographical references and index.
    ISBN 0-87630-740-3
    1. Pediatric psychopharmacology.   I. Holttum, John.   II. Gershon,
Samuel.   III. Title.
    [DNLM: 1. Psychotropic Drugs—therapeutic use.   2. Psychotropic
Drugs—pharmacology.   3. Mental Disorders—drug therapy.   4. Mental
Disorders—in infancy & childhood.   5. Mental Disorders—in
adolescence.   QV 77 R8134t 1994]
RJ504.7.R68   1994
618.92′8918—dc20
DNLM/DLC
for Library of Congress   94-6401
                                                                        CIP

Published by
BRUNNER/MAZEL, INC.
19 Union Square West
New York, New York 10003

Manufactured in the United States of America

10 9 8 7 6 5 4 3 2 1

Contents

Foreword

Less that 30 years ago, it was possible to write a foreword to a monograph on psychopharmacology stating that the subject had come of age, and that it was appropriate to have an overall perspective on psychopharmacology in adulthood. Now the time has come for the publication of a comprehensive, yet appropriately skeptical, first textbook on pediatric psychopharmacology. One might ask, "Do we know enough about psychiatric disorders in childhood and adolescents? Are sufficient diagnostic criteria available in these areas? Is there a critical mass of clinical trials and overall empirical data to justify such an effort?" The answers to these questions are resoundingly Yes.

Drs. Rosenberg, Holttum, and Gershon have developed a seminal book on psychopharmacology in childhood and adolescents. They have provided in this textbook a first opportunity for childhood specialists to find in one place the necessary and essential guidelines for psychopharmacologic intervention in childhood and adolescent disorders. The authors are to be complimented on their appropriate level of skepticism in compiling such a comprehensive manual. As they indicate, this area of clinical research is undergoing a developmental phase, but it would be one's hope that such a book will stimulate further investigation and clinical use of psychopharmacologic agents in these populations.

Since the diagnostic rubric has been substantial enough in these areas, clinicians should feel more comfortable with utilizing these agents in their treatment approaches. I found this book so interesting that I am already awaiting the next edition. I am convinced that just as in the adult disorders, further progress in psychopharmacology will be stimulated when researchers realize the extent of the work that has already taken place. In the next decade, it is likely that we will learn much more about the psychopharmacologic agents currently available and their application, and also that newer agents designed primarily for childhood and adolescent disorders will become available. It is that recognition that leads one to be optimistic about the future successful treatment of these disorders. The range of psychotropic drugs covered in this review is extensive, and includes psychostimulants, tricyclic antidepressants, monoamine oxidase inhibitors, antipsychotics, lithium carbonate, anticonvulsants, anxiolytics, and antihypertensive medications when utilized for psychotropic reasons. In a similar fashion, a number of other adjunctive agents are covered.

In summary, the reader will find this book user friendly, easy to follow, and clearly a resource that one will want to keep chained to one's desk so that colleagues are not tempted to borrow it permanently. Those who can benefit by reading it include all physicians working with childhood and adolescence disorders, as well as all clinical specialists who are involved in the diagnosis and treatment of such disorders.

David J. Kupfer, M.D.

Preface

Although psychotropic medications have been a major therapeutic tool in the treatment of adults with mental illness for the past four decades, the use of these agents in the treatment of children and adolescents with psychiatric disorders is as young as the patients themselves. One reason is that, until recently, specific psychiatric diagnoses were not well defined or characterized in the pediatric population. However, we now know that the presentation in children of many psychiatric illnesses, such as mood disorders, is quite similar to that seen in adults. We also know that these disorders, if seen first in childhood or adolescence, are likely to respond to the same treatments that are effective in adults, with appropriate modifications.

A second reason that pediatric psychopharmacology is still very much in the developmental stages is the potency of the therapeutic agents and their potential side effects. When prescribed appropriately, these agents can do great good, restoring many incapacitated individuals to normal, productive lives. However, the appropriate administration of psychoactive medications requires training, skill, and ongoing interaction with the patient and family throughout the course of treatment. This is particularly true of young patients, whose continuing growth and development may necessitate frequent therapeutic adjustments.

Finally, the treatment of children with medications that exert their primary action on the brain must be approached with great care for social, ethical, and legal reasons. Most experiments that carry the potential of great benefit also carry the risk of some harm. The controversy surrounding the use of methylphenidate to treat children with attention-deficit hyperactivity disorder has brought home the lesson that the administration of psychotropic agents to children is ground that must be trod slowly and carefully.

We now have had roughly 40 years' experience, however, in administering these drugs to adults, as well as some limited experience with children, and their therapeutic efficacy and associated risks are well characterized. And medications with more specific indications and fewer side effects are on the market or in the pipeline. More investigators, particularly those who have come of age in the era of pharmacotherapy, feel comfortable exploring the use of these agents through controlled clinical trials in child patients, and more clinicians, faced with a child in psychological distress, are willing to consider their careful clinical use. Although the picture is by no means complete, we felt that enough sound information and clinical experience were now available to enable us to prepare a clinically useful *Textbook of Pharmacotherapy for Child and Adolescent Psychiatric Disorders*.

This manual is meant to serve as a practical guide to the use of modern psychiatric drugs in patients age 18 and under. Although it is written primarily for the prescribing psychiatrist, the book can be used by other health-care professionals involved in the management of children and adolescents with major psychiatric disorders, including psychologists, social workers, therapists, nursing staff and students, medical students, pediatricians, and family practitioners. We have focused on the major classes of agents currently used in clinical practice. Those agents whose use is primarily of historic interest, such as the older sedative-hypnotics, are not included.

We have delineated what is known on the basis of a critical review of controlled clinical trials as the highest standard of evaluation of pharmacotherapeutic efficacy. Since child and adolescent psychiatry continues to be plagued by a paucity of such trials, however, where there is little systematic evidence to guide clinical decision making, we have attempted to synthesize the limited available data and to offer a proposed "best resolution" of current scientific insights into these still-developing areas of psychopharmacology. Often these recommendations are based on the best clinical judgment of the authors and of the consultants to the development of this manual. In other situations where little is known, we discuss necessary areas for future investigation, and attempt to provide suggestions for dispensing such medications as safely and effectively as possible.

We wish to thank the following for their critical reviews of various chapters and their assistance in the production of this manual: Drs. Patrick Burke, Duncan Clark, Rohan Ganguli, Matcheri Keshavan, Howard Moss, William Pelham, Neal Ryan, J. John Mann, and D. Richard Martini, all of the University of Pittsburgh School of Medicine, and Dr. Magda Campbell of the New York University Medical Center.

Textbook of Pharmacotherapy for Child and Adolescent Psychiatric Disorders

Section I

Introduction to Psychopharmacology

C h a p t e r 1

Historical Perspective on Child and Adolescent Psychopharmacology

Any historical discussion of child and adolescent psychopharmacology is destined to be brief. Child psychiatry as a distinct area of study is just over a century old, developing in parallel with the psychological study of normal child development, and the concept of biological psychiatry as applied to child and adolescent mental disorders is even younger.[1,12] That is not to say that psychopharmacology is a new concept. Feldman[4] cites several antiquated examples of drug treatment for psychiatric illness. In the 1600s, a 24-year-old woman was treated with copious amounts of fresh apple cider, "borage," and "bugloss" (meant to produce the emesis, diuresis, diaphoresis, and diarrhea necessary for purging). This was followed by shaving her head and applying a moist pack of herbal extracts and "the warm lungs of lambs, sheep, young whelps or pigeons alive." The patient failed to recover from her "madness."[4] By the next century, several true psychotropics were available. Amyl nitrite was felt to be indicated for catatonia, opium and stramonium (an anticholinergic agent) for psychosis, and cannabis for depression. Of these, opium was considered the most remarkable of cures.[4]

Ironically, these agents and the study of other psychotropics remained the exclusive domain of medicine and neurology for many years. Psychiatry, or at least the mental illness with which psychiatrists now concern themselves, was more a topic of philosophy than of science. The concept of insanity as a spiritual and thereby nonphysical illness dominated the late 18th and early 19th centuries, perhaps contributing to the dominance of psychotherapeutic treatments. German physician Johann Christian Reil has been credited with the first systematic practice of such therapy, and in his "Rhapsodies About the Application of Psychotherapy to Mental Disturbances" (1803), he voiced the opinion that emotional illness could not be cured by physical treatments.[1]

Although the lay press often deems him the founder of psychotherapy, Sigmund Freud (1856–1939) was simply the first of the Germanic psychiatrists to successfully integrate psychotherapy into a medical community that was dominated by the experimental methods of neurologists and psychologists in Germany and France. Freud's German elder, Wilhelm Griesinger (1817–1868), was one of the first to merge psychiatry with the burgeoning field of experimental neurology, advocating that all mental illness was ultimately attributable to dysfunction of the brain. His treatments focused on proper mental hygiene and symptomatic drug treatment, but disdained the "trickery" of psychotherapy.[1]

The practice of psychopharmacology served, in some ways, to unite these two divergent approaches to mental illness. Prior to the 1950s, psychotropic drugs were used for nonspecific results: amphetamines and other stimulants for alertness or to alleviate depression; barbiturates and other sedatives for calming or sleep. Chlorpromazine was developed accidently by the French pharmaceutical firm Rhone-Poulenc, in an attempt to synthesize antihistamines with fewer side effects.[9] Its first psychiatric use in 1952 yielded remarkable and unexpected effectiveness for the excitement and psychosis of mania.[7] Simultaneously, the monoamine oxidase inhibitor iproniazid was used for the treatment of tuberculosis and had an unexpected antidepressant effect.[16] With the discovery of these drugs, an era of specific pharmaceutical treatment for mental illness began and psychiatrists began to consider both psychotherapy and pharmacotherapy as standard treatment.

If psychiatry was somewhat slow to make use of drug treatment, child psychiatry virtually dawdled. Leo Kanner wrote the first textbook on the subject, *Child Psychiatry*, a thorough and scholarly work whose later editions were maligned for giving rise to the concept of the "schizophrenogenic mother."[10] The fourth edition of this 735-page text, released in 1972, devotes only two pages to the psychopharmacology of childhood disorders.[11] Discussed are Bradley's early studies of amphetamine for the treatment of behavioral disorders,[2,3] the use of anticonvulsants for behavioral disruption,[13] and several open trials of chlorpromazine for severely disturbed children.[5,6,8] Notably absent are clear diagnostic categories of subjects and a critique of research methods used in these studies. Kanner closed the discussion with a quote from Bender,[11] who said: "We appear to be in the beginning of a new era of understanding the use of drugs in psychiatric practice."

In truth, by 1972 psychiatry was already well into this new era, with child psychiatry at least a decade behind. The early reports of Bradley were replicated several times between 1937 and 1970, but only in the past two decades have researchers established specific indications, outcome measures, pharmacokinetics, and dose/response relationships for stimulant medications (Chapter 3).[17] Reports of the successful use of neuroleptics in children were common between 1953 and the late 1960s, but were invariably performed on heterogeneous diagnostic groups using poorly controlled designs.[17] The work of Magda Campbell and colleagues from the early 1980s to the present represents the definitive studies of neuroleptic therapy in childhood psychosis, autism, and aggression, as well as the careful analysis of the short- and long-term side effects of these drugs in youngsters (see Chapter 7). Finally, the existence of major affective illness, and, therefore, its treatment, in prepubertal children was not widely accepted until the late 1970s, and was pioneered by Puig-Antich and others in the past decade.[14,15]

In reading the current textbook, it may become apparent that definitive studies of most psychopharmacologic approaches to child and adolescent mental illness have yet to be performed. It is the authors' hope that a critical review of current knowledge in this area will both prove useful to practicing physicians and serve to highlight the limitations of our current knowledge in pediatric psychopharmacology. Similarly, it is the authors' opinion that the treatment of child and adolescent mental illness, both pharmacologic and nonpharmacologic, represents the highest priority for new research and funding.

References

1. Alexander, F.G., Selesnick, S.T. (1966). *The History of Psychiatry*. New York: Harper & Row.

2. Bradley, C. (1937). Behavior of children receiving Benzedrine. *Am. J Psychiatry, 94*, 577–585.

3. Bradley, C., Bowen, M. (1941). Amphetamine (Benzedrine) therapy of children's behavior disorders. *Am. J Orthopsychiat, 11*, 92–103.

4. Feldman, P.E. (1965). Ancient psychopharmacotherapy. *Bull Menninger Clin, 65*, 256–263.

5. Freed, H., Pfeifer, C.A. (1956). Treatment of hyperkinetic emotionally disturbed children with prolonged administration of chlorpromazine. *Am. J Psychiat, 113*, 22–26.

6. Gatski, R.L. (1955). Chlorpromazine in the treatment of emotionally maladjusted children. *JAMA, 157*, 1298–1300.

7. Hamon, J., Paraire, J., Velluz, J. (1952). Remarques sur l'action de 4560 RP sur l'agitation maniaque. *Ann Med Psychol, 110*, 332–335.

8. Hunt, B.R., Frank, T., Krush, T.P. (1956). Chlorpromazine in the treatment of severe emotional disorders of children. *Am. J Dis Child, 91*, 268–277.

9. Jacobsen, E. (1986). The early history of psychotherapeutic drugs. *Psychopharmacology, 89*, 138–144.

10. Kanner, L. (1935). *Child Psychiatry*. Springfield, Ill.: CC Thomas.

11. Kanner, L. (1972). *Child Psychiatry* (4th ed.). Springfield, Ill.: CC Thomas.

12. Parry-Jones, W.L. (1989). Annotation: The history of child and adolescent psychiatry: Its present day relevance. *J Child Psychol Psychiatry, 30*, 3–11.

13. Pasamanick, B. (1951). Anticonvulsant drug therapy of behavior problem children with abnormal electroencephalograms. *Arch Neurol Psychiatry, 56*, 752–766.

14. Petti, T.A., Law, W. (1982). Imipramine treatment of depressed children: A double-blind pilot study. *J Clin Psychopharmacol, 2*, 107–110.

15. Puig-Antich, J. (1980). Affective disorders in childhood. *Psychiatr Clin North Am, 3*, 403–434.

16. Selikoff, J.J., Robitzak, E.H., Orustain, G.G. (1952). Treatment of pulmonary tuberculosis with hydrazine derivatives of isonicotinic acid. *JAMA, 150*, 973–982.

17. Wiener, J.M. (1984). Psychopharmacology in childhood disorders. *Psychiatr Clin North Am, 7*, 831–843.

Chapter 2

Characteristics of Drug Disposition During Childhood

Robert A. Branch, M.D.

The therapeutic benefits of any drug therapy and the risks of toxicity depend on the relationship between the delivery of the drug to the patient (dose and dose interval), the disposition of the drug to determine drug concentration at the effector site (pharmacokinetics), and the drug's action at the effector site and the end response (pharmacodynamics). Intersubject variations in response, and specifically variations in therapeutic outcome among adults and children of varying ages, are a consequence of the balance among these variables. It is clear that a child is not simply a small adult, and that physiologic differences in any of the determinants of kinetics and dynamics will influence this balance. There are numerous examples of what appears to be a true difference in the dynamic response to a given plasma concentration. These include drugs where higher doses can be achieved with less toxicity (such as digoxin),[1] where therapeutic levels in adults can be associated with toxicity or even sudden death in children (such as the tricyclic antidepressants),[2] or where lower plasma levels are required to achieve a desired therapeutic effect (for example, haloperidol).[3] In addition, child maturation results in sequential changes in a number of physiologic determinants of drug disposition. Thus there is a need to identify both the pharmacokinetic and pharmacodynamic interrelationships for each drug. The physiologic determinants of drug disposition will be discussed in greater detail in this chapter, while individual kinetic–dynamic interrelationships will be discussed with respect to individual drugs in later chapters.

Regardless of the age of a child receiving a drug, the dispositional characteristics of the drug will depend on the interaction between the physicochemical properties of the drug and the physiologic process in the patient. Physical properties of the drug include molecular size, charge, pK_a or ionic disassociation constant, and lipid solubility. These factors will determine the drug's distribution, as well as the route of elimination. In general, water-soluble drugs have a small volume of distribution and can be eliminated unchanged in urine, while lipid-soluble drugs have a large volume of distribution and require metabolism to more water-soluble moieties prior to elimination. Depending on the physical characteristics of any given drug, the balance of physiologic factors influencing that drug's disposition will vary. These physiologic factors have the potential to be altered during childhood development and by disease states. Thus the influence of any one of these processes can be complex; it can be mediated by a variety of factors and can determine the disposition of different drugs to a variable extent.

Distribution

The major aspects of distribution affected by aging are volume of distribution (V_d) and plasma protein binding. Conceptually, the apparent volume of distribution is the volume into which a drug distributes in the body when the body is at equilibrium, and is related to the pool from which the drug concentration is measured. It is a theoretical concept and reflects the partitioning of drug between the fluid compartments in the body, such as plasma, interstitial fluid, and intracellular fluid. It is calculated by

$$V_d = \frac{D}{C_p} \tag{1}$$

where D represents the fraction of the dose absorbed and C_p is drug concentration at equilibrium. In general, apart from the newborn infant, the volume of distribution relates linearly to body weight. Thus the common practice of modifying initial loading dose regimens to achieve a given initial plasma concentration rapidly by factoring in weight is rational for many drugs.

Most drugs in plasma are reversibly bound to proteins, such as albumin, which has specific binding sites for acidic drugs, such as globulin and alpha-1-acid glycoprotein, and generally is more important for basic drugs. The extent of binding is pharmacologically relevant, as only unbound drug is available for distribution into tissues and is capable of evoking a pharmacologic response. The extent of protein binding is, therefore, important in determining both pharmacologic response and drug disposition.

In general, serum albumin concentrations do not change from early childhood through child development; however, decreased numbers of binding sites per molecule can be found in neonatal hyperbilirubinemia,[4] and thus reduce the binding of an acidic drug. The situation for alpha-1-acid glycoprotein is more complex. In general, higher concentrations of this acute-phase acting protein are found in children,[5] and this increase has been observed to increase the protein binding of basic psychotropic drugs such as haloperidol to result in reduced free-drug concentrations. In addition, intercurrent infections and physical stress are common in children and can be expected to be associated with further rises in the concentration of this protein, a decrease in free-drug concentration, and a reduced pharmacodynamic response.

Age-related changes in distribution due either to small body mass or to altered drug binding can be expected to influence a drug's half-life independently of factors influencing drug elimination. The reason for this change is apparent from the dependence of the half-life ($t_{1/2}$) on both its total clearance from the blood (Cl) and its apparent volume of distribution (V_d), according to the equation:

$$t_{1/2} = \frac{0.693\ V_d}{Cl} \tag{2}$$

This relationship indicates that the smaller the child, the smaller is the V_d and the shorter is the half-life. As an extreme illustration, in adults, both propranolol and indocyanine green (ICG) have similar systemic clearances of approximately 1000 ml/min. Propranolol is a lipophilic compound with an extensive volume of distribution, while ICG is confined essentially to the vascular compartment. As a consequence of distributional differences alone, propranolol has an average half-life of about 150 minutes in comparison with ICG's half-life of about 3 minutes.[6] Volume of distribution differences within a single drug as related to age differences will not be as dramatic. However, even drugs with relatively long half-lives, such as imipramine, have a shorter half-life in 5- to 12-year-olds (11–42 hours) than in 13- to 16-

year-olds (14–89 hours).[7] Thus it can be anticipated that a drug with a narrow therapeutic window may need more frequent dosing intervals to remain within that therapeutic window because of its shorter half-life, even if clearances are comparable to those of other drugs.

In addition to influencing drug distribution, changes in protein binding have a potential to influence drug elimination. A change in the free fraction of a drug in the blood can lead to an increase in the amount of drug available to the drug-metabolizing enzymes, and, therefore, to an increase in the total clearance of some drugs. This increase can shorten the half-life of a drug in the absence of any change in the activity of drug-metabolizing enzymes. An example of this phenomenon is provided by the decrease in the half-life of tolbutamide in acute viral hepatitis. This decrease has been attributed solely to a decrease in its binding to plasma proteins, since it has been shown that even though the total (free plus bound) clearance of tolbutamide increases, protein binding decreases and free clearance remains unchanged.[8] Thus the combination of decreased body mass and increased binding in the same young individual both would be expected to contribute independently to a shorter drug half-life irrespective of factors that modify drug clearance. This contribution to reductions in half-life, in conjunction with efficient metabolic clearance, may have led to the erroneous conclusion that children are "superefficient" in drug elimination as compared with adults.

Elimination

Drug elimination is defined as the irreversible loss of a drug from the site of measurement; this includes both metabolism and excretion. Clearance is an important parameter that is worth discussing in a general context that is pertinent to both adults and children, before focusing on physiologic variables that can be influenced by childhood development. Clearance relates drug concentration to the rate of elimination, thereby providing a measure of efficiency of the elimination process. By definition, total or systemic clearance is a measure of the amount of plasma cleared of drug per unit time. This measure can be obtained from measurements of drug concentration in plasma after bolus doses (equation 2) or at steady state (equation 3):

$$Cl = \frac{I}{Cp_{ss}} \tag{3}$$

where I is the rate of drug administration and Cp_{ss} is the steady-state plasma concentration. Clearance is independent of the mechanism of elimination involved, and if multiple routes of elimination occur concurrently, it provides an estimate of the sum of these processes.

When the rate of elimination is proportional to the amount of drug present, it is a first-order process; a good example is theophylline kinetics in childhood.[9] Under first-order conditions, the clearance of a drug is constant over a range of concentrations. Not all drugs undergo first-order kinetics, however; in some instances, dose-dependent or zero-order elimination occurs as a result of the saturation of an energy-requiring process. Clearance in these cases is nonlinear and will vary depending on the achieved concentration of drug. Diphenylhydantoin provides a classic example.[10] The major practical implication of the difference between first-order and zero-order kinetics is that in the former instance, dosing increments can be expected to be associated with proportionate increases in steady-state plasma concentrations (i.e., are predictable); in the latter instance, dosing increments result in exponential increases in steady-state plasma concentrations for equal dose increments. Alternatively, smaller and smaller dosing increases are required to provide equivalent changes in plasma concentration. This is more difficult, but still possible, to predict. Both concepts are practically applied in the therapeutic drug monitoring of theophylline and diphenylhydantoin, respectively, in clinical practice,[11,12] and require consideration for any therapeutic agent in which a relationship is defined between measured level of drug and the dynamic response.

Clearance can also be described as the efficiency of removal of drugs across an organ of elimination, the two major organs being the liver and the kidney. Extraction by the liver provides an explanation for the so-called first-pass effect in which drugs with high hepatic clearances have low oral systemic availability. Hepatic clearance (Cl_H) reflects the efficiency with which the liver irreversibly removes drug from the blood. It is determined by both the fraction of drug removed or extracted (E) from the blood during passage through the liver and the liver blood flow (Q_H). The relationship between these parameters is given by

$$Cl_H = Q_H E \qquad (4)$$

Drugs that are given orally must pass through the liver before reaching the systemic circulation. If hepatic enzymes (or enzymes in the intestinal mucosa) extract drug from the blood as it passes through, then the fraction (F) of the total dose entering the general circulation is reduced. For drugs that are completely absorbed from the gastrointestinal (GI) tract, this fraction F (or systemic availability) is determined by the drug's extraction (E) by the liver according to the equation:

$$F = 1 - E \qquad (5)$$

Thus, as E approaches unity, the amount of drug that reaches the systemic circulation becomes a very small fraction of the dose given, and little drug effect can be anticipated.

Intersubject variations in drug clearance, and the influence of childhood development on the average clearance, as well as the extent of intersubject variations at any age, largely depend on the physiologic process involved in drug clearance. The two major routes of elimination for most drugs are renal excretion and biotransformation, although pulmonary exhalation or direct secretion to bile can be a major route for certain drugs.

Renal excretion can be due to filtration or by anion or cation renal tubule cell transport. Irrespective of the mechanism, renal excretion has been found to relate closely to measures of the glomerular filtration rate (GFR), such as creatinine clearance or even serum creative concentrations for most drugs.[13] The GFR is low in proportion to body weight or surface area in the neonatal period up to 6 months postnatal, but thereafter meets total body requirements by more nearly reflecting surface area, rather than body weight.[14]

In general, intersubject variations in the clearance of drugs that undergo renal clearance in modest and steady-state plasma concentration during chronic therapy are a predictable function of GFR. Thus dosage modification with drugs like aminoglycosides, vancomycin, penicillins, and cephalosporins in childhood is relatively easy and predictable.[13]

In contrast to renal clearance mechanisms, biotransformation is a much more variable process. The 10-fold to 100-fold intersubject variation for most metabolic routes in adults is reflected by an equivalent extent of variation in childhood. When using mean clearances of drugs at varying ages, it is clear that for drugs with first-order kinetics, the dose required to achieve a given steady-state plasma concentration is not predicated on the basis of normalization by age or weight. Even the common practice of normalizing by surface area tends to result in lower plasma concentrations than those anticipated from predictions based on adults. Examples of this phenomenon include digoxin,[15] phenobarbital,[16] diphenylhydantoin,[17] carbamazepine,[18] haloperidol,[19] and desipramine.[20] This has led to the suggestion that drug metabolizing activity is increased in childhood. A more likely explanation is that children are exposed to similar ingestions of naturally occurring xenobiotics that are the normal substrates and regulators of drug metabolizing activity. Thus a child requires and acquires a drug metabolizing capability related to physiologic need that is comparable to that of adults, rather than based on an age-related maturation in function. But whatever the mechanisms involved, the consequence is that a wide dosage range can be anticipated to achieve any given plasma concentration of drug, and a flexible range is needed to enable a required therapeutic response.

A further factor contributing to intersubject variations in drug response is the complexity of drug metabolism. It is well recognized that several different families of drug metabolizing enzymes may contribute to either oxidative (phase I) or conjugative (phase II) metabolism, and that any one drug may be a substrate for different enzyme systems, with the balance between alternative metabolic routes varying among individuals. Oxidative metabolism, predominantly by members of the cytochrome P-450 family of enzymes, results in a minor structural change, generally making the compound slightly more hydrophilic, but a more suitable substrate for phase II metabolism. The product may be an unstable electrophyl capable of causing cellular damage or an active drug with comparable or even greater potency than the parent drug, or it may be inactive. Thus the dynamic response relationship can be complex.

The enzymes in the P-450 family have very selective substrate configuration requirements, yet each of the identified enzymes has been shown to metabolize numerous substrates, and there is no way of predicting which drug will be metabolized by which enzyme. However, if two drugs are characterized as substrates for the same enzyme, competitive mutual inhibition of drug metabolism can be anticipated to cause a drug interaction when the drugs are coadministered. Each enzyme also has specific regulatory mechanisms, differential organ distribution, or even differential distribution within the hepatic acinus. In addition, some enzymes—like cytochrome P-4503A4, which is responsible for the metabolism of such widely differing drugs as nifedipine, erythromycin, midazolam, cyclosporin A, and dapsone—exhibit a broad-based unimodal distribution of activity.[20] In contrast, others—like cytochrome P-4502D6, which is responsible for the metabolism of debrisoquine, sparteine, nortriptyline, dextromethorphan, and many other drugs—exhibit a genetically based polymorphism in which a subgroup in the normal population has a total defect in synthesis of this protein.[21] A single nucleic acid deletion with a subsequent frame shift in genetic coding is responsible for 80% of the defects in this protein's synthesis.[22] The frequency of this defect varies among ethnic groups, being about 8% in Caucasians and less than 1% in Asians.[23] The implication of this phenomenon is that the subpopulation with a defect of P-4502D6 can be expected to have different pharmacokinetic and pharmacodynamic responses to any drug that is predominantly metabolized by this enzyme, as compared with subjects with high expression of this enzyme.

Conjugative metabolism involves adding a chemical group to the drug molecule, which almost always results in a marked loss of drug activity and a considerable increase in hydrophilicity. Numerous alternative enzyme systems are involved, some of which, like glucuronidation and sulfation, tend to be unimodally distributed. Others, like acetylation and demethylation, exhibit genetic polymorphism. In some instances, the situation can be exceedingly complex, as the metabolite can be hydrolyzed back to the parent drug, creating a shuttle or equilibrium phenomenon.

Given the complexity of drug metabolism, it is not surprising that each drug must be considered as a unique entity. Considerable effort in the drug-discovery process is spent on characterizing this information. Unfortunately, up to the present time, this characterization tends to be performed for adults, rather than children. There is, therefore, an urgent need, with both newly developing drugs and drugs developed in adults, to acquire information that can be used to rationalize and anticipate variations in drug disposition in children. In the meantime, the paucity of available information makes it imperative that the clinician be cautious, starting with low doses and dose ranges to achieve the desired end point.

References

1. Morselli, P.L., Assael, B.M., Gomeni, R., et al. (1975). Digoxin pharmacokinetics during human development. In P.L. Morselli, S. Garattini, and F. Sereini (Eds.), *Basic and Therapeutic Aspects of Perinatal Pharmacology* (pp. 377–392). New York: Raven Press.

2. Riddle, M.A., Nelson, J.C., Kleinman, C., et al. (1991). Sudden death in children receiving norpramin: A review of three reported cases and commentary. *J Am Child Adolesc Psychiatry, 30*, 104–108.

3. Teicher, M.H., Glod, C.A. (1990). Neuroleptic drugs: Indications, guidelines for their rational use in children and adolescents. *J Child Adolesc Psychopharmacol, 1*, 33–56.

4. Rane, A., Lunde, P.K.M., Jalling, B., et al. (1971). Plasma protein binding of diphenylhydantoin in normal and hyperbilirubinemic infants. *J Pediatr, 78*, 877–882.

5. Schley, J., Muller-Oerlinghausen B. (1983). The binding of chemically different psychotropic drugs to alpha-1-acid glycoprotein. *Pharmacopsychiatria, 16*, 82–85.

6. Branch, R.A., James, J., Read, A.E. (1986). A study of factors influencing drug disposition in chronic liver disease using the modelling drug (+)-propranolol. *Bri J Clin Pharmacol, 3*, 243–249.

7. Williams, R.L., Blaschke, T.F., Meffin, P.J., et al. (1977). Influence of acute viral hepatitis on disposition and plasma binding of tolbutamide. *Clin Pharmacol Ther, 21*, 301–309.

8. Levy, G. (1974). Pharmacokinetic control of theophylline therapy. In *Clinical Pharmacokinetics*. Washington, D.C.: American Pharmaceutical Association.

9. Garrettson, L.K., Kim, O.K. (1970). Apparent saturation of diphenylhydantoin metabolism in children. *Pediatr Res, 4*, 455.

10. Levy, G., Kogsooko, R. (1975). Pharmacokinetic analysis of the effect of theophylline on pulmonary function in children. *J Pediatr, 86*, 789–793.

11. Rane, A., Wilson, J.T. (1975). Plasma level monitoring of diphenylhydantoin and carbamezepine in the pediatric patient. International Symposium on Clinical Pharmacy and Pharmacology. *Excepta Medica*, Amsterdam.

12. Maher, J.F. (1988). Pharmacokinetic alterations with renal failure and dialysis. In B. Chernow (Ed.), *The Pharmacological Approach to the Critically Ill Patient* (pp. 47–68). Baltimore: Williams and Wilkins.

13. West, J.R., Smith, H.W., Chasis, H. (1948). Glomerular filtration rate, effective renal blood flow and maximal excretory capacity in infancy. *J Pediatr, 32*, 10–18.

14. Krusula, R.W., Pellegrino, P.A., Hastreiter, A.R., Soyka, L.F. (1972). Serum levels of digoxin in infants and children. *J Pediatr, 81*, 566–569.

15. Svensmark, O., Buchthal, F. (1964). Diphenylhydantoin and phenobarbital. Serum levels in children. *Am J Dis Child, 108*, 82–87.

16. Jalling, B., Boreus, L.O., Rane, A., Sjogvist, F. (1970). Plasma concentrations of diphenylhydantoin in young infants. *Pharmacol Clin, 2*, 200–202.

17. Rane, A., Hojer, B., Wilson, J.T. (1976). Kinetics of carbamazipine into its 10, 11 episode metabolism in children. *Clin Pharmacol Ther, 19*, 276–279.

18. Nebert, D.W., Nelson, D.R., Coon, M.J., et al. (1991). The P-450 superfamily: Update on new sequence, gene mapping, and recommended nomenclature. *DNA Cell Biol, 10*, 1–14.

19. Gualtieri, C.T., Golden, R., Evans, R.W., Hicks, R.E. (1984). Blood level measurement of psychoactive drugs in pediatric psychiatry. *Ther Drug Monitor, 6*, 127–141.

20. Breimer, D.D., Schellens, J.H.M., Soons, P.A. (1989). Nifedipine: Variability in its kinetics in man. *Pharmacol Ther, 44*, 445–454.

21. Jacqz, E., Hall, S., Branch, R.A. (1986). Genetically determined polymorphisms in oxidative drug metabolism. *Hepatology, 6*, 1020–1032.

22. Gough, A.C., Miles, J.S., Spurr, N.K., et al. (1990). Identification of the primary gene defect at the cytochrome P-450 *CYP2D* locus. *Nature, 347,* 773–776.

23. Nakamura, K., Goto, F., Ray, W.A., et al. (1985). Interethnic differences in genetic polymorphisms of debrisoquine and mephenytoin hydroxylation between Japanese and Caucasian populations. *Clin Pharmacol Ther, 38,* 402–408.

Classes of Medication

C h a p t e r   3

Psychostimulants

The psychostimulants methylphenidate (Ritalin), dextroamphetamine sulfate (Dexedrine), and magnesium pemoline (Cylert) are the most commonly prescribed medications in all of child psychiatry, despite the fact that they have been approved by the Food and Drug Administration (FDA) only for attention-deficit hyperactivity disorder (ADHD) in children, adolescents, and adults, and for narcolepsy.[7,12,21] Nearly 2% of the school-age population receive stimulant medication for ADHD symptoms.[7] These medications remain controversial, however, because of their side effects and concern about their potential for abuse and addiction, leading certain special-interest groups to press for their immediate recall and removal from the market.

Currently, methylphenidate and dextroamphetamine sulfate are classified by the FDA as Schedule II drugs, the most restrictive classification for drugs felt to be medically useful.[15,21] Magnesium pemoline is classified as a Schedule IV drug. The authors wish to emphasize, however, that in the field of child psychiatry, and in psychiatry in general, the use of stimulant medications is not considered controversial. These medications are solid, first-line, bread-and-butter–type medications with a remarkably benign side-effect profile. The disorder that they are most commonly used to treat, ADHD, is one with marked functional impairment, long-term morbidity, and enormous consequences for the child and family. Although more long-term studies are needed, the drugs have demonstrated efficacy (see below). It is true that children and adolescents with ADHD exhibit a twofold to fourfold increased risk for substance abuse, but current data show no evidence that the use of prescribed stimulant medication results in the increased use, or abuse of, and dependence on, recreational or prescription drugs, or in dependence on and addiction to the stimulants themselves.[7,12,43] Nonetheless, close supervision and monitoring of the child or adolescent and his or her family members for the potential for abuse are required when stimulants are prescribed. When used properly, the stimulants are beneficial and safe, as well as cost-effective, in decreasing hyperactivity, distractibility, impulsivity, and fidgetiness, and in increasing attention span. State-dependent learning is not a problem when stimulants are used.[7] Cognitive effects may respond optimally to relatively modest doses of stimulant medications, while behavioral symptoms may require larger doses.[23–25] No normative clinical or laboratory values have been elucidated at this time.

Carlson and associates[48] compared the effects of methylphenidate with those of placebo on the performance of ADHD boys following their success or failure at tasks assigned to them. They provided evidence for a "salutary" effect of methylphenidate on the boys' performance and perceptions after attempting to solve both solvable and unsolvable puzzles. Boys exposed to unsolvable puzzles demonstrated increased persistence on a subsequent generalization task when receiving methylphenidate as compared with placebo. No differences were found between placebo and a "no pill" condition on the Posner letter-matching task and four other measures of phonologic processing in an attempt to isolate the effects of methylphenidate to parameter estimates of selective attention, the basic cognitive process of retrieving name codes from permanent memory, and a constant term that represented nonspecific aspects of information processing. Responses to the letter-matching stimuli were found to be more rapid with methylphenidate than with placebo.[49] It is important to note that this improvement in performance was isolated to the parameter estimate that reflected nonspecific aspects of information processing.

A lack of active medication effect was found on the other measures of phonologic processing, supporting the Posner task finding suggesting that methylphenidate exerts beneficial effects on academic processing through general rather than specific aspects of information processing.[49]

Chemical Properties

For the chemical properties of the psychostimulants, see Table 3-1 and Figures 3-1 through 3-3.

Table 3-1
Pharmacokinetics of CNS Stimulants in Children and Adolescents

Generic Name (Brand Name)	Onset of Action	Peak Plasma Concentration	Plasma Half-Life	Metabolism and Excretion	Comments
Methylphenidate (Ritalin)	30–60 minutes, up to 3 hours for SR	1–2 hours, 4–5 hours for SR	1–2 hours	Metabolized by hepatic microsomal enzymes	Drug concentrations higher in brain than in blood
Dextroamphetamine sulfate (Dexedrine)	30–60 minutes, 1–2 hours for spansule	2 hours, 8–10 hours for spansule	6–8 hours	Metabolized partly by liver and partly excreted unchanged in urine	Excretion increased by acidification of urine, decreased by alkalinization. Develops high concentration in brain
Magnesium pemoline (Cylert)	Variable, acute, and delayed effects	2–4 hours	8–12 hours	Metabolized 60% by the liver and excreted 40% unchanged in urine	Without significant sympathomimetic activity, half-life increased with chronic administration

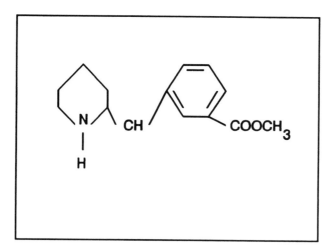

Figure 3-1
Methylphenidate (Ritalin)

The stimulants used in child and adolescent psychiatry are sympathomimetic amines that may be administered orally.[7,12,15,21] They are then absorbed from the GI tract, and cross the blood–brain barrier. The onset of action for methylphenidate and dextroamphetamine is generally observed within 20 minutes to one hour, with a three- to six-hour duration of action.[7,12] Stimulants of the central nervous system (CNS) exert their maximum effect when they are being most rapidly absorbed, and clinical efficacy is probably related to the rate of rise of the blood level.[12] This is when the

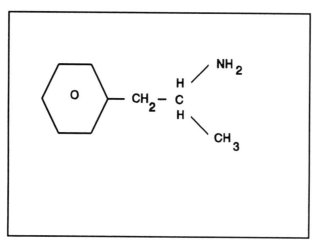

Figure 3-2
Amphetamine

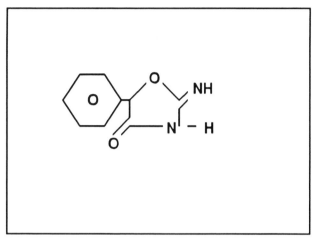

Figure 3-3
Pemoline

target symptoms, including hyperactivity, distractibility, inattentiveness, impulsivity, and fidgetiness, are most susceptible to the stimulants' effects. The clinical effectiveness of the stimulants has not been shown to correlate with absolute or peak blood levels,[12] and no therapeutic window has as yet been delineated for any of them.[7,12] Sustained-release methylphenidate's onset of action can be delayed for as long as three hours, with a shorter overall duration of action and more day-to-day variability than two doses of regular methylphenidate given around breakfast and lunchtime.[27,28]

Pelham and associates[27] compared the relative efficacy of standard methylphenidate, sustained-release methylphenidate, sustained-release dextroamphetamine, and pemoline in 22 ADHD children in a double-blind, placebo-controlled crossover evaluation. They found that sustained-release dextroamphetamine and pemoline produced the most consistent beneficial effects and were recommended for 10 of the 15 children who were responders to medication. The continuous-performance task results demonstrated that all four medications had an effect within two hours of ingestion, and the effects lasted for nine hours.[28]

Indications

Indications for use are shown in Table 3-2.

ADHD Children and Adolescents

Over 600,000 children per year are treated with stimulants for ADHD symptoms.[7] ADHD which is most often considered a disorder of catecholamine un-

Table 3-2
**Indications for CNS Stimulants in Childhood
and Adolescent Psychiatry**

FDA-approved indications
- ADHD in childhood and adolescence
- Narcolepsy (methylphenidate and dextroamphetamine)
- Exogenous obesity (dextroamphetamine)

Possible indications
- ADHD in preschool children
- Undifferentiated attention-deficit disorder
- ADHD in intellectually subaverage children and adolescents
- ADHD symptoms in children and adolescents with Fragile X syndrome
- ADHD symptoms in children and adolescents with PDD (autism)
- ADHD symptoms in children and adolescents with head trauma and/or organic brain disease
- ADHD in children and/or adolescents with tic disorders (i.e., Tourette's syndrome)
- Potentiation of narcotic analgesia

---

deractivity. The therapeutic effect of stimulants, sympathomimetic agents that increase catecholamine levels by inhibiting their reuptake, provides indirect evidence for this concept. Up until recently, stimulant medications were predominantly prescribed to children 6 to 10 years of age, and generally were discontinued around the onset of puberty and adolescence. Many practicing clinicians believed that ADHD remitted at puberty, but further investigation has demonstrated that its course is extremely variable, and that symptoms can and do persist into adolescence and adulthood.[9,32] Stimulants have been found effective in treating ADHD symptoms throughout life,[32,50,51] which has led to a dramatic increase in their use for both adolescents and adults. Approximately one million persons with ADHD have been treated with stimulants thus far;[7,32] nonetheless, they frequently are not prescribed correctly.

Case History
A 10-year-old boy was referred for child psychiatric evaluation because of "problem school behavior." He was found to have a history of disruptive behavior since the age of 2, and, according to his mother, had since become more "hyper." She and her husband had hoped that the child would "grow out of it," but instead his behavior deteriorated. He was failing all of his fifth-grade courses, despite school psychoeducational assessment that revealed that he functioned in the above-average range. The school was threatening to expel him for his disruptive behavior, which included an inability to stay seated in the classroom and to wait in line with the other children, high levels of motoric activity, easy distractibility, an inability to attend to tasks, and impulsivity. His

parents confirmed similar behavior at home. There was no evidence for mood disorder, psychosis, or drug and alcohol use. The family history was noncontributory.

A comprehensive behavioral management program was implemented. This, however, proved to only be minimally effective. High rates of hyperactivity were still observed as measured by Parent and Teachers Conner's Questionnaires. A methylphenidate trial was initiated. The patient was started on a drug A/B trial: methylphenidate versus placebo. Doses of methylphenidate included 5 mg b.i.d., 10 mg b.i.d., 10/15 mg, 15 mg b.i.d., 20/15 mg, 20/20 mg, and placebo. The patient, his family, and his teachers all were blind to the patient's medication status. The parents and teachers were asked to fill out the Conner's Questionnaire forms, and the teachers also filled out a daily report card assessing his behavior during each class period. Only the treating psychiatrist knew the dose of medication the patient was receiving. It was determined that the patient responded best (greatest reduction in target symptoms with fewest side effects) to a dose of methylphenidate 15 mg b.i.d. Combined with the comprehensive behavioral program, he was maintained on this dose of methylphenidate. At six months, he continued to show good improvement, was no longer failing all of his classes, and his homeroom teacher described him as "being a different child."

Clinical Efficacy

Hyperactivity

The stimulants significantly reduce hyperactivity in children and adolescents with ADHD.[7,12] It should be noted that while the increased activity during structured settings such as the classroom is decreased, the child still is appropriately active during periods of recreation and play.

Distractibility

The stimulants are also quite effective in decreasing distractibility and increasing attention span. This is particularly evident in structured settings such as the classroom.[49–52]

Social Interactions

Stimulants have been shown to significantly increase a child's responsiveness to and compliance with parental commands.[33] The children also do better interpersonally with both peers and adults.[34] Stimulant use has been shown to improve impulsivity, aggression, and noncompliance associated with ADHD,[6,7] but not in children who have pure oppositional defiant disorders or conduct disorders without ADHD. In children who carry both diagnoses, the aggression and impulsivity may decrease when the ADHD has been effectively treated.[53,55,57]

Motivation

Motivation may be improved since there are fewer impediments to allowing the child to perform required tasks.[12] This is an area of active investigation, and the stimulants' exact effects on motivation remain unclear. Further study is necessary.

Academic Achievement

By decreasing the interfering behaviors associated with ADHD, stimulant use would be expected to result in the enhancement of academic achievement. Nonetheless, up until very recently, it was believed that there was only minimal or no improvement in academic performance.[35] Recent investigation, however, has revealed that the use of methylphenidate does significantly improve accuracy and productivity in the academic setting.[29,36,37] These studies had the advantage over previous studies and reviews[35] of utilizing written assignments given by the child's teachers as opposed to standardized achievement tests to measure academic performance. Moreover, Pelham[25] has argued that stimulants improve accuracy and speed most significantly in those areas that have already been partially learned, but require practice in such subjects as math and spelling. It must be emphasized that stimulant-induced learning has not been demonstrated to be state dependent,[3,52] so that allowing ADHD children to go on medication-free holidays is not likely to result in either short- or long-term disruption of learning.

Mood and Emotion

In contrast to adults, children rarely experience mood elevations or euphoric effects when taking stimulants,[30] although they may precipitate a worsening of mood and/or irritability (see "Side Effects"). Nonetheless, children and adolescents treated with stimulants consistently rate themselves as "happier" as compared with when they receive placebo.[48] Currently, stimulants are not recommended for treating dysphoria and depression, as they sometimes are in adult depression.

Clinical Concern

Before initiating a stimulant trial, behavioral interventions such as social skills training, problem-solving skills, behavioral modification, and family therapy should be tried.[7,21] In addition, see Table 3-3. If these are insufficient or untenable, then stimulant medications can be used to help ameliorate the behavior. Stimulants should not be used in place of or as an alternative to behavioral interventions, since the few available studies of their long-term effectiveness have failed to demonstrate such effectiveness when used alone.[44,54,56,58] Unfortunately, these studies suffer from a lack of rigorous methodology, and currently there are no prospective studies of the long-term outcome for children with ADHD in randomly assigned to medication versus placebo. No one has studied children on stimulants over several years to determine the long-term effects of these medications as these children progress into adulthood. It does appear that since neither stimulant medication nor behavioral therapy alone is adequate to control the ADHD symptoms, a combination of both modalities should be the treatment of choice.[26] It is also not possible to predict whether or not a child will respond to a particular stimulant trial.[22]

Trials of a medication should be performed to assess whether or not a child truly needs the medication. Methylphenidate and dextroamphetamine sulfate are short-acting and lend themselves well to a placebo versus medication trial (called drug A/B trials), wherein the patient serves as his or her own control.[22] In this way, the medication's efficacy can be assessed at various dosages, leading to a determination of the dose that produces the most benefit and fewest side effects.[22] When a multimodality treatment approach is utilized in the treatment of ADHD, the likelihood of a good clinical outcome is increased. Children who do not receive proper treatment are at a greatly increased risk of having Axis I and II diagnoses (i.e., substance abuse and antisocial personality disorder).[32,44] See Tables 3-4 and 3-5 for ADHD symptoms targeted by stimulant medications and schema for pharmacologic intervention in ADHD.

Narcolepsy

Narcolepsy is a disorder of excessive daytime sleepiness in which the person experiences sudden-onset rapid-eye-movement (REM) sleep attacks.[16] Cata-

Table 3-3
Important Considerations When Prescribing Stimulants

Use with caution in children and adolescents with:
- Conduct disorders
- History of substance abuse/dependence
- Antisocial family members
- Substance-abusing/dependent family members
- Tic disorders (i.e., Tourette's syndrome)
- Psychosis
- Failure to thrive (i.e., physical retardation)
- Liver impairment (especially magnesium pemoline)

27

Table 3-4
Stepwise Progression in the Pharmacologic Treatment of ADHD

Document baseline behaviors medication-free by parents and teacher Iowa Conner's Questionnaire for at least one week and by clinical evaluation.
Behavioral therapy with social skills training, parent management training, education services, classroom instruction.
If not sufficient . . .
Stimulant Trial First choice—Methylphenidate (Ritalin): Check blood pressure, pulse, height, weight. May want to consider starting with clonidine if patient or family history of tic disorders (i.e., Tourette's) or substance abuse/dependence, or patient has failure to thrive. Second choice—Dextroamphetamine (Dexedrine): Same pretreatment screening. Third choice—Pemoline (Cylert): Also check LFTs. Fourth choice—Desipramine (Norpramin): Need to monitor cardiac function. Probably preferable to imipramine (Tofranil) since it has fewer side effects. Fifth choice—Clonidine (Catapress): Need to monitor cardiac function closely. Side effects can be problematic. Sixth Choice—Bupropion (Wellbutrin): Still preliminary.

plectic attacks consisting of the total or partial collapse of skeletal muscle tone are commonly observed in narcolepsy. It is usually diagnosed in the second decade of life. Polysomnographic studies are required to make a definitive diagnosis, with behavioral and educational interventions generally attempted first.[16] These consist of looking into the sleep habits and hygiene of the patient and family and having the patient avoid irregular sleep schedules. Patients are often advised to take short naps to determine whether these will ameliorate the condition, and this approach can preclude the need for pharmacologic intervention. If behavioral and educational methods are inadequate, and particularly when the child falls asleep in school, the CNS stimulants methylphenidate (Ritalin) and dextroamphetamine sulfate (Dexedrine) can effectively treat the symptoms of these sleep problems.[15,16,21] High dosages of both methylphenidate and dextroamphetamine sulfate (20–200 mg/day each in divided doses) are required. However, tolerance often develops, making it even more important to encourage the patient to continue to try to take brief naps, and to take drug holidays from the medications whenever possible. This may serve to minimize the development of tolerance. It should be noted that cataplectic attacks are often refractory to treatment with stimulants. The tricyclic antidepressants (e.g., imipramine 75–150 mg/day) have been found useful in some patients with cataplexy[15] (see Chapter 4). Monoamine oxidase inhibitors (MAOIs) (e.g., phenelzine 30–75 mg/day) have also been effective in the treatment of sleep attacks in narcolepsy, but are ineffective in treating cataplexy (see Chapter 6).

Table 3-5
How to Do an Outpatient Medication Assessment

1. Begin behavioral intervention first; after stabilized and if insufficient, then proceed with medication assessment. Note that using other interventions first and adding medication only if they are insufficient is now recommended in the PDR and by most experts in the field.
2. Include in the behavioral intervention components that can serve as dependent measures in medication assessment (e.g., daily living report card or task sheet or teacher frequency counts with the child's individual target behavior, both academic and social, monitored).
3. Talk with the child's pediatrician/primary practitioner about the assessment and elicit cooperation. The child should have a recent physical exam to rule out conditions that preclude an assessment with stimulants. Emphasize that the evaluation will provide objective information that can be used in long-term treatment planning and will protect both the child's and the practitioner's best interests.
4. Select type and doses of medication. Standard protocol utilized in our ADHD clinic includes placebo, 0.3 mg/kg methylphenidate b.i.d., and 0.6 mg/kg methylphenidate b.i.d. (reduced to 0.15 and 0.3 mg/kg for low and high doses, respectively, for overweight children, for older and therefore heavier children, and for children who do not have behavior problems). Other preparations could be employed for a variety of reasons (e.g., need long-acting preparation because school will not administer midday dose). If using d-amphetamine, halve the dose, and if using pemoline, use six times a single methylphenidate dose with a.m. administration only. Ensure that times of the day during which the child exhibits problems with overlap with peak medication times.
5. Establish a random schedule in which medication condition changes daily, but limit randomization to ensure that each dose is given at least once per week (e.g., week 1: P, 0.3, P, 0.6, 0.3). Have each dose occur between five and 10 times or until stable data have been obtained and a pattern or lack thereof is clear.
6. Have the pharmacist package medication and placebo in identical, self-locking opaque capsules in dated, individual envelopes in random order.
7. Let everyone, including the child, know that the assessment is occurring, but keep everyone who will provide any information regarding the child's response blind to the conditions.
8. Have teacher rate child on IOWA Conner's Daily (as a measure of main effect) and have parent complete Abbreviated Conner's nightly (as a measure of rebound), along with a brief side-effects rating scale.
9. Also gather daily objective information from the school regarding the child's major behavioral and academic problems.
10. If no. 9 is too difficult for the teacher, use daily report card record (already established for the behavioral intervention) and teacher ratings to assess response.
11. After the assessment has been completed, break blind and compute means and standards deviations for dependent measures within each condition.
12. Giving most weight to the child's major problem areas, determine whether or not the incremental improvement obtained with medication outweighs any side effects observed. Consider variability and final level of functioning when assessing response.

From Pelham, W.E., Milich, R. (1991). Individual differences in response to Ritalin in classwork and social behavior. In B.P. Osman, L. Greenhill (Eds), *Ritalin: Theory and Patient Management* (pp. 203–221). New York: Mary Ann Liebert, Inc.

Exogenous Obesity

The *Physicians' Desk Reference* (PDR) lists dextroamphetamine sulfate as indicated for use as a "short-time (a few weeks) regimen of weight reduction based on caloric restriction for patients refractory to alternative therapy. . . ."[21] Other stimulants have been used to inhibit appetite, but since tolerance develops to their anorectic effects within two weeks, they are generally too short-term to be of any true value in weight loss programs.[15,16] Fluoxetine (Prozac) is expected to be approved for the short-term treatment of exogenous obesity, and may have certain characteristics (longer half-life) that may make it more effective in weight-loss programs and clinics (see Chapter 4).

Attention-Deficit Disorder Without Hyperactivity

This disorder was referred to in the third edition of the *Diagnostic and Statistical Manual of Mental Disorders* (DSM-III) as attention-deficit disorder without hyperactivity and in DSM-III-R as undifferentiated attention-deficit disorder. This is a residual category reserved for disturbances in which the primary feature is "problems with initiating and maintaining attention." Barkley and associates[59] demonstrated that methylphenidate can decrease distractibility and improve attention span, interpersonal interactions, and responsiveness to instructions and commands, resulting in more productive and accurate academic performance for these children.

Attention-Deficit Hyperactivity Disorder

In Preschool Children

Only dextroamphetamine sulfate (Dexedrine) is FDA approved for children under 6 years of age (but not for children under 3 years of age).[21] Currently, there are no controlled studies demonstrating whether or not stimulants are beneficial in these populations. Barkley[8] found that preschoolers treated with methylphenidate exhibited significantly more side effects than did older children and adolescents. The efficacy of methylphenidate in this population was observed to be equivalent to that in older children, but somewhat more variable.

Differentiating between what is and what is not pathologic behavior in preschool children can be extremely difficult. Stimulant therapy, therefore, should be utilized only where other treatment modalities (behavioral modification therapy, parent management and education training, social skills training, structured preschool programs, etc.) have been unsuccessful. When implementing a stimulant medication in this population, it is important to start at a very low dose and to increase the dose gradually, as these children appear to be exquisitely sensitive to side effects.

In Intellectually Subaverage Children and Adolescents

In the past, clinicians were loath to prescribe stimulants for children with intellectual handicaps, such as mental retardation (MR). It was feared that such centrally acting stimulants would exacerbate preexisting CNS anomalies and predispose the children to severe side effects, especially seizures. McBridge and colleagues[20] demonstrated that methylphenidate in therapeutic doses did not lower the seizure threshold. This was confirmed by Crumrine and colleagues,[11] who found that therapeutic doses of methylphenidate in children with seizures and ADHD did not increase the likelihood of seizures. Although the data here are still scarce, recent studies appear to support the cautious use of stimulants in this population.

Aman and colleagues[1-5] studied the clinical effects of methylphenidate and thioridazine in 30 children with below-average IQs who had been diagnosed with ADHD and/or conduct disorder. They found that methylphenidate, but not thioridazine, resulted in a consistent and significant reduction in problem behavior as documented by teacher, but not parent, ratings. Moreover, it was noted that higher functioning children in the sample (IQs greater than 45) typically showed a favorable response to methylphenidate, while children of low functional levels (IQs less than 45 and mental ages less than 4.5 years) generally experienced adverse clinical responses or no improvement. Their data further suggested that mental age and IQ might be important determinants of stimulant response and side-effect sensitivity. It is important to note that it should not be concluded that retarded children with an IQ below 45 cannot respond to stimulant medication; replication of this work is required before such a determination can be made.

Handen and colleagues[14] demonstrated that MR children with ADHD may be at a significantly greater risk of developing side effects from stimulant use than nonretarded children. They evaluated the adverse side effects of two doses of methylphenidate (0.3 mg/kg, 0.6 mg/kg) in a placebo-controlled, double-blind study of 27 children with ADHD and IQs of 48–74. While methylphenidate was shown to significantly decrease the rates of irritability, anxiety, moodiness, and activity level when compared with placebo, medication for six of the children (22%) had to be discontinued due to the appearance of intolerable side effects, including motor tics and severe social withdrawal.

With Fragile X Syndrome

This is the second most common known genetic cause of MR, and many children with this disorder have symptoms of ADHD that do respond to stimulants.[12]

With Pervasive Developmental Disorder

The DSM-III-R states that ADHD cannot be diagnosed in the presence of pervasive developmental disorder (PDD, autism).[45] Nonetheless, children and adolescents with PDD often exhibit the classic ADHD symptoms of hyperactivity, impulsivity, distractibility, fidgetiness, and so on. Stimulants have been found to be effective and safe when used properly in this population.[12] Particular care must be used in monitoring side effects, as motor and behavioral side effects may be difficult to document. The recommendation is to start at a low dose and increase it very gradually.

With Head Trauma and/or Organic Brain Disease

Brain-damaged children and adolescents often experience ADHD symptoms, including hyperactivity, difficulty in attending, distractibility, and impulsivity, and may benefit from stimulant medication.[12] Seizures secondary to stimulant use are not felt to be a greater hazard in this population.

With Tic Disorders (Tourette's Syndrome)

Most authorities advise against using stimulants in children and adolescents with tic disorders.[7] It is known that stimulant medication can exacerbate preexisting motor tics or result in the de novo onset of tics, including those observed in Tourette's syndrome. Most neuropsychiatrists recommend against the use of stimulants in patients with Tourette's syndrome, and instead recommend antipsychotics, clonidine, or antidepressants. It should be noted, however, that simple motor tics are not infrequently seen in patients treated with stimulants, and their onset may not mandate that the stimulant be discontinued. In this case, it is important to compare the degree to which the medication is benefiting the patient with the magnitude of the side effects. If there has been a significant reduction in the patient's behavioral problems, and the tics do not interfere with the child's functioning or concern the parents, stimulant use may be continued, with close monitoring of the tics' course. The parents and child should be informed that simple tics, such as the "bunny rabbit nose," buccal lingual tics, and simple picking behavior, may be transient and nonproblematic. If the decision is made to proceed with the stimulant trial, careful observation is necessary, and the subsequent development of additional tic behavior and/or coprolalia usually requires that the stimulant be discontinued.

When a child develops outright Tourette's syndrome, the stimulants should be discontinued immediately, and the child's parents advised to inform any other clinician whom they might contact that the child should not receive stimulant medication. Stimulants are not, however, absolutely contraindicated in a child with a family history positive for Tourette's syndrome or other prominent tic disorders. Methylphenidate remains the drug of choice in children with ADHD. It is imperative to remember that it is the child who is being treated, not the family history. Therefore, avoidance of all stimulants in favor of an alternative medication, such as desipramine, is not indicated. However, the child should be monitored very closely for tics while on stimulants, and if they develop, the stimulant stopped. The clinician's threshold for continuing the medication in such a patient is necessarily lower, and the development of simple motor tics may warrant immediate discontinuation.

Some clinicians have suggested combining neuroleptics and stimulants for these patients, but this has not been widely endorsed. This combination therapy would result in both stimulation and inhibition of dopamine transmission, although its success has been reported in some cases.[12] It may be considered when a child's hyperactivity is severe and has failed to respond to any other intervention but the stimulant. A risk/benefit analysis must be conducted by the clinician, patient, and family. If the improvement in ADHD symptoms outweighs the motor tic side effects and the family agrees, cautious implementation of a stimulant trial with or without a neuroleptic or clonidine might be considered.

Gadow and colleagues[47] offer some recent preliminary data on using methylphenidate to treat hyperactive children with comorbid tic disorder. They treated 11 hyperactive prepubertal boys with a concomitant tic disorder with placebo and three doses of methylphenidate (0.1, 0.3, and 0.5 mg/kg) for two weeks each, under double-blind conditions in school settings. Short-term behavioral effects noted included decreased hyperactive/disruptive behaviors in the classroom and less physical aggression in the lunchroom and on the playground. Interestingly, methylphenidate also decreased the occurrence of vocal tics in the classroom and the lunchroom, while all but two children exhibited either no change or a reduction in motor tics.[47] Despite the fact that these findings are encouraging, the authors point out that the study was specific to the school setting, and that it is possible that at those times when drug rebound effects are more likely to occur (i.e., after school and in the evening), the tics may manifest as rebound phenomena, or have been "saved up," only to reoccur at a higher frequency. Moreover, four boys studied experienced worsening of tics at doses that were higher than the minimally effective dose. Obviously, further study, including the assessment of long-term behavioral effects, is necessary. Again, this is a highly controversial area and most authorities recommend that stimulants be immediately and permanently discontinued when Tourette's syndrome is observed or multiple motor tics occur.

Reduction of Narcotic Analgesic Needs and Narcotic-Induced Side Effects

The addition of stimulants has been found to be useful in adult patients with severe cancer pain who require very high dosages of narcotics that result in intolerable sedation.[13] Dextroamphetamine sulfate, in particular, in doses of 5–20 mg/day, has been found effective in lowering the narcotic dosage requirements and resulting side effects. The dosage needs to be adjusted according to the patient's needs, taking into account when the pain is most acute and when it is most important for the patient to be alert. Therefore, dextroamphetamine sulfate can be given either in a single early-morning dose or in divided doses, depending on the patient's requirements. We were unable to find any published evidence of stimulants being used to reduce narcotic requirements and narcotic-induced side effects in children. This may be an area worthy of future investigation.

Contraindications

For contraindications, see Table 3-6.

Psychosis

In general, stimulants are contraindicated when the patient is psychotic or has a history of psychosis, since they can induce a psychosis or exacerbate a preexisting one.[7,12,21] In fact, amphetamine-induced psychosis is the model used to explain the dopamine hypothesis of schizophrenia.[16] Indeed, the two conditions are best treated with an antipsychotic such as haloperidol. Stimulant medications should be avoided in psychotic children and adolescents.

Table 3-6
Stimulant Contraindications

Absolute:
• None
Relative:
• Psychosis
• Pregnancy
• History of substance abuse in patient and/or family
• Tic disorders (Tourette's syndrome) in child and/or family
• History of adverse reaction to stimulants
• Height/growth retardation
• Cardiac/blood pressure anomalies
• Impaired liver functioning (magnesium pemoline)
• Patient being treated with MAOI (infrequent in children and adolescents)

Pregnancy

As stimulants cross the placenta, they are virtually never indicated during pregnancy.[12,15,21]

History of Substance Abuse

Since amphetamines have long been a popular drug of abuse with potentially severe consequences, including psychosis, concern has been voiced over their use. Many children with ADHD have a coexisting oppositional defiant disorder or conduct disorder, which is associated with a significantly increased risk for recreational drug abuse.[16] It is, therefore, essential to monitor both the patient and family closely when stimulants are prescribed. Nevertheless, there are no data to support the view that stimulants, when prescribed correctly, lead to the increased use/abuse of recreational drugs.[43] Antidepressants such as desipramine may be preferable, however, if the patient or family members are at particularly high risk for abusing or selling stimulants. Still, antidepressants are not without their own risks, and they may have significant disadvantages as a first-line treatment for children and adolescents (see Chapter 4).

Tic Disorders (Tourette's Syndrome)

Before initiating a stimulant trial, it is important to screen for the presence of tics in both the child and family. While a positive family history for tic disorders does not preclude the use of psychostimulants in children and adolescents, it does mandate closer monitoring for evidence of tics while the patient is receiving stimulant medication (see "Indications").

History of Adverse Reactions

As with any medication, stimulants generally should not be used in children and adolescents who have a history of adverse reactions to their use.

Height/Growth Retardation

Reports from the early 1970s indicated that methylphenidate and dextroamphetamine could suppress a child's height and weight.[38,39] Subsequent clinical investigation has demonstrated that stimulant use does not result in a significant decrease in the ultimate height of most children,[19] although it is very common to observe a reduction in weight gain. Some children do, however, experience delayed height gain while taking stimulants, which apparently is related to both the medication dose and the length of time that the child is receiving it.[7,12]

35

Dextroamphetamine appears to suppress growth more than methylphenidate or pemoline does, and this effect most often is seen during the first year of treatment. The eventual height and weight of children treated with these medications are not significantly affected, however, and a rebound growth or habituation to the growth-suppressing effect produced in the first year is usually noted.[19,40] On the other hand, it should be pointed out that adolescents between 15 and 18 years of age, the period of epiphyseal closing, who continue to receive stimulant medication may experience a permanent decrease in their ultimate height of over 1 inch.[12] This height loss seems to occur more commonly in taller children, possibly as the result of an alteration in cartilage metabolism rather than in growth hormone production and metabolism.[12,19] The risk can, in large part, be minimized by choosing an alternative medication for children who fail to thrive, monitoring their weight and height very carefully, and stopping the stimulant if any significant delay is noted. The use of drug holidays (summer vacation, Christmas vacation, etc.) is recommended, as is using the minimum required dose necessary to improve behavior.

Cardiac/Blood Pressure Anomalies

Stimulants should not be prescribed for children with baseline hypertension and/or tachycardia.[7,12] Instead, a medication such as clonidine, which has antihypertensive effects, is preferable. When tachycardia and/or hypertension occurs after the initiation of a stimulant trial, the effects on pulse and blood pressure are usually not clinically significant, and often do not require that the medication be discontinued.[12] Careful monitoring is, of course, necessary, and additional investigation, including an electrocardiogram (ECG) and/or cardiology consultation, is recommended. It should be noted that increased heart rate is a direct effect of these agents, and thus is present in virtually all medicated children. Increases to levels that are clinically significant and of concern to the patient and physician are uncommon.

Impaired Liver Functioning

Impaired liver functioning has been observed only with the use of pemoline.[7] Hepatitis with elevated liver function tests (LFTs) is observed in nearly 3% of children receiving this drug. Unfortunately, this complication does not always remit upon discontinuation of the medication, and so it is essential that LFTs be checked in all children for whom pemoline use is being considered. If the baseline LFTs are abnormal, pemoline should not be prescribed. An antidepressant trial is warranted in this case, if the child has failed a methylphenidate and dextroamphetamine trial.

Patients on MAOIs

Children and adolescents are very rarely prescribed MAOIs due to the strict dietary restrictions and the lack of documented efficacy in this population. Nonetheless, stimulants should not be used within one week to 10 days of the discontinuation of an MAOI.

Seizures

There is no increased frequency of seizures with the use of stimulants.[11] Careful monitoring is required when coadministering stimulants and anti-convulsants as stimulants tend to increase the blood levels of these medications. Nevertheless, stimulants can be administered safely and with good success in children with seizure disorders. (Refer to Table 3-5.)

Side Effects

Side effects are listed in Table 3-7.

Table 3-7
Stimulant Side Effects

Common: • Insomnia   • Decreased appetite   • Gastrointestinal pain   • Irritability   • Increased heart rate (clinically insignificant)   • Paradoxical worsening of behavior
Uncommon: • Psychosis   • Sadness/isolation   • Major depressive episodes   • Cognitive impairment   • Growth retardation   • Tic disorders (i.e. Tourette's syndrome)   • Increased heart rate (clinically significant)   • Impaired liver functioning (pemoline only)   • Increased blood pressure   • Dizziness, lethargy, fatigue   • Nausea, constipation   • Rash/hives   • Hyperacusis   • Formication   • Necrotizing angitis brain (IV amphetamine)

Insomnia

Insomnia is the most common side effect observed with stimulant use. Barkley et al.[41] found that over 50% of 82 ADHD children receiving methylphenidate, 0.3 mg/kg and 0.5 mg/kg, developed insomnia, a decrease in appetite, nervousness, irritability, and increased crying on both doses. Fortunately, these side effects are usually transitory and mild. In fact, in the Barkley study, many of these "side effects" were present during the placebo phase of the trial. The differences in side effects between the two phases was not reported as being significant. These side effects may be a manifestation of the underlying disruptive behavior disorder, a rebound drug effect, a direct drug effect, or a primary sleep disturbance. If the sleep disturbance dissipates, the stimulant can be continued. On the other hand, if the insomnia does not reverse, further clinical and/or laboratory investigation is necessary, and the stimulant may have to be discontinued.

Anorexia/Weight Loss

Anorexia and weight loss are common, but usually are short-term side effects. Dextroamphetamine appears to suppress weight more than methylphenidate or pemoline does. The anorexia and weight loss are said to be minimized by giving the stimulants after meals. But this recommendation should be weighed against the reported pharmacokinetics of the stimulants, which suggest that since these medications are best absorbed at an acid pH and that alkaline substances, such as lactose in milk, are known to interfere with their absorption, they should actually be given a half hour before meals. It should be noted, however, that current practice holds that the risks of side effects outweigh the benefits of giving the medications before meals, so they are usually prescribed after meals. It should also be kept in mind that children with ADHD were notoriously poor eaters prior to receiving stimulant medication.

Irritability

Irritability is also a frequent short-term side effect. It is not always easy to tell whether the irritability is a side effect of the medication or a manifestation of the underlying disorder, since the presentation is usually the same in both cases. Drug A/B trials to determine whether or not the child is more irritable on stimulant medication are often informative. If this is not possible, observing the patient while off the medication and being monitored by teachers and parents can be helpful.

Dysphoria/Social Isolation

Children on stimulants very commonly are reported as looking "sadder." This may be due to a drug effect, or may simply arise from the fact that the child at baseline was so hyperactive that the less hyperactive behavior may lead others to think that he or she might be depressed. This state requires careful monitoring since, although dysphoria with tearfulness and intermittent sadness is usually a short-term side effect, it may persist during treatment or after long-term treatment has been discontinued.

Abdominal Pain

Children frequently report abdominal pain while initially on stimulants, but this usually disappears with time. When using pemoline, however, LFTs must be drawn to rule out a chemical hepatitis.

Decreased Cognitive Ability

Impairment in cognitive ability is typically observed only when stimulants are used at high doses (e.g., methylphenidate dosages greater than 1 mg/kg/day). Standard dosages of between 0.3 mg/kg/day and 0.69 mg/kg/day have not been shown to cause cognitive depression.[22]

Increased Hyperactivity

While between 70% and 80% of children treated with stimulants exhibit a significant improvement in their behavior, up to one third of such children will become more hyperactive on stimulants, exhibiting what has been referred to as "behavioral rebound." Johnston and colleagues[42] found that this effect is quite variable during the time the children are on medication, and that this rebound rarely results in the stimulant's having to be discontinued. Each case must be considered separately. One option is to decrease the lunchtime or early-afternoon dose. Another option is to decrease the dose to the previously tolerated dose and observe whether that dose is sufficient to ameliorate the target symptoms. It should be noted that just because a child shows this effect with one stimulant (e.g., methylphenidate), this does not mean that the child will exhibit the same behavior rebound with another stimulant.

Motor Tics, Tourette's Syndrome

These side effects are uncommon, but potentially severe. Prior to starting a stimulant, all patients and their families must be screened for the presence of tics, adventitious movements, Tourette's, and so on.

Growth Suppression

See Contraindications.

Hypertension/Tachycardia

Brown and Sexson[10] observed that black adolescents treated with methylphenidate may be at increased risk for diastolic blood pressure elevation. The effects on blood pressure were statistically but not clinically significant. Blood pressure and pulse changes in children are extremely variable, and frequently, with careful monitoring, do not require cessation of the stimulant medication. Since this effect almost always produces tachyphylaxis, monitoring of all vital signs is essential. It is, however, rare that the stimulant will have to be discontinued, and often the symptoms do not persist.

Psychosis

Paranoid psychotic complications in adults ingesting large doses of amphetamines have been well documented. Ney[18] first reported the occurrence of psychotic phenomena, including auditory, visual, and tactile hallucinations, in an 8-year-old child receiving therapeutic dosages of dextroamphetamine. Moreover, Lucas and Weiss[17] observed methylphenidate hallucinosis in both a 10-year-old boy receiving therapeutic dosages of methylphenidate and a 15-year-old girl who took an excess of methylphenidate. Whenever stimulants are administered, careful monitoring for thought disorder/psychosis is mandatory. If psychosis occurs, the stimulant must be discontinued and a different class of medication utilized (such as antipsychotics or antidepressants).

Chemical Hepatitis

Impaired liver functioning is seen only with pemoline, and the resulting chemical hepatitis is not always reversible upon discontinuing the medication. Thus it is essential to check LFTs prior to starting pemoline. After it is started, LFTs should be checked every three months for the first year, and then at least every six months. If the patient exhibits any side effects, such as jaundice or abdominal pain, stat LFTs should be drawn and the medication suspended. Abnormal LFTs mandate that the pemoline be held. If the clinician is suspicious of the validity and reliability of the results of the LFTs, they may be repeated. Consistent alterations in LFTs, however, preclude pemoline's use.

Rare Side Effects

Nausea/vomiting, constipation, dizziness, lethargy, fatigue, nightmares, anxiety, rash/hives, hyperacusis, formication, and fearfulness may be observed, though rarely, as a result of stimulant use. Necrotizing angiitis is a very rare complication resulting from intravenous (IV) amphetamine abuse.[21]

Decreased Seizure Threshold

There is no evidence that stimulants lower the seizure threshold.[11]

Increased Recreational Use/Abuse of Drugs

There is no evidence that stimulants, when prescribed correctly, result in an increased propensity to use/abuse recreational drugs or other prescription drugs, or that they increase physical and psychological dependence on stimulants.[12,43]

Overdose

An overdose of stimulants is less dangerous than overdosing with some other psychotropic medications, such as the tricyclic antidepressants and lithium. Nonetheless, children and adolescents with ADHD and/or conduct disorders have a higher rate of suicide attempts than do children and adolescents without these disorders. Thus careful monitoring is required when these medications are prescribed. Overdosing with stimulants results in autonomic hyperactivity secondary to their sympathomimetic effects, with resulting hypertension, hyperthermia, and tachycardia. Psychosis and/or toxicity may also occur. An overdose may result in death because of hypertensive, hyperthermic, cardiovascular, or epileptic complications.

Stimulant overdose is a medical emergency and requires urgent treatment. Paranoid psychosis is usually best treated with the antipsychotic chlorpromazine, 50 mg PO/intramuscularly (IM) four times a day, since it blocks both dopamine and alpha-adrenergic receptors, thereby serving as both an antipsychotic and an antihypertensive.[15] Severe hypertension and tachycardia are best treated with propranolol, 1 mg intravenously (IV) every 5 minutes, with a maximum dose of 8 mg.[15]

When the hypertension is mild, haloperidol, 5 mg b.i.d., is probably a better choice, since it has fewer anticholinergic and sedating properties than does chlorpromazine. On the other hand, if extra sedation is necessary because of the psychosis, the benzodiazepines are an excellent, safe alternative. Lorazepam, 1–2 mg PO/IM, is the best choice since it is the only benzodiazepine that can be given IM, and is relatively short-acting.[15] Any psychosis and delirium should clear within a few days, if properly treated.

Finally, if the patient is unconscious or having seizures, maintaining an adequate airway, breathing, and circulation (ABCs) is crucial. High fevers require appropriate medical management. Seizures can be treated with lorazepam or diazepam.

Abuse

The practicing clinician should be cognizant of the significant abuse potential of the stimulants. Dextroamphetamine has the highest risk for abuse, with methylphenidate having a lower risk and pemoline the lowest risk for abuse of all the stimulants. Amphetamine abuse, both orally and IV, has been reported, with severe consequences (necrotizing angiitis of the brain).

The stimulants produce a sense of euphoria that initially may be quite pleasing to adolescents with ADHD and/or conduct disorders, who commonly suffer from feelings of low self-esteem. It is important to note that persons taking methylphenidate and dextroamphetamine quickly become tolerant of their euphorigenic and sympathomimetic effects. Tolerance is not seen in children and adolescents treated therapeutically for ADHD. Stimulant abusers who become tolerant to high doses of stimulants can tolerate doses that could seriously harm or kill persons without such tolerance. The practicing clinician should be alert for the following signs and symptoms when stimulants are taken in *large nontherapeutic* quantities.

1. Sympathomimetic overload (hypertension, tachycardia, dry mouth, pupillary dilation)

2. Stereotyped behaviors

3. Irritability/emotional lability

4. Paranoia/formication

Chronic abuse looks much like schizophrenia. Characteristic signs and symptoms include:

1. Psychosis

2. Auditory/visual/tactile hallucinations

3. Ideas of reference

Psychological withdrawal after stimulants have been abused is common, although physical withdrawal does not occur. Careful monitoring for a resulting dysphoria and/or major depressive episode with feelings of hopelessness and suicidal ideation is important.

Drug Interactions

See Tables 3-8 and 3-9.

The interaction of pemoline with other medications has not been studied in humans. Careful monitoring of patients receiving pemoline while on other drugs, particularly drugs with CNS activity, is required.

Table 3-8
Methylphenidate Drug Interactions

Inhibits metabolism of:
• Anticoagulants (i.e., warfarin [Coumadin])
• Anticonvulsants (phenobarbital, phenytoin [Dilantin], primidone [Mysoline])
• Phenylbutazone (Butazolidin)
• Heterocyclic antidepressants (i.e., amitriptyline, Elavil)
Decreases hypotensive effect of:
• Guanethidine
In combination with Imipramine can cause:
• Confusion
• Mood lability
• Aggression
• Agitation
• Psychosis
Potentiates effect of:
• All sympathomimetic medications (i.e., ephedrine)
• Recreational stimulants (cocaine)
Metabolism is slowed by:
• MAOIs

Initiating and Maintaining Treatment

Available preparations of psychostimulants and their costs are shown in Table 3-10.

Prior to initiating the psychostimulants, children and adolescents should have a physical examination, with special attention paid to heart rate, blood pressure, height, and weight. A baseline screen for abnormal involuntary movements, including tics, should be performed. It is important to elicit any family history of motor movement tic disorders. As the stimulants do cross the placenta, they should not be prescribed during pregnancy, and so a pregnancy test and evaluation for adequate contraceptive use are essential in all women of childbearing age. When prescribing methylphenidate or dextroamphetamine, laboratory tests are generally not necessary. When pemoline therapy is to be initiated though, LFTs are mandated, as nearly 3% of patients placed on pemoline will develop a chemical hepatitis that is not always reversible upon discontinuing the medication.

When children and adolescents are treated with stimulants, they should be monitored at each visit for any involuntary movements/tics by observation and/or history. Whenever the dose is increased, it is important to check blood pressure, pulse, height, and weight. In addition, it is advisable to re-

43

Table 3-9

Dextroamphetamine Drug Interaction

Inhibits: • Beta-adrenergic blockers (propranolol)
In combination with TCAs, MAOIs, inhibiting antidepressants, narcotics: • Effects of both medications increased
Delays absorption of: • Phenytoin • Phenobarbital • Ethosoximide
Decreases hypotensive effect of: • Guanethidine
Absorption lowered by: • GI-acidifying agents
Absorption increased by: • GI-alkalinizing agents
Renal clearance increased by: • Urine-acidifying agents
Renal clearance decreased by: • Urine-alkalinizing agents (i.e., thiazides)
Increases: • Plasma corticosteroid levels
May alter: • Urinary steroid measurements • Insulin requirements

cord height and weight at regular three-to four-month intervals. When using pemoline only, LFTs should be drawn every six months. Children and adolescents should have an annual physical examination by their pediatrician or family practitioner.

Specific Agents and Indications

Methylphenidate

Methylphenidate remains the drug of choice in the treatment of ADHD in children and adolescents. It is one of the safest medications in all of child psychiatry, with a quick onset of action and a short half-life. It is effective in 70–80% of children and adolescents.

Table 3-10

Available Preparations and Cost of Psychostimulants

	Commercially Available Preparations	**Dosage Form**	**Average Cost/Day**
Dextroamphetamine	Generic (dextroamphetamine sulfate)	5 mg (scored), 10 mg (scored) tablets	$0.12
	Dexedrine	5 mg (unscored), 10 mg (unscored) tablets; 5 mg/5 ml elixir	$0.72
	Dexedrine spansules (sustained release)	5 mg, 10 mg, 15 mg capsules	$0.82
Methylphenidate	Generic	5 mg, 10 mg, 20 mg* tablets	$0.77
	Ritalin	5 mg (unscored), 10 mg (unscored), and 20 mg* (unscored) tablets	$1.02
	Ritalin - SR (sustained release)	20 mg tablet	$1.06
Pemoline	Cylert	18.75 mg, 37.5 mg, 75 mg (scored) tablets, 37.5 mg chewable (scored) tablets	$1.89

*Methylphenidate/Ritalin 20 mg often not carried by pharmacies.
Source: Red Book Annual Pharmacist Reference 1989–1990. Oradell, NJ: Medical Economics.

Methylphenidate-SR, 20mg, can take up to three hours to have any effect. Sustained-release methylphenidate is, in theory, comparable to 10 mg methylphenidate after breakfast and 10 mg after lunch. In reality, however, regular methylphenidate is superior for individual children in almost every case.[27,28] Moreover, the sustained-release form does not last as long as would a second dose of regular methylphenidate. Increased day-to-day variability is also observed. A single daily dose of sustained-release methylphenidate is almost never adequate in ameliorating the target symptoms, so that once-daily dosing is rarely, if ever, successfully achieved. A further disadvantage of sustained-release methylphenidate is that when it is chewed instead of swallowed, very high blood levels can result, with toxic side effects. Finally, tolerance to sustained-release methylphenidate after several months of therapy has been documented, but has not been demonstrated when the other stimulants are used therapeutically. Therefore, we believe that sustained-release methylphenidate is not a particularly useful medication for the child psychopharmacologist.

Dosage and Administration
See Tables 3-11A and 3-11B.

The starting dose of methylphenidate is usually 0.3 mg/kg/dose. Whenever possible, a simple drug A/B trial is ideal for determining whether or not the child truly benefits from the medication and what the most effective dose is (Table 3-4 shows how to perform a drug A/B trial). When it is not possible to perform such a trial, initiating treatment at a dose of 0.15 mg/kg and increasing it gradually, monitoring closely for efficacy versus toxicity, is recommended. In general, a dose exceeding 1 mg/kg is not recommended since laboratory tests have shown cognitive impairment at such high doses. Optimal doses are usually achieved between 0.3 and 0.7 mg/kg given three times per day.[12] If this range is unsuccessful and the child suffers no side effects, the dose may be gradually increased to a maximum of 1 mg/kg/dose. Dosages greater than 1 mg/kg are not recommended because of unacceptable side effects.

Table 3-11A
Clinician's Guide to Using Stimulants for ADHD in Children and Adolescents

Methylphenidate schedule: • Not approved for children < 6 years old.   • Six years and older: Start with 5 mg twice a day, increase by 5–10 mg/week to maximum dose not to exceed 60 mg.   • Optimal dose 0.3–0.7 mg/kg two to three times per day (total daily dose: 0.9–2.1 mg/kg/day). Do not exceed 1 mg/kg/dose.
Dextroamphetamine schedule: • Not approved for children < 3 years.   • 3–5 years: Start with 2.5 mg/day increased by 2.5 mg/week, adjust to best tolerated dose.   • 6 years and older: Start with 2.5 mg twice a day increased by 5 mg/week to maximum dose not to exceed 40 mg.   • Optimal dose 0.15–0.5 mg/kg two to three times daily (total daily dose: 0.3–1.5 mg/kg/day).
Pemoline schedule: • Not approved for children < 6 years old.   • 6 years and older: Start with 37.5 mg/day, increase by 18.75 mg/week to maximum daily dose of 112.5 mg/day.

Table 3-11B
Dose Ranges

Drug	Therapeutic Dose Range	Usual Dose Range	Extreme Dose Range
Methylphenidate	0.15–0.6 mg/kg/day	20–40 mg/day	40–60 mg/day or higher
Dextroamphetamine	0.08–0.3 mg/kg/day	10–20 mg/day	30–40 mg/day
Pemoline	0.6–4 mg/kg/day	37.5–112.5 mg/day	> 112.5 mg/day

For the practicing clinician, this generally translates into treating children who weigh less than 30 kg with 5 mg after breakfast and 5 mg after lunch. For very young children, the tablets can be broken in half, so that 2.5 mg b.i.d. is given. In children who weigh more than 30 kg, a starting dose of 10 mg after breakfast and 10 mg after lunch should be given. Single doses above 20 mg are generally not recommended. Adolescents and children often require similar absolute amounts since adolescents frequently need lower weight-adjusted doses.

Doses are increased in the morning and at lunchtime every other week, so that five full days of the child's daily report card and parent–teacher Conner's Rating Scales can be assessed. Individual adjustment of the dose is often required. For instance, if the child is having problems with hyperactivity on the school bus, a dose 30 minutes before he or she gets on the bus is suggested. On the other hand, if the problems with behavior do not manifest themselves until the first school period or shortly after it, it may be best to give the child his or her dose when he or she gets to school. In addition, if the effect of the methylphenidate seems to be wearing off at about 10:30 or 11:00 a.m., raising the morning dose or giving the second dose at 10:00 or 11:00 a.m. may be advisable. Thus it is crucial to determine when the behavior is most problematic and in what setting. Sometimes, a small afternoon dose is required. This should not be given later than 4:00 p.m. since exacerbation of behavior may result. Many physicians prescribe a smaller dose at this time than the two earlier doses.

Determination of whether or not the child requires medication on weekends or after school can be difficult, but is important. If the main problems are in school and the parents feel that the behavior at home is not a problem, then weekend doses may not be necessary. On the other hand, if significant problems with behavior are occurring after school and/or on weekends, medication may be indicated during these times. In some cases, p.r.n. doses of the stimulant may be warranted, if, for instance, the family is going to a function where the child has typically had significant difficulty in the past.

Reassessment of medication needs is essential on at least a yearly basis, if not more often. Taking the child off medication over summer and Christmas vacations is a good way to assess the continued need for stimulants, as well as to minimize the risk of developing tolerance. A drug A/B trial can also be performed a year after the initiation of the stimulant, particularly if there is a question as to whether the stimulant is needed or whether the dosage should be altered.

Dextroamphetamine

When methylphenidate is unsuccessful, dextroamphetamine is usually the next line of treatment. As with methylphenidate, 70–80% of children and adolescents will respond to dextroamphetamine. Unfortunately, there is no way to predict which child will respond to which medication. Moreover, the fact that a child does not respond to methylphenidate does not mean that he or she will not respond to another stimulant.

Dextroamphetamine, like methylphenidate, is a safe medication with relatively few side effects and a half-life that is longer than that of methylphenidate, but still fairly short. Growth suppression with dextroamphetamine is greater than with methylphenidate, but rebound growth after cessation of dextroamphetamine treatment is greater (see Table 3-12 for a comparison of psychostimulant properties). Anorexia and weight loss caused by dextroamphetamine is also greater than with methylphenidate. The amphetamines are believed to be the most potentially addictive of the psychostimulants, although when prescribed therapeutically, abuse/dependence has not been shown to occur.[7,12]

Dosage and Administration
See Tables 3-11A and 3-11B.

The therapeutic dose range for dextroamphetamine is half that for methylphenidate (i.e., 0.15–0.5 mg/kg/day). This translates into a starting dose of 2.5 mg dextroamphetamine (half of the smallest dextroamphetamine capsule) after breakfast and lunch. It is particularly important to ensure that the medication is given after meals whenever possible, since dextroamphetamine is more anorectic than either methylphenidate or pemoline. For very small or very young children, the dextroamphetamine elixir may be advisable. Doses of 5 mg dextroamphetamine after breakfast and lunch are recommended for children who weigh more than 30 kg. Dose adjustment and assessment are similar to those described for methylphenidate.

Pemoline

Pemoline is used far less commonly than the other stimulants. It can be useful, however, since it lacks significant sympathomimetic activity and is some-

Table 3-12
Comparison of Some Properties of Psychostimulants

	Methylphenidate	Dextroamphetamine	Pemoline
Sustained-release form	Yes	Yes	No (no need—half-life same as sustained release for methylphenidate and dextroamphetamine)
Anorexia	Less	Most	Less
Growth suppression	Less	Most	Less
Addictive potential	Less	Most	Least
Sympathomimetic arousal	Yes	Yes	Less
Can cause chemical hepatitis	No	No	Yes
Can cause increase in heart rate/blood pressure	Yes	Yes	Less

times helpful when the other, more commonly used psychostimulants have caused intolerable side effects. It must be noted that when the other stimulants have caused a psychosis or severe tic/movement disorder, pemoline should probably not be used.

Dosage and Administration
See Tables 3-11A and 3-11B.

Pemoline has the advantage of usually being given one time per day. It is usually started at a dose of 37.5 mg in the morning and then increased gradually to 0.5–3 mg/kg/day. When the child is obese and particularly large, an initial dose of 37.5 mg/day may be implemented. The maximum dose is 112.5 mg/day. Older adolescents will sometimes require higher doses, up to 2.2 mg/kg/day.

In contrast to the other stimulants, pemoline does not cause an increase in heart rate or blood pressure, but it can cause a chemical hepatitis (Table 3-12), so that LFT monitoring is required when it is used.

Sallee and colleagues[31] found that the acute initial administration of a single dose of pemoline 2 mg/kg resulted in a significant improvement in atten-

49

tion to task within two to three hours after the dose in 20 6- to 12-year-old children with ADHD. Of these children, 25% developed abnormal involuntary movements of the extremities, trunk, face, and mouth.[31,46] On repeated doses, however, these movements dissipated in all but one of the children. Increasing the dose of pemoline sooner than recommended may, however, expose children to unpleasant and potentially debilitating side effects and cannot be recommended at this time.

References

1. Aman, M.G., Marks, R.E., Turbott, S.H., et al. (1991). Methylphenidate and thioridazine in the treatment of intellectually subaverage children: Effects on cognitive-motor performance. *J Am Acad Child Adolesc Psychiatry, 30*, 816–824.

2. Aman, M.G., Marks, R.E., Turbott, S.H., et al. (1991). Effects of methylphenidate and thioridazine in intellectually subaverage children. *J Am Acad Child Adolesc Psychiatry, 30*, 246–256.

3. Aman, M.G. (1982). Stimulant drug effects in developmental disorders and hyperactivity—toward a resolution of disparate findings. *J Autism Dev Disord, 12*, 385–398.

4. Aman, M. (1988). The use of methylphenidate in autism (Letter to the Editor). *J Am Acad Child Adolesc Psychiatry, 27*, 821–822.

5. Aman, M.G., Singh, N.N. (1982). Methylphenidate in severely retarded residents and the clinical significance of stereotypic behavior. *Appli Res in Men Retardation, 3*, 345–358.

6. Barkley, R.A. (1977). A review of stimulant drug research with hyperactive children. *Child Psychol Psychiatry, 18*, 137–165.

7. Barkley, R.A. (1990). *Hyperactive Children: A Handbook for Diagnosis and Treatment*. New York: Guilford Press.

8. Barkley, R.A. (1988). The effects of methylphenidate on the interactions of preschool ADHD children with their mothers. *J Am Acad Child Adolesc Psychiatry, 27*, 336–341.

9. Barkley, R.A., Anastopoulos, D.C., Guevremont, D.C. (1991). Adolescents with ADHD: Patterns of behavioral adjustment, academic functioning, and treatment utilization. *J Am Acad Child Adolesc Psychiatry, 30*, 752–761.

10. Brown, R.T., Sexson, S.B. (1989). Effects of methylphenidate on cardiovascular responses in ADHD adolescents. *J Adoles Health Care, 10*, 179–183.

11. Crumrine, P.K., Feldman, H.M., Teodori, J., et al. (1987). The use of methylphenidate in children with seizures and attention deficit disorder. *Ann Neurol, 48*, 112–114.

12. Dulcan, M.K. (1990). Using psychostimulants to treat behavioral disorders of children and adolescents. *Child Adolesc Psychopharmacol, 1*, 7–22.

13. Forrest, W.H., Brown, B., Brown, C.R., et al. (1977). Dextroamphetamine with morphine for the treatment of postoperative pain. *N Engl J Med 296*, 712.

14. Handen, B.L., Feldman, H., Gosling, A., et al. (1991). Adverse side effects of methylphenidate among mentally retarded children with ADHD. *J Am Acad Child Adolesc Psychiatry, 30*, 241–245.

15. Arana, G.W., Hyman, S.E. (1991). *Handbook of Psychiatric Drug Therapy* (2nd ed., pp. 162–170). Boston: Little Brown.

16. Kaplan, H.I., Sadock, B.J. (1991). *Synopsis of Psychiatry* (6th ed., pp. 658–660). Baltimore: Williams & Wilkins.

17. Lucas, A.R., Weiss, M. (1971). Methylphenidate hallucinosis. *JAMA, 217*, 1079–1081.

18. Ney, P.G. (1967). Psychosis in a child associated with amphetamine administration. *Can Med Assoc J, 97*, 1026–1029.

19. Klein, R.G., Mannuzza, S. (1988). Hyperactive boys almost grown up: III. Methylphenidate effects on ultimate height. *Arch Gen Psychiatry, 45*, 1131–1134.

20. McBridge, M.C., Wang, D.D., Torres, C.F. (1986). Methylphenidate in therapeutic doses does not lower seizure threshold. *Ann Neurol, 20*, 428.

21. *Physicians' Desk Reference* (45th ed.) (1991). Oradell, N.J.: Medical Economics Co.

22. Pelham, W.E., Milich, R. (1991). Individual differences in response to ritalin in classwork and social behavior. In B.P. Osman, L. Greenhill (Eds.), *Ritalin: Theory and Patient Management* (pp. 203–221). New York: Mary Ann Liebert.

23. Pelham, W.E. (1989). Behavior therapy, behavioral assessment, and psychostimulant medication in the treatment of ADD: An interactive approach. In L. Bloomingdale, J. Swanson, & R. Klorman (Eds.), *Attention Deficit Disorders: New Directions* (vol. 4) (pp. 169–195). New York: Spectrum.

24. Pelham, W.E., Hoza, J. (1987). Behavioral assessment of psychostimulant effects on ADD children in a summer day treatment parogram. In R.

Prin (Ed.), *Advances in Behavioral Assessment of Children and Families* (vol. 3) (pp. 3–33). Greenwich, Conn.: JAI Press.

25. Pelham, W.E. (1986). The effects of stimulant drugs on learning and achievement in hyperactive and learning disabled children. In J.K. Torgesen & B. Wong (Eds.), *Psychological and Educational Perspectives on Learning Disabilities* (pp. 259–295). New York: Academic Press.

26. Pelham, W.E., Murphy, H.A. (1986). Attention deficit and conduct disorders. In M. Hersen (Ed.), *Pharmacological and Behavioral Treatment: An Integrative Approach* (pp. 108–147). New York: Wiley.

27. Pelham, W.E., Sturges, J., Hoza, J., et al. (1987). The effects of sustained release 20 and 10 mg Ritalin bid on cognitive and social behavior in children with ADD. *Pediatrics, 80,* 491–501.

28. Pelham, W.E., Greenslade, K.E., Vodde-Hamilton, M.A., et al. (1990). Relative efficacy of long-acting CNS stimulants on children with ADHD: A comparison of standard methylphenidate, sustained-release methylphenidate, sustained-release dextroamphetamine, and pemoline. *Pediatrics, 86,* 226–237.

29. Pelham, W.E., Bender, M.E., Caddell, J., et al. (1985). Methylphenidate and children with ADD. *Arch Gen Psychiatry, 42,* 948–952.

30. Rapoport, J., Buchsbaum, M., Weingartner, H., et al. (1980). Dextroamphetamine: Cognitive and behavioral effects in normal and hyperactive boys and normal adult males. *Arch Gen Psychiatry, 37,* 933–943.

31. Sallee, F., Stiller, R., Perel, J., et al. (1989). Pemoline-induced abnormal involuntary movements. *J Clin Psychopharmacol, 9,* 125–129.

32. Wender, P. (1987). *The Hyperactive Child, Adolescent, and Adult: Attention Deficit Disorder Through the Lifespan.* New York: Oxford University Press.

33. Barkley, R.A. (1985). The social interactions of hyperactive children: Developmental changes, drug effects, and situational variation. In R. McMahon & R. Peters (Eds.), *Childhood Disorders: Behavioral-Developmental Approaches* (pp. 218–243). New York: Brunner/Mazel.

34. Whalen, C.K., Henker, B., Buhrmester, D., et al. (1989). Does stimulant medication improve the peer status of hyperactive children? *J Consult Clin Psychol, 57,* 545–549.

35. Barkley, R.A., Cunningham, C.E. (1978). Do stimulant drugs improve the academic performance of hyperkinetic children? *Arch Gen Psychiatry, 36,* 201–208.

36. Douglas, V.I., Barr, R.G., O'Neill, M.E., et al. (1988). Dosage effects and individual responsivity to methylphenidate in attention deficit disorder. *Child Psychol Psychiatry, 29*, 453–475.

37. Rapport, M.D., DuPaul, G.J., Stoner, G., et al. (1986). Comparing classroom and clinic measures of attention deficit disorder: Differential, idiosyncratic, and dose-response effects of methylphenidate. *J Consult Clin Psychol, 54*, 334–341.

38. Safer, D.J., Allen, R.P., Barr, E. (1972). Depression in growth in hyperactive children on stimulant drugs. *N Engl J Med, 287*, 217–220.

39. Safer, D.J., Allen, R.P. (1973). Factors influencing the suppressant effects of two stimulant drugs on the growth of hyperactive children. *Pediatrics, 51*, 660–667.

40. Mattes, J.A., Gittelman, R. (1983). Growth of hyperactive children on maintenance regimen of methylphenidate. *Arch Gen Psychiatry, 40*, 317–321.

41. Barkley, R.A., McMurray, M.B., Edelbrock, C.S., et al. (1990). The side effects of methylphenidate: A systematic placebo controlled evaluation. *Pediatrics, 86*, 184–192.

42. Johnston, C., Pelham, W.E., Hoza, J., et al. (1988). Psychostimulant rebound in attention deficit disordered boys. *J Am Acad Child Adolesc Psychiatry, 27*, 806–810.

43. Gadow, K.D. (1981). Prevalence of drug treatment for hyperactivity and other childhood behavior disorders. In K.D. Gadow & J. Loney (Eds.) *Psychosocial Aspects of Drug Treatment for Hyperactivity* (pp. 13–70). Boulder, Col.: Westview Press.

44. Weiss, G., Hechtman, L., Milroy, T., et al. (1985). Psychiatric status of hyperactives as adults: A controlled prospective 15 year follow up of 63 hyperactive children. *J Am Acad Child Psychiatry, 23*, 211–220.

45. *Diagnostic and Statistical Manual of Mental Disorders* (3rd ed., revised). (1987). Washington, D.C.: American Psychiatric Association.

46. Sallee, F., Stiller, R., Perel, J., et al. (1985). Oral pemoline kinetics in hyperactive children. *Clin Pharmacol Ther, 37*, 606–609.

47. Gadow, K.D., Nolan, E.E., Sverd, J. (1992). Methylphenidate in hyperactive boys with comorbid tic disorder: II. Short-term behavioral effects in school settings. *J Am Acad Child Adolesc Psychiatry, 31(3)*, 462–471.

48. Carlson, C.L., Pelham, W.E., Milich, R., et al. (1993). ADHD boys' performance and attributions following success and failure: Drug effects and individual differences. *Cog Ther Res, 17*, 269–287.

49. Balthazor, M.J., Wagner, R.K., Pelham, W.E. (1991). The specificity of the effects of stimulant medication on classroom learning-related measures of cognitive processes for attention deficit disorder children. *J Abnorm Child Psychol, 19*, 35–52.

50. Pelham, W.E., Hamilton, M.V., Murphy, D.A., et al. (1991). The effects of methylphenidate on ADHD adolescents in recreational, peer group, and classroom settings. *J Clin Psychol, 20*, 293–300.

51. Evans, S.W., Pelham, W.E. (1991). Psychostimulant effects on academic and behavioral measures for ADHD junior high school students in a lecture format classroom. *J Abnorm Child Psychol, 19*, 537–552.

52. Stephens, R.S., Pelham, W.E., Skinner, R. (1984). State-dependent and main effects of methylphenidate and pemoline on paired-associate learning and spelling in hyperactive children. *J Consult Clin Psychol, 52*, 104–113.

53. Hinshaw, S.P., Henker, B., Whalen, C.K., et al. (1989). Aggressive, prosocial, and nonsocial behavior in hyperactive boys: Dose effects of methylphenidate in naturalistic settings. *J Consult Clin Psychol, 57*, 636–643.

54. Gittelman, R., Abikoff, H. (1989). The role of psychostimulants and psychosocial treatments in hyperkinesis. In T. Sagvolden & T. Archer (Eds.), *Attention Deficit Disorder: Clinical and Basic Research* (pp. 167–180). Hillsdale, N.J.: Erlbaum.

55. Klorman, R., Brumaghim, J.T., Salzman, L.F., et al. (1988). Effects of methylphenidate on attention-deficit hyperactivity disorder with and without aggressive/noncompliant features. *J Abnorm Psychol, 97*, 413–422.

56. Gittelman, R., Mannuzza, S. (1985). Diagnosing ADD-H in adolescents. *Psychopharmacol Bull, 21*, 237–242.

57. Murphy, D.A., Pelham, W.E., Lang, A.R. (1992). Aggression in boys with attention deficit disorder: Methylphenidate effects on naturalistic observations of aggression, response to provocation in the laboratory, and social information processing. *J Abnorm Child Psychol, 20*, 1–16.

58. Gittelman, R., Mannuzza, S., Shenker, R., et al. (1985). Hyperactive boys almost grown up. *Arch Gen Psychiatry, 42*, 937–947.

59. Barkley, R.A., DuPaul, G.J., McMurray, M.B. (1991). Attention deficit disorder with and without hyperactivity: Clinical response to three dose levels of methylphenidate. *Pediatrics, 87(4)*, 519–531.

C h a p t e r 4

Tricyclic Antidepressants

The antidepressant drugs are a heterogeneous group of compounds that, in adults, have been found to be effective in the treatment of major depressive disorder, generalized anxiety disorder, panic disorder, and a variety of other conditions. In this section, we will focus on the tricyclic antidepressants (TCAs). Novel and atypical antidepressants, such as fluoxetine, sertraline, bupropion, and trazadone, are discussed in Chapter 5.

The TCAs have long been the first-line antidepressants used by most clinicians for adults because of their established efficacy, safety, and ease of administration.[1,108] However, they have been far less successful in the treatment of child and adolescent conditions. This is particularly true of child and adolescent depression, where there is no conclusive evidence that TCAs are superior to placebo. Nonetheless, investigation has revealed other potential roles for TCAs in the treatment of child and adolescent psychiatric conditions, which will be discussed here. We will also explore the present status of psychopharmacology in child and adolescent major depression and suggest possible future directions.

Chemical Properties

See Table 4-1.

The TCAs, such as imipramine, desipramine, clomipramine, amitriptyline, and nortriptyline, are dibenzapine derivatives. Because they undergo significant first-pass metabolism by the liver and are less bound to proteins,[4] these agents are metabolized significantly more rapidly in children and adolescents than in adults. This faster metabolism is true of all compounds with primary hepatic metabolism because of the greater liver mass in relation to body size in children and adolescents. Children and adolescents, like adults, can show a more than 30-fold difference in heterocyclic blood levels at a particular dose,[8–10] and steady-state TCA levels can vary widely in children receiving fixed daily doses of medication.[11] Liver biotransformation of TCAs primarily involves oxidation, aromatic hydroxylation, and demethylation. Approximately 5% of the population are "slow hydroxylators" and will have significantly longer half-lives and higher plasma blood levels.[12] These are persons who metabolize TCAs slowly and may develop CNS side effects, which need to be differentiated from worsening of depression or ADHD.[13] As severe cardiotoxicity and deaths have been reported,[13] close monitoring of TCA blood levels is required.

The mechanism by which TCAs are effective in the treatment of adult depression and other disorders has not been clearly established. There is, however, evidence that these agents affect monoamine neurotransmitter systems in the CNS, such as serotonin and norepinephrine.[1] The TCAs block the reuptake of norepinephrine and serotonin, potentiating their action. It has been suggested that antidepressants work by increasing noradrenergic and/or serotonergic transmission, compensating for a presumed deficiency.[1]

Indications

See Table 4-2.

Depression

Diagnosis
Child and adolescent depression appears to be a valid diagnostic entity. Studies have established evidence corroborating its validity.[14–22]

Symptom Frequency and Severity
Ryan and colleagues[14] compared symptom frequency and severity in two sequential samples of 95 prepubertal children and 92 adolescents, aged 6–18 years, all assessed according to the Schedule for Affective Disorders and Schizophrenia for School-Aged Children.[14] All met the research diagnostic criteria (RDC) for major depressive disorder (MDD). No significant differ-

Table 4-1
Relative Neurotransmitter Effects of Tricyclic Antidepressants

	Noradrenergic	**Serotonergic**	**Dopaminergic**
Imipramine	+ +	+ +	0
Amitriptyline	+ +	+ +	0
Desipramine	+ + +	+/–	0
Nortriptyline	+ + +	+/–	0
Fluoxetine	0	+ + +	0
Trazodone	0	+	0
Maprotiline	+ + +	0	0
Bupropion	0	0	+ + +

Source: Ryan, N.D. (1990). Heterocyclic antidepressants in children and adolescents. *J Child Adolesc Psychopharmacol, 1(1)*, 21–31.

Table 4-2
Clinical Indications for TCAs

FDA-approved indications: • Enuresis
Established indications: • Enuresis • ADHD in children and adolescents
Probable indications: • ADHD in adults • School absenteeism / school phobia • OCD • Depression

ences between the two groups in the majority of depressive symptoms were noted. Adolescents were, however, observed to have greater anhedonia, hopelessness, hypersomnia, weight change, drug and alcohol use, and lethality of suicide attempt, whereas prepubertal children had more depressed appearance, somatic complaints, agitation, separation anxiety, phobias, and hallucinations. Children and adolescents whose depression had lasted at least two years had significantly higher rates of suicide attempts, ideation, and lethality than those with depressions of shorter duration (Table 4-3).

Table 4-3
Prepubertal Versus Adolescent Depression

Depressive Signs and Symptoms	Prepubertal Children	Adolescent
Anhedonia	Less	More
Hopelessness	Less	More
Sleep	Hyposomnia	Hypersomnia
Weight	Less likely to change	Often changes
Suicide	Decreased lethality of attempt	Increased lethality of attempt
Appearance	More depressed	Less depressed
Somatic complaints	More	Less
Separation anxiety, phobias, hallucinations	More	Less

Source: Rosenberg, D.R., Wright, B.A., Gershon, S. (1992). Depression in the elderly. *Dementia, 3,* 157–173.

Endogenous and Anxious Factors in Depression

Ryan and colleagues[14] also studied a discrete population of 296 children who met DSM-III diagnoses of any Axis I disorder. Factor analysis revealed both an "endogenous" and an "anxious" factor, as has been found in many adult depression studies (Table 4-4).[23–25] Ryan and associates also observed three other factors: (1) negative life conditions, (2) appetite and weight changes, and (3) conduct disturbance. They concluded that relatively few differences are seen between children and adolescents with MDD, and these are overshadowed by the similarities.[23–25]

Table 4-4
Factors Associated with Child and Adolescent Depression

- Endogenous
- Anxious
- Negative life conditions
- Appetite and weight changes
- Conduct disturbance

Source: Rosenberg, D.R., Wright, B.A., Gershon, S. (1992). Depression in the elderly. *Dementia, 3,* 157–173.

Family History

As reported by Puig-Antich and colleagues,[26] a family history of mood disorders in parents is associated with a much greater likelihood of a mood disorder in their children. This, in turn, is associated with an increase in the lifetime risk for mood disorders.[27–30]

Recently born individuals have a greater probability than have their grandparents of developing a mood disorder. Both longitudinal and cross-sectional studies using population and family study samples have demonstrated an increased prevalence of mood disorders in adults.[31]

Biological Abnormalities

Biological abnormalities have been identified in children with depression (Table 4-5). Puig-Antich[31] reported increased growth hormone (GH) secretion during sleep in depressed children. These children also secrete less GH in response to insulin-induced hypoglycemia. This abnormality persists after resolution of the depression and cessation of the pharmacologic intervention. This is an important finding since identification of this GH abnormality could serve as a marker of depression even after the depression has resolved.[31–33]

Kutcher and associates[102] observed increased nocturnal GH secretion at midnight and 1:00 a.m. in nine depressed adolescents, as compared with nine normal controls. Another study examining unstimulated GH secretion in adolescents found blunted nocturnal GH in those depressed adolescents who were suicidal, as compared with normal controls.[103] The nonsuicidal depressed adolescents had normal nocturnal GH secretion. Ryan and associates[104] have shown blunted GH response to desmethylimipramine in depressed suicidal adolescents, as compared with normal controls, but not in depressed nonsuicidal adolescents. Jensen and Garfinkel[105] did not show differences in GH response to oral clonidine or L-dopa in adolescent boys, but the number of subjects in the study was small (eight MDD versus five normals). Meyer and associates[106] found significantly lower 24-hour mean GH

Table 4-5

Biological Abnormalities in Child and Adolescent Depression

- *Increased* GH secretion during sleep
- Secrete *less* GH in response to insulin-induced hypoglycemia
- 50% *do not* suppress cortisol when given DST
- EEG *not* helpful

Source: Rosenberg, D.R., Wright, B.A., Gershon, S. (1992). Depression in the elderly. *Dementia, 3,* 157–173.

concentration in depressed boys than in normal boys, and significant blunting was found in both the 8:00 a.m. to 8:00 p.m. period and the 8:00 p.m. to 8:00 a.m. period. More recently, Ryan and colleagues failed to demonstrate any difference in nocturnal GH secretion between prepubertal MDD and normal control children (unpublished data). Thus, according to Ryan and Dahl,[107] the question of abnormalities of unstimulated GH secretion in depressed children and adolescents appears to be complicated by maturational changes, and its interpretation remains unclear.

Other measurements of biological abnormalities in children and adolescents with MDD include the dexamethasone suppression test (DST) and sleep electroencephalography. As with GH secretion, some findings are similar to those found in adults, but there do appear to be some major related differences. The reader is referred to Mann and Kupfer's textbook *The Biology of Depressive Disorders*[107] for a more complete review of the various biological markers and abnormalities observed throughout development in MDD patients.

Abnormal Dexamethasone Suppression Test.   Recent studies adjusted for the age, weight, and faster rate of metabolism in children reveal that 50% of depressed children and adolescents do not suppress cortisol upon being given the DST.[32,34] Weller and associates[35] showed that children who do not suppress cortisol secretion after the DST are at higher risk of relapse of their mood disorder. Birmaher and colleagues,[36] however, recently reported a study of 24-hour serial cortisol determinations measured during baseline and after the administration of 0.25 and 0.5 mg of dexamethasone in a sample of outpatient children with MDD, nonaffective psychiatric controls, and normal controls.[36] The 24-hour baseline cortisol measurement and the DST did not distinguish among the three groups. The authors also measured 24-hour serum dexamethasone levels; no significant group differences were observed. *These results raised serious questions as to the usefulness of this test in the diagnosis of mood disorders in children.*[36]

Electroencephalography.   Unlike adults, sleep electroencephalography has not proved helpful in delineating childhood and adolescent depression.

Indications for Pharmacotherapy.   See Table 4-6.

Major Depressive Disorder

Controlled studies have failed to demonstrate that TCAs are superior to placebo in the treatment of childhood and adolescent depression. In a five-week double-blind study of clinical efficacy, Puig-Antich and colleagues[37] observed that imipramine was comparable to placebo in treating major depression in

Table 4-6
Pharmacotherapy of Depression in Different Age Groups

Child	Ineffective
Adolescent	Ineffective
Middle aged	Very effective
Elderly	Appears to be effective

Source: Rosenberg, D.R., Wright, B.A., Gershon, S. (1992). Depression in the elderly. *Dementia, 3,* 157–173.

children 6 to 12 years of age. Geller and colleagues[38] observed similar results in a double-blind, placebo-controlled study of nortriptyline in children using a "fixed plasma level" design. While overall group comparisons of imipramine versus placebo demonstrated no superiority of active medication, analyses of a subgroup of medication responders showed that the plasma drug levels correlated significantly with treatment response. In their study of 30 children, a plasma level greater than 150 ng/ml of imipramine plus desipramine best discriminated between responders (85%) and nonresponders (30%). They also observed several predictors of a therapeutic response, including pretreatment severity (negative), MDD and RDC psychotic type (negative), and plasma level (positive). They could find no predictors of placebo response. They recommended prior placebo washout periods when conducting future antidepressant trials. Clinicians continue to prescribe these agents in the belief that future studies will show that higher plasma levels or correctly adjusted doses of antidepressants will be effective.[4]

The TCAs also have not been shown to be superior to placebo in the treatment of depressed adolescents. Kramer and Feiguine[39] conducted a double-blind, placebo-controlled study of amitriptyline and failed to demonstrate superiority over placebo. In a double-blind, placebo-controlled study of nortriptyline in adolescents with major depression, Geller et al.[40] observed no superiority over placebo. Ryan and colleagues[41] treated depressed adolescent outpatients with imipramine in an "open-label" study and failed to find a relationship between imipramine plasma levels and clinical response. Strober[42] evaluated the effects of imipramine, lithium, and fluoxetine in the treatment of adolescent major depression and failed to demonstrate a significant relationship of clinical response to plasma antidepressant level. As with childhood depression, clinicians continue to prescribe TCAs to depressed adolescents.

Lack of Efficacy of TCAs in Children and Adolescents

Because controlled studies have failed to demonstrate that TCAs are superior to placebo, it is crucial to determine whether this is due to problems in the design, the methodology, and/or the conduct of the studies.[43] It is also possible that because of the developmental plasticity of the nervous system, children and adolescents may respond differentially to antidepressants than do adults. For example, children and adolescents might respond in a pharmacologically different manner because of quantitative and/or qualitative developmental differences in their neurotransmitter systems.[43] It is also possible that only a subgroup of antidepressants is effective in this population and/or that DSM-III-R or RDC criteria or treatment-outcome measures for MDD do not delineate those children and adolescents whose depressions respond to antidepressant therapy.[4]

Before it is concluded that TCAs are ineffective in childhood and adolescent depression, it is important to consider several relevant issues. During the 1960s, there was concern that some of the first critical studies of imipramine and MAOIs in adults failed to demonstrate superiority over placebo.[43] As recently as 1974, Morris and Beck[44] reviewed the then-available literature and observed that one third of the controlled trials of antidepressants demonstrated no significant difference from placebo. This is relevant to children and adolescents because the total number entered into controlled studies is still too small to declare an outcome.[4] Fewer than 250 children and adolescents have been enrolled in placebo-controlled, double-blind trials.[43] But although the high level of placebo response in child and adolescent studies has been problematic, it is not limited to this population, and it is also causing significant problems in current adult studies assessing psychopharmacologic and psychotherapeutic effectiveness in the treatment of depression.[45] Predictors of placebo response have not been identified. One possibility is that patients and families enrolled in placebo-controlled studies receive more education about their illness than do typical clinically treated patients. Some treatments of adult depression that have proved effective (such as cognitive and behavioral therapy) involve educating patients about their illness as an important first step in dealing with and ameliorating their depression. It is said that such recognition can lead to a better understanding of one's disease.

It is imperative that multisite studies carefully define depressive symptomatology such as depressive mood and suicidal ideation.[43] Studies to date have been plagued by significant differences in nosology, diagnosis, and methodology. It may be important (and possible) in future drug studies to assess both psychopharmacologic and psychosocial interventions in each respective group so that treatment-resistant cases can be switched to another cell.[43] It is vital to distinguish depressive syndromes not just from normal controls, but also from other psychiatric conditions in both clinic-referred and nonreferred (i.e., normal) populations.[43,46]

There is, of course, the possibility that TCAs simply do not work in children and adolescents, in which case it would be necessary to determine whether there is an age shift. In other words, at what age do young adults begin to respond to TCAs? For example, is there a difference in response to these agents between 17-year-olds and 18-, 19-, or 20-year-olds? Currently, there are no controlled studies to answer this question.

If there is a particular time at which a shift occurs, it would be important to identify maturational factors that might account for this age shift. We do know that estrogen effects peak in adolescence and that alterations in the noradrenergic system are particularly prominent during that time. Moreover, mania is much more common in adolescents and adults than in prepubertal children. In addition, stimulant-induced euphoria has not been observed in prepubertal children, whereas it has been seen in adolescents and adults treated with stimulant medication.[2]

The current clinical impression is that these children and adolescents do not "grow out of their depression." Instead, it is believed that when they are followed longitudinally, they are seen to continue to suffer depressive episodes. It is also possible that younger children and adolescents diagnosed with MDD and treated with TCAs represent a particularly refractory group of depressive patients who "dilute" the effects of the antidepressants. That is, these children and adolescents are analogous to (and may become) those adults who have refractory depressions unresponsive to standard pharmacologic intervention. There are data that strongly indicate continuity from child and adolescent depression to adult forms of the disorder. The clinical syndrome appears similar throughout this age span. There also seem to be similarities in psychobiological correlates. Therefore, in some ways, the surprising thing is that the studies so far have not demonstrated the efficacy of TCAs in depressed children and adolescents. It is, of course, possible that these agents do not work because of developmental differences. On the other hand, it is also possible that TCAs are effective in some children and adolescents, although perhaps not many, and it is simply harder to discern. It would be remarkable to learn that, even considering development, these drugs do not work in any children and adolescents, given the other similarities between childhood and adolescent and adult depression, and given most reasonable models of development.

Electroconvulsive Therapy

Because the antidepressants have not yet been shown to be effective in the treatment of child and adolescent depression, and because of their not insignificant side effects, it is necessary to consider alternative therapies. Electroconvulsive therapy (ECT) has not been systematically studied in child and adolescent depression, but in adults, it remains the most potent treatment for MDD, and is often used as the treatment of choice after a failure of tricyclic therapy.[109–112] It has also been shown to be safe, and its side-effect profile compares quite favorably with that of the antidepressants. Treatment with ECT may prove effective in refractory depression. Currently, there is no significant evidence establishing the efficacy of this treatment modality in child and adolescent MDD.

Current Practice

Despite the fact that TCAs have not been proved effective in the treatment of MDD, their use for children and adolescents is widespread, and is even considered standard practice in many clinical settings. Many clinicians feel compelled to try these agents, particularly when other behavioral/psychosocial interventions have been unsuccessful. There are, of course, children and adolescents who may be more likely to respond to TCAs. A child or adolescent, for example, with a family member who has responded well to a particular TCA, probably merits a trial of the same agent, since this means that he or she also may have a favorable response. Therefore, we have delineated the following guidelines.

As in adults with MDD, antidepressant treatment is typically maintained for nine to 12 months before a gradual tapering off is initiated. It should be noted that Kupfer and associates[100] have found that in adults with MDD, maintenance therapy at doses comparable to those used to treat peak depressive symptoms can reduce the risk of relapse of a depressive episode. There are no data for children and adolescents. This option may be considered in children or adolescents who have demonstrated a dramatic response to TCA therapy and who have not experienced any undue side effects. Discussion with the patient and family is indicated. Standard dosing regimens for specific agents can be found in Table 4-7.

Attention-Deficit Hyperactivity Disorder

Up to 30% of children treated with stimulants for ADHD do not improve, necessitating alternative treatments.[47,48] Imipramine, DMI and amitriptyline have been shown to be superior to placebo in treatment of ADHD.[49–52] It should be noted, however, that although these studies have demonstrated antidepressants to be more effective than placebo, most studies find stimulants to be superior to antidepressants.[53–55] Many clinicians consider TCAs, such as desipramine and imipramine, to be the next drug choices when a patient fails to respond to stimulant medication. Wender[56] has observed that when used to treat ADHD, TCAs improve mood and hyperactivity, but they do not improve concentration, and they may be sedating. In a double-blind,

Table 4-7
Dosage and Regimen of TCAs in Major Depressive Disorder (MDD)

Imipramine:
- Used at doses up to 5.0 mg/kg/day.
- Preskorn et al. [11]: Among children responders, serum levels of 125-250 ng/ml.
- Puig-Antich et al. [91]: Serum levels in children >150 ng/ml optimal.
- Start with dose 75 mg/day [91].
- After 7–10 days draw serum desipramine and imipramine levels.
- Formula [91]: New dose = (initial dose/intial plasma level) × desired level.
- Adolescents: No significant relationship between serum level and clinical response.
- Generally raised to serum levels > 150 ng/ml (adult levels).
- Carefully monitoring required (see Table 4.10).

Desipramine:
- Doses up to 5 mg/kg/day.
- No evidence of relationship between plasma level to clinical response.
- Children and adolescents treated with serum levels effective in adult MDD.
- Usually increased to achieve serum levels > 150 ng/ml as in adults.
- Serum levels >150ng/ml may increase risk for ECG abnormalities
  (i.e., increased heart rate, conduction abnormalities)(may be of more statistical than clinical significance).
- Careful monitoring required (see Table 4.10).

Nortriptyline:
- Titrate to give serum levels between 75–100 mg/ml. [2,4]
- Usually requires daily doses of 0.5-2.0 mg/kg.
- Careful monitoring required (see Table 4-10).

Amitriptyline:
- Typically used at doses up to 5.0 mg/kg/day.
- Serum levels not useful in monitoring efficacy or toxicity.
- Careful monitoring required (see Table 4-10).
- High anticholinergic and sedating side effects make problematic.

Clomipramine:
- Experimental.
- No standardized guidelines.
- Dugas et al. [58]: Open trial doses 0.24–2.93 mg/kg/day effective in 12/26 children and adolescents with "depressive" symptoms.
- Double-blind, placebo-controlled studies needed.
- Relatively unfavorable side-effect profile.
- Careful monitoring required (Table 4-10).

Doxepin:
- Available in oral solution.
- More water-soluble (free of alcohol) than nortriptyline.
- Not studied in children and adolescents.
- Unfavorable side-effect profile.
- Not recommended for use.

Maprotilene:
- Antidepressant most associated with seizure induction.
- Not recommended for use in children and adolescents.

65

placebo-controlled crossover study of 12 prepubertal male children with ADHD comparing the efficacy of methylphenidate, desipramine and clomipramine, it was seen that while methylphenidate was significantly better than desipramine and clomipramine in improving classroom functioning, clomipramine was more effective than desipramine in decreasing aggressive, impulsive, and depressive/mood symptoms.[49] Further study of clomipramine in treating children and adolescents with ADHD is clearly warranted. Desipramine is, however, still considered the first-line antidepressant to treat ADHD because it is the most studied of the antidepressants. It also has a relatively favorable anticholinergic and sedating side-effect profile as compared with other TCAs, including clomipramine. It is likely, however, that any TCA would be similarly effective in the treatment of ADHD.[4] It is important to point out, though, that the long-term efficacy of TCAs has not been established (i.e., more than a few months).

There are no guidelines as to how long to maintain ADHD patients on TCAs. With recent investigation showing that adults continue to exhibit ADHD symptoms and can benefit from stimulant medication (see Chapter 3), we recommend using the same principles for medication management as described for treating ADHD children and adolescents with stimulants. Frequent assessment of the need for medication is warranted. Trials off medication (e.g., over the summer, weekends, and holidays) may also be helpful. Finally, placebo-controlled, double-blind studies may help to determine whether or not the medication is truly benefiting the child. Standard dose regimens can be found in Table 4-8.

In Adults

Until recently, many practicing clinicians believed that ADHD remitted at puberty, but further investigation has shown that its course is extremely variable and that symptoms can persist into adolescence and adulthood.[5] Stimulants have been found to be effective in treating ADHD symptoms throughout life. There are no data on adults, but this is an area worthy of investigation. Adult patients with ADHD who fail to respond to stimulant medication may benefit from a TCA trial (e.g., desipramine). Comorbid diagnoses of depression are also not uncommon in patients with ADHD.

And Coexisting Tics

The existence of tic symptoms may warrant a TCA trial. These agents have the advantage that they are effective in the treatment of ADHD, but do not exacerbate tics. For a full discussion about stimulant-induced tics or how to manage patients with a family history of tic disorders, refer to Chapters 3 and 7.

We recommend using desipramine as the first antidepressant in the treat-

Table 4-8
Dosage and Regimen of TCAs for ADHD

Desipramine:
- Optimal doses 2.5-5 mg/kg/day.
- Should not exceed serum levels > 300 ng/ml.
- No significant correlation between serum level, dosage, and clinical response.
- Serum levels >150 ng/ml and doses > 3.5 mg/kg/day associated with increased risk heart rate and altered cardiac conduction.
- Serum levels <300 ng/ml, ECK PR < 200 ms and QRS < 120 ms advocated.
- Daily doses >5 mg/kg/day may be needed clinically to achieve serum levels >150 ng/ml.
- Doses >3.5 mg/kg may be too much for some children.
- Careful monitoring required (see Table 4-13).
- Heterocyclic of choice.

Imipramine:
- More effective than placebo.
- Less effective than stimulants.
- Used when desipramine is ineffective and/or if patient has difficulty falling or staying asleep.
- Dosing and administration guidelines similar to desipramine
- More anticholinergic and sedating side effects than desipramine.
- Careful monitoring necessary (see Table 4-13).

Nortriptyline:
- Has not systematically been studied.
- Anecdotal reports of efficacy.
- Favorable anticholinergic and sedative side-effect profile.
- May be considered if imipramine, desipramine, other "more standard" agents unsuccessful or contraindicated.
- Careful monitoring required (see Table 4-13).

Amitriptyline:
- Has not been systematically studied.
- Unfavorable anticholinergic and sedative side-effect profile.
- No recommended for use.

Clomipramine:
- Shown to be less effective.
- Less effective than methylphenidate in improving overall classroom functioning.[43, 49]
- More effective than desipramine in reducing scores reflecting aggressivity.[43]
- More anticholinergic and sedative side effects than desipramine.
- Less studied than desipramine.
- Careful monitoring required (see Table 4-13).

Doxepin:
- Not recommended for use in children and adolescents.

Maprotilene:
- Not recommended for use in children and adolescents.

ment of ADHD and tics. This antidepressant has a relatively favorable side-effect profile, and there is some literature to support its use.[6] It should be noted that it is not an effective treatment of tic disorders.

We recommend a trial of desipramine in a child or adolescent who develops or shows worsening of tic behaviors when treated with stimulants and whose ADHD necessitates pharmacologic treatment. It is important to emphasize, however, that if tics do not dissipate to a tolerable level after stimulant medication is discontinued, alternative therapy may be necessary, such as clonidine, which targets both ADHD and tic symptoms. On the other hand, clonidine is often associated with more side effects in children and adolescents, such as sedation, and is generally more unpleasant for these patients. Further study is necessary to determine whether or not desipramine or other TCAs are safe and effective in treating ADHD with coexistent tics.

Enuresis

Enuresis remains the only FDA-established indication for the use of TCAs in children and adolescents. Their efficacy in treating this disorder has been demonstrated in over 40 double-blind studies.[4] It is important to note that patients may become tolerant to the antienuretic effect, and it may wear off after several weeks. Many patients relapse once the medication is withdrawn. It also should be noted, however, that unlike TCA therapy of other psychiatric conditions, the antienuretic effect is seen without delay once treatment is initiated. Desipramine and imipramine, which are equally efficacious,[4] are the only antidepressants that have been approved by the FDA for the treatment of enuresis. Imipramine has more side effects (sedating and anticholinergic), but is less expensive.[4] It is recommended that desipramine be reserved for patients who have both diurnal and nocturnal enuresis, or for those whose nocturnal enuresis has not responded to conservative behavioral measures.[57]

Clomipramine has also been used to treat enuresis, with a therapeutic effect observed at plasma concentrations of 20–60 ng/ml.[58,59] It must be emphasized that these pharmacologic approaches should not be employed until all organic etiologies are ruled out by physical and laboratory examination. Moreover, behavioral therapy (such as the bell-and-pad apparatus) is the treatment of choice for nonorganic functional enuresis. The TCAs are used as a supplement, or when the child is away overnight. Children may become tolerant to these medications after approximately six months, and discontinuation of TCA therapy often results in symptom recurrence. These agents are recommended only after all other behavioral approaches have failed, and are likely to be effective only for short-term use. Standard dosing regimens can be found in Table 4-9.

Table 4-9
Dosage and Regimen of TCAs for Enuresis

Desipramine:
- Equally effective as imipramine.[57]
- Typical doses 1–2.5 mg/kg/day.
- Doses of 50–75 mg/day usually sufficient.
- Antienuretic effects occur soon after treatment initiated.
- Relationship of serum level to clinical outcome not clear.
- Routine clinical practice: ECGs not usually done since final daily dose, usually ≤2.5 mg/kg/day.
- Risk of cardiotoxicity low at these doses.
- We recommend baseline ECGs and serial ECG rhythm strips after each dose increase with recent reports of sudden cardiac death.

Imipramine:
- Similar dosing and administration guidelines as for desipramine.
- Titrated to give serum levels imipramine plus desipramine >60 ng/ml.
- Desipramine preferred because of more favorable side-effect profile.
- Has same antienuretic effects as desipramine.
- Antienurectic effect not related to anticholinergic mechanism.

Nortriptyline:
- Has not been studied.
- Does not have FDA approval.
- Not recommended for use.

Amitriptyline:
- Has not been studied.
- Unfavorable anticholinergic and sedative side-effect profile
- Not recommended for use.

Clomipramine:
- Shown to be effective.[58,59]
- Targeted plasma concentrations: 20–60 ng/ml.
- Use only if desipramine and imipramine ineffective.
- Side-effect profile less favorable than desipramine.
- Plasma levels <20 ng/ml and >60 ng/ml associated with lack of efficacy.[58,59]

Doxepin:
- Has not been studied.
- Not recommended for use.

Maprotilene:
- Has not been studied.
- Not recommended for use.

Case History

Alex, a 12-year-old boy, was referred for an evaluation of his learning disability and possible attention-deficit disorder. At the time of his evaluation, there was marked marital discord between the parents, indicating that separation was imminent, which would eventually end in divorce. Alex was very large for his age, very awkward, and poorly coordinated. He exhibited many specific learning disabilities affecting reading comprehension, auditory decoding, and penmanship. His poor fine motor control contributed to an almost illegible handwriting. Printed words were also very difficult to identify because of reversals, indicating severe visuomotor integration problems.

During the course of the history taking, his mother indicated that Alex had always been severely enuretic, never having achieved nighttime bladder control for longer than six months. There were two six-month periods, when he was 8 and 10 years old, respectively, when he was substantially continent. But even during these periods, he would be incontinent three to four times each month. Since the age of 5, he had had complete bladder control during the daytime. There were no episodes of soiling reported.

On examination, Alex appeared as a 12-year-old boy who looked somewhat older, primarily because of his obesity. There were no positive findings on the standard mental status examination. He appeared mildly dysphoric and had very low self-esteem. He did not meet any other criteria for an affective disorder. He related that he was overly active, distractible, impulsive, and restless. He also had a number of temper outbursts each week. He was very evasive and used much denial when describing his bed-wetting. He indicated that all forms of help, including alarms, changes in drinking habits, and parental awakenings in the first few hours of sleep, were ineffective.

Alex was started on 50 mg of imipramine at bedtime, and required an eventual dose of 200 mg before there was a moderate cessation of his enuresis. Wet nights decreased from nightly to three to four times per month. His parents agreed that they did not want any further treatment for the enuresis, since they felt that this was a sufficient improvement. They also noted good improvement in Alex's behavior, as well as a positive change in his affect and self-esteem.

Source: Garfinkel, B.D. (1990). The elimination disorders. In B.D. Garfinkel, G.A. Carlson, E.B. Welles (Eds.), *Psychiatric Disorders in Childhood and Adolescence* (pp. 329–330). Philadelphia: W.B. Saunders.

1-Deamino-8-d-Arginine-Vasopressin (DDAVP)

Pediatricians not uncommonly use DDAVP as the medication treatment of first choice in enuretic children, while using TCAs less frequently (see Chapter 5).

School Absenteeism/School Phobia/Separation Anxiety

Gittelman-Klein and Klein[113] showed a superiority of imipramine over placebo in combination with a psychosocial treatment program in 20 children and adolescents aged 7 to 15 years with anxiety-related school absenteeism. This has not been confirmed in other studies. Klein and colleagues[60] suggest that imipramine can be effective in ameliorating separation anxiety, but that anticipatory anxiety often continues to be problematic. They observed that doses of 75–200 mg/day were effective for school-phobic children and adolescents, whereas patients with severe separation anxiety without school phobia sometimes responded to doses of 25–50 mg/day. School-phobic children and adolescents who responded to imipramine showed at least minimal improvement when doses of 125 mg/day were achieved. When clinical improvement occurred, further dose increments usually resulted in increased improvement.[60] Maximal response most often was seen within six to eight weeks. Klein and colleagues[60] recommended continuing the effective imipramine dose for at least eight weeks after symptom remission, and then gradually tapering and withdrawing the medication.

Klein and colleagues[61] recently assessed the efficacy of imipramine in children and adolescents aged 6 to 15 years with separation anxiety disorder. They were treated for a month with behavioral therapy. If they did not respond, they entered a double-blind, randomized, six-week trial of imipramine or placebo. Of 45 patients accepted, 21 (47%) entered the trial. Approximately half of the children improved with either treatment, and imipramine revealed no superiority.

Berney and colleagues,[62] using low-dose clomipramine, showed no superiority of medication over placebo. Further study is required to determine the role of TCAs in these conditions.

Anxiety/Panic Disorder/Phobic Disorders

Ballenger and associates[63] reported that three children with panic disorder and severe separation anxiety and agoraphobia improved while receiving imipramine. It should be noted, however, that these children were also being treated with the anxiolytic alprazolam. There are very limited data on the treatment of panic disorder, phobic disorders, and anxiety disorders in children and adolescents. A placebo-controlled study is necessary.

Obsessive-Compulsive Disorder

Clomipramine is an antiobsessional drug that has been found effective in the treatment of adult obsessive-compulsive disorder (OCD), and it also may be effective in child and adolescent OCD, although the evidence is less robust. Clomipramine inhibits serotonin reuptake, thereby potentiating its effects, and its primary metabolite, desmethylclomipramine, inhibits norepinephrine uptake.[115] In adults, it is believed to be even more effective than the pure serotonin reuptake inhibitor fluoxetine in the treatment of OCD. It is, however, also believed that blocking serotonin reuptake is crucial to clomipramine's anti–obsessive-compulsive actions.

There are limited studies on the use of clomipramine in child and adolescent OCD. High pretreatment levels of platelet serotonin have been found to be a positive predictor of favorable clinical response to clomipramine therapy, which results in a substantial reduction in platelet serotonin concentration.[64]

In a double-blind, placebo-controlled study of 19 OCD children and adolescents 10 to 18 years of age, clomipramine was shown to be superior to placebo. This antiobsessional effect appears to be distinct, at daily doses of 100 to 200 mg, from the antidepressant effect.[64] In a follow-up study, Flament and associates[65] showed the continued superiority of clomipramine over placebo.

Clomipramine has been shown to be superior to other TCAs in the treatment of OCD. Leonard and colleagues[66] found clomipramine to be superior to desipramine in the treatment of 49 children and adolescents with severe OCD in a 10-week crossover design. When desipramine was given to those patients who improved on clomipramine, they experienced a relapse of their obsessive-compulsive symptoms at rates similar to those for placebo in a prior study.[64]

Children and adolescents with OCD were studied in an eight-week multicenter, double-blind, parallel group trial of clomipramine versus placebo.[67] Efficacy assessments included the NIMH Global Rating Scale and the child version of the Yale-Brown Obsessive-Compulsive Scale. After eight weeks, clomipramine-treated patients showed a mean reduction in Yale-Brown Obsessive Compulsive Scale scores of 37% versus 8% treated with placebo.[67] Side effects were typical of those seen with TCAs. In a one-year open-label treatment, clomipramine therapy continued to be effective and well tolerated.

Fluoxetine and other specific serotonin reuptake inhibitors (SSUIs), which also appear to be useful in OCD, although less effective than clomipramine, have fewer side effects. Simeon and associates,[68] in an attempt to maximize therapeutic effects and minimize adverse effects, treated six adolescents with OCD with a clomipramine–fluoxetine combination. The patients were first treated with clomipramine alone. If this was not effective or if side effects developed, fluoxetine was added to the regimen. Clinical global improvement with clomipramine alone was rated as moderate in three patients and minimal in three others. Clinical global improvement with the clomipramine–fluoxetine combination was rated as marked in five patients and moderate in one. These improvements were achieved with relatively low daily doses of clomipramine, 25–50 mg, and fluoxetine, 20–40 mg. The drug combination was well tolerated. Side effects were greater and less tolerable with clomipramine alone than with the clomipramine–fluoxetine combination. The authors concluded that relatively low doses of the clomipramine–fluoxetine combination may potentiate the therapeutic effects and minimize the side effects in patients with OCD. They did not report that any of the patients experienced akathisia. This side effect of fluoxetine treatment may be more common than was initially believed (see "Side Effects"). It is possible that clomipramine–fluoxetine combinations may increase this risk. Larger controlled trials are warranted. Standard dose regimens can be found in Table 4-10.

Case History

Jane, who is 17 years old, remembers vividly that at age 5 or 6, she repeatedly washed her hands. She said that she needed to "cover each spot" and would wash her hands again and again because of an inner urge to be certain that her hands were clean. This gradually improved over the next few years, but by age 7 or 8, the obsession and compulsion had changed. Jane had enuresis at night until well into the third grade. She would shower, but would not feel clean, and would have to take two or three more baths per day. The subjective feeling of a lack of cleanliness and of being contaminated did not wash away. As a result, she also had to change her clothes two or three times a day.

When she was 9 years old, Jane experienced a specific precipitating event. While approaching the end of a book, she would feel uncertain about whether she understood it. As she finished the last paragraph, she would have a terrible feeling that she had not read the book correctly and would begin to slowly reread it. She would read and reread each paragraph carefully, going over and over sentences, paragraphs, chapters, and the entire book. Her schoolwork was especially impaired if she had to read out loud. Her pervasive thoughts were that she was not doing her work correctly.

In the summer following the ninth grade, Jane attempted to make herself read and socialize more. She, however, became increasingly more anxious and uncertain. She decided to lose weight so that she would become more acceptable to others. She became markedly depressed. She noticed that her heart would beat fast, that she was short of breath,

Table 4-10
Dosage and Regimen of TCAs in Child and Adolescent OCD

Clomipramine:
- Drug of choice.
- Superior to other antidepressants.
- Side effects can be problematic.
- Slighly more effective than fluoxetine.
- Initial dose: 25 mg/day for children <25 kg, 50 mg/day if >25 kg.
- Increase dosage weekly by amount equal to subject's initial dose.
- Maximum daily dose should not exceed 5 mg/kg or 250 mg.
- Addition of fluoxetine can reduce clomipramine dose, enhance efficacy, and decrease side effects.
- Combination of fluoxetine 20–40 mg/day and clomipramine 25–50 mg/day may be best.
- Combination therapy may exacerbate problematic fluoxetine side effects (i.e., akathisia).
- Careful monitoring required (see Table 4-13).

Other TCAs not recommended

and that she felt desperate and suicidal. During the early fall of the 10th grade, she found herself overwhelmed with anxiety, unable to concentrate at all on her work, and completely unable to function at school. She was hospitalized in a psychiatric hospital for six months. The first three months of that hospitalization were in a "short-term" acute-care ward. She was told that her diagnosis was "free-floating anxiety." She said that talking in group and individual therapy did little to help. She was placed on haloperidol, 5 mg twice daily, with no improvement. Nortriptyline and imipramine were both given brief clinical trials. She reported that while the drugs helped with the anxiety, they did not ameliorate her major depression, suicidal thoughts, thoughts of guilt, and listlessness. The medication did not help the almost constant thoughts with which she struggled. Finally, she was referred to a behavioral medicine clinic during the last three months of the hospital stay, where a therapist gave her cognitive behavioral therapy. She was told to focus on her feelings, instead of her thoughts, and this appeared to help in distracting her from the obsessions. By January of the 10th-grade year, at age 16, she was back in school and seeing her therapist weekly for individual cognitive therapy.

The therapy continued for a year and a half, with more family-oriented focused therapy. The family history included a ruminative, obsessive father. The father, who had impulsive temper outbursts, would often physically assault the mother, twisting her arm, kneeing her in the chest, throwing crystal in the house, and forcing himself on his wife sexually. Jane had been very frightened of him, and had been "kidnapped" by him when she was 6 years old. However, he was also a very hard-working studious person who was at times quite likable.

At the time that Jane was seen for an evaluation for clomipramine, her main obsession continued to be with reading. She would often stop, repeat the reading, and not be able to go on. There was an almost constant preoccupation with checking her schoolwork that required her to spend two or three times longer than necessary doing her homework or schoolwork. She became afraid that she would hurt the children for whom she was baby-sitting, although she had spent the previous summer baby-sitting from 12 to 13 hours per day. She would ruminate about suicide and what she was doing to prevent self-destruction. As she remembered her wrongdoings, she became more certain that she might harm herself; while having these distressing thoughts, she found that her heart was beating fast and that she could not breathe. She attempted to control these thoughts, although she had very little control. Compulsions were limited to reading and rereading. She said that she became very distressed if anyone interrupted her.

Jane responded poorly to a clinical trial of clomipramine. She continued to have marked difficulty with obsessions and compulsions. Plans for treatment included a trial of exposure in vivo and response prevention, as well as a medication trial with fluoxetine. Jane and her mother were very depressed that the clomipramine had not been successful. Day hospitalization was arranged while the cognitive therapy and new medication trial were arranged. Her symptoms were so distressing that she continued to have occasional suicidal ideation of a moderate to severe degree.

Source: Jensen, J.B. (1990). Obsessive-compulsive disorder in children and adolescents. In B.D. Garfinkel, G.A. Carlson, E.B. Welles (Eds.), *Psychiatric Disorders in Childhood and Adolescents* (pp. 93–94). Philadelphia: W.B. Saunders.

Bulimia Nervosa

The use of antidepressants in the treatment of bulimia nervosa remains controversial. The routine use of TCAs is not recommended, but Mitchell and Groat[70] recommend them for patients with significant depression. In view of the fact that TCAs have not been shown to be superior to placebo in the treatment of childhood and adolescent depression, we do not recommend their use in bulimic patients either with or without depression. The risk-versus-benefit ratio does not favor their use.

Anorexia Nervosa

The TCAs have not been found effective in treating anorexia nervosa.

Drug Craving

See Chapter 14.

Night Terrors and Somnambulism

Pesikoff and Davis[71] reported that four children with night terrors, two children with somnambulism, and one child with both disorders experienced complete remission of their sleep disorders when treated with imipramine (10–50 mg at bedtime). The routine use of imipramine or other TCAs is not recommended as these disorders are often self-limited in children. Pharmacologic intervention should be reserved for patients who prove refractory to behavioral interventions and whose sleep disorders result in a threat to physical safety, such as sleepwalking out of the house or falling down stairs.

Borderline Personality Disorder

The TCAs (and other psychotropic agents, including neuroleptics, fluoxetine, and MAOIs) have been proposed as a possibly effective pharmacologic intervention in borderline personality disorders. Although the data to support this claim are limited, there are some minimal data to suggest the efficacy of TCAs for this condition. The clinician is reminded that an overdose of a TCA can result in death, even if the adolescent arrives at the hospital promptly.[4] Moreover, the dangers of antidepressant toxicity are greater in adolescents than in adults. Borderline personality patients, who are characteristically impulsive and not infrequently make attention-seeking suicide gestures, therefore, should not routinely be placed on an agent whose ability to relieve their symptoms is questionable and whose potential to cause harm is great.

Conduct Disorder

Antidepressant therapy has been proposed for conduct-disordered children and adolescents, especially those with an affective conduct disorder. There are limited data demonstrating the effectiveness of antidepressants in this population. Conduct-disordered patients, like patients with borderline personality disorder, are notoriously impulsive and make suicide attempts approximately as often as do depressed patients (but not as many actually kill themselves). Therefore, TCAs are not the first- (or second-) line treatment for conduct disorders.

Dysthymia

Although TCAs have been reported to be helpful in treating some cases of dysthymia in adults, they are more effective in the treatment of depression.

Antidepressants can improve a major depressive episode, but not affect the dysthymia ("double depression"). Given the lack of evidence of the efficacy of TCAs in dysthymic children and adolescents, many clinicians recommend psychosocial interventions as the first-line treatment of this disorder.

Undifferentiated Attention-Deficit Disorder

Undifferentiated ADD (ADD without hyperactivity) is a diagnostic entity that has been added in DSM-III-R. Wender[56] has reported that when used to treat ADHD, TCAs improve mood and decrease hyperactivity, but usually are sedating and do not improve concentration. Therefore, firm guidelines regarding the administration of TCAs to ADD patients without hyperactivity cannot be established. Prescribing a nonheterocyclic antidepressant such as bupropion may merit consideration as it appears not to adversely affect cognition and to be less sedating (see discussion of bupropion below).

Trichotillomania and Other Compulsive Impulse Control Disorders

Swedo and colleagues[69] performed a double-blind comparison of clomipramine and desipramine in the treatment of trichotillomania and found mean daily doses of 180 mg clomipramine to be effective. This condition is believed to be related to OCD. Significantly, desipramine was not found to be effective in the treatment of trichotillomania. McDougle and colleagues[71] treated five autistic outpatients aged 13, 24, 27, 20, and 33 years with clomipramine. Four of the patients (including the 13-year-old) showed significant improvement in disturbances of social relatedness, OCD symptoms, and/or aggressive and impulsive behavior when treated with open-label clomipramine. The fifth patient remained unchanged. Among the four patients who responded, three improved after six to eight weeks, and one required up to 12 weeks of treatment with clomipramine before significant changes occurred. Mean doses of clomipramine were 185 ± 74 mg/day. Clomipramine blood levels were not obtained during treatment, but each patient lived with responsible parents or group home staff members who administered the medication as prescribed. The authors were not able to determine from this study whether or not the reduction in social withdrawal and aggressivity was a direct effect of the clomipramine or an indirect result of the decrease in OCD symptoms.[71]

Garber and associates[3] conducted an open clinical trial of clomipramine for chronic stereotypic and self-injurious behaviors in 11 consecutive patients ranging in age from 10 to 20 years and who had concomitant developmental disorders. Ten patients (91%) showed marked decreases in rates of target behaviors. It is important to note that no seizures occurred despite the fact that six of the patients had histories of epileptic events, and improvement was evident regardless of the level of mental retardation. Placebo-controlled study is necessary to determine the true role of clomipramine in treating impulse control disorders such as trichotillomania.

Substance-Abuse Disorders

There are reports that desipramine is more effective than placebo or lithium in decreasing cocaine craving and increasing cocaine abstinence[72] (see Chapter 14). There are still very limited data on adults, and even less on the child and adolescent population. Kaminer[73] reported the case of a 16-year-old male who was dependent on cocaine while being treated for ADHD with dextroamphetamine, and who developed symptoms of severe depression with suicidal behavior. While an inpatient, he was treated with desipramine for cocaine craving, depression, and ADHD, and experienced significant improvement in all three. The Minnesota Cocaine Craving Scale was used to monitor cocaine craving. Further study in this area is clearly warranted (see Chapter 14).

Posttraumatic Stress Disorder

There are no truly effective treatments for the core symptoms of posttraumatic stress disorder (PTSD). In adults, when there is coexistent depression, anxiety, panic symptoms, and so on, antidepressants are frequently used, with some reports of success in decreasing the coexistent symptomatology. There are no data on children and adolescents. Because of the lack of conclusive evidence of the efficacy of TCAs in the treatment of child and adolescent depression, anxiety, and panic symptoms, we do not recommend their routine use in PTSD patients with these comorbid diagnoses.

Chronic Pain Syndromes

The overlap of physical and psychiatric symptoms in chronic pain syndromes often creates diagnostic and therapeutic difficulty. In adults, TCAs have been shown to be beneficial in the treatment of chronic pain syndromes. Imipramine has been shown in animal studies to potentiate morphine analgesia. In adults, imipramine and amitriptyline have been effective in reducing chronic pain associated with diabetic neuropathy.[74] Analgesic effects of amitriptyline are seen with antidepressant levels lower than those usually effective in the treatment of adult MDD. Low-dose therapy (i.e., 100–150 mg of imipramine/day) is recommended for the initial treatment of chronic pain, although doses can be increased to the 150–300 mg range.[1] There are no data on children and adolescents.

Table 4-11
Contraindications to TCA Therapy

Absolute:
- Pregnancy
- Prior hypersensitivity reaction
- Currently on MAOI

Relative:
- Epilepsy
- Psychosis (i.e., schizophrenia)
- Cardiac
- Thyroid
- Diabetes?

Contraindications

See Table 4-11.

Pregnancy

In general, TCAs should not be administered during pregnancy, although there may be exceptional cases, such as a woman who has been shown to clearly respond to a particular TCA and who is known to decompensate (i.e., become suicidal) when the medication is withdrawn. This is a decision that requires a great deal of consideration, and it is imperative that the risks versus benefits be fully discussed. We recommend trying to taper the TCA whenever possible, but if the family and/or patient is unwilling and/or the clinician believes this to be a direct threat to the patient's life, medication can be continued with close monitoring, such as with ultrasound or physical examination.

Since TCAs are secreted in breast milk, mothers should be discouraged from breast-feeding if they are taking TCAs.

Allergy

A history of hypersensitivity to TCAs is a contraindication to TCA therapy.

Cardiac Conduction Anomalies

Cardiac disorders must be approached cautiously when TCA therapy is being considered (see "Side Effects").

MAOI Therapy

A TCA should not be administered while a patient is receiving an MAOI, and should not be initiated until the patient has been off of the MAOI for at least two weeks. It should be noted that an MAOI can be added to an ongoing TCA regimen that has only been partially effective[7] (see Chapter 6). Adding an MAOI to a TCA is relatively safe for desipramine and nortriptyline, provided there is careful monitoring, but it is contraindicated when imipramine or amitriptyline is being administered. Pare and colleagues[114] argue that a TCA–MAOI combination may provide relative protection against tyramine-induced hypertension.

Epileptic Patients

For patients with epilepsy, TCAs can lower the seizure threshhold. Such patients are vulnerable to mood disorders, including depression (see Chapter 9). When a patient is on a stable anticonvulsant regimen, this is generally not problematic. Careful monitoring of anticonvulsant and antidepressant levels is necessary, and dose adjustment may be necessary.

Psychosis

As TCAs can induce or exacerbate psychosis,[4] we do not advocate their use for psychotic children and adolescents. The risk/benefit ratio does not favor their use in view of their lack of demonstrated efficacy in child and adolescent depression.

Thyroid Dysfunction

The use of TCAs in patients with thyroid dysfunction must be approached cautiously, because this condition can induce cardiac arrhythmias.[116]

Diabetes

Theoretically, TCAs could increase glucose levels.[4] However, many adult diabetics who are depressed are treated with TCAs. Careful monitoring of blood glucose levels is recommended.

Side Effects

See Table 4-12.

Cardiac

Mild increases in PR and QRS intervals are common in children and adolescents treated with TCAs.[4] A mild increase in the pulse rate of up to 120 beats a minute is not uncommon, and is frequently asymptomatic.[4] Large in-

Table 4-12
Side Effects of TCAs in Children and Adolescents

- Cardiac
- Anticholinergic
- Psychosis
- Mania
- Seizures
- Hypertension
- Confusion
- Insomnia/nightmares
- Rash
- Tics
- Tremor
- Incoordination
- Anxiety
- Sexual dysfunction
- Photosensitization

creases in cardiac conduction slowing (i.e., PR > 0.21 and QRS > 0.12) can be dangerous, and can result in arrhythmias and/or heart block.

Cardiovascular side effects are of particular concern in children and younger adolescents because of the efficiency with which they convert TCAs to potentially toxic 2-hydroxy metabolites.[75,76] They appear to be more sensitive to cardiac toxicity than are older adolescents and adults.[75] In an attempt to minimize cardiac side effects associated with peak TCA plasma levels in children, Dugas and associates[77] recommend giving divided doses—b.i.d.–t.i.d. dosages for total daily doses of over 1 mg/kg. Administering the total daily dose at one time, as at bedtime, is not recommended for children. Ryan and associates[76] did, however, observe that, once the dosage was stabilized, the total daily dose of imipramine could be safely given to adolescents at bedtime without increasing the risk of cardiac side effects.

Sudden Death

Of greatest concern are the reports of sudden cardiac deaths of children on TCAs. Three of the cases involved desipramine and one involved imipramine. Saraf and colleagues[78] reported the case of a 6-year-old girl receiving imipramine for separation anxiety disorder and school phobia who died three days after the dose had been raised to 300 mg at bedtime, or almost 15 mg/kg. Treatment guidelines for the use of TCAs recommend not exceeding daily doses of 5 mg/kg.[79] This death is believed to have been directly due to treatment with an excessive dose of imipramine and inadequate monitoring.

81

Sudden cardiac death has also been reported in three children treated with desipramine.[80] Suprisingly, little is known about these cases. These deaths have been presumed by many to be due to cardiac abnormalities. It is not known, however, whether the patients had preexisting medical and/or cardiac abnormalities, how they were monitored, and whether dosages had recently been increased (as was the case for the girl treated with imipramine).[80]

One death was that of an 8-year-old boy who had been treated for ADHD with unknown desipramine doses for two years and who had no known cardiac disease. Another 8-year-old boy with ADHD died of sudden cardiac arrest after being treated with desipramine at 50 mg/day for six months. The third case was that of a 9-year-old boy who was treated with desipramine for an unknown time and with unknown dosages. Levels of desipramine drawn after cardiac arrest were reportedly "therapeutic or subtherapeutic" in all three cases.

These sudden deaths have generated concern regarding the safety of TCAs in young children, especially at daily doses greater than 3.5 mg/kg. Winsberg and colleagues[81] found that three of seven children (43%) receiving imipramine at daily doses of 5 mg/kg developed asymptomatic prolongation of the PR interval of up to 180 ms without a significant relationship to steady-state blood levels of the medication. Preskorn and associates[82] noted that with imipramine at daily doses of up to 5 mg/kg decreased conduction efficiency (as measured by an electrocardiogram [ECG] was found when imipramine plus DMI levels were greater than 250 ng/ml. Biederman and colleagues[84-86] have studied the cardiovascular effects of desipramine in nearly 200 children and adolescents, evaluating associations among dose, plasma levels, and cardiac complications. They have consistently found small, clinically asymptomatic, but statistically significant increases in heart rate, diastolic blood pressure, and ECG conduction parameters associated with desipramine therapy at daily doses of up to 5 mg/kg. Documented ECG evidence of atrioventricular (AV) block (i.e., PR $\geq$ 200 ms) was observed in only 0.5% of cases. Complete AV conduction defect of the right bundle branch type (i.e., QRS $\geq$ 120 ms) was observed in 3% of the cases. Eighteen percent of the patients at drug-free baseline examination and 35% of the cases with new manifestations on desipramine showed evidence of sinus tachycardia (heart rate $\geq$ 100 beats/minute), and 10% of baseline patients and 23% of new cases on desipramine showed evidence of incomplete right bundle branch block (i.e., QRS 100–120 ms). It is important to note that Biederman and colleagues' data[86-88] do not confirm the hypothesis that prepubertal children may be at increased risk for cardiac side effects.[84-86] Biederman and colleagues[80,86] emphasize that since 10% of healthy children meet

ECG criteria for incomplete right bundle branch block and 18% for sinus tachycardia, it is vital to obtain ECGs in these patients at baseline while medication-free.

The clinical significance of the aforementioned cardiovascular findings remains unclear. TCA-induced sinus tachycardia and delays in intracardiac conduction rarely appear to be clinically significant in noncardiac adult and child patients.[82,84,89-94] Prolongation of the PR interval in the absence of AV conduction block is generally not clinically significant and does not result in hemodynamic compromise.[80,86] In fact, incomplete right bundle branch block is a normal ECG finding in children up to 10 years of age. Nonetheless, the development of incomplete right bundle branch block in children being treated with TCAs necessitates close clinical and ECG monitoring, especially at doses greater than 3.5 mg/kg/day.[80,86] Complete right bundle branch block in a child with a healthy heart does not necessarily imply impaired cardiac function. Its development does, however, necessitate assessment of cardiac ejection fraction and cardiac output, since it decreases the electromechanical function of the right ventricle.[80,86] It is important to note that right bundle branch block in the presence of preexisting cardiac disease has more serious implications. It is, therefore, recommended that in patients who have congenital heart disease, murmurs, acquired heart impairment, rhythm disturbances, a family history of serious cardiac disease (sudden cardiac death), or diastolic hypertension (greater than 90 mmHg), or when the cardiac status of the child is uncertain, additional cardiac evaluation be undertaken.[80,86] The evaluation should include a 24-hour Holter monitor and echocardiogram.[86] This can help in assessing the potential benefits versus the risks of treating patients with TCAs.

It must also be emphasized that sinus tachycardia, which is not uncommon in children treated with TCAs, was found in 20% of Biederman and colleagues'[84-86] patients at drug-free baseline evaluation. In older children and adolescents, however, a heart rate that remains persistently above 130 beats per minute is of concern and should prompt further noninvasive cardiac evaluation, including Doppler echocardiography, to assess ventricular ejection fraction and cardiac output.[86]

It is known that toxic concentrations of TCAs (i.e., after an overdose) can significantly depress myocardial conduction (see "Overdose"). Therapeutic doses of these agents, however, appear to be safe and have little adverse effect on left ventricular ejection fraction in adults, even in those with diagnosed cardiac disease.[93,94] It also appears that cardiovascular changes associated with imipramine and desipramine are rapidly reversible when the TCA dose is decreased or discontinued.[91,92] But it should be noted that this issue has not been evaluated adequately in children treated with TCAs, and that the reversibility of such cardiac complications in children has not been systematically assessed.[80,86]

Treatment with TCAs at doses above 3.5 mg/kg or at plasma levels greater than 150 ng/ml may increase the risk of asymptomatic ECG changes, particularly a slight prolongation of the PR interval and moderate increases in the QRS duration.[80,86] Delayed cardiac conduction and minor increases in diastolic blood pressure and heart rate can also be seen.

It is not known whether or not children treated with TCAs have a higher risk for sudden death than do untreated children or children receiving different treatments. It should be noted that this is not the first time that concern has been raised regarding a possible association between the use of TCAs and sudden cardiac death. Coull and colleagues[95] reported that six of 53 patients with cardiac disease died suddenly after receiving amitriptyline, while there were no sudden cardiac deaths in control patients. The Boston Collaborative Drug Surveillance Program[96] monitored adverse reactions to TCA drugs and failed to confirm this finding.

At the present time, no causal link between sudden cardiac death and TCA use has been established. It is important to remember that adverse, idiosyncratic reactions can be seen with any medication.[80,86] It is not known how many children have been treated with TCAs, although the number is believed to be quite large. This suggests that if such a risk exists, it most likely is small.[80,86] Utilizing an epidemiologic approach, Biederman and associates have generated some new data on the "sudden death" phenomenon in children and adolescents on TCAs. Their results suggest that sudden death from TCAs is an extraordinarily rare event when therapeutic plasma levels are used (personal communication). Nonetheless, this potential risk and other side effects need to be taken into account when TCA therapy is considered. For example, in depressed children with known cardiovascular impairment, we recommend that these agents be avoided since they have not been demonstrated to be superior to placebo in the treatment of child and adolescent depression. On the other hand, a child with ADHD who has not responded to stimulant medication, and whose disruptive behavior causes severe problems for the patient, family, school, and peers, may warrant a desipramine trial since this agent has been shown to be superior to placebo in the treatment of ADHD.

Although clinicians should not be so alarmed that they refuse to prescribe these medications, careful monitoring is essential in these patients. See Table 4-13 for ECG and blood pressure guidelines for the use of TCAs.

Table 4-13

ECG and Blood Pressure Guidelines for the Use of TCAs in Children and Adolescents

---

A. ECG

Baseline ECG must be done in all patients before starting treatment with TCAs (for ECG, BP, and pulse parameters, see below).

For doses greater than 25 mg/day, ECG rhythm strip should be obtained before each TCA dose increase or when TCA reaches the steady state (three–five days).

During maintenance, ECGs or rhythm strips will be repeated at least once every three months.

Tricyclic antidepressants will be reduced or discontinued if:

PR interval: Patient is ≤10 years of age and PR interval is >0.18. Patient is >10 years old and PR interval is >0.20.

QRS interval: >0.12 second or widening more than 50% over baseline QRS interval.

Corrected QT: ≥0.48 second.

Heart rate: Patient is ≤10 years of age and *resting* heart rate is >110. Patient is >10 years of age and *resting* heart rate is >100.

B. Blood pressure (BP)*

The child should be in a comfortable, sitting position and *sufficient time should be allowed for recovery from recent activity or apprehension.*

For inpatients, BP and pulse should be measured at least three times a week.

For outpatients, during dose titration, BP and pulse should be done at least once a week. During maintenance, BP and pulse should be taken at least once a month (if it is possible, we recommend that the school nurse take more frequent BP and pulse readings and call us if the patient has questionable readings or they meet the criteria for lowering or discontinuing TCAs).

The manometer must be well calibrated and proper cuff size should be used (long enough to completely encircle the circumference of the arm—with or without overlap—and wide enough to cover approximately 75% of the upper arm between the top of the shoulder and the olecranon).

Tricyclic antidepressants will be reduced or discontinued if:

Patient is ≤10 years of age and *resting* BP ≥140/90 or if BP is persistently greater than 130/85 (50% of the time during three weeks).

Patient is >10 years of age and *resting* BP ≥150/95 or persistently greater than 140/85 (50% of the time during three weeks).

C. Patients who must continue treatment with TCAs and have questionable or borderline BP and/or ECG or they meet the above criteria for lowering or discontinuing TCAs will be referred to the pediatric cardiology department at Children's Hospital for further evaluation and Holter monitoring.

D. Lying and standing BP and pulse may be obtained to assess possible orthostatic hypotension at the discretion of the physician.

These criteria were developed by Dr. James Zuberbuhler and Dr. Lee Beerman (Children's Hospital of Pittsburgh). These guidelines are empirical and subject to change.

Note: These BP guidelines were made under the assumption that patients will remain on treatment with TCAs for six to nine months.

Anticholinergic

Dry mouth and constipation are frequently seen in both children/adolescents and adults. Fortunately, these side effects are usually dose-limiting and often dissipate with time. Blurred vision and urinary retention are believed to be less common in children and adolescents than in adults.[4]

Psychosis/Mania

Psychosis is an uncommon but potentially serious adverse side effect of TCA therapy.[4] Antidepressant-induced mania is a well-described, albeit uncommon, side effect.[97–99]

Seizures

All of the antidepressants can decrease the seizure threshhold, although this side effect is uncommon. The risk of seizures is highest in children and adolescents with neurologic disorders, abnormal electroencephalograms (EEGs), and/or abnormal neurologic examination.[4] Maprotilene is the tricyclic antidepressant most associated with increasing the risk of seizures, especially at doses greater than 300 mg/day. This has led many investigators to call for its withdrawal. Great caution should be employed in its use.

Hypertension

Hypertension is an uncommon side effect. It is usually clinically significant only when there is preexisting hypertension.[4]

Confusion

Confusion most often is secondary to anticholinergic toxicity, and has been reported with higher tricyclic plasma levels.[82] Preskorn and colleagues[83] did observe cognitive toxicity in children that was associated with subtherapeutic plasma TCA levels.

Insomnia/Nightmares

Nightmares and insomnia are relatively uncommon side effects of TCAs in children and adolescents.[4]

Rash

An allergic reaction to TCA therapy is relatively rare. Such a reaction may be caused by tartrazine, the FD&C Yellow No. 5 dye used in some TCA formulations.[4] It should be noted, however, that some allergic reactions do appear to result from the active ingredients as well.

Tics/Incoordination/Tremor/Anxiety/Photosensitization

Tics, incoordination, tremor, anxiety, and photosensitization are occasional side effects of TCAs.[4]

Sexual Dysfunction

Breast enlargement and galactorrhea have been reported occasionally in females treated with TCAs.[4] Gynecomastia in males has also been reported. Increased libido, decreased libido, and impotence have been observed as well.

Overdose

The TCAs have a very high potential for causing death when taken in overdose,[4] even if the child is taken to the hospital immediately after the event. When a patient overdoses on more than 1 gram of a TCA, toxicity often results and death can occur.[1] Heart arrhythmias, seizures, hypotension, and so on can result in death.[1] It should be noted that, as in adults, plasma antidepressant levels often do not reflect the severity of the overdose.[4] Fatal arrhythmias can occur in patients with therapeutic and relatively modest TCA blood levels. Almost all symptoms develop within 24 hours of the overdose.[1]

Central-nervous-system side effects ranging from drowsiness to coma are common.[1] These side effects can be exacerbated and potentiated if the patient has also ingested other CNS depressants, such as benzodiazepines, alcohol, or barbiturates.[1] Antimuscarinic side effects are frequent and often pronounced, and include dry mucous membranes, warm dry skin, blurred vision, and mydriasis;[1] cardiovascular toxicity may also occur. Respiratory arrest and uncontrolled seizures can result from a severe overdose.[1]

Treatment of Overdose

In the event of an overdose, it is essential to provide close cardiac and respiratory monitoring. When decreased ventilation is noted, ventilatory assistance is indicated. Hypotension may necessitate the administration of fluids. Pressors such as epinephrine may be necessary if hypotension is severe or does not abate with simple fluid replacement. Epinephrine is the medication of choice in this situation because it can counteract the anti-alpha-adrenergic side effects of the TCA.[1] Continuous cardiac monitoring in the intensive-care setting is required for any patient with arrhythmia and/or QRS duration greater than 0.12. Serum antidepressant levels should be closely monitored, and cardiac monitoring should be continued until the arrhythmias and the QRS have normalized and plasma antidepressant levels are no longer toxic. We wish to reemphasize that antidepressant levels do not always reflect the severity of tricyclic overdose, and fatal arrhythmias can occur in patients with modest plasma TCA levels.[4]

Sinus tachycardia often does not necessitate treatment.[1] Direct-current cardioversion may be indicated for supraventricular tachycardia causing hypotension or myocardial ischemia.[1] Propranolol is safe and effective in the treatment of recurrent supraventricular tachycardia, but digoxin is contraindicated because it can precipitate or exacerbate heart block.[1] In those patients with ventricular tachycardia or ventricular fibrillation, cardioversion is the treatment of choice. Administration of a loading dose of lidocaine and a drip of 2 mg per minute may decrease the risk of recurrence.[1] It should be noted that doses of lidocaine higher than 2 mg per minute may increase the risk for seizures. If lidocaine is unsuccessful in alleviating arrhythmias, propranolol and bretylium are then indicated. Quinidine, disopyramide, and procainide are contraindicated for patients who have overdosed on TCAs because they may prolong the QRS and precipitate heart block. Physostigmine also is not effective in treating TCA-induced arrhythmias.[1] Temporary pacemakers may be necessary in cases of second- and third-degree heart block.

If the patient is alert, emesis induction is indicated.[1] Intubation and gastric lavage are necessary if the patient is not alert. In addition, 30 grams of activated charcoal with 120 cc of magnesium citrate should be given to reduce the absorption of residual drug, since bowel motility may have been slowed.[1]

Seizures can be problematic in patients who have overdosed on TCAs, particularly maprotilene. Benzodiazepines such as diazepam or lorazepam are the first-line treatment for TCA-induced seizures. Diazepam should be administered in doses of 5–10 mg IV at a rate of 2 mg/minute.[1] This may be repeated every 5–10 minutes until the seizures are controlled. The risk of respiratory decompensation secondary to benzodiazepine use can be minimized by administering IV benzodiazepines slowly. Lorazepam should be administered in doses of 1–2 mg IV over several minutes.[1] Lorazepam's advantages over diazepam include its longer effect when administered acutely (hours versus minutes), a possible lower risk of respiratory depression, and IM availability. Intravenous administration can be problematic in youngsters, and the problem can be exacerbated if the patient is thrashing about. If benzodiazepines are unsuccessful in treating seizures, phenytoin is indicated. A loading dose of 15 mg/kg not exceeding 50 mg/minute is recommended.[1] When phenytoin is given too rapidly (more rapidly than 50 mg/minute), severe hypotension may result.

We also wish to emphasize that forced diuresis and dialysis are not helpful because of the tissue binding of TCAs. Indeed, these interventions may increase hemodynamic compromise.[1]

Abuse

The TCAs have a low risk for abuse. Anticholinergic side effects are very rarely used to induce an altered mind state.[4]

Drug Interactions

See Table 4-14.

Available Preparations and Costs

See Table 4-15.

Table 4-14
Drug Interactions of TCAs

May increase effect of:
- CNS stimulants
- CNS depressants
- MAOIs
- Sympathomimetics (i.e., ephedrine)
- Alcohol
- Antipsychotics
- Benzodiazepines
- Barbiturates
- Anticholinergic agents
- Thyroid medications (cardiac effects)
- Seizure-potentiating drugs
- Phenytoin

May decrease effect of:
- Clonidine
- Guanethidine

Effects may be increased by:
- Phenothiazines
- Methylphenidate
- Oral contraceptives (estrogen)
- Marijuana (tachycardia)

Effects may be decreased by:
- Lithium
- Barbiturates
- Chloral hydrate
- Smoking

Table 4-15
Available Preparations and Cost of TCAs

Drug	Commercially Available Preparation	Dosage Forms	Average Cost/Day
Imipramine	Generic	10, 25, 50 mg tablets 75, 100, 125, 150 mg capsules	$0.23
	Tofranil	10, 25, 50 mg unscored tablets	
	Imipramine pamoate (Tofranil-PM)	25 mg/2 ml IM injection (rarely, if ever, used in child and adolescent psychiatry)	
Desipramine	Norpramin	10, 25, 50, 75, 100,150 mg unscored tablets	$2.22
	Pertofrane	25, 50 mg capsules	
Amitriptyline	Generic	10, 25, 50, 75, 100, 150 mg tablets	$0.16
	Elavil	10, 25, 50, 75, 100, 150 mg unscored tablets	
	Endep	10, 25, 50, 75, 100, 150 mg scored tablet (Injectable form rarely, if ever, used in child and adolescent psychiatry)	
Nortriptyline	Pamelor	10, 25, 50, 75 mg capsules Oral solution (equivalent to 10 mg/5 ml)	$2.11
Maprotilene	Generic	25, 50, 75 mg tablets	$2.31
	Ludiomil	25, 50, 75 mg scored tablets	

Source: *Red Book Annual Pharmacist Reference, 1991–1992.* Oradell, N.J.: Medical Economics Co.

Initiating and Maintaining Treatment

Before Starting Medication

Prior to initiating a TCA trial, children and adolescents should have a physical examination, with special attention paid to heart rate, blood pressure, weight, and height.

To detect a preexisting cardiac conduction defect, a baseline ECG is required.[4] Thereafter, an ECG rhythm strip should be obtained in children younger than 16 years of age at each dose increase and at frequent intervals during the period of dose elevation.[4] We recommend that older adolescents receive close monitoring as well. In fact, we advocate using the same guidelines as recommended for initiating and maintaining TCAs therapy in children younger than 16 years of age. As they are relatively noninvasive tests that are not particularly unpleasant or painful, the benefits of obtaining ECGs outweigh any minor inconveniences, especially in view of the potentially devastating consequences of failing to pick up a previously undetected cardiac anomaly. With reports of sudden cardiac death, the clinician cannot be faulted for exercising caution when prescribing these medications. It is also important to elicit any family history of cardiac disease.

The TCAs do cross the placenta so that a pregnancy test and evaluation for adequate contraceptive use is advised in females of childbearing age, since these medications should not be prescribed during pregnancy. Oral contraceptives containing estrogen can increase the effects of TCAs. Indeed, toxicity can occur via inhibition of antidepressant metabolism. Patients should also be observed for tics and involuntary movements on starting medication. A complete blood count and differential should generally be obtained at baseline. Liver function should also be checked since TCAs are metabolized by the liver.

It is vital that the clinician prescribing TCAs take a thorough substance-abuse history. When these agents are taken in combination with marijuana, sinus tachycardia may become prominent (see Chapter 14). Nicotine may decrease the effects of the TCAs by increasing their metabolism, thereby lowering plasma levels. The TCAs can also increase the CNS effects of alcohol (see "Drug Interactions").

When Treatment Is Initiated

When children and adolescents are treated with TCAs, it is important to check blood pressure, pulse, and ECG rhythm strip at each dose increase (see Table 4-13 for cardiac guidelines). Plasma antidepressant levels should be drawn five to seven days after the last dose increase, and 12 hours after the most recently administered dose. Children and adolescents should have an annual physical examination by their pediatrician or family practitioner.

Dry mouth is a frequently encountered side effect, and it may be ameliorated by reducing the dose, or by using sugar-free gum or candy. Rarely, bethanechol, a cholinergic agonist, can be used in doses of 10 mg q.i.d. to 50 mg q.i.d. to reduce this symptom when conservative measures are unsuccessful. The only common side effect of bethanecol therapy is stomach cramps, which necessitates lowering the dose.[4]

Constipation, another commonly encountered anticholinergic side effect of TCA therapy, can often be managed with Colace or Metamucil. Laxatives should not be used. Bethanechol would also help, but we recommend using stool softeners or bulk first.

When the more serious anticholinergic complication of delayed urination occurs (which is rare in children and adolescents), dose reduction and/or bethanechol treatment is warranted.

Confusion is often a sign of anticholinergic toxicity and requires prompt intervention. This requires dosage reduction or the giving of physostigmine.

If a seizure occurs, immediate discontinuation of the medication is advised until a seizure workup has been completed.[4] If a neurologic workup concludes that the seizure was drug-induced, then an anticonvulsant may be added to the regimen. Anticonvulsant prophylaxis permits the antidepressant to be restarted and eventually returned to full dosage.

Finally, if an allergic reaction occurs during TCA therapy, discontinuation of the medication is advised until a complete medical workup has been completed. Lowering the dose temporarily and consulting a dermatologist or switching to a structurally unrelated antidepressant is recommended.[4]

Interference with Diagnostic Blood Tests

These agents can interfere with a number of diagnostic tests, such as increasing the blood levels of cholesterol, aspartate transaminase (SGOT), alanine transaminase (SGPT), bilirubin, lactate dehydrogenase (LDH), alkaline phosphatase, eosinophils, catecholamines, and glucose. They can also decrease blood glucose levels, granulocytes, and platelets.

Dispensing TCAs

As discussed earlier, these agents have a potential for causing death, either in accidental or deliberate overdose. Therefore, it is absolutely essential that they be kept under careful supervision. Locking them away in child-protective containers, especially if there are infants or young children in the household, is advised. With regard to adolescents, it is vital that both the parents and physician assess whether the patient is capable of reliably and safely taking his or her own medication. In cases where the adolescent is known to be impulsive, it may be advisable to have the parents dispense the medications until the adolescent has demonstrated that he or she can take them responsibly. We also advocate prescribing no more than a two-week supply of medication at one time. If the patient visits are scheduled at intervals longer than two weeks, writing a prescription for a two-week supply with one or two refills is recommended.

Treatment Duration

There are no firm guidelines as to how long to continue treatment with TCAs for children and adolescents with psychiatric disorders. They are currently FDA approved for treating depression in patients at least 12 years of age and enuresis in children at least 6 years of age (Table 4-16). Thus it is difficult to offer definitive guidelines on the use of these agents. Our recommendations are based on a review of the available literature and on clinical experience.

Table 4-16
FDA Advertising Guidelines

Drug Name	Age Limit	Dose Limit	Indications
Imipramine	6 years for enuresis	2.5 mg/kg/day for children	Depression in adults and adolescents; enuresis in children
Desipramine	Not recommended for children	150 mg/day	Depression in adults and adolescents
Amitriptyline	12 years	300 mg/day	Depression in adults and adolescents
Nortriptyline	Not recommended for children	150 mg	Depression in adults and adolescents
Maprotiline	18 years	225 mg	Major depression
Trazadone	18 years	600 mg	Major depression
Fluoxetine	No mention	80 mg	Major depression
Buproprion	No mention	450 mg/day	Major depression

Source: Physicians' Desk Reference, 1992.

Withdrawal of Medication

Children are at a higher risk than adults for experiencing withdrawal symptoms when TCAs are discontinued because they metabolize these medications more rapidly than do adults.[4] In fact, children commonly show daily withdrawal effects on regular once-daily dosing, and these agents often need to be given in two or three divided doses daily for prepubertal children and younger adolescents.[4] Withdrawal symptoms of TCAs are similar in children and adults, including anxiety, agitation, disrupted sleep, behavioral activation, and somatic or GI distress.[101] The symptoms often give the overall impression of a flu-like syndrome and are largely related to the anticholinergic effects.[4] On withdrawal of TCAs, the anticholinergic effects are responsible for the resultant withdrawal effects. These can be avoided or minimized by gradually tapering the medication over a period of two weeks. If withdrawal symptoms do occur, they can be treated by restarting the medication and/or tapering it more gradually.[4]

Clinical Practice

For the dosing and administration of specific agents, see Tables 4-8, 4-9, and 4-10.

For therapy combining TCAs with antipsychotics, see Chapter 7.

References

1. Arana, G.W., Hyman, S.E. (Eds.) (1991). *Handbook of Psychiatric Drug Therapy (second edition)* (pp. 38–78). Boston: Little Brown.

2. Rapoport, J.L., Buchsbaum, M.S., Weingartner, H., et al. (1980). Dextroamphetamine: Its cognitive and behavioral effects in normal and hyperactive boys and normal men. *Arch Gen Psychiatry, 37*, 933–943.

3. Garber, H.J., McGonigle, J.J., Slomka, G.T., et al. (1992). Clomipramine treatment of stereotypical behaviors and self-injury in patients with developmental disorders. *J Am Acad Child Adolesc Psychiatry, 31(6)*, 1157–1160.

4. Ryan, N.D. (1990). Heterocyclic antidepressants in children and adolescents. *J Child Adolesc Psychopharmacol, 1*, 21–30.

5. Wender, P. (1987). *The Hyperactive Child, Adolescent, and Adult: ADD Through the Lifespan.* New York: Oxford University Press.

6. Riddle, M.A., Hardin, M.T., Cho, S.C., et al. (1988). Desipramine treatment of boys with ADHD and tics: Preliminary clinical experiences. *J Am Acad Child Adolesc Psychiatry, 27*, 811–814.

7. Ryan, N.D., Puig-Antich, J., Rabinovich, H., et al. (1987). MAOIs in adolescent major depression unresponsive to tricyclic antidepressants. *J Am Acad Child Adolesc Psychiatry, 26*, 400–406.

8. Sjoquist, F., Bertilsson, L. (1984). Clinical pharmacology of antidepressant drugs: Pharmacogenetics. *Adv Biochem Psychopharmacol, 39*, 359–372.

9. Preskorn, S.H., Weller, E.B., Weller, R.A., et al. (1983). Plasma levels of imipramine and adverse effects in children. *Am J Psychiatry, 140*, 1332–1335.

10. Ryan, N.D., Puig-Antich, J., Cooper, T.B., et al. (1987). Relative safety of single versus divided dose imipramine in adolescent major depression. *J Am Acad Child Adolesc Psychiatry, 26*, 400–406.

11. Preskorn, S.H., Bupp, S.J., Weller, E.B., et al. (1989) Plasma levels of imipramine and metabolites in 68 hospitalized children. *J Am Acad Child Adolesc Psychiatry, 28*, 373–375.

12. Potter, W.Z., Calil, H.M., Suftin, T.A., et al. (1982). Active metabolites of imipramine and desipramine in man. *Clin Pharmacol Ther, 31*, 393–401.

13. Preskorn, S.H., Jerkovich, G.S., Beber, J.H., et al. (1989). Therapeutic drug monitoring of tricyclic antidepressants: A standard of care issue. *Psychopharmacol Bull, 25*, 281–284.

14. Ryan, N.D., Puig-Antich, J., Ambrosini, P., et al. (1987). The clinical picture of major depression in children and adolescents. *Arch Gen Psychiatry, 44*, 854–861.

15. Weinberg, W.A., Rutman, J., Sullivan, L., et al. (1973). Depression in children referred to an educational diagnostic center: Diagnosis and treatment: Preliminary report. *J Pediatr, 83*, 1065–1072.

16. Puig-Antich, J., Blau, S., Marx, N., et al. (1978). Prepubertal major depressive disorder: A pilot study. *J Am Acad Child Adolesc Psychiatry, 17*, 695–707.

17. Carlson, G.A., Cantwell, D.P. (1979). A survey of depressive symptoms in child and adolescent psychiatric population: Interview data. *J Am Acad Child Adolesc Psychiatry, 18*, 587–599.

18. Strober, M., Green, J., Carlson, G. (1981). Phenomenology and subtypes of major depressive disorder in adolescence. *J Affect Disord, 3*, 281–290.

19. Kovacs, M., Feinberg, T.L., Crouse-Novak, M.A., et al. (1984). Depressive disorders in childhood: A longitudinal prospective study of characteristics and recovery (Part 1). *Arch Gen Psychiatry, 41*, 229–237.

20. Cytryn, L., McKnew, D.H., Bunney, W.E., et al. (1972). Diagnosis of depression in children: A reassessment. *Am J Psychiatry, 35*, 773–782.

21. Chambers, W.J., Puig-Antich, J., Paez, P., et al. (1985). The assessment of affective disorders in children and adolescents by semistructural interview: Test-retest reliability of the schedule for affective disorders and schizophrenia for school-age children, present episode version. *Arch Gen Psychiatry, 42*, 696–702.

22. Orvaschel, H., Puig-Antich, J., Chambers, W., et al. (1982). Retrospective assessment of prepubertal major depression with the kiddie SADS-E. *J Am Acad Child Adolesc Psychiatry, 21*, 392–397.

23. Young, M.A., Scheffner, W.A., Klerman, G.L., et al. (1986). The endogenous subtype of depression: A study of its internal construct validity. *Br J Psychiatry, 148*, 257–267.

24. Young, M.A. (1983). Evaluating diagnostic criteria: A lucent class paradigm. *Psychiatry Res, 17*, 285–296.

25. Nelson, J.C., Charney, D.S. (1981). The symptoms of major depressive disease. *Am J Psychiatry, 138*, 1–13.

26. Puig-Antich, J., Blau, S., Marx, N., et al. (1978). Prepubertal major depressive disorder: Pilot study. *J Am Acad Child Adolesc Psychiatry, 17*, 695–707.

27. Joyce, P.R., Oakley-Brocone, M.A., Wells, W., et al. (1990). Birth cohort trends in major depression: Increasing rates and earlier onset in New Zealand. *J Affect Disord, 18*, 83–89.

28. Robins, L.N., Helzer, J.E., Weissman, M.M., et al. (1984). Lifetime prevalence of specific psychiatric disorders in three sites. *Arch Gen Psychiatry, 41*, 949–958.

29. Hagrell, O., Lanke, J., Rorsman, R., et al. (1982). Are we entering an age of melancholy? Depressive illness in a prospective epidemiologic study over 25 years: The Lundby Study, Sweden. *Psychol Med, 12*, 279–289.

30. Ryan, N.D., Williamson, D.E., Iyenger, S., et al. (1992). A secular increase in child and adolescent onset affective disorder. *J Am Acad Child Adolesc Psychiatry, 31*, 600–605.

31. Puig-Antich, J. (1987). Affective disorders in children and adolescents: Diagnostic validity and psychobiology. In H.Y. Meltzer (Ed.), *The Third Generation of Progress* (p. 843). New York: Raven Press.

32. Weller, E.B., Weller, R.A. (1990). Depressive disorders in children and adolescents. In B.D. Garfinkel, G.A. Carlson, E.B. Weller (Eds.), *Children and Adolescents* (pp. 3–20). Philadelphia: Harcourt, Brace, Jovanovich.

33. Kaplan, H.I., Sadock, B.J. (Eds.) (1988). *Synopsis of Psychiatry, Behavioral Sciences, Clinical Psychiatry* (5th ed.) (pp. 631–647). Baltimore: Williams & Wilkens.

34. Casta, C.D., Arana, G.W., Powell, K. (1989). The DST in children and adolescents with major depressive disorder. *Am J Psychiatry, 146*, 503–507.

35. Weller, E.D., Weller, R.A., Fristad, M.A., et al. (1986). Dexamethasone suppression test and clinical outcome in prepubertal depressed children. *Am J Psychiatry, 143*, 1469–1470.

36. Birmaher, B., Ryan, N.D., Dahl, R. (1992). DST in children with MDD. *J Am Acad Child Adolesc Psychiatry, 31(2)*, 291–297.

37. Puig-Antich, J., Perel, J.M., Lupatkin, W., et al. (1987). Imipramine in prepubertal major depressive disorders. *Arch Gen Psychiatry, 44*, 81–89.

38. Geller, B., Cooper, T.B., McCombs, H.G., et al. (1989). Double-blind, placebo-controlled study of nortriptyline in depressed children using a "fixed plasma level" design. *Psychopharmacol Bull, 25*, 101–108.

39. Kramer, A.D., Feiguine, R.J. (1981). Clinical effects of amitriptyline in adolescent depression: A pilot study. *J Am Acad Child Psychiatry, 20*, 636–644.

40. Geller, B., et al. (1989). A double-blind, placebo-controlled study of nortriptyline in adolescents with major depression. Washington, D.C.: National Institute of Mental Health New Clinical Drug Evaluation Unit (NCDEU) Annual Meeting (abstract).

41. Ryan, N.D., Puig-Antich, J., Cooper, T.B., et al. (1986). Imipramine in adolescent major depression: Plasma level and clinical response. *Acta Psychiatr Scand, 73*, 275–288.

42. Strober, M. (1989). Effects of imipramine, lithium, and fluoxetine in the treatment of adolescent major depression. Washington, D.C. National Institute of Mental Health New Clinical Drug Evaluation Unit (NCDEU) Annual Meeting (abstract).

43. Jensen, P.S., Ryan, N.D., Prien, R. (1992). Psychopharmacology of child and adolescent major depression: Present status and future direction. *J Child Adolesc Psychopharmacol, 2(1)*, 31–45.

44. Morris, J.B., Beck, A.T. (1974). The efficacy of antidepressant drugs. *Arch Gen Psychiatry, 30*, 667–674.

45. Robinson, L.A., Berman, J.S., Neimeyer, R.A. (1990). Psychotherapy for the treatment of depression: A comprehensive review of controlled outcome research. *Psychol Bull, 108*, 30–49.

46. Angold, A., Weissman, M.M., John, K., et al. (1987). Parent and child reports of depressive symptoms in children at low and high risk of depression. *J Child Psychol Psychiat, 28*, 901–915.

47. Rapoport, J.L., Zametkin, A. (1980). ADD. *Psychiatr Clin N Am, 3*, 425–442.

48. Barkley, R.A. (1977). A review of stimulant drug research with hyperactive children. *J Child Psychol Psychiatry, 18*, 137–165.

49. Garfinkel, B.D., Wender, P.H., Sloman, L., et al. (1983). Tricyclic antidepressants and methylphenidate treatment of ADD in children. *J Am Acad Child Psychiatry, 22*, 343–348.

50. Biederman, J., Baldessarini, R.J., Wright, V., et al. (1989). A double-blind, placebo-controlled study of desipramine in the treatment of ADD: I. Efficacy. *J Am Acad Child Adolesc Psychiatry, 28*, 777–784.

51. Donnelly, M., Zametkin, A.J., Rapoport, J.L., et al. (1986). Treatment of childhood hyperactivity with desipramine: Plasma drug concentration, cardiovascular effects, plasma and urinary catecholamine levels, and clinical response. *Clin Pharmacol Ther, 39*, 72–81.

52. Gittelman-Klein, R. (1987). Pharmacotherapy of childhood hyperactivity: An update. In H.Y. Meltzer (Ed.), *The Third Generation of Progress* (pp. 1215–1284). New York: Raven Press.

53. Campbell, M., Grega, D.M., Green, W.H., et al. (1985). *Child and Adolescent Psychopharmacology*. Beverly Hills, Calif.: Sage.

54. Rapoport, J.L., Mikelson, E.J. (1978). Antidepressants. In J.S. Werry (Ed.), *Pediatric Psychopharmacology: The Use of Behavior Modifying Drugs in Children* (pp. 208–233). New York: Brunner/Mazel.

55. Rapoport, J.L., Quinn, P.O., Bradbard, G., et al. (1974). Imipramine and methylphenidate treatment of hyperactive boys. *Arch Gen Psychiatry, 30*, 789–798.

56. Wender, P.H. (1988). ADHD. In J.G. Howells (Ed.), *Modern Perspectives in Clinical Psychiatry* (pp. 149–169). New York: Brunner/Mazel.

57. Shaffer, D. (1985). Enuresis. In M. Rutter, I Hersov (Eds.), *Child and Adolescent Psychiatry: Modern Approaches* (pp. 465–481). Oxford: Blackwell Scientific Publications.

58. Dugas, M., Zarifian, E., Lehevzey, M.F., et al. (1980). Preliminary observations of the significance of monitoring tricyclic antidepressant plasma levels in the pediatric patient. *Ther Drug Monit, 2*, 307–314.

59. Morselli, P.L., Branchetti, G., Dugas, M. (1983). Therapeutic drug monitoring of psychotropic drugs in children. *Pediatr Pharmacol, 3,* 149–156.

60. Klein, D.F., Gittelman, R., Quitkin, F., et al. (1980). *Diagnosis and Drug Treatment of Psychiatric Disorders: Adults and Children.* Baltimore: Williams & Wilkins.

61. Klein, R.G., Koplewicz, H.S., Kanner, A. (1992). Imipramine treatment of children with separation anxiety disorder. *J Am Acad Child Adolesc Psychiatry, 31(1),* 21–28.

62. Berney, T., Kolvin, I., Bhate, S.R., et al. (1981). School phobia: A therapeutic trial with clomipramine and short-term outcome. *Br J Psychiatry, 138,* 110–118.

63. Ballenger, J.C., Carek, D.J., Steele, J.J., et al. (1989). Three cases of panic disorder with agoraphobia in children. *Am J Psychiatry, 146,* 922–924.

64. Flament, M.F., Rapoport, J.L., Murphy, D.L., et al. (1985). Clomipramine treatment of childhood obsessive-compulsive disorder: A double-blind controlled study. *Arch Gen Psychiatry, 42,* 977–983.

65. Flament, M.F., Rapoport, J.L., Murphy, D.L., et al. (1987). Biochemical changes during clomipramine treatment of childhood obsessive-compulsive disorder. *Arch Gen Psychiatry, 44,* 219–225.

66. Leonard, H.L., Swedo, S.E., Rapoport, J.L., et al. (1989). Treatment of obsessive-compulsive disorder with clomipramine and desipramine in children and adolescents: A double-blind crossover comparison. *Arch Gen Psychiatry, 46,* 1088–1092.

67. DeVeaugh-Geiss, J., Moroz, G., Biederman, J. (1992). Clomipramine hydrochloride in childhood and adolescent OCD—A multicenter trial. *J Am Acad Child Adolesc Psychiatry, 31(1),* 45–49.

68. Simeon, J.G., Thatte, S., Wiggins, D. (1990). Treatment of adolescent obsessive-compulsive disorder with a clomipramine-fluoxetine combination. *Psychopharmacol Bull, 26(3),* 285–290.

69. Swedo, S.E., Leonard, H.L., Rapoport, J.L., et al. (1989). A double-blind comparison of clomipramine versus desipramine in the treatment of trichotillomania (hairpulling). *N Engl J Med, 321,* 497–501.

70. Mitchell, J.E., Groat, R. (1984). A placebo-controlled double-blind trial of amitriptyline in bulimia. *J Clin Psychopharmacol, 4,* 186–193.

71. McDougle, C.J., Price, L.H., Volkmar, F.R., et al. (1992). Clomipramine

in autism: Preliminary evidence of efficacy. *J Am Acad Child Adolesc Psychiatry, 31(4),* 746–750.

72. Gawin, F.H., Kleber, H.D., Byck, R., et al. (1989). Desipramine facilitation of initial cocaine abstinence. *Arch Gen Psychiatry, 46,* 117.

73. Kaminer, Y. (1992). Desipramine facilitation of cocaine abstinence in an adolescent. *J Am Acad Child Adolesc Psychiatry, 31(2),* 312–317.

74. Kuinesdal, B., Molin, J., Roland, A., et al. (1984). Imipramine treatment of painful diabetic neuropathy. *JAMA, 251,* 1727.

75. Baldessarini, R.J. (1990). Drugs and the treatment of psychiatric disorders. In A.F. Gilman, T.W. Roll, A.S. Nies, P. Taylor (Eds.), *Goodman and Gilman's The Pharmacological Basis of Therapeutics* (8th ed.) (pp. 383–435). New York: Pergamon Press.

76. Ryan, N.D., Puig-Antich, J., Cooper, T.B., et al. (1987). Relative safety of single versus divided dose imipramine in adolescent major depression. *J Am Acad Child Adolesc Psychiatry, 26,* 400–406.

77. Dugas, M., Zarifan, E., Lehevzey, M.F., et al. (1980). Preliminary observations of the significance of monitoring tricyclic antidepressant plasma levels in the pediatric patient. *Ther Drug Monit, 2,* 307–314.

78. Saraf, K.P., Klein, D.F., Gittelman-Klein, R., et al. (1974). Imipramine side effects in children. *Psychopharmacologia (Berlin), 37,* 265–274.

79. (1990). Sudden death in children treated with a tricyclic antidepressant. *Med Lett Drug Ther, 32,* 53.

80. Biederman, J. (1991). Sudden death in children treated with a tricyclic antidepressant. *J Am Acad Child Adolesc Psychiatry, 30,* 495–498.

81. Winsberg, B.G., Goldstein, S., Yepes, L.E. (1975). Imipramine and EKG abnormalities in hyperactive children. *Am J Psychiatry, 132,* 542–547.

82. Preskorn, S.H., Weller, E.B., Weller, R.A., et al. (1983). Plasma levels of imipramine and adverse side effects in children. *Am J Psychiatry, 140,* 1332–1335.

83. Preskorn, S.H., Weller, E., Jerkovich, G., et al. (1988). Depression in children: Concentration dependent CNS toxicity of tricyclic antidepressants. *Psychopharmacol Bull, 24,* 275–279.

84. Biederman, J., Gastfriend, D., Jellinek, M.S., et al. (1985). Cardiovascular effects of desipramine in children and adolescents with ADD. *J Pediatr, 106,* 1017–1020.

85. Biederman, J., Baldessarini, R.J., Wright, V., et al. (1989). A double-

blind placebo controlled study of desipramine in the tratment of ADD: I. Efficacy. *J Am Acad Child Adolesc Psychiatry, 28*, 772–784.

86. Biederman, J., Baldessarini, R.J., Wright, V., et al. (1989). A double-blind placebo controlled study of desipramine in the treatment of ADD: II. Serum drug levels and cardiovascular findings. *J Am Acad Child Adolesc Psychiatry, 28*, 903–911.

87. Hayes, T.A., Panitch, M.L., Barker, E. (1975). Imipramine dosage in children: A comment on imipramine and electrocardiographic abnormalities in hyperactive children. *J Am Acad Child Psychiatry, 132*, 545–547.

88. Silber, E.N., Katz, L.N. (1975). *Heart Disease*. New York: Macmillan.

89. Glassman, A.H., Bigger, J.T. (1981). Cardiovascular effects of therapeutic doses of tricyclic antidepressants: A review. *Arch Gen Psychiatry, 38*, 815–820.

90. Glassman, A.H., Johnson, L.L., Giardina, E.V., et al. (1983). The use of imipramine in depressed patients with congestive heart failure. *JAMA, 250*, 1997–2001.

91. Puig-Antich, J., Perel, J.M., Lupatkin, W., et al. (1979). Plasma levels of imipramine (IMI) and desmethylimipramine (DMI) and clinical response in prepubertal major depressive disorder. *J Am Acad Child Psychiatry, 18*, 616–627.

92. Puig-Antich, J., Perel, J.M., Lupatkin, W., et al. (1987). Imipramine in prepubertal major depressive disorders. *Arch Gen Psychiatry, 44*, 81–89.

93. Roose, S.P., Glassman, A.H. Gardina, E.V., et al. (1987). Tricyclic antidepressants in depressed patients with cardiac conduction disease. *Arch Gen Psychiatry, 44*, 273–275.

94. Veith, R.C., Raskind, M.A., Caldwell, J.H., et al. (1982). Cardiovascular effects of therapeutic doses of tricyclic antidepressants in depressed patients with chronic heart disease *N Engl J Med, 306*, 954–957.

95. Coull, D.C., Crooks, J., Dingwall-Fordyce, I., et al. (1970). Amitriptyline and cardiac disease: Risk of sudden death identified by monitoring system. *Lancet, 2*, 590–591.

96. Boston Collaborative Drug Surveillance Program. (1972). Adverse reactions to the tricyclic antidepressant drugs. *Lancet, 1*, 529–531.

97. Bunney, W.E., Jr., Goodwin, F.K., Murphy, D.I., et al. (1972). The switch process in manic-depression illness II: Relationship to catecholamines, REM sleep and drugs. *Arch Gen Psychiatry, 27*, 304–309.

98. Lensgraf, S.J., Favazza, A.R. (1990). Antidepressant induced mania (Letter). *Am J Psychiatry, 11*, 1569.

99. Wehr, T.A., Goodwin, F.K. (1981). Rapid cycling of manic depressives induced by tricyclic antidepressants. *J Clin Psychopharmacol, 1*, 235–265.

100. Kupfer, D.J., Frank, E., Perel, J.M., et al. (1992). Five-year outcome for maintenance therapies in recurrent depression. *Arch Gen Psychiatry, 49*, 769–773.

101. Dilsaver, S.C., Greden, J.F. (1984). Antidepressant withdrawal phenomena. *Biol Psychiatry, 19*, 237–256.

102. Kutcher, S.P., Williamson, P., Silverberg, J., et al. (1988). Nocturnal growth hormone secretion in depressed older adolescents. *J Am Acad Child Adolesc Psychiatry, 27*, 751–754.

103. Dahl, R.E., Ryan, N.D., Williamson, D.E., et al. (1992). The regulation of sleep and growth hormone in adolescent depression. *J Am Acad Child Adolesc Psychiatry, 31*, 615–621.

104. Ryan, N.D., Puig-Antich, J, Rabinovich, H., et al. (1988). Growth hormone response to desmethylimipramine in depressed and suicidal adolescents. *J Affect Disord, 15*, 323–337.

105. Jensen, J.B., Garfinkel, B.D. (1990). Growth hormone dysregulation in children with major depressive disorder. *J Am Acad Child Adolesc Psychiatry, 29*, 295–301.

106. Meyer, W.J. III, Richards, G.E., Cavallo, A., et al. (1991). Depression and growth hormone. *J Am Acad Child Adolesc Psychiatry, 30*, 335.

107. Ryan, N.D., Dahl, R.E. (1993). The biology of depression in children and adolescents. In J.J. Mann, D.J. Kupfer (Eds.), *The Biology of Depressive Disorders*. New York: Plenum.

108. Glassman, A.H., Roose, S.P. (1990). Tricyclic treatment: What is adequate and who is refractory? In A. Tasman, S.M. Goldfinger, C.A. Kaufmann (Eds.), *American Psychiatric Press Review of Psychiatry (vol. 9)* (p. 60). Washington, D.C.: American Psychiatric Press.

109. Crowe, R.R. (1984). Electroconvulsive therapy—A current perspective. *N Engl J Med, 311*, 163–167.

110. Fink, M. (1985). Convulsive therapy: Fifty years of progress. *Convulsive Ther, 1*, 204–216.

111. Kendell, R.E. (1981). The present status of electroconvulsive therapy. *Br J Psychiatry, 139*, 265–283.

112. Zorumski, C.F., Rutherfore, J.L., Burke, W.J., et al. (1986). ECT in primary and secondary depression. *J Clin Psychiatry, 47*, 298–300.

113. Gittelman-Klein, R., Klein, D.F. (1971). Controlled imipramine treatment of school phobia. *Arch Gen Psychiatry, 25*, 204–207.

114. Pare, C.M.B., Kline, N., Hallstrom, C., et al. (1982). Will amitriptyline prevent the "cheese" reaction of monoamine oxidase inhibitors? *Lancet,* 183–186.

115. Davis, J.M., Glassman, A.H. (1991). Antidepressant drugs. In H.I. Kaplan, B.J. Sadock (Eds.), *Comprehensive Textbook of Psychiatry* (5th ed.) (p. 1644). Baltimore: Williams & Wilkins.

116. Kaplan, H.I., Sadock, B.J. (Eds.). (1991). *Synopsis of Psychiatry* (p. 660). Baltimore: Williams & Wilkins.

Novel (Atypical) Antidepressants

The serotonin reuptake inhibitor fluoxetine (Prozac) has become popular, and is often a drug of choice, because of its lack of anticholinergic and cardiac side effects and of withdrawal symptoms. Although recent reports of its possible association with inducing suicidal and homicidal ideation have made some patients and practitioners reluctant to use it, subsequent investigation has revealed that, when compared with other antidepressants, it does not pose an increased risk of self- or other-directed violence. In addition, new specific serotonin reuptake inhibitors (SSUI), sertraline (Zoloft) and paroxetine (Paxil), which have shorter half-lives and fewer side effects than fluoxetine, have been introduced. Other SSUIs, such as fluvoxamine, have not yet been approved for use in the United States. Bupropion (Welbutrin) and trazadone (Desyrel), antidepressants that are not chemically related to the TCAs or the SSUIs, are approved for treating depression in adults. Finally, this chapter briefly covers the adjuvant treatment of depression with thyroid hormones.

Fluoxetine

Although fluoxetine has been on the market for a relatively short time, it is a very popularly prescribed antidepressant. An SSUI, it has virtually no direct effect on other neurotransmitter systems or receptor sites.[9] In adults, it has been shown to have different and fewer side effects than TCAs. These SSUIs are relatively safe in overdose. And unlike the TCAs, they are not associated with weight gain. The starting and maintenance dose of 20 mg/day, which is given once a day, facilitates patient compliance. Efficacy and safety have not yet been established for children and adolescents, but its clinical use in this population has been increasing.

Reports of a possible association of fluoxetine with suicide and the emergence of other violent behavior recently received a great deal of attention in the scientific and lay press. Subsequent study, however, has revealed that fluoxetine is no more likely than any other antidepressant to induce suicidal or homicidal behavior.

Sertraline

Another SSUI, sertraline, which recently become available in the United States, has the advantage of a much shorter half-life and fewer side effects than fluoxetine. Unlike fluoxetine, sertraline does not increase plasma levels of other psychotropic medications.[3] Its efficacy has also been demonstrated in MDD and OCD in adults.[4–6] Indeed, the agents most effective in the treatment of OCD—clomipramine, fluoxetine, sertraline, and fluvoxamine—all inhibit serotonin reuptake (clomipramine also inhibits norepinephrine reuptake).

Paroxetine

Paroxetine, like sertraline, is an SSUI that also has a much shorter half-life and fewer side effects than fluoxetine.

In this chapter, we focus primarily on fluoxetine since this agent has been the most extensively used both in adult and in child and adolescent psychiatry. Because of the recent introduction of sertraline and paroxetine into the U.S. market, there are no available data for children and adolescents. We will discuss differences between fluoxetine and sertraline/paroxetine where applicable (Table 5-1). Because fluvoxamine has not been approved for use in the United States, we will not discuss this agent here. The same principles as in prescribing fluoxetine and sertraline apply.

Chemical Properties

See Table 5-2 and Figures 5-1, 5-2, and 5-3.

Table 5-1

Comparison of Fluoxetine, Sertraline, and Paroxetine Clinical Profiles

	Fluoxetine	Sertraline	Paroxetine
Long half-life	Yes	No	No
Increases plasma levels of other psychotropic medications	Yes	No	No
Overall side effects	More	Less	Less
Increased anxiety and restlessness	More	Less	Less

In contrast to the TCAs, fluoxetine selectively blocks serotonin reuptake, with no effect on norepinephrine uptake. It also has no effect on norepinephrine or dopamine reuptake.[10] Its site of action is believed to be the serotonin reuptake pump as opposed to the neurotransmitter receptor site. Chemically, it is unrelated to the TCAs.

Fluoxetine is metabolized primarily by the liver. Active and inactive metabolites are excreted in the urine by the kidneys. When administered at standard doses of 20 mg/day, fluoxetine achieves peak plasma levels after six to eight hours. It has a longer elimination half-life than standard TCAs of two to three days. Moreover, its primary active metabolite, norfluoxetine, has a half-life of seven to nine days. Although it may take six to eight weeks for steady-state plasma levels to be achieved, once they occur, they remain steady thereafter. Fluoxetine is highly protein bound (95%).

Sertraline and paroxetine, like fluoxetine, are also chemically unrelated to the other TCAs. Like fluoxetine, their mechanism of action is believed to be linked to its inhibition of CNS neuronal uptake of serotonin. In humans, sertraline and paroxetine have been observed to block the uptake of serotonin into platelets. They do not affect norepinephrine or dopamine uptake.

Mean peak plasma concentrations occur between five and nine hours in adults. The half-life of sertraline is approximately 26 hours, and the half-life of paroxetine is approximately 14 hours, considerably less than that of fluoxetine. Steady-state sertraline levels are generally achieved within one week of daily dosing, while steady-state paroxetine levels are attained within 10 days. Both undergo extensive first-pass metabolism. In contrast to fluoxetine, their principal metabolites have been shown to be significantly less active than the parent compounds. Sertraline and paroxetine, like fluoxetine, are highly protein bound (95–98%).

Table 5-2
Pharmacokinetics of Serotonin Reuptake in Children and Adolescents

Generic Name (Brand Name)	Onset of Action	Peak Plasma Concentration (hours)	Plasma Half-Life	Metabolism and Excretion	Comments
Fluoxetine (Prozac)	Usually within 2–4 weeks	6–8	2–3 days; 10 metabolite norfluoxetine 7–9 days	Liver; active and inactive metabolites excreted by kidney	May take up to 6–8 weeks for clinical response.
Sertraline (Zoloft)	2–3 weeks	4.5–8.4	26 hours	Extensive first-pass metabolism	May take up to 6–8 weeks for clinical response. More study needed.
Paroxetine (Paxil)	2–3 weeks	3–8	14 hours	Extensive first-pass metabolism	May take up to 6–8 weeks for clinical response. More study needed.

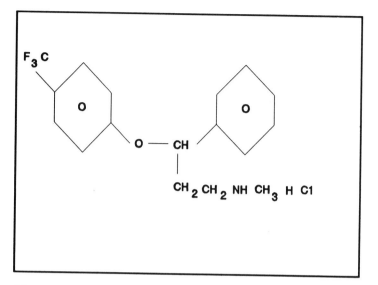

Figure 5-1
Fluoxetine

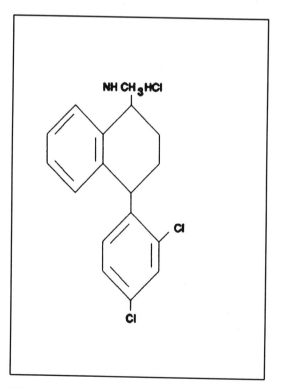

Figure 5-2
Sertraline

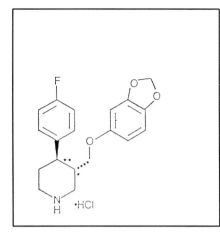

Figure 5-3
Paroxetine

Indications

See Table 5-3.

Major Depressive Disorder

In adults, placebo-controlled studies have shown fluoxetine's therapeutic effectiveness in outpatients to be similar to that of the TCAs.[11] There are no placebo-controlled studies demonstrating its effectiveness in the treatment of childhood and adolescent depression. Reports of fluoxetine-induced improvement in depressed children and adolescents thus far have been limited to a few, small open-label studies.[18,19] These agents have certain characteristics that may make them worth a trial in childhood and adolescent depression. Impulsivity, suicidal behavior, and aggression have been associated with reduced cerebrospinal fluid (CSF) levels of the serotonin metabolite 5-hydroxyindoleacetic acid (5-HIAA).[12–15]

Recent neuroendocrine studies of depressed adolescents suggest that abnormal CNS serotonin function may be present,[16] which means that SSUIs that increase CNS serotonin levels may be particularly beneficial in this population.[16,17] Depression in children and adolescents is frequently characterized by impulsivity and comorbid disruptive behavior disorders, so that the SSUIs may be attractive to clinicians because they increase CNS serotonin levels, and hence may reduce impulsivity. Nonetheless, at present, their value here is simply speculative.

In an open trial of fluoxetine in which 15 depressed adolescents and young adults 16 to 24 years of age were treated, Boulos and colleagues[19] found that a starting daily dose of 20 mg was often tolerated poorly, and that patients did better on 5–10 mg daily for the first week. Indeed, some of the patients exhibited antidepressant responses on doses as low as 5–10 mg/day. The au-

Table 5-3

**Indications for SSUIs (Fluoxetine, Sertraline, and Paroxetine)
in Child and Adolescent Psychiatry**

FDA-established indications: • None
Probable indications: • None
Possible indications: • MDD/dysthymia • ADHD • OCD • Trichotillomania • Compulsive impulse control disorders • Panic disorder • Anorexia nervosa • Bulimia nervosa • Prader-Willi Syndrome • Self-injurious behavior • Borderline personality disorder • PTSD • Drug craving

thors concluded that fluoxetine, in doses ranging from 5 to 40 mg/day, when used in combination with psychosocial treatments, may be an effective antidepressant for adolescents or young adults who have been refractory to standard TCA therapy. Schweizer and associates[22] found that in adults daily 20 mg doses of fluoxetine were as effective as 60–80 mg/day in achieving improvement in depressive symptoms, and that little was gained by raising the daily dose of fluoxetine above 20 mg. They did note that a trial of six to eight weeks may be required before resistance to fluoxetine treatment is inferred. Further study is clearly needed in children and adolescents.

Because sertraline and paroxetine have shorter half-lives than fluoxetine, and thus may have more benign side-effect profiles, we advocate double-blind, placebo-controlled studies with these agents as well, to better determine the role of SSUIs in treating childhood and adolescent MDD. Since placebo-controlled studies of antidepressants in depressed children and adolescents so far have been rather discouraging, the potential usefulness of these agents mandates further careful study.

Obsessive-Compulsive Disorder

A recent double-blind, crossover trial of fixed-dose fluoxetine (20 mg q.d.) and placebo in 14 children and adolescents, ages 8 to 15 years, with OCD suggested that it is a generally safe and effective in the short-term treatment of such patients. The study took 20 weeks, with a crossover at eight weeks. The severity of OCD symptoms as measured on the Yale-Brown Obsessive Compulsive Scale (CY-BOCS) decreased 44% after the initial eight weeks of fluoxetine treatment, as compared with a 27% decrease after placebo.[2] During the initial eight weeks, the magnitude of improvement for the fluoxetine group significantly exceeded that for the placebo group as measured by the Clinician's Global Impression-Obsessive Compulsive Disorder Scale, but not by the CY-BOCS. The most common medication side effects were well tolerated.

Fluoxetine may also be useful in combination with clomipramine (see "Obsessive-Compulsive Disorder," Chapter 4, and Table 5-10.[68] There are very limited data available, and further study is necessary before this strategy can be endorsed.

Sertraline has also been found to be effective in the treatment of adult OCD.[7] There are no data on children or adolescents. Further study is necessary to define sertraline's role in the treatment of OCD with and without clomipramine.

Attention-Deficit Hyperactivity Disorder

Barrickman and colleagues[24] used fluoxetine to treat 19 children and adolescents with ADHD. It was administered in open-label fashion for six weeks, and nearly 60% of the patients were rated as being at least moderately improved. All patients received between 20 and 60 mg of fluoxetine per day. Adverse effects were noted to be minimal, and most of them resolved spontaneously or with dosage adjustment. Interestingly, almost all of the subjects responded within one week after achieving the therapeutic dose.

This finding, is important because, although other antidepressants (such as desipramine and imipramine) have been found effective in the treatment of ADHD, some patients respond only partially, or not at all, to stimulants and TCAs. This underscores the need for additional medication options, since up to 30% of patients treated with stimulants fail to respond. Fluoxetine has the additional advantage of once-a-day dosing, thus avoiding the patient's having to take the medication during school hours. Moreover, its long half-life may be beneficial in that, not uncommonly, teachers observe more improvement in children on stimulants than do parents, because their effects have often worn off by the time the child returns home from school. Because of fluoxetine's long half-life, its efficacy may continue while the child is at home.

Sertraline and paroxetine should also be investigated to determine their potential role in the treatment of ADHD. With their favorable side-effect profiles, they may have utility for this condition.

Self-Injurious Behavior

King[25] reported a single case in which fluoxetine, 40 mg/day, reduced self-injurious behavior (SIB), including head banging and biting, in a 19-year-old with moderate mental retardation. This reduction in SIB lasted about 60 to 70 days. The consensus of the treatment team was that the incidence of SIB then approached that of pre–fluoxetine treatment.

On the other hand, Bass and Beltis[97] observed a significant and sustained reduction in SIB in a 17-year-old male with severe to profound mental retardation who was treated openly with fluoxetine. They reported a 40–50% reduction in SIB accompanied by improvement in mood stability, motor capacities, and social activity. No adverse effects or decreased therapeutic effects were observed during two years of treatment at daily doses of 40 mg. Twelve weeks before being started on fluoxetine, the patient had been unresponsive to naltrexone, an opiate receptor blocker, in a double-blind, placebo-controlled trial.

This study supports the hypothesis that SIB may have an obsessional and compulsive quality, and thus may be expected to respond to alterations in the serotonin system. This is further supported by previous reports of the partial efficacy of the treatment of SIB in children with Lesch-Nyhan syndrome with the serotonin precursor L-5-hydroxytryptophan.[26,27]

An open trial of fluoxetine, in doses ranging from 20 mg q.i.d. to 80 mg/day, resulted in a significant improvement in Clinical Global Impressions ratings of clinical severity in 15 of 23 patients with DSM-III-R diagnoses of autistic disorder and in 10 of 16 patients with mental retardation.[28] It should be noted, however, that six of the 23 patients with autistic disorder and three of the 16 patients with mental retardation experienced side effects that significantly interfered with functioning, consisting primarily of restlessness, hyperactivity, agitation, decreased appetite, or insomnia. Mentally retarded patients (and perhaps autistic patients, as well) may be more susceptible to the side effects of psychotropic medications, and have, in fact, been found to be more susceptible to methylphenidate-induced side effects.[28,29] Lower doses of fluoxetine may be warranted, with very gradual increments (see "Dosing and Administration"). This area deserves more investigation, but future study should utilize double-blind, placebo-controlled trials and stringent behavioral measures. As it is difficult to diagnose psychopathology in patients with autism and mental retardation, therapy is difficult, and the accurate quantification of therapeutic effect can be enormously challenging. Nonetheless, this population has enormous needs.

Sertraline and paroxetine, which have more favorable side-effect profiles than fluoxetine, may be especially helpful in patients with SIB, particularly in those with obsessive and/or compulsive manifestations.

Drug Craving
See Chapter 14.

Panic Disorder
Fluoxetine has been shown to be effective in the treatment of adults with panic disorder. However, there are no data on children and adolescents. This area merits further study, since TCAs have not been shown to be superior to placebo. Moreover, fluoxetine, in contrast to the benzodiapazines, is not addictive.

Sertraline and paroxetine also merit study in children and adolescents with panic disorder because of their favorable side-effect profiles. As yet, there are no data on either adults or children and adolescents.

Trichotillomania and Other Compulsive-Impulsive Control Disorders
The serotonergic agent clomipramine has been found effective in the treatment of trichotillomania (a disorder believed to have an obsessive-compulsive component) and in the treatment of autistic children with disturbances in social relatedness, obsessive-compulsive symptoms, impulse control problems, and/or aggressive behaviors.[8] (See "Indications" in Chapter 4.) Although there are no data on fluoxetine, it makes sense that this agent may be helpful for some of these patients. Combination therapy with clomipramine may enhance efficacy and allow the use of lower doses of each agent, while minimizing toxicity.

Anorexia Nervosa
Fluoxetine has been observed to decrease obsessional symptoms in patients with OCD. Anorexics' preoccupation with their body weight has often been referred to as obsessional. Moreover, a high incidence of mood disorders in anorexia nervosa patients and their families has been reported.[40] Thus far, however, the TCAs, including clomipramine and other psychotropic agents such as lithium, diazepam, metoclopramide, sulpiride, cyproheptadine, and pimozide, have failed to produce significant improvement.[31-39] Weltzin and colleagues[30] observed that 10% of 16 anorexia patients treated with fluoxetine in an open trial after inpatient weight restoration maintained their weight gains and experienced a significant decrease in anorexic symptoms and obsessions.

There are no data on the use of sertraline or paroxetine in patients with anorexia. These agents have the advantage of causing weight loss less frequently than does fluoxetine (see "Side Effects"), which could be a significant consideration for anorexics, who frequently have very low body weights. We believe that SSUIs should be a last resort in treating anorexic patients, and cannot endorse their generalized use in patients whose weight loss is already a major concern. Placebo-controlled study is necessary. If they are employed, close monitoring is essential.

Bulimia Nervosa

The SSUIs may be ideal agents for this disorder.[41–47] The cycle of bingeing and purging in bulimia has often been characterized as having a compulsive and/or obsessive quality, for which the SSUIs may be especially effective. Moreover, as with anorexia, mood disorders are prominent. In addition, bulimic patients are notoriously prone to impulsive acts, such as suicide attempts. The SSUIs are less lethal in overdose than are the TCAs (see "Overdose").

Foss and associates[48] conducted a double-blind, placebo-controlled study of six weeks' duration, with a double-blind extension period of 18 weeks, of patients judged to be treatment responders. Fluoxetine or placebo was randomly administered to 40 women with bulimia. All received placebo on a single-blind basis during the second week of the study. The investigators defined success as the patient's no longer meeting the DSM-III-R criteria for bulimia nervosa or the frequency of bingeing and purging decreasing to less than 50%. In the fluoxetine group, 18 patients completed the initial six-week study and 16 the entire study. In the placebo group, however, 18 completed six weeks, and then 15 withdrew because of lack of therapeutic effect. Two patients stopped after 12 weeks, and only one patient was able to complete the entire 24 weeks. Foss and associates concluded that fluoxetine at 60 mg/day was significantly more effective in the treatment of bulimia than was placebo.

Fava and colleagues[49] studied the long-term effectiveness of fluoxetine in the treatment of 19 outpatients with bulimia nervosa who had been treated with fluoxetine for more than three months. Retrospective analysis was conducted to gather data regarding three distinct periods in the course of the illness: (1) before treatment, i.e., patient baseline; (2) six to eight weeks into treatment; and (3) at the end of treatment, i.e., on discontinuation, or at the time of data collection if the patient was still on fluoxetine. At follow-up, 13 of 19 patients were on fluoxetine, whereas six patients had discontinued. The frequency of binges per week significantly decreased during fluoxetine treatment in all patients. The authors concluded that fluoxetine was shown to have produced a significant improvement in binge and purge frequency at follow-up.

It is important to reiterate that the short-term efficacy of fluoxetine is no greater than that reported for TCAs and MAOIs.[50] The chief advantage of fluoxetine lies in its relative safety as compared with these other medications. Nonetheless, patients who improve on any of these drugs often have persistent bulimic symptoms. Additional study is necessary to determine the long-term effectiveness of fluoxetine and other SSUIs, such as sertraline, in the treatment of bulimia. Bulimics frequently exhibit significant shifts in their body weight. Since sertraline may not be as likely to cause weight loss as fluoxetine, it may have particular usefulness in this population.

Prader-Willi Syndrome

The Prader-Willi syndrome (PWS) is a congential disorder characterized by obesity, small stature, hypogonadism, hyperphagia, and mental retardation, and it occurs in one in 10,000–15,000 live births.[51-53] Psychiatric complications are common, including aggression, behavioral disturbances, and depression. The patient's hoarding of and preoccupation with food often takes on an obsessional and ritualistic character, and desperate parents may be forced to padlock their refrigerators and keep all food out of reach of these children. Behavioral and psychotherapeutic interventions have been largely unsuccessful, as have pharmacologic approaches, including neuroleptics, standard antidepressants, lithium, carbamazepine, and methylphenidate. These agents have the added disadvantage (except for methylphenidate) of either causing weight gain or increasing appetite craving. The initial excitement regarding a role for opiate receptors in the pathology of the illness and the potential utility of naloxone and naltrexone has largely dissipated as these agents have been shown to be ineffective.

Recent excitement has been generated, however, regarding the SSUIs. These agents do not cause weight gain, and they may suppress appetite. In addition, they are effective in the treatment of OCD. Since the hoarding and overeating behavior exhibited by PWS patients has often been described as obsessional in nature, these medications may be useful in these patients as well. Of depressed patients being treated with fluoxetine, 13% experienced some weight loss (this does not appear to occur with sertraline). A recent report by Dech and Budow[54] described a 17-year-old female with PWS, including mild mental retardation, compulsive eating with gross obesity, and trichotillomania and trichophagia. The patient had a long history of multiple cognitive, behavioral, and pharmacologic treatments, including several inpatient hospitalizations that had met with only limited success. She demonstrated a marked improvement in weight control and a moderate improvement in hair pulling over a six-month period of observation at a dose of 80 mg/day. This also coincides with the available data that suggest that obsessive-compulsive patients require higher doses of fluoxetine than do depressed patients without OCD.

Selikowitz and associates[55] provided further evidence of a possible role for serotonergic agents in the treatment of this disorder. They conducted a double-blind, placebo-controlled trial to determine the effect of fenfluramine on the weight and behavior of patients with PWS. Fenfluramine treatment was associated with significant weight loss, an improvement in food-related behavior, and a decrease in aggressive behavior directed toward others. Skin picking and other self-mutilation were, however, unaffected. None of the patients suffered any side effects of the medication.

Thus fluoxetine, sertraline, paroxetine, and fenfluramine may have an important role to play in the treatment of some patients with PWS. In addition, antiobsessional agents such as clomipramine also may have a role. The disadvantage of using clomipramine is that in general it does not curb appetite or result in weight loss, but it is possible that certain PWS patients with obsessional and compulsive symptoms contributing to their obesity and overeating may lose weight and experience a decreased desire to overeat. Further study is clearly warranted. We suggest trying fluoxetine, sertraline, paroxetine, or fenfluramine in preference to clomipramine because of their more favorable side-effect profiles and their relative safety when taken in overdose. Patients with PWS often have impulse control problems that may make the administration of TCAs such as clomipramine potentially dangerous.

Borderline Personality Disorder

Although there have been no controlled studies of SSUIs in the treatment of borderline personality disorder, they are not uncommonly prescribed. These patients often exhibit impulsivity and aggression, and may make suicidal gestures, such as cutting themselves, and exhibit prominent shifts in mood. As CNS serotonin deficiency has been associated with impulsivity, aggression, and severity of suicide attempts, and with suicide completions as evidenced in postmortem brains, these agents may be of theoretical value in the treatment of this disorder. Moreover, because of their relative safety when taken in overdose and their benign side-effect profile, their risk/benefit ratio is favorable. In addition, patients with borderline personality disorder often have comorbid mood disorders for which these agents may be helpful.

Posttraumatic Stress Disorder

There is no known effective pharmacologic therapy for the treatment of PTSD. When symptoms of depression, anxiety, panic, psychosis, or significant agitation or aggression are present, psychotropic medications may help, and SSUIs may be beneficial in some cases. These medications are relatively safe in these patients, and may ameliorate depressive or panic symptoms. There are no data on children and adolescents, and further study is warranted.

Contraindications

See Table 5-4.

Table 5-4
Contraindications to Using Fluoxetine, Sertraline, and Paroxetine

- Known hypersensitivity reaction
- On MAOI within past five weeks (fluoxetine) or past two weeks (sertraline)
- Pregnancy
- Liver disease

History of Allergic Reaction

A known hypersensitivity to fluoxetine or sertraline is an absolute contraindication to their use.

Patients on MAOIs

Fluoxetine and sertraline should not be prescribed to any patient who has received an MAOI within two weeks. Conversely, an MAOI should not be started within five weeks of using fluoxetine (see Chapter 6). In patients receiving both fluoxetine and an MAOI, there have been reports of severe, sometimes fatal, reactions. Some cases had features resembling those of the neuroleptic malignant syndrome.

Pregnancy

There is virtually no indication for administering fluoxetine, sertraline, or paroxetine during pregnancy. These medications can cross the placenta. Nursing mothers should also avoid these medications. Exceptions occur when life-threatening psychiatric processes are evident and are clearly ameliorated by this treatment.

Liver Disease

These medications should be given cautiously in patients with liver disease.

Side Effects

See Table 5-5.

Gastrointestinal Complaints

Gastrointestinal complaints, including nausea, diarrhea, and dyspepsia, are very common side effects in patients treated with SSUIs. Nausea was observed in 33% of 15 adolescents treated with fluoxetine.[19] Tolerance to nausea often develops after one to two weeks on the drug.[56]

Weight Loss

Weight loss and decreased appetite are fairly common side effects with fluoxetine. A weight loss greater than 5% of body weight was seen in 13% of pa-

Table 5-5
Side Effects of Fluoxetine, Sertraline, and Paroxetine

Common:
- GI (nausea, diarrhea, dyspepsia)
- Decreased appetite
- Weight loss (fluoxetine only)
- Nervousness
- Insomnia
- Excess sweating
- Sedation
- Dream Intensification (fluoxetine > sertraline and paroxetine)
- Motor restlessness
- Dry mouth
- Male sexual dysfunction, anorgasmia

Occasional:
- Social disinhibition
- Subjective sensation of excitation
- Hypomania/mania
- Rash/allergic reactions
- Seizure
- Hair loss

Side effects of heterocyclic agents not seen:
- Anticholinergic
- Cardiovascular

There is no evidence that self-destructive phenomena (i.e., suicidal ideation/attempts) are more common with fluoxetine than with other antidepressants.

tients treated with fluoxetine, as compared with 4% of patients treated with placebo and 3% of patients treated with tricyclics.[94] Moreover, 9% of patients experienced anorexia, but patients rarely discontinue the treatment because of weight loss. Boulos and colleagues[19] noted that five of 15 adolescents on fluoxetine had anorexia. It should be pointed out, however, that the weight gain associated with TCAs is frequently a distressing side effect.

Nervousness and Insomnia
Nervousness and insomnia are common side effects of SSUIs. Unpublished data on 117 patients at McLean Hospital treated with fluoxetine show that patients with these symptoms before fluoxetine therapy do slightly better than those without these symptoms at baseline.[56] Changing the time of drug administration often fails to affect the insomnia. Riddle and colleagues[61] found that sleep disturbances occurred in 11 of 24 patients treated with fluoxetine, 20 or 40 mg/day, for depressive or obsessive-compulsive symptoms. Of 15 adolescents treated with fluoxetine, 20% reported feeling tense and

13% had difficulty sleeping while receiving the medication.[19] In adults, trazadone, 25–50 mg at bedtime, has proved helpful for fluoxetine-induced insomnia.[1] It should be noted, however, that some patients receiving trazadone and fluoxetine exhibit cognitive impairment. There are no data on the use of a trazadone–fluoxetine combination for children and adolescents. In general, polydrug therapy should be avoided. Nonetheless, in a patient whose depression appears to be responding to fluoxetine, but who continues to have problems with insomnia, the cautious addition of low-dose trazadone may be helpful. In contrast to the benzodiapazines, trazadone is sedating without being addictive. In a patient suffering from insomnia, the clinician should be alert for possibly evolving hypomania/mania, particularly if other maniclike symptoms become evident.

Excess Sweating
One third of all patients treated with fluoxetine by Boulos et al.[19] had increased sweating, a relatively common side effect with SSUIs.

Sedation
Although these agents are primarily thought to be activating agents, sedation is considered a common side effect. Moreover, changing the timing of drug administration often fails to affect the sedation.[56] Nonetheless, we recommend that if a patient experiences sedation after receiving fluoxetine, sertraline, or paroxetine in the morning, administration should be tried at bedtime.

Dreaming
Having abnormal dreams is a frequent side effect of fluoxetine. Early and sustained dreaming in four dysthymic adult patients on fluoxetine has been reported.[57] These patients spontaneously described these dreams as "newly" vivid. Interestingly, this intensification of dreams was not experienced as unpleasant, but more as a curiosity. The dreams became more memorable, although they did not change in content or form. The dreams returned to baseline in two patients who discontinued fluoxetine, and subsequently increased in one case upon rechallenge with the medication. According to the author, this "vibrant" dreaming preceded antidepressant response. There is no other literature regarding this claim.

It is known that fluoxetine suppresses REM sleep less than do most antidepressants.[58] In addition, fluoxetine produces less sedation than do other serotonergic agents, such as trazadone.[59] While this fact may explain the increased dream intensity and better dream recall on awakening, polysomnographic studies[58,60] have not described this dream phenomenon. There is a paucity of other available literature on this subject.

Motor Restlessness/Akathisia

Riddle and colleagues[61] observed motor restlessness, a relatively common side effect of SSUIs, in 46% of children and adolescents treated with fluoxetine, 20–40 mg/day, for depressive or obsessive-compulsive symptoms.[56] Indeed, three children with ADHD actually showed an exacerbation of symptoms while on fluoxetine.

Neuromuscular restlessness can approximate neuroleptic-induced akathisia, and may respond to dosage reduction or temporary benzodiazepine therapy.[1] Clonazepam, 0.25–0.5 mg b.i.d., has proved useful in treating this akathisia-like syndrome.[1] As mentioned, the incidence of akathisia with fluoxetine use is being reported more frequently.

Social Disinhibition

Social disinhibition may be a relatively common side effect of fluoxetine. Six of 24 children and adolescents treated with fluoxetine, 20–40 mg/day, experienced this side effect.[56]

Subjective Sensation of Excitation

Behavioral side effects characterized by a subjective sensation of excitation were observed in three of 24 patients treated with fluoxetine at daily doses of 20–40 mg.[56]

Dry Mouth

Dry mouth is reported as being a common side effect of sertraline. It was also noted in 40% of 15 depressed adolescents on fluoxetine.[19]

Male Sexual Dysfunction

In adults, male sexual dysfunction, primarily ejaculatory delay, is considered a relatively common side effect of sertraline. Pfizer Inc., the manufacturer of sertraline (Zoloft), has reported that sexual dysfunction occurred in 15.5% of males treated with sertraline, as opposed to 2.2% treated with placebo.[94] Anorgasmia has been reported to affect approximately 5% of patients treated with fluoxetine.[20] This side effect may respond to cyproheptadine taken PO four to eight hours before sexual activity is planned.[21] There are no data on children and adolescents, although it is believed that this side effect is less common in this population. Nonetheless, the practicing clinician must be aware of the side effect, particularly when administering sertraline to adolescent (and possibly sexually active) males.

Emergence of Self-Destructive Phenomena

Recently, Teicher and colleagues[62,63] published reports that generated a great deal of publicity and controversy in the scientific and lay communities, when they suggested that the emergence of intense suicidal preoccupation in six adult patients may have been induced by fluoxetine. The evidence for this was far from conclusive, since the majority of these patients had previously experienced suicidal ideation and had been treated with a variety of psychotropic medications. Prior to this report, Gorman and colleagues[64] had noted that, in an open trial of fluoxetine in the treatment of panic attacks, two nonresponders who dropped out of the study because of adverse side effects became depressed and developed suicidal ideation. Only one of the two had a prior history of depression.

King and associates[65] reported that self-injurious ideation or behavior appeared de novo or was intensified in six patients, 10–17 years of age, among 42 children and adolescents receiving fluoxetine for OCD. Before receiving fluoxetine, four of the patients had significant risk factors for self-destructive behavior, including depression and suicidal ideation or attempt. Indeed, several recent reports have failed to show any association between fluoxetine treatment and suicidality.[66–68] Boulos and colleagues[19] treated 15 adolescents with treatment-resistant depression with fluoxetine doses of 5–40 mg/day for six to seven weeks without observing any increase in suicidal ideation, suicide gestures, or self-inflicted injuries either in the month prior to or during the fluoxetine treatment period. It should be noted that depressed patients have a significantly increased rate of attempting and completing suicide, with 10–15% actually killing themselves, and significantly more making suicidal gestures and attempts. Bipolar depression is associated with an even higher suicide risk, up to 20%. Depression is a serious illness with life-threatening consequences. But, as with all psychotropic medications, careful monitoring for toxicity, lack of treatment efficacy, and worsening of the depression is most important.

Mania/Hypomania

Various reports describing mania induced by fluoxetine have surfaced.[69–79] Achamallah and Decker[80] were the first to describe a case of mania in an adolescent that was induced by fluoxetine. Rosenberg and colleagues[81] reported the evolution of hypomania and mania in a 13-year-old boy treated with low-dose fluoxetine (10 mg/day), necessitating its discontinuation and subsequent stabilization with lithium and carbamazepine. Boulos and colleagues[19] noted that one patient in their study of 15 depressed adolescents and young adults developed a full-blown mania at eight weeks, after an initial positive response to the medication. After discontinuation of fluoxetine, she was stabilized on valproic acid, and has since remained euthymic. Any patient being treated by an antidepressant must be carefully monitored for the evolution of mania/hypomania.

Rash/Allergic Reactions

In the initial studies on fluoxetine, 4% of the patients developed a rash and/or urticaria,[94] and almost a third were withdrawn from treatment as a result. All patients recovered completely upon the discontinuation of the fluoxetine—although in some cases, treatment with antihistamines or steroids was required. Any patient being treated with an antidepressant must be carefully monitored for hypersensitivity reactions.

Seizures

Twelve patients among more than 6000 evaluated (0.6%) experienced events described as seizures, a rate comparable to that observed with other antidepressants.[94] Thus it is important that fluoxetine be introduced with care in patients with a history of seizure disorder. Although antidepressants have been reported to lower the seizure threshold, this does not preclude their use, particularly for the treatment of disorders for which fluoxetine is efficacious. Ensuring that the patient is on a stable anticonvulsant regimen, and adjusting the dosage accordingly in the event of impaired seizure control, is recommended. There are no data on sertraline or paroxetine, but similar precautions are recommended.

Hair Loss

A case of severe hair loss in an adult treated with fluoxetine was reported by Jenike.[82] In a multicenter trial of approximately 600 patients, he reported a rate of less than 1%, suggesting that true hair loss as a fluoxetine side effect is negligible.[82] In the study by Boulos and associates[19] in which 15 depressed adolescents and young adults were treated with fluoxetine, two patients reported hair thinning. This effect was transient, however, and did not require medication withdrawal.

Anticholinergic Effects

Fluoxetine, sertraline, and paroxetine have essentially no anticholinergic side effects.

Cardiovascular Effects

Most notable about fluoxetine, sertraline, and paroxetine is the general absence of adverse cardiovascular side effects.

Overdose/Toxicity

In contrast to the TCAs, overdoses with SSUIs have a low lethality. This makes it easier for clinicians to prescribe these agents for impulsive patients suffering from a wide variety of psychopathologic processes who are prone to making suicidal gestures. The chances of surviving without severe toxicity and sequelae are far greater with the SSUIs.

There has been only one report of a lethal overdose when fluoxetine was taken by itself, but there have been several reports of lethal overdose when it was taken with other psychotropic drugs. Thus it is essential in cases of fluoxetine overdose that the clinician determine what other drugs were taken. Symptoms of fluoxetine overdose can include agitation, nervousness, restlessness, nausea, vomiting, insomnia, seizures, hypomania/mania, and other signs of CNS excitation.[94]

The management of fluoxetine overdose involves establishing and maintaining an airway to ensure adequate oxygenation and ventilation.[94] Activated charcoal with sorbitol may be more effective than emesis or lavage. It is important that cardiac and vital signs be monitored during the acute period of the overdose. When managing fluoxetine (or sertraline, or paroxetine) overdose, it is essential that the possibility of multiple drug involvement be considered. Thus, in addition to questioning the patient and family, urine and serum drug screens must be performed to adequately gauge what substances the patient ingested.

There have been no reported deaths with sertraline or paroxetine overdose thus far. Management is similar to that recommended for fluoxetine.

Abuse

There is little potential for abuse with these agents.

Drug Interactions

See Table 5-6.

Table 5-6
Drug Interactions—Fluoxetine*

Coadministration can result in dangerous side effects for patients on:
<ul><li>MAOIs</li><li>Heterocyclics</li><li>L-tryptophan</li><li>Lithium</li></ul>
When used with these agents, increases plasma levels of:
<ul><li>Heterocyclic antidepressants</li><li>Benzodiazepines (i.e., diazepam)</li></ul>
Coadministration can result in decreased therapeutic effect of:
<ul><li>Buspirone</li></ul>

*Side effects of sertraline and paroxetine are likely similar, although in some cases they may be less severe or prolonged due to its shorter half-life.

Available Preparations

See Table 5-7.

Initiating and Maintaining Treatment

Prior to initiating treatment, children and adolescents should have a physical examination, with special attention to vital signs, height, weight, and liver function. As these agents do cross the placenta, a pregnancy test and evaluation for adequate contraceptive use may be warranted in females of childbearing age. It is also advisable to discern the sexual history of adolescent males, since these agents occasionally have been reported to cause anorgasmia in adults. This may be an important compliance issue. Extensive laboratory testing is generally unnecessary.

It is also important to take a careful substance-abuse history. The patient and family need to be warned about the potential danger of taking fluoxetine, sertraline, and paroxetine in combination with drugs and alcohol. A case of mania as a result of a fluoxetine–marijuana interaction has been reported in an adult.[72]

If the patient is on another psychotropic agent, particularly a TCA, it should be tapered off prior to starting fluoxetine, since fluoxetine can increase TCA levels significantly. In those cases where it is decided to use fluoxetine (or sertraline, or paroxetine) with a TCA, careful monitoring of TCA levels is

Table 5-7
Available Preparations and Costs of Antidepressants (Atypical Agents)

Drug	Commercially Available Preparations	Dosage Forms	Average Cost/ Day
Trazadone	Generic	50, 100 mg tablets	$1.15
	Desyrel	50, 100 mg scored tablets 150 and 300 mg "Dividose" tablets that divide into thirds	
Bupropion	Welbutrin	75, 100 mg unscored tablets	$1.44
Fluoxetine	Prozac	20 mg Pulvules (capsules)	$1.44
Sertraline	Zoloft	50, 100 mg scored tablets	$0.54

Source: Red Book Annual Pharmacist Reference, 1991–1992. Oradell, N.J.: Medical Economics.

necessary. The measurement of fluoxetine, sertraline, or paroxetine levels is not helpful in assessing or targeting clinical response.

Because of the substantial publicity regarding fluoxetine and its alleged association with suicidal behavior, we recommend confronting this issue with the patient and family, if it is decided the patient may benefit from this agent. Emphasis on close monitoring and active participation by the patient and family so that any behavioral side effects are immediately noted and acted upon can provide reassurance. We have found it helpful to give the parents and patient a drug information sheet on fluoxetine, in nonmedical jargon. It describes what fluoxetine is, how the medication can help, how the physician will monitor treatment, what the side effects are, and the possible drug interactions (Table 5-8). In our experience, confronting the issues directly frequently reassures the patient and family.

Patients on SSUIs should be monitored at each visit for involuntary movements and CNS excitation (mania/hypomania). It is also advisable to record height and weight at regular three- to four-month intervals. Children and adolescents should have an annual physical examination.

Treatment Duration
There are no firm guidelines as to how long treatment with SSUIs in children and adolescents should last. The reader is referred to the guidelines on treatment duration discussed in Chapter 4.

Withdrawal
In contrast to the TCAs, withdrawal flu-like syndromes and other sequelae do not generally occur with the SSUIs. Thus tapering is not necessary, and immediate discontinuation of even high-dose therapy is safe.

With the advent of sertraline and paroxetine, it has become important to know whether intolerance to one SSUI means that the patient will be intolerant to all others. Recent findings in adults suggest that this does not happen.[82] A multicenter trial that studied how patients who experienced intolerable side effects from fluoxetine would respond to sertraline included 100 patients who met the DSM-III-R criteria for MDD, and who had discontinued fluoxetine because of the side effects.[82] After a washout of at least four weeks following fluoxetine discontinuation and an additional one-week, single-blind placebo period, patients were switched to open treatment with sertraline. They began treatment with 50 mg per day, and, based on their response, doses were titrated upward as necessary. The maximum daily dose was 200 mg/day. Weekly assessments included administration of the HAM-D and the recording of adverse effects and laboratory values. Based on an interim analysis of the first 60 patients completing at least six weeks of treat-

Table 5-8
Parent Information on Prozac

What is Prozac?

Prozac (generic name fluoxetine) is a new medication that was developed as an antidepressant. It is chemically different from other antidepressant medications, and works in a different way. It is available in capsules (called Pulvules) and in a liquid form.

How can this medication help?

Because Prozac is so new, there has not been much research on its use with children and adolescents, although a great deal is known about its use with adults. It is being used on a trial basis to help children and adolescents who suffer from depression, OCD, or obsessions or compulsions as part of Tourette's syndrome. It may be effective for patients who have tried other medications, but do not get better or develop side effects.

How will the doctor monitor this medicine?

The doctor will want you to have regular visits to evaluate how Prozac is working, to adjust the dose, to watch for side effects, and to see if other treatment is needed.

What side effects can this medicine have?

Any medication may have side effects. Because each patient is different, your doctor will work with you to get the most positive effects and the fewest negative effects from the medicine. This list may not include rare or unusual side effects. Please talk to the doctor if you suspect the medicine is causing a problem. In general, Prozac has fewer and less troublesome side effects than other antidepressants.

Common nuisance side effects:

Nausea; weight loss or gain; anxiety or nervousness; insomnia (trouble sleeping); excessive sweating; headaches.

Some persons may become restless or agitated, with increased activity and rapid speech, and an uncomfortable feeling of being "speeded up." This is worse at first, and may improve if the dose is lowered.

There has been a lot of publicity suggesting that Prozac may cause suicidal thoughts. This is very rare, if it occurs at all, and may be due to the depression itself rather than Prozac. In any case, if suicidal thoughts or actions appear or worsen, call the doctor right away.

What else should I know about this medicine?

It can be dangerous to take Prozac at the same time or within five to six weeks of taking a type of antidepressant called an MAO inhibitor (Nardil, Parnate, or Marplan).

Prozac interacts with many other medications. Be sure each doctor knows all of the medications that are being taken, or have been taken in the past several months.

Source: Dulcan, M.K. (1992). Information for parents and youth on psychotropic medications. *J Child Adolesc Psychopharmacol, 2*(2), 81–101.

ment, 75% were rated as being very much or much improved. These results suggest that, as with the TCAs, patients who are unable to tolerate one SSUI may be treated successfully with another.

Finally, to provide information on the use of sertraline for the continuation of maintenance therapy, Turner and associates[83] reported that, in a placebo-controlled study of maintenance sertraline therapy for 44 weeks, sertraline helped to prevent the relapse of an index episode of depression and the recurrence of further episodes, with few side effects.

Clinical Practice

Dosing and Administration
Tables 5-9 through 5-12.

For lithium augmentation of fluoxetine nonresponsiveness, see Chapter 8.

For the use of antipsychotics and fluoxetine, see Chapter 7.

For the use of benzodiazepines, see Chapter 10.

Table 5-9
Dosage and Administration of Fluoxetine, Sertraline, and Paroxetine in Child and Adolescent MDD

Fluoxetine:
- Not proven effective by controlled study.
- Open-label studies indicate possible efficacy.[18,19]
- To minimize side effects, low-dose therapy is recommended.
- Therapeutic response may be seen at doses as low as 5 mg/day.
- Initiate dose at 5 mg/day and increase by 5 mg every seven to 10 days to maximum dose of 20 mg/day.
- Lowest effective dose should be prescribed.
- Medication trial of six to eight weeks necessary before treatment resistance can be determined.
- Once treatment response occurs, must be maintained on medication for nine to 12 months.
- Still experimental.
- Careful monitoring required.

Sertraline:
- Not proven effective by controlled study.
- No open-label studies.
- Doses over 100 mg should be given b.i.d.
- Six- to eight-week trial is necessary before treatment resistance can be determined.
- If treatment response occurs, maintain on medication nine to 12 months.
- Consider maintenance medication therapy.
- Experimental.
- Careful monitoring required.

Paroxetine:
- Not proven effective by controlled study.
- No open-label studies.
- Initiate dose at 10 mg/day and increase by 10 mg every seven days to maximum dose of 50 mg/day.
- Six- to eight-week trial is necessary before treatment resistance can be determined.
- If treatment response occurs, maintain on medication nine to 12 months.
- Consider maintenance medication therapy.
- Experimental.
- Careful monitoring required.

Table 5-10

Dosage and Administration of Fluoxetine, Sertraline, and Paroxetine in OCD and Conditions with Obsessive-Compulsive Symptoms (i.e., Trichotillomania)

Fluoxetine:
- Effective treatment.
- Combination therapy with clomipramine may enhance efficacy, decreases doses of both, and minimizes side effects.
- Have to monitor closely for possible increased risk of fluoxetine side effects (i.e., akathisia).
- Start with fluoxetine 20 mg q.o.d. and clomipramine 25 mg.
- If no response after 10–14 days, increase fluoxetine to 20 mg and clomipramine to 50 mg: May after 10–14 days, increase fluoxetine to 20 mg b.i.d. if no response.
- Carefully monitor clomipramine levels and signs of toxicity.
- If clomipramine contraindicated, start with fluoxetine 20 mg q.o.d. and increase every 10–14 days to a maximum daily dose of 80 mg/day, i.e., 20 mg q.i.d.

Sertraline:
- Not known to be effective.
- May be effective in adults.
- Controlled study is necessary before this can be recommended for routine use.

Paroxetine:
- Not known to be effective.
- Not recommended for routine use.

Table 5-11

Dosage and Administration of Fluoxetine, Sertraline, and Paroxetine in ADHD

Fluoxetine:
- No controlled studies documenting efficacy.
- One open-label study suggests may be effective.
- Only use after other standard medications fail.
- Start with doses 20 mg q.o.d.
- If no improvement after seven to 10 days, increase dose by 20 mg q seven to 10 days until symptom relief or maximum dose of 80 mg/day (i.e., 20 mg q.i.d.).
- Careful monitoring required.

Sertraline and Paroxetine:
- No controlled or open-label studies demonstrating efficacy.
- Not recommended for use until further studied.

Table 5-12
Dosage and Administration of Fluoxetine, Sertraline, and Paroxetine in Self-injurious Behavior

---

Fluoxetine:
- No controlled studies showing effective.
- Anecdotal and open-label case studies indicate potential role.
- Should only be used after nonchemical restraint found to be unsuccessful.
- Need to start with very low doses and increase very gradually because of possible increased sensitivity of these patients to side effects.
- Starting doses of 5 mg/day are suggested.
- If no improvement, can increase dose by 5 mg every 10–14 days until symptom relief or toxicity.
- Would not exceed 80 mg (i.e., 20 mg q.i.d.).
- Monitor closely for efficacy versus toxicity.

Sertraline and Paroxetine:
- No controlled or open-label studies showing effective.
- Not recommended for use until further studied.

Trazadone

Trazadone is an atypical antidepressant that is chemically unrelated to the TCAs. It differs from TCAs in having almost no anticholinergic side effects. In adults, this agent has been used primarily to treat depression, although recent experience demonstrates its potential value in other areas as well. It is not considered a first-line antidepressant, but may be considered when other agents are unsuccessful or cause incapacitating side effects.

Trazadone is best known for its sedative effect, and is often chosen when insomnia or other sleep disturbance is prominent. It is very effective in improving sleep quality, increasing total sleep time, decreasing the number of nighttime awakenings, decreasing REM sleep, and, unlike the TCAs, not decreasing stage IV sleep.[85]

There are very limited data on children and adolescents. In fact, the American Academy of Child and Adolescent Psychiatry's *Textbook of Child and Adolescent Psychiatry*[84] does not even mention trazadone. In this section, we will briefly discuss some of its possible applications in this population.

Chemical Properties

See Table 5-13 and Figure 5-4.

Trazadone is rapidly absorbed from the GI tract following oral administration and reaches peak plasma concentrations in one to two hours. These

Table 5-13
Pharmacokinetics of Trazadone and Bupropion

Generic Name (brand name)	Peak Plasma Concentrations (hours)	Plasma Half-Life (hours)	Metabolism and Excretion	Comments
Trazadone (Desyrel)	1–2	6–11	Liver—active metabolite m-chlorophenyl-piperazine excreted by kidneys.	Inhibits serotonin reuptake; no anticholinergic effects.
Bupropion (Welbutrin)	2	8–24	Liver—metabolites hydroxybupropion and threohydrobupropion excreted in urine.	Hydroxybupropion concentrations > 1250 ng/ml associated with lack of clinical response.

peak plasma levels are achieved more rapidly on an empty stomach. It has a relatively short half-life of six to 11 hours. Trazadone is metabolized by the liver, and its active metabolite, m-chlorophenyl-piperazine, is excreted by the kidneys.

Indications

We do not recommend trazadone's routine use in children and adolescents at this time.

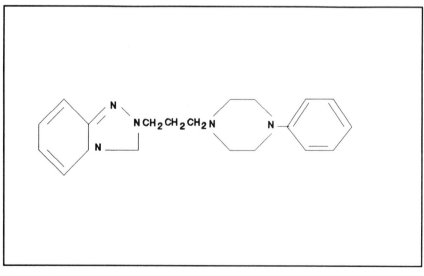

Figure 5-4
Trazadone

Side Effects

See Table 5-14.

Sedation

Sedation is a very common side effect of trazadone,[86] but can be lessened if the medication is taken in divided doses. Children and younger adolescents may be especially susceptible. Starting the medication at low doses and increasing it very gradually is recommended. In time, some patients may tolerate this medication with fewer problems. It should be noted that even though trazadone is often given at bedtime to facilitate sleep, occasionally patients report sedation the next day.

Orthostatic Hypotension

In adults, orthostatic hypotension can occur. This is believed to be mediated, in part, by its alpha-1-adrenergic antagonism.[95] This effect can be decreased if the trazadone is taken with food, which slows its absorption. This side effect may be less common in children and adolescents, although the data are limited on trazadone's efficacy and toxicity in this population.

Dizziness

Dizziness is a common, often transient side effect of trazadone.

Headache

The occurrence of headache may be related to trazadone's sedative effect.

Nausea and Vomiting

Disturbances of the GI tract such as nausea and vomiting can be problematic, but can be minimized, or even prevented, by taking the medication in

Table 5-14
Side Effects of Trazadone

Common: <ul><li>Sedation</li><li>Orthostasis (in adults, children?)</li><li>Dizziness</li><li>Headache</li><li>Nausea/vomiting</li></ul>
Rare but important: <ul><li>Priapism</li></ul>
No cardiac, anticholinergic side effects

divided doses and with meals. Taking the medication with meals slows
its absorption.

Priapism

Priapism, a rare side effect of trazadone therapy, is a prolonged erection in
the absence of any sexual stimulation. Males taking trazadone must be told
to report any prolonged erections immediately. The occurrence of priapism
constitutes a medical emergency, and the immediate discontinuation of trazadone is warranted. The priapism that occurs on trazadone, unlike idio-
pathic priapism, frequently results in permanent erectile dysfunction, even
when prompt treatment is received. Because there are no data demonstrating trazadone's efficacy in treating child or adolescent psychiatric conditions, we advocate against using it for adolescent males. If this side effect
appears, it precludes trazadone's use in the future, even after the condition
has stabilized.

Anticholinergic Effects

Anticholinergic side effects are generally not seen with trazadone.

Cardiac Effects

Trazadone does not have the antiarrhythmic effects of the TCAs. It does not
appear to exert a major effect on cardiac conduction.

Overdose/Toxicity

One great advantage of trazadone is its relative lack of toxicity in overdose.
There have been no reported lethal overdoses when trazadone was taken
alone. However, fatalities have occurred when trazadone was taken with
other drugs, and thus it is important to ask the patient and family what
other drugs were ingested. Urine and serum drug screens are also
necessary.

Abuse

There is virtually no risk for abuse of trazadone.

Available Preparations

See Table 5-7.

Drug Interactions

See Table 5-15.

Table 5-15
Trazadone Drug Interactions

Increases serum levels:
- Digoxin
- Pheytoin
- CNS depressants

Initiating and Maintaining Treatment

We do not recommend trazadone's use for children and adolescents at this time.

Bupropion

Bupropion is an atypical antidepressant unrelated to the TCAs. Its approval by the FDA was delayed because of concern about the incidence of seizures associated with its use, but specific guidelines have been adopted to decrease the risk of untoward effects, and it is now available in the United States. In adults, it is FDA approved only for MDD, and it is not approved for use in patients under 18 years of age. There are very limited data on children and adolescents. Thus far, ADHD is the only disorder in this population where some evidence for bupropion's efficacy exists. This may be due in part to the fact that bupropion is structurally related to amphetamine and the sympathomimetic diethylpropion. It has few anticholinergic effects, and does not alter cardiac conduction or cause orthostasis. Bupropion requires further study in children and adolescents. It is not a first-line agent for treating psychopathology in this population. Nonetheless, its properties make it a potentially attractive agent for use in a variety of disorders, and it clearly merits further investigation.

Chemical Properties

See Table 5-13 and Figure 5-5.

Bupropion is rapidly absorbed from the GI tract after oral administration. It is primarily metabolized by the liver, and its metabolites, hydroxybupropion and threohydrobupropion, are excreted in the urine. These metabolites may have particular clinical relevance. Golden and associates[87] found that plasma hydroxybupropion concentrations greater than 1250 ng/ml were correlated with a lack of positive clinical response to bupropion therapy. Peak plasma concentrations are achieved within two hours. The half-life of bupropion ranges from eight to 24 hours.

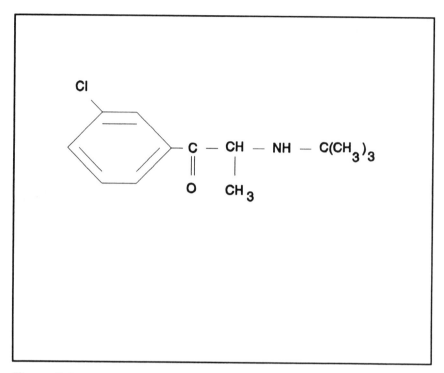

Figure 5-5
Bupropion

Indications

See Table 5-16.

Attention-Deficit Hyperactivity Disorder
Simeon and colleagues[88] treated 17 male patients ranging in age from 7 to
13 years with ADHD and/or conduct disorders in an open clinical trial with
a baseline placebo period of four weeks, eight weeks of bupropion therapy,
and two weeks of a postdrug placebo. Evaluations included clinical assessments, parents' and teachers' ratings, self-ratings, cognitive tests, and blood-
level measurements of bupropion. Fifteen patients received a daily maximum dose of 150 mg, one received 100 mg, and one received 50 mg. Clinical
global improvement with bupropion therapy was marked in five patients,
moderate in seven, and mild in two, and no improvement was observed in
three patients. The authors did note that, overall, bupropion appeared to be
less effective in improving the core symptoms of ADHD, such as poor attention span, distractibility, and impulsivity, although half of their patients
had been nonresponders to previous therapy. Bupropion was found to be
both safe and effective in the patients they treated.

Table 5-16
Indications for Bupropion in Children and Adolescents

Established indications:
• None
Probable indications:
• None
Possible indications:
• ADHD
• MDD

Clay and colleagues[89] used bupropion to treat 30 prepubertal children with diagnoses of ADHD in a double-blind, placebo-controlled study, and found it to be safe and effective. In addition, as did Simeon and associates,[88] these authors found that children with prominent conduct disorder symptoms responded especially well to bupropion. Optimal doses ranged from 3 to 7 mg/kg/day (100–250 mg/day). In addition, some of the children who had failed to respond to stimulant medications had a good response to bupropion. Interestingly, some patients who had never received stimulants, and who did not respond well to bupropion, responded well when methylphenidate was prescribed openly at a later time.

Finally, Casat and colleagues[90] administered bupropion to 20 ADHD children and placebo to 10 ADHD children. Significant improvement was observed in the bupropion-treated group.

These studies offer hope that an alternative medication to those already mentioned might exist. This is important because ADHD is a very common disorder in this country, and although stimulants are very effective, a significant proportion of patients fail to respond to these medications. It should be noted, however, that confirmation of these findings is needed.

Major Depressive Disorder
In adults, bupropion has been found to be as effective as standard antidepressant therapies in the treatment of MDD. There are no data on children and adolescents. Based on its preliminary success in treating some patients with ADHD, investigation into the role it might play in the treatment of child and adolescent MDD is warranted. (See below regarding guidelines to minimize risk for seizures.)

Contraindications

See Table 5-17.

135

Table 5-17

Contraindications to Bupropion Therapy for Children and Adolescents

Absolute:
• Known hypersensitivity
• Pregnancy
• On MAOI
• Past or current history of bulimia or anorexia nervosa
• Seizure disorder
• Organic brain disease
• History of head trauma
• CNS tumor
• EEG abnormalities
• Recent withdrawal from benzodiazepines or alcohol
Relative:
• Concomitant administration of psychotropics known to lower seizure threshold
• Hepatic disease
• Renal disease

Hypersensitivity Reaction

A history of hypersensitivity to bupropion is an absolute contraindication to its use.

Pregnancy

It is not advisable to administer this agent during pregnancy, as it crosses the placenta and is secreted in breast milk. For exceptions, see TCA contraindications, Chapter 4.

Bulimia/Anorexia Nervosa

A current or prior diagnosis of bulimia or anorexia nervosa contraindicates the use of bupropion. A higher incidence of seizures has been reported when bupropion is administered to these patients.

Patient on MAOIs

Bupropion should not be prescribed to patients on MAOIs. The patient should be off the MAOI for at least two weeks prior to the initiation of bupropion therapy.

Seizure Disorder

Bupropion should probably be avoided in children and adolescents with seizure disorders until more is known about the medication.

Organic Brain Disease

Because of its significantly increased association with seizures, we do not recommend using bupropion in children and adolescents with a history of head trauma, CNS tumor, or other organic brain disease. Electroencephalo-gram abnormalities probably contraindicate its use at this time, although consultation with a neurologist is advised.

Recent Withdrawal from Benzodiazepines or Alcohol

Although children and adolescents appear to be far less susceptible to severe withdrawal phenomena, including seizures, when alcohol and benzodiaze-pines are abruptly withdrawn (see Chapter 14), we do not recommend bu-propion in such patients because of its increased association with seizures, and because little is known about this medication in treating children and adolescents.

Patients on Other Psychotropics

The concomitant ingestion of other psychotropics, such as haloperidol and lithium, that may affect the seizure level is a relative contraindication to prescribing bupropion.

Hepatic/Renal Disease

Bupropion should be given cautiously to patients with liver or kidney disease because of the potential for the accumulation of the medication in the body.

Side Effects

See Table 5-18.

Seizures

Seizures are the side effect of most concern with bupropion, having been found to occur in 0.4% of all patients treated with doses of 450 mg/day or less, which is a four-fold increased incidence as compared with other antidepressants. Moreover, the incidence of seizures increases at higher doses of bupropion, so that at doses of 450–600 mg/day, the risk is approximately 4%.[91] Because of this increased risk, it is recommended that daily doses not exceed 450 mg. In addition, no individual dose should be greater than 150 mg. Finally, doses of 150 mg should be given no more frequently than every six hours.

Agitation/Restlessness/Irritability

These are relatively common side effects seen with bupropion therapy.[94] They may dissipate as therapy continues, but if they do not, dosage reduc-tion may be necessary.

Table 5-18
Side Effects of Bupropion Therapy

- Seizures
- Agitation
- Weight loss
- Headache
- Nausea
- Upper respiratory complaints

Does not:
- Impair cognition
- Cause daytime sleepiness
- Cause orthostasis
- Cause anticholinergic effect
- Cause weight gain
- Cause cardiac effects

Weight Loss

As mentioned earlier, this agent has a structural similarity to amphetamine. Weight loss may occur in approximately 25% of patients.[92]

Headache and Other Effects

Headache, insomnia, nausea, upper respiratory complaints, tremor, and constipation are common side effects with bupropion therapy.[92]

Cognitive Effects

Clay and colleagues[89] noted in their study of children with ADHD that bupropion had positive effects on memory performance, which may be unique among the antidepressants. Other antidepressants either have no effect or a negative effect in this regard. It should be noted, however, that Ferguson and Simeon[93] observed no adverse or positive effects on cognition on a cognitive battery in 17 children with ADD or conduct disorders who were in an open trial with bupropion.

Daytime Drowsiness

Daytime drowsiness is not observed with bupropion.

Anticholinergic Effects

Bupropion is not associated with significant anticholinergic effects.

Cardiac Effects

Bupropion is not associated with significant cardiac side effects. Nonetheless, adequate study of bupropion in patients with cardiac disease has not been performed, so caution is necessary when prescribing this medication to such patients.

Orthostatic Hypotension
Drug-induced orthostatic hypotension is not seen with bupropion.

Overdose
Bupropion is significantly safer than the TCAs when taken in overdose. Overdoses of bupropion when taken alone have not been fatal.

Abuse

There is no evidence that bupropion, when prescribed correctly, results in an increased propensity to use/abuse recreational drugs, to use/abuse other prescription drugs, or to increase physical and psychological dependence on bupropion.

Drug Interactions

See Table 5-19.

Available Preparations

See Table 5-7.

Initiating and Maintaining Treatment

Choosing to use bupropion in the treatment regimen of children and adolescents can be difficult, since there are no current FDA-established indications for its use in psychiatric disorders in this population. This agent is not considered a first-line treatment, and is indicated in child and adolescent psychiatry only when other, more standard treatments have proved unsuccessful.

Prior to initiating a bupropion trial, children and adolescents should have a physical examination, with special attention paid to vital signs and height and weight. A baseline screen for abnormal involuntary movements, including tics, should be performed. It is important to elicit any family history of motor movement tic disorders. Bupropion does cross the placenta, and so a pregnancy test and evaluation for adequate contraceptive use is essential in all females of childbearing age, as bupropion should not be prescribed during pregnancy.

A thorough drug and alcohol evaluation should be conducted, since bupropion should not be started after recent withdrawal from alcohol or ben-

Table 5-19
Drug Interactions—Bupropion

Acute toxicity may be increased by: • MAOIs
Increases adverse experiences when administered concurrently with: • L-dopa
Use caution when administering with: • Drug metabolized by liver   • Phenytoin   • Barbiturates   • Carbamazepine   • Cimetidine

zodiazepines. The use of drugs and alcohol while on bupropion should
be discouraged.

It is also important to determine the eating habits of patients being considered for bupropion therapy. It is contraindicated for patients with a current
or past history of bulimia or anorexia nervosa, because of the increased risk
of suicide in this population.

Careful neurologic screening is warranted as well. Bupropion therapy is contraindicated for patients with a history of organic brain disease, including a
seizure disorder, EEG abnormalities, a history of head trauma, or a CNS tumor. We recommend a baseline laboratory screen to include a complete
blood count with differential, electrolytes (these may be abnormal in patients with bulimia or anorexia), LFTs and renal function tests (i.e., BUN/
creatinine to assess liver and kidney status), and a urine drug screen. We
also recommend obtaining a baseline EEG to make sure there are no underlying EEG irregularities. Nonepileptic abnormalities probably preclude bupropion's use at this time, but consultation with a neurologist is
recommended. A baseline ECG is recommended, even though bupropion is
not believed to cause cardiac side effects. It has not been adequately studied
in patients with cardiac disease, so caution is necessary. If the ECG is normal, ECGs do not need to continue to be monitored during therapy.

When children and adolescents are treated with bupropion, they should be
monitored at each visit for any involuntary movements/tics by observation
and history. Whenever the dose is increased, it is important to check blood
pressure, pulse, height, and weight. In addition, it is advisable to record
height and weight at regular three- to four-month intervals. Plasma concentrations of bupropion have not been found too helpful, although one study
on adults found that plasma hydroxybupropion concentrations above 1.250

ng/ml were associated with a lack of clinical response.[87] Therefore, if access to a laboratory that analyzes bupropion's metabolites is available, ordering these plasma concentrations may be of some use.

Clinical Practice

Initiating and Maintaining Treatment
See Table 5-20.

Thyroid Hormones

The use of thyroid hormones in psychiatry is based on a premise similar to that for augmenting antidepressant therapy with lithium.[96] L-triiodothyronine (T3 or L-triiodothyronine; Cytomel), the most commonly used thyroid hormone, is employed as an adjuvant to an antidepressant medication in an attempt to convert a nonresponder or a partial responder into an antidepressant-responsive patient.[96] More rarely, thyroxine (T4 or levothyroxine; Levoxine, Levothroid, and Synthroid) is sometimes used for the same purpose. Endogenous and exogenous T4 is converted in the body into triiodothyronine.[96]

Table 5-20
**Dosage and Administration of Bupropion for Children
and Adolescents**

ADHD:
- Some open-label and controlled studies show possible efficacy.
- Start with test dose 100 mg/day.
- If this is tolerated well, increase dose to 100 mg b.i.d.
- Do not administer individual doses >150 mg.
- Increase doses by 100 mg every seven to 10 days to a maximum of 450 mg/day.
- Doses of 150 mg should be given at least six hours apart.

MDD:
- No studies demonstrating efficacy.
- Adult studies show effective.
- Use adult guidelines.
- Only use if standard agents fail (e.g., TCAs, fluoxetine).
- Start with dose 100 mg/day.
- If tolerated, increase dose to 100 mg b.i.d.
- Increase dose by 100 mg every seven to 10 days until symptoms relieved, toxicity, or maximum dose of 450 mg/day.
- Do not administer individual dose >150 mg.
- Give doses of 150 mg at least six hours apart.

Chemical Properties

Thyroid hormones undergo variable absorption by the GI tract after oral absorption.[96] Absorption can be decreased by food, and is increased when administered on an empty stomach. The half-life of T3 is one to two days, and that of T4 is six to seven days. The mechanism of action for thyroid hormone effects on increasing antidepressant effectiveness is unknown.

Indications

Adjuvant to Antidepressants

There is only one indication for thyroid hormone treatment in psychiatry, and that is to augment the action of antidepressants. It is important to point out that there is no association between thyroid function tests (i.e., thyroid-stimulating hormone) and the response to T3 or T4 supplementation of an antidepressant regimen. Such supplementation, like the lithium augmentation of antidepressant therapy, is indicated if a patient has been nonresponsive or only partially responsive to a six-week course of antidepressant therapy at appropriate doses. (For information on lithium augmentation, see Chapter 8.) The use of T3 is believed to be more effective than using T4. In standard clinical practice, lithium is generally added to an antidepressant regimen before T3 augmentation is instituted. Several controlled studies have indicated that T3 converts 33% to 75% of antidepressant responders, while several other studies have failed to find such a relationship.[96] There are no data on children and adolescents, and further study is necessary before we can recommend this treatment for this population.

Contraindications

Cardiac Disease

Thyroid hormones should not be given to patients with cardiac disease or hypertension.[96]

Diabetic Patients

Thyroid hormones may increase the insulin requirements of diabetic patients.[96] Thus diabetes is a relative contraindication to their administration.

Side Effects

Weight loss, palpitations, nervousness, diarrhea, abdominal cramps, sweating, tachycardia, increased blood pressure, tremors, headache, and insomnia are the most common side effects of thyroid hormone therapy.[96]

Overdose

Overdoses can lead to cardiac failure and death.[96] Immediate emergency and ICU monitoring is required.

Abuse

Thyroid hormones are sometimes abused in an effort to lose weight (particularly by medical personnel).

Drug Interactions

See Table 5-21.

Clinical Practice

Dosage and Administration

For an adult who has failed to respond to antidepressants after six weeks of therapy, 25–50 μg/day of T3 may be added to the patient's regimen.[96] It can be used as an adjunct to all of the TCAs and trazadone in adults, but there are very limited data on its use with bupropion or fluoxetine, and no information on its use with sertraline or paroxetine. An adequate trial of T3 supplementation is seven to 14 days.[96] If it is successful, it should be continued for two months, and then tapered at the rate of 12.5 μg per day every three to seven days.

There are no data on children and adolescents. Because of the potentially severe side effects, we are hesitant to recommend its use. This is especially true since we have not even shown what antidepressants, if any, are effective in child and adolescent depression. Perhaps if a child has a family member who showed a positive response at some point to T3 therapy, it might be considered. We recommend against routinely adding T3 to antidepressants for children and adolescents who have not responded. As we have mentioned, this may encompass the majority of children and adolescents. We advocate instead trying a different, safer antidepressant, such as fluoxetine.

Table 5-21
Drug Interactions—Thyroid Hormones

Potentiate effects of:
• Anticoagulants
• Warfarin
Increase:
• Insulin requirements in diabetics
Should not be coadministered with:
• Sympathomimetics—increase risk of cardiac decompensation

143

References

1. Arana, G.W., Hyman, S.E. (Eds.) (1991). *Handbook of Psychiatric Drug Therapy* (2nd ed.) (pp. 38–78). Boston: Little, Brown.

2. Riddle, M.A., Scahill, L., King, R.A., et al. (1992). Double-blind, crossover trial of fluoxetine and placebo in children and adolescents with obsessive compulsive disorders. *J Am Acad Child Adolesc Psychiatry, 31(6)*, 1062–1069.

3. Berman, I., Sapers, B.L., Saltzman, C. (1992). Sertraline: A new sertonergic antidepressant. *Hosp Community Psychiatry, 43*, 671–672.

4. Cohn, C.K., Shrivastava, R., Mendels, J., et al. (1990). Double-blind, multicenter comparison of sertraline and amitriptyline in elderly depressed patients. *J Clin Psychiatry, 51(suppl. B)*, 28–33.

5. Doogan, D.P., Calliard, V. (1988). Sertraline: A new antidepressant. *J Clin Psychiatry, 49(suppl.)*, 46–51.

6. Reimherr, F.W., Chouinard, G., Cohn, C.K., et al. (1990). Antidepressant efficacy of sertraline: A double-blind, placebo- and amitriptyline-controlled, multicenter comparison study in outpatients with major depression. *J Clin Psychiatry, 51(suppl. B)*, 18–27.

7. Chouinard, G., Goodman, W., Greist, J., et al. (1990). Results of a double-blind placebo-controlled trial of a new serotonin uptake inhibitor, sertraline, in the treatment of obsessive compulsive disorder. *Psychopharmacol Bull, 26*, 279–284.

8. McDougle, C.J., Price, L.H., Volkmar, F.R., et al. (1992). Clomipramine in autism: Preliminary evidence of efficacy. *J Am Acad Child Adolesc Psychiatry, 31(4)*, 746–750.

9. Bardeleben, U.V., Steiger, A., Gerken, A., et al. (1989). Effects of fluoxetine upon pharmacoendocrine and sleep-EEG parameters in normal controls. *Int Clin Psychopharmacol, 4*, 1–5.

10. Bergstrom, R.F., Lemberger, L., Farid, N.A., et al. (1988). Clinical pharmacology and pharmacokinetics of fluoxetine: A review. *Br J Psychiatry, 153(suppl. 3)*, 47–50.

11. Benfield, P., Heel, R.C., Lewis, S.P. (1986). Fluoxetine: A review of its pharmacodynamic and pharmacokinetic properties, and therapeutic efficacy in depressive illness. *Drugs, 32*, 481–508.

12. Traskman, L., Asberg, M., Bertilsson, L., et al. (1981). Monoamine metabolites in CSF and suicidal behavior. *Arch Gen Psychiatry, 38*, 631–636.

13. Roy, A., DeJong, R.A., Linnoila, M. (1981). Cerebrospinal fluid mono-amine metabolites and suicidal behavior in depressed patients. *Arch Gen Psychiatry, 38*, 631–636.

14. Virkkunen, M., DeJong, J., Bartko, J., et al. (1989). Relationship of psychobiological variables to recidivism in violent offenders and impulsive fire setters: A follow-up study. *Arch Gen Psychiatry, 46*, 604–606.

15. Mann, J.J., McBride, P.A., Brown, R.P., et al. (1992). Relationship between central and peripheral serotonin indexes in depressed and suicidal psychiatric inpatients. *Arch Gen Psychiatry, 49*, 442–446.

16. Kutcher, S.P., Makin, D., Silverberg, J., et al. (1991). Nocturnal cortisol, thyroid stimulating hormone and growth hormone secretory profiles in depressed adolescents. *J Am Acad Child Adolesc Psychiatry, 30*, 407–414.

17. Ryan, N.D., Puig-Antich, J., Rabinovich, H., et al. (1988). MAOIs in adolescent major depression unresponsive to tricyclic antidepressants. *Am Acad Child Adolesc Psychiatry, 27*, 755–758.

18. Joshi, P.T., Walkup, J.T., Capozzoli, J.A., et al. (1989). The use of fluoxetine in the treatment of major depressive disorder in children and adolescents. Paper presented at the 36th Annual Meeting of the American Academy of Child and Adolescent Psychiatry, October 11–15, New York, N.Y.

19. Boulos, C., Kutcher, S., Gardner, D., et al. (1992). An open naturalistic trial of fluoxetine in adolescents and young adults with treatment-resistant major depression. *J Child Adolesc Psychopharmacol, 2*, 103–111.

20. Herman, J.B., Brotman, A.W., Pollack, M.H., et al. (1990). Fluoxetine-induced sexual dysfunction. *J Clin Psychiatry, 51*, 25.

21. Kaplan, H.I., Sadock, B.J. (1991). Biological therapies. In H.I. Kaplan, B.J. Sadock (Eds.), *Synopsis of Psychiatry* (6th ed.) (p. 650). Baltimore: Williams & Wilkins.

22. Schweizer, E., Rickels, K., Amsterdam, J.D., et al. (1992, October). What constitutes an adequate antidepressant trial of sertraline? *Psychiatric Times*, 17.

23. Riddle, M.A., Hardin, M.T., King, R., et al. (1990). Fluoxetine treatment of children and adolescents with Tourette's and obsessive compulsive disorders: Preliminary clinical experience. *J Am Acad Child Adolesc Psychiatry, 29*, 45–48.

24. Barrickman, L., Noyes, R., Kuperman, S., et al. (1991). Treatment of ADHD with fluoxetine: A preliminary trial. *J Am Acad Child Adolesc Psychiatry, 30(5)*, 762–767.

25. King, B.H. (1991). Fluoxetine reduced self-injurious behavior in an adolescent with mental retardation. *J Child Adolesc Psycopharmacol, 1,* 321–329.

26. Anders, T.F., Cann, K.M., Ciaranello, R.D., et al. (1978). Further observations on the use of 5-hydroxytryptophan in a child with Lesch-Nyan syndrome. *Neuropediatric, 9,* 157–166.

27. Custells, S., Chakrabarti, C., Winsberg, B.G., et al. (1979). Effects of L-5-hydroxytryptophan on monoamine and amino acids turnover in the Lesch-Nyan syndrome. *J Autism Dev Disord, 9,* 95–103.

28. Handen, B.L., Feldman, H., Gosling, A., et al. (1991). Adverse side effects of methylphenidate among mentally retarded children with ADHD. *J Am Acad Child Adolesc Psychiatry, 30,* 241–245.

29. Aman, M.G., Marks, R.E., Turbott, S.H., et al. (1991). Clinical effects of methylphenidate and thioridazine in intellectually subaverage children. *J Am Acad Child Adolesc Psychiatry, 30,* 246–256.

30. Weltzin, T.E., Hsu, L.K.G., Kaye, W.H. (1990). An open trial of fluoxetine in anorexia nervosa: Maintenance of body weight and reduction of obsessional features. Abstract. Presented at the Fourth International Conference on Eating Disorders, April 28, New York, N.Y.

31. Crisp, A.H., Lacey, J.H., Crutchfield, M. (1987). Clomipramine and "drive" in people with anorexia nervosa: An inpatient study. *Br J Psychiatry, 150,* 355–358.

32. Lacey, J.H., Crisp, A.H. (1980). Hunger, food intake and weight: The impact of clomipramine on a refeeding anorexia nervosa population. *Postgrad Med J, 56,* 79–85.

33. Biederman, J., Herzog, D.B., Rivins, T.M., et al. (1985). Amitriptyline in the treatment of anorexia nervosa: A double-blind, placebo-controlled study. *J Clin Psychopharmacol, 5,* 10–16.

34. Halmi, K.A., Eckert, E., LaDo, T.J., et al. (1986). Treatment efficacy of cyproheptadine and amitriptyline. *Arch Gen Psychiatry, 43,* 177–181.

35. Halmi, K.A., Eckert, E., Falk, J.R. (1982). Cyproheptadine for anorexia nervosa. *Lancet, 1,* 1357–1358.

36. Vandereycken, W. (1984). Neuroleptics in the short-term treatment of anorexia nervosa: A double-blind placebo-controlled study with sulpirid. *Br J Psychiatry, 144,* 288–292.

37. Goldberg, S.G., Halmi, K.A., Eckert, E.D., et al. (1979). Cyproheptadine in anorexia nervosa. *Br J Psychiatry, 134,* 67–70.

38. Vanderegcken, W., Pierloot, R. (1982). Pimozide combined with behavior therapy in the treatment of anorexia nervosa. *Acta Psychiatr Scand, 66*, 445–450.

39. Gross, H.A., Ebert, M.H., Faden, V.B. (1981). A double-blind controlled trial of lithium carbonate in primary anorexia nervosa. *J Clin Psychopharmacol, 1*, 376–381.

40. Pope, H.G., Hudson, J.I. (1985). *New Hope for Binge Eaters: Advances in the Understanding and Treatment of Bulimia.* New York: Harper & Row.

41. Kennedy, S.H., Piran, N., Garfinkel, P.E. (1985). Monoamine oxidase inhibitor therapy for anorexia nervosa and bulimia: A preliminary trial of isocarboxazid. *J Clin Psychopharmacol, 5*, 279–285.

42. Wermuth, B.M., Davis, K.L., Hollister, L.E., et al. (1977). Phenytoin treatment of the binge eating syndrome. *Am J Psychiatry, 134*, 1249–1253.

43. Pope, H.G., Hudson, J.I., Jonas, J.M., et al. (1983). Bulimia treatment with imipramine: A double-blind placebo-controlled study. *Am J Psychiatry, 14*, 554–558.

44. Mitchell, J.E., Groat, R. (1984). A placebo-controlled double-blind trial of amitriptyline in bulimia. *J Clin Psychopharmacol, 4*, 186–193.

45. Hughes, P.L., Wall, L.A., Cunningham, C.J., et al. Treating bulimia with desipramine. *Arch Gen Psychiatry, 43*, 182–186.

46. Walsh, B.T., Stewart, J.M., Roose, S.P., et al. (1984). Treatment of bulimia with phenelzine. *Arch Gen Psychiatry, 41*, 1105–1109.

47. Kennedy, S., Piran, N., Garfinkel, P.E. (1986). Isocarboxazide in the treatment of bulimia. *Am J Psychiatry, 143*, 1495–1496.

48. Foss, I., Trygstad, O., Jettestad, S. (1990). Double-blind study of fluoxetine and placebo in treatment of bulimia nervosa. Abstract. Presented at the Fourth International Conference on Eating Disorders, April 28, New York, N.Y.

49. Fava, M., Herzog, D.B., Hainburger, P., et al. (1990). A retrospective study of long-term use of fluoxetine in bulimia nervosa. Abstract. Presented at the Fourth International Conference on Eating Disorders, April 28, New York, N.Y.

50. Herzog, D.B. (1992, October). Serotonin uptake inhibitors. *Psychiatric Times*, 17.

51. Prader, A., Labhart, A., Willi, H. (1956). Ein syndrom von adiposita kleinwuchs, kryptorchismus und oligophrence. *Myotonicartigern Zustand in Neurgeborenaher Schwer Med Wochenschr, 86*, 1260–1261.

52. Cassidy, S.B. (1987). Prader-Willi syndrome. *Curr Probl Pediatr, 14,* 1–55.

53. Cassidy, S.B. (1987). Recurrence risk in Prader-Willi syndrome. *Am J Med Genet, 28,* 59–60.

54. Dech, B., Budow, A. (1991). The use of fluoxetine in an adolescent with Prader-Willi syndrome. *J Am Acad Child Adolesc Psychiatry, 30,* 298–302.

55. Selikowitz, M., Sunman, J., Pendergast, A., et al. (1990). Fenfluramine in Prader-Willi syndrome: A double-blind, placebo controlled trial. *Arch Dis Child, 65,* 112–114.

56. Cole, J.O., Bodkin, J.A. (1990). Antidepressant drug side effects. *J Clin Psychiatry, 51(suppl. 1),* 21–26.

57. Markowitz, J.C. (1991). Fluoxetine and dreaming (Letter). *J Clin Psychiatry, 52,* 432.

58. Bernstein, J.G. (1988). *Handbook of Drug Therapy in Psychiatry* (2nd ed.) (p. 140). Littleton, Mass.: PSG Publishing.

59. Scharf, M.B., Sachais, B.A. (1990). Sleep laboratory evaluation of the effects and efficacy of trazadone in depressed insomniac patients. *J Clin Psychiatry, 51(suppl. 9),* 13–17.

60. Nicholson, A.N., Pascoe, P.A. (1988). Studies on the modulation of the sleep-wakefulness continuum in man by fluoxetine, a 5-HT uptake inhibitor. *Neuropharmacology, 27,* 597–602.

61. Riddle, M.A., King, R.A., Hardin, M.T., et al. (1990). Behavioral side effects of fluoxetine in children and adolescents. *J Child Adolesc Psychopharmacol, 1,* 193–198.

62. Teicher, M.H., Glod, C., Cole, J.O. (1990). Emergence of intense suicidal preoccupation during fluoxetine treatment. *Am J Psychiatry, 147,* 207–210.

63. Teicher, M.H., Glod, C., Cole, J.O. (1990). Suicidal preoccupation during fluoxetine treatment (Letter). *Am J Psychiatry, 147,* 1380–1381.

64. Gorman, J.M., Liebowitz, M.R., Fyer, A.J., et al. (1987). An open trial of fluoxetine in the treatment of panic attacks. *J Clin Psychopharmacol, 5,* 329–332.

65. King, R.A., Riddle, M.A., Chappell, P.B., et al. (1991). Emergency of self-destructive phenomena in children and adolescents during fluoxetine treatment. *J Am Acad Child Adolesc Psychiatry, 30,* 179–186.

66. Ayd, F.J., Jr. (1990). In defence of fluoxetine. *Int Drug Ther News, 25,* 29–30.

67. Beasley, C.M., Dornserf, B.E., Bosomworth, J.C., et al. (1991). Fluoxetine and suicide: A meta-analysis of controlled trials of treatment of depression. *Br Med J, 303*, 685–692.

68. Fava, M., Rosenbaum, J.F. (1991). Suicidality and fluoxetine: Is there a relationship? *J Clin Psychiatry, 52*, 108–111.

69. Settle, E.C., Jr., Settle, G.P. (1984). A case of mania associated with fluoxetine. *Am J Psychiatry, 141*, 280–281.

70. Sholomskas, A.J. (1990). Mania in a panic disorder patient treated with fluoxetine. *Am J Psychiatry, 141*, 1090–1091.

71. Steiner, W. (1991). Fluoxetine-induced mania in a patient with obsessive compulsive disorder (Letter). *Am J Psychiatry, 152*, 280–281.

72. Stoll, A.L., Cole, J.O., Lukas, S.E. (1991). A case of mania as a result of fluoxetine–marijuana interaction. *J Clin Psychiatry, 52*, 280–281.

73. Turner, S.M., Jacob, R.G., Beidel, D., et al. (1985). A second case of mania associated with fluoxetine (Letter). *Am J Psychiatry, 142*, 274–275.

74. Wong, D.T. Horng, J.S., Bymaster, F.P., et al. (1974). A selective inhibitor of serotonin uptake: Lilly 110140 3-(p-trifluoromethylphenoxy)-N-methyl-3-phenylpropylanine. *Life Sci, 15*, 47.

75. Hon, D., Preskorn, S.H. (1989). Mania during fluoxetine treatment for recurrent depression (Letter). *Am J Psychiatry, 146*, 1638–1639.

76. Lebegue, B. (1987). Mania precipitated by fluoxetine (Letter). *Am J Psychiatry, 144*, 1620.

77. Nakra, B.R.S., Szwabo, P., Grossberg, G.T. (1989). Mania induced by fluoxetine (Letter). *Am J Psychiatry, 146*, 1515–1516.

78. Chouinard, G., Steiner, W. (1986). A case of mania induced by high-dose fluoxetine treatment (Letter). *Am J Psychiatry, 143*, 686.

79. Feder, R. (1990). Fluoxetine-induced mania. *J Clin Psychiatry, 51*, 524–525.

80. Achamalla, N.S., Decker, D.H. (1991). Mania induced by fluoxetine in an adolescent patient. *Am J Psychiatry, 148*, 1404.

81. Rosenberg, D.R., Johnson, K., Sahl, R. (1992). Evolution of hypomania and mania in an adolescent treated with low dose fluoxetine. *J Child Adolesc Psychopharmacol, 2*, 299–305.

82. Jenike, M.A. (1991). Severe hair loss associated with fluoxetine use. *Am J Psychiatry, 148*, 392.

83. Turner, S., et al. (1992, October). *Psychiatric Times*, 17.

84. Wiener, J.M. (Ed.) (1991). *Textbook of Child and Adolescent Psychiatry.* Washington, D.C.: American Psychiatric Press.

85. Mouret, J., Cemoine, P., Minuit, M.P., et al. (1988). Effects of trazadone on the sleep of depressed subjects: A polysomnographic study. *Psychopharmacology, 95,* 537.

86. Newton, R. (1981). The side effect profile of trazadone in comparison to an active control and placebo. *J Clin Psychopharmacol, 1(suppl. 6),* 895.

87. Golden, R.N., Rudorfer, M.V., Sherer, M.A., et al. (1988). Bupropion in depression. I. Biochemical effects and clinical response. II. The role of metabolites and clinical outcomes. *Arch Gen Psychiatry, 45,* 139, 145.

88. Simeon, J.G., Ferguson, H.B., Fleet, J.W. (1986). Bupropion effects in attention deficit and conduct disorders. *Can J Psychiatry, 31,* 581–585.

89. Clay, T.H., Gaultieri, C.T., Evans, R.W., et al. (1988). Clinical and neuropsychological effects of the novel antidepressant bupropion. *Psychopharmacol Bull, 24,* 143–148.

90. Casat, C.D., Pleasants, D.Z., Schroeder, D.H., et al. (1989). Bupropion in children with attention deficit disorder. *Psychopharmacol Bull, 25,* 198–201.

91. Davidson, J. (1989). Seizures and bupropion: A review. *J Clin Psychiatry, 50,* 256.

92. Lineberry, C.G., Johnson, J.A., Raymond, R.N., et al. (1990). A fixed dose (300 mg) efficacy study of bupropion and placebo in depressed outpatients. *J Clin Psychiatry, 51,* 194.

93. Ferguson, H.B., Simeon, J.G. (1984). Evaluating drug effects on children's cognitive functioning. *Prog Neuropsychopharmacol Biol Psychiatry, 8,* 683–686.

94. *Physicians' Desk Reference* (45th ed.) (1991). Oradell, N.J.: Medical Economics Co.

95. Davis, J.M., Glassman, A.H. (1991). Antidepressant drugs. In H.I. Kaplan & B.J. Sadock (Eds.), *Comprehensive Textbook of Psychiatry* (5th ed.) (p. 1644). Baltimore: Williams & Wilkins.

96. Kaplan, H.I., Sadock, B.J. (Eds.) (1991). *Synopsis of Psychiatry: Behavioral Sciences* (p. 660). Baltimore: Williams & Wilkins.

97. Bass, J.N., Beltis, J. (1991). Therapeutic effect of fluoxetine on naltrexone-resistant self-injurious behavior in an adolescent with mental retardation. *J Child Adolesc Psychopharmacol, 1,* 331–340.

Monoamine Oxidase Inhibitors

Monoamine oxidase inhibitors (MAOIs) are a class of antidepressant defined by function rather than structure. All drugs in this class either reversibly or irreversibly inhibit the enzyme monoamine oxidase (MAO). Although these agents have been the focus of intensive biochemical and clinical research over the past 50 years, their popularity in psychiatric practice has varied tremendously. By the late 1960s, several indications had emerged, and new agents were put into use for the treatment of depression and anxiety disorders. Soon thereafter, the prototype MAOI, iproniazid, was removed from the market when it was associated with hepatic failure.[47] Phenelzine and tranylcypromine fell from favor when cases of hypertensive crisis were recognized and their efficacy based on early trials was questioned.[60,155]

However, MAOIs remained important investigative tools despite their decline in clinical use, perhaps because of the central role of MAO in neurophysiology.[128,155] The emergence of new and more stringently controlled clinical trials, the ability to manage hypertensive reactions through dietary restriction of tyramine, and the synthesis of several new MAOIs that are less sensitive to tyramine have again brought these agents to the forefront of clinical research. In particular, a great deal of work has been devoted to defining subtypes of depression that may respond preferentially to MAOIs.[116]

Although MAOIs are not yet considered first-line therapy for any disorder, they are the most frequent second choice for the treatment of depressed adults with anxious or atypical symptoms.[90] Since TCAs are widely studied and historically have been viewed as being of lower risk, MAOI use in young people has been especially limited. But recent concern over the cardiotoxic side effects of TCAs in children, with rare cases of sudden death, suggests a reconsideration of MAOIs in child psychiatry. Among the disorders that may respond to MAOIs are several of specific interest to child and adolescent psychiatrists, including major depressive disorder (MDD), anorexia and bulimia, ADHD, and social and school phobia. These findings, and the pending availability of new MAOIs that do not require dietary restriction, greatly increase the importance of these agents to child and adolescent psychiatry. Nevertheless, MAOI therapy represents a target for future research in preadolescent children. *No MAOI compound is currently FDA approved for psychiatric indications in children under 16 years of age.*

Chemical Properties

The discovery that MAOIs "elevate" mood predates the same discovery for tricyclic compounds, making MAOIs the oldest class of antidepressant in current use. Iproniazid was noted to cause euphoria during investigational use for tuberculosis in the early 1950s, an effect that was not shared by the related (weak MAOI) compound isoniazid.[14] Several reports of success with iproniazid in the treatment of depression followed.[59,71,149] Since that time, three MAOI compounds have been marketed in the United States for psychiatric indications: phenelzine (Nardil), tranylcypromine (Parnate), and isocarboxazid (Marplan) (Figure 6-1). Two other compounds, furazolidone (Furoxone) and procarbazine (Matulane), are marketed as antimicrobial and antineoplastic agents respectively. However, several others are in use internationally or are under investigation (Table 6-1). The MAOIs have been chemically classified as hydrazine (phenelzine) and nonhydrazine agents (tranylcypromine), although many compounds under current investigation are structurally unique.

Absorption and Metabolism

Peak levels of both phenelzine and tranylcypromine are reached within two hours after a single oral dose. Maximum enzyme inhibition is achieved after seven to 14 days of chronic administration.[82] The elimination half-lives of phenelzine and tranylcypromine are less than three hours.[5] However, since

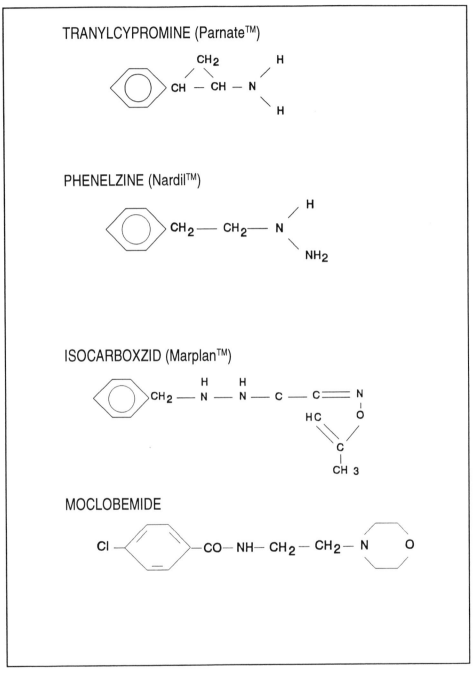

Figure 6-1
Chemical Structures of Some MAOI Drugs

Table 6-1
FDA Approval and Indications for MAOIs

MAO Inhibitor	Kinetics	FDA Approval	Indications
Nonselective			
Iproniazid (Marsalid)	IRR	Withdrawn	Antidepressant
Isocarboxazid (Marplan)	IRR	Probable (≥ 16+ years)	Refractory depression
Phenelzine (Nardil)	IRR	APP (≥ 16+ years)	Atypical depression
Tranylcypromine (Parnate)	IRR*	APP (adult)	Major depression w/o melancholia
Selective MAO-A			
Clorgyline	IRR†	NA	Similar to nonselective MAOIs
Moclobemide	REV	NA	Probably for depressive disorders
Selective MAO-B			
l-Deprenyl (selegiline)	IRR†	NA	Possible use in Parkinson's disease
Pargyline (Eutonyl)	IRR†	Withdrawn	Antihypertensive
Uncharacterized			
Furazolidone (Furoxone)	?	APP (≥ 1 month)	Antimicrobial
Procarbazine (Matulane)	?	APP (any age)	Stage III–IV Hodgkin's disease

*Partially reversible in vitro.
†Nonselective at higher doses.
Abbreviations: NA—not approved in the United States; APP—approved (age range);
IRR—irreversible MAOI; REV—reversible competitive MAOI.
Source: References 32, 75, 92.

both are irreversible inhibitors, once the drug binds to MAO, the enzyme is effectively removed from the system. The resulting reduction in MAO activity persists for as long as two weeks after the drug has been metabolized, while new enzyme is synthesized.[63,76,82] Amrein and colleagues[5] demonstrated the pharmacodynamic distinction between reversible and irreversible MAOIs by comparing the activities of tranylcypromine (irreversible, nonspecific) and moclobemide (reversible MAOI-A). Both are eliminated quickly, with half-lives of approximately two hours, but MAO activity returns to normal 24 hours after the discontinuation of moclobemide. The elimination half-lives of reversible MAOIs vary to a greater degree than do those of currently approved agents, and may be as long as 12 to 15 hours.[5]

Acetylation Rate

The metabolism rates of some MAOIs are influenced by acetylation phenotype. In the late 1950s, it was recognized that the rate of isoniazid metabolism showed a bimodal population distribution.[35] Slow or fast metabolism proved to be a genetic trait characterized by activity of the hepatic enzyme acetyltransferase. Phenelzine metabolism is particularly dependent on acetylation trait, and some early studies found that individuals with the slow acetylation trait showed superior clinical response and increased side effects with phenelzine.[89] However, several contradicting studies have found no predictive value of acetylation trait.[26,110] In bipolar depression, clinical response correlates with peak plasma levels of tranylcypromine, but not with the rate of elimination.[72] The relationship between percent MAO inhibition and clinical response (discussed below) may have been the basis for early studies showing poorer response in fast acetylators. No study has examined the predictive value of acetylation trait when platelet MAO inhibition is controlled at over 80%. Preliminary experience with moclobemide suggests that its metabolism is not greatly influenced by acetylation phenotype.[120]

Mechanism of Action

The common site of action for MAOIs is the ubiquitous mitochondrial enzyme monoamine oxidase. This enzyme deaminates a variety of substrates, including serotonin, epinephrine, norepinephrine, tyramine, and dopamine. Monoamine oxidase exists in at least two forms (A and B), which differ in substrate preference, systemic distribution, and sensitivity to specific MAOIs. Although both forms metabolize tyramine and dopamine, MAO-B predominates in the CNS and accounts for most of the dopamine metabolism in the striatum. Cortical dopamine is primarily metabolized by MAO-A.[73]

The three agents commonly prescribed in the United States are nonselective, inhibiting both forms of the enzyme. However, experimental use of selective inhibitors such as moclobemide, clorgyline (MAOI-A), and L-deprenyl (selegiline, MAOI-B) has revealed functional differences between MAO subtypes. Selective MAO-B inhibitors are less effective in depression and are not sensitive to dietary tyramine. Therefore, the antidepressant and pressor effects of MAOIs[93] are mediated by MAO-A inhibition. This was demonstrated by Mann and associates[73] in a controlled trial of L-deprenyl. At low doses, L-deprenyl is a selective MAO-B inhibitor, and shows no greater antidepressant effect than placebo. At higher doses, the drug is less selective, inhibiting both MAO-A and MAO-B, and does show significant antidepressant properties.[73]

As with all antidepressants, the precise mechanism of action of MAOIs is limited by our understanding of the pathophysiology of affective disorders. In its simplest form, the amine hypothesis attributes depressive symptoms to underactivity of serotonin and/or norepinephrine, which may be treated by either blocking the reuptake of amine neurotransmitters (via TCAs) or by slowing their metabolism (via MAOIs).[6] Yet, both tricyclic compounds and MAOIs require two to four weeks of administration before producing clinical

155

benefit, despite immediate neurotransmitter changes. Administration of an MAOI initially increases the intracellular levels of both CNS and peripheral substrates. The MAO-A inhibitors cause a rise in serotonin and norepinephrine levels preferentially, while MAO-B inhibitors have a greater effect on systemic dopamine levels.[63] Chronic administration is associated with the return of these neurotransmitters levels to baseline, but with long-term changes in receptor populations.[76] It is this latter change in receptor density that is thought to mediate the clinical effects of MAOIs. Interestingly, TCAs have also been shown to weakly inhibit MAO, suggesting that MAO inhibition may represent a common therapeutic mechanism for both categories of drug.[138]

Platelet MAO Assays

Some data suggest that a threshold level of MAO inhibition is required for these drugs to be effective for depression, as measured by percent inhibition of platelet MAO. Biochemical studies detect significant changes in neurotransmitters and metabolites, with greater than 80% inhibition of platelet MAO,[40] and correlations with symptom response suggest a clinical threshold at 80–90% platelet enzyme inhibition.[28,98] This threshold is further supported by Ravaris and colleagues'[103] demonstration that phenelzine was not superior to placebo at 60% inhibition, but was superior at a mean platelet MAO inhibition of 83%. The use of platelet MAO activity to assess adequate central MAO inhibition is not applicable to newer, selective MAO-A inhibitors, since platelet MAO is type B.[152]

Indications

See Table 6-2.

General Issues in Children and Adolescents

Although not approved for younger children, the indications for MAOI prescription appear to be widening in recent years. Current agents are approved for children 16 years and older. In this population, adult guidelines for depressive, anxiety, and eating disorders may be applied, with additional care paid to the issues of compliance and dietary restrictions.[114,115] Preliminary studies of MAOIs for ADHD are promising, and eventually may lead to the inclusion of these agents among accepted therapies for younger children. Since selective, reversible agents such as moclobemide may soon become available in the United States, the risk factors that traditionally limited the prescription of MAOIs for younger children may become irrelevant. Therefore, child and adolescent psychiatrists should be familiar with most indications for MAOIs, regardless of current approval.

Table 6-2
Psychiatric Indications for MAOI Drugs

Approved	"Atypical" depression Major depression without melancholia ("nonendogenous") Depressive disorders refractory to TCAs
Probable	Major depression (all types) Panic disorder with or without agoraphobia Social phobia/agoraphobia without panic Borderline personality disorder with depression
Experimental	Attention-deficit hyperactivity disorder Childhood depression (<16 years) Anorexia and bulimia Borderline personality disorder without depression Separation anxiety/school phobia

Depressive Disorders

Subtypes of Depression

The primary indication for MAOIs is depression. Although there is evidence that these agents may be superior to TCAs in treating some subtypes of depression, the clinical distinction of subtypes remains difficult, especially in children and adolescents. The current diagnostic system in the United States (DSM-III-R) organizes affective disorders into major categories distinguished by symptom criteria (Table 6-3).[4] Recognized subtypes of unipolar major depression include seasonal, psychotic, and melancholic. Prior to the adoption of this system, classification differed among investigators, depending on their theoretical basis. Therefore, early drug trials may compare "endogenous and reactive," "primary and secondary," or "psychotic, neurotic, and anxious" subtypes. Of these, endogenous depression most closely corresponds to the DSM-III-R criteria for major depression.[4] The definition of melancholia, a current subtype of major depression, has remained fairly stable. However, other subtypes have been variably defined across research sites, producing heterogenous samples in most early studies.

It may be argued that DSM-III-R classifications should not be the sole construct for clinical trials of antidepressants, since these classifications undoubtedly do not represent the "last word" on pathophysiologic subtypes of depression. The preferable method is statistical grouping of symptom clusters and differential responses to treatment without a priori constructs, an approach used in only a few important studies.

Table 6-3

DSM-III-R Diagnostic Categories for Depressive Illness and Subtypes

Major depression
• with or without seasonal pattern
• with or without melancholia
• with or without psychotic features
Dysthymia (or depressive neurosis)
• primary or secondary type
Depressive disorder, NOS

Source: Reference 4.

Atypical Depression

After MAOIs fell out of favor in the 1960s, one of the few persistent indications was atypical depression.[149] After more than 30 years, this term remains difficult to define. In the broadest sense, atypical refers to any depressive disorder that does not exhibit classic signs of endogenous or melancholic depression. So defined, this subtype could include patients from any of the current DSM-III-R categories. The original and most common definition of atypical depression is *a subtype of major depression* with "reversed" neurovegetative signs: weight gain rather than loss, hypersomnia rather than insomnia, mood reactivity, and mood worsening in the evening rather than the morning.[149] This subtype is not included in DSM-III-R, but is the only approved indication for MAOI therapy. Other definitions have included patients who may not meet the criteria for major depression, such as hysteroid dysphoria (see "Borderline Personality Disorder"), depression with prominent anxiety, and neurotic, nonendogenous, or reactive depression.

Several early studies reported a preferential response of atypical depression to MAOIs.[24,88,102,117,119,149] However, patient samples included subjects with prominent anxiety symptoms, a separate indication for MAOIs. One early placebo-controlled study found amitriptyline to be superior to phenelzine on global measures of depressive and neurotic symptoms.[54] Another study found that the prospective division of depressive patients into neurotic, psychotic, and schizophrenic subtypes failed to predict phenelzine response.[101] These early trials were limited not only by heterogeneous patient samples, but also by simultaneous treatment of the patients with other medications and variable dosing strategies.[65,79] Analysis of specific symptom response was often narrow, using global ratings of neurosis or anxiety. This liability was addressed in one early double-blind comparison of phenelzine and amitriptyline in 130 depressed outpatients. Ravaris and colleagues[104] used structured interviews to rate improvement and to derive a "diagnostic index" to distinguish endogenous from nonendogenous depression. The medications produced equal improvement on global scales, with no difference between endogenous and nonendogenous classifications. However, those with mood reactivity, as an isolated feature, responded significantly better to phenelzine, while sleep disturbance responded better to amitriptyline.[104]

Later attempts to predict the response to MAOIs were more discriminating in both symptom definition and patient selection. Parsons and colleagues[86] studied a large number of subjects with atypical depression who were defined as patients "meeting DSM-III-R criteria for major depression or dysthymia who have reactive mood and any associated atypical symptoms (hyperphagia, hypersomnolence, rejection sensitivity, or leaden paralysis)." Forty-seven percent of these subjects also met the criteria for borderline personality disorder (discussed below). In three reports of this large data set, they found that the number of atypical symptoms is a strong positive predictor of response to phenelzine and a negative predictor of response to imipramine.[66,70,86,135] Similarly, Kayser and colleagues[56] used structured symptom inventories to evaluate the response to phenelzine and amitriptyline in 169 depressed outpatients. The results were analyzed both on the basis of depressive subtypes (melancholic and nonmelancholic major depression, minor depression, and atypical depression) and on the basis of symptom groups (depressive, somatic, anxiety, and interpersonal sensitivity). Atypical depression was defined as having mood reactivity plus two or more of the following: hypersomnia, hyperphagia or weight gain, leaden paralysis, and high interpersonal insensitivity. In symptom-based analysis, phenelzine was found superior to amitriptyline for phobic anxiety, general anxiety, and interpersonal sensitivity symptoms, accounting for a significant overall superiority of phenelzine after six weeks of therapy. However, response was statistically equivalent when patients were grouped by predefined subtypes, including atypical depression.[56] In contrast to the majority of studies, Davidson and associates[29] did not find atypical symptoms to be significant positive predictors of MAOI response. One possible explanation is that atypical symptoms may predict a negative response to tricyclic agents, rather than a strong positive response to MAOIs.

In summary, the recent data indicate that specific atypical depressive and anxiety symptoms are more useful in predicting response to MAOIs than is the categorical diagnosis of currently defined subtypes. The MAOIs may be superior for, as yet, poorly defined subtypes of depression, which include reversed neurovegetative signs, mood reactivity, interpersonal sensitivity, anxiety, and phobia. It is unclear whether this differential response indicates the existence of subtypes with distinct pathophysiologic bases, or simply a differential response to side effects and overall antidepressant efficacy.[52,151,161] No controlled trials exist that compare MAOIs with SSUIs or bupropron, both of which have seen use for atypical depression (see Chapter 4).

Major Depression (Unipolar)

A number of early reports suggested that heterocyclic compounds were more effective than MAOIs in the treatment of severe or endogenous depression, especially when accompanied by melancholia[24,149] (see Chapter 4), while several others concluded that MAOIs were probably equally effective on global outcome measures.[97,104,106] Ravaris and associates'[104] study cited above suggests that any difference is probably slight, and may be limited to the symptom of insomnia.

More recent studies support the effectiveness of MAOIs for classic major or endogenous depression. Tranylcypromine has been used successfully in open[77] and controlled[39,111] trials. L-Deprenyl is superior to placebo at doses that inhibit MAO-A.[73] Isocarboxazid has been less well studied than phenelzine and tranylcypromine, but appears to have equal efficacy.[25,27,46] In direct comparison with TCAs, MAOIs generally show equal efficacy for major depression, although comparison is difficult in many studies owing to inadequate doses of one or both agents. Under double-blind conditions, high-dose phenelzine (75 mg/day) was as effective as imipramine in 32 cases,[142] and was both more effective and better tolerated than amitriptyline in 29 cases.[98] Georgotas and associates[43,44] compared phenelzine with nortriptyline in elderly patients with major depression, verifying adequate dosing of nortriptyline with plasma levels. After six weeks, phenelzine was found to be as effective as nortriptyline (57.1% versus 54.5% responders), but after 12 weeks, phenelzine (80.9%) was superior to nortriptyline (68.2%).[43,44] In the study by Kayser and associates,[56] melancholic and nonmelancholic major depression responded equally well to phenelzine and amitriptyline, although patients with anxiety and interpersonal sensitivity responded better to phenelzine.

Recently, moclobemide has seen more intensive study than traditional MAOIs. In a large, multicenter controlled study of major depression, moclobemide was shown to be at least equal in efficacy and superior in tolerance to imipramine,[11,19,141,144] desipramine,[39] and clomipramine.[21,34,38,64]

In further attempts to find pretreatment markers for antidepressant specificity, abnormal baseline MAO activities have been detected in many psychiatric disorders. Platelet MAO activity has been shown to be higher than normal in unipolar depression and lower than normal in bipolar depression.[33,107] It has been suggested that high baseline platelet MAO may predict a positive response to MAOIs. However, this effect does not appear to be specific, as Georgotas and colleagues[45] found that among elderly depressed patients, higher baseline platelet MAO activity predicted antidepressant response to both phenelzine and nortriptyline. Therefore, high baseline platelet MAO activity may be associated with the severity or manifestation of depression, but does not seem to predict antidepressant specificity.

In summary, current evidence indicates that under research conditions, MAOIs are an effective treatment for major or endogenous depression in adults, although TCAs may be more effective at alleviating insomnia. However, MAOIs have not become first-line therapy due to the additional liability of dietary tyramine restriction and the risk of the tyramine pressor reaction. Moclobemide has undergone controlled comparisons with tricyclic agents internationally, and appears to be equal to or superior in efficacy, while not conferring a significant risk of hypertensive reactions, but is not yet available in the United States. Again, MAOIs have not been directly compared with newer antidepressant agents, such as SSUIs and bupropion.

Bipolar Depression

The depressed phase of bipolar affective disorder is often resistant to treatment with standard TCAs. As noted above, bipolar depression is most often associated with decreased baseline platelet MAO activity, and since elevated MAO activity is purported to be a positive predictor of MAOI response, bipolar depression might be expected to respond poorly. This is not the case. Furthermore, high platelet MAO activity has also been detected in some bipolar depressed patients who responded to MAOI therapy.[108] Reversed neurovegetative signs are common in bipolar depression, leading to the proposal that bipolar depression should respond to the same agents as atypical depression.[49]

Quitkin and associates[96] reported the successful treatment of bipolar depressed patients in an open trial with MAOIs. However, few placebo-controlled trials of MAOIs are available. Thase and colleagues[49,139] compared the efficacy of tranylcypromine with that of imipramine as a first-line agent for bipolar depression, and examined the effect of crossing nonresponders over to the opposite medication condition. In the first phase of this study, 56 subjects with bipolar depression were treated under double-blind conditions with tranylcypromine or imipramine. Tranylcypromine proved significantly better for both symptom reduction and tolerance.[49] In the second phase, 18 patients who had not responded to the initial agents were crossed over to the opposite medication condition. Nine of 12 patients who had failed imipramine responded to tranylcypromine, and one of the four patients who had failed tranylcypromine responded to imipramine.[139]

These data make a strong case for the treatment of bipolar depressed patients with MAOIs if they have failed tricyclic treatment. In the studies above, no increased risk of manic induction was noted with tranylcypromine, but this remains a risk of antidepressant therapy in bipolar patients, and has been reported with MAOIs (see "Adverse Reactions").

Child and Adolescent Depression

Very little has been written about the use of MAOIs in child and adolescent depression. This lack of use is largely attributable to the risk of tyramine pressor reactions and the difficulty, especially in older children, of maintaining strict dietary control. In addition, depression was not recognized as a significant mental health problem in children until the mid-1970s and Rutter's Isle of Wight studies,[112] delaying testing of all antidepressant agents in children behind that in adults.[95]

Despite the lack of research, strong arguments exist for testing MAOIs in child and adolescent depression. The frequency of atypical depressive symptoms in adolescents and young adults has led to the proposal that atypical depression may, in fact, be the primary manifestation of major depression in young people.[20,114,115] Furthermore, controlled studies of tricyclic agents have not supported their efficacy for adolescent depression,[61,113] and only partially support their efficacy for preadolescent children (see Chapter 4).[95]

The only two studies of MAOIs in child and adolescent depression are favorable, albeit inconclusive. Frommer[37] conducted a double-blind, placebo-controlled study of phenelzine combined with chlordiazepoxide in 16 depressed and 15 phobic children aged 9 to 15 years. The clinical descriptions appear to meet the criteria for major depression in the first group and for separation anxiety/school phobia in the second, although the presence of neurovegetative signs and their nature were not mentioned. Although the groups were merged for analysis, the phenelzine–chlordiazepoxide combination was seen to be superior to placebo–chlordiazepoxide overall.[37] In the only other published series, Ryan and associates[115] conducted a retrospective study of 23 cases of adolescent major depression treated with an MAOI. In each case, the child had failed a trial of a tricyclic compound and was subsequently treated with either phenelzine or tranylcypromine. If the tricyclic had shown no benefit, an MAOI was used alone. If there had been incomplete response, an MAOI was prescribed in combination with the TCA. When used in this manner, 74% of children responded to treatment, but only 57% both responded and maintained dietary restrictions.[115] Of the seven adolescents who became noncompliant with dietary restrictions, one experienced a pressor response, but none had serious consequences.

Conclusions

The MAOIs are effective therapy for most forms of depression, including major depression with or without melancholia and bipolar depression. Additionally, MAOIs appear to be superior to TCAs for the treatment of depression with prominent anxiety symptoms, especially panic attacks or phobia, and depression with reversed neurovegetative signs. Only two clinical trials of MAOIs in child and adolescent depression have been carried out, and few conclusions may be drawn from these data alone. However, on the basis of experience in adults and the frequency of atypical symptoms in young people, it seems likely that MAOIs will work as well in adolescents as in young adults. Trials for other disorders have demonstrated the safety of MAOIs in both children and adolescents, provided dietary compliance and the availability of prompt medical attention are assured. If these conditions can be met, and a child or adolescent has failed treatment with tricyclic agents and SSUIs, MAOIs should be considered. Recent concern over the cardiotoxicity of TCAs in children and the pending availability of MAOIs that do not require dietary restrictions should give rise to new clinical trials in this age group, and may eventually place MAOIs ahead of TCAs in the pharmacologic treatment of child and adolescent depression. Currently, sensitivity to dietary tyramine may be reduced by the *cautious* combination of MAOIs with TCAs (see "Dosage and Administration").[115]

Anxiety Disorders

Depression with prominent anxiety or phobia appears to respond better to MAOIs than to TCAs (discussed above). However, since anxiety and phobia are independent indications for MAOI treatment, it is difficult to determine whether this represents a depressive subtype or two comorbid conditions that both respond to MAOIs. Clinical trials in patients with comorbid depression and panic attacks show that phenelzine is superior to amitriptyline, but that the superiority may be restricted to anxiety symptoms, with roughly equal effects on depression.[56] As with other indications, MAOIs are effective therapy for anxiety disorders, but have seen far less use than heterocyclic antidepressants and benzodiazepines (see Chapter 10).

Panic Disorder

Reports of the successful treatment of panic attacks with MAOIs date back to the late 1950s.[118] However, few studies have focused on simple panic (without agoraphobia) as a separate clinical entity. Platelet MAO activity has been tested and found to be significantly lower in panic disorder patients,[7] although the clinical significance of this finding is unknown. Buigues and Vallejo[18] treated 35 outpatients with panic disorder or panic disorder with agoraphobia in an open trial of phenelzine. This study is particularly interesting for its stringent definition of drug response. A panic disorder patient was considered a responder only if panic attacks and "subpanic" symptoms ceased completely. Agoraphobics were considered responders if they stopped experiencing anticipatory anxiety and started confronting avoidant

163

behavior *without* behavioral intervention. If additional behavioral treatment was required for success, they were termed partial responders. According to these criteria, 34 of 35 patients had remission within six months. The last was considered a partial responder.[18]

Agoraphobia/Social Phobia

In contrast to simple panic, both panic disorder with agoraphobia and social phobia have been comparatively well studied. Agoraphobia may also present without a history of panic attacks, and in such cases is difficult to distinguish from social phobia (Table 6-4).[4] Apart from the presence or absence of panic attacks, all three of these phobic disorders are phenomenologically similar to the childhood diagnosis of separation anxiety, formerly called school phobia. All are frequently associated with depressive and somatic symptoms; each may lead to avoidant behavior aimed at averting a phobic situation; and the severity of each is judged by the degree to which avoidant behavior interferes with normal functioning.

Early clinical trials of iproniazid noted its success in treating panic disorder with agoraphobia (then termed phobic anxiety).[117,149] Case studies of other MAOIs report success in the treatment of various phobic states.[57,60,131] Mountjoy and associates[80] studied 30 subjects with social phobia, and found the combination of diazepam and phenelzine to be superior to diazepam and placebo. Sheehan and associates[122] noted that, compared with imipramine, phenelzine showed a superior trend, but was statistically equal in reducing phobic symptoms. In a four-cell design comparing phenelzine and behavioral

Table 6-4

Comparison of DSM-III-R Diagnostic Criteria for Agoraphobia Without Panic Attacks and Social Phobia

Agoraphobia Without Panic Attacks	Social Phobia
A fear of being in places or situations from which escape might be difficult (or embarrassing) or in which help might not be available in the event of suddenly developing symptoms that could be incapacitating or extremely embarrassing.	A persistent fear of one or more situations in which the person is exposed to possible scrutiny by others and fears that he or she may do something or act in a way that will be humiliating or embarrassing.
Examples of fears include: dizziness or falling, depersonalization or derealization, loss of bladder or bowel control, vomiting, or cardiac distress. Common agoraphobic situations include being outside the home alone, being in a crowd or standing in line, being on a bridge, and traveling in a bus, train, or car.	Examples of fears include: being unable to continue talking while speaking in public, choking on food when eating in front of others, being unable to urinate in a public lavatory, hand trembling when writing in the presence of others, and saying foolish things or not being able to answer questions in social situations.

Source: Reference 4.

exposure therapy, Solyom and colleagues[130] found that all three treatment conditions were superior to placebo. The fact that patients who also received behavioral therapy showed higher self-rated improvements and lower relapse rates than those who received only phenelzine highlights the importance of nonpharmacologic treatment for phobic states.[130] Of interest to child psychiatrists is the early study by Frommer[37] cited above. One of the two groups successfully treated with phenelzine plus chlordiazepoxide appears to meet current criteria for separation anxiety/school phobia.[37] However, no other trials of MAOIs in separation anxiety are available.

Most of these early trials were conducted on patients with phobic symptoms plus comorbid generalized anxiety, dysthymia, major depression, or substance abuse. Only recently have studies been restricted to relatively homogeneous phobic syndromes. In open trials, moderate to marked improvement of social phobic symptoms was observed in 79% of 29 subjects treated with tranylcypromine[143] and 100% of 11 subjects treated with phenelzine.[69]

Two placebo-controlled studies used current criteria of social phobia. Liebowitz and associates[68] compared phenelzine with atenolol (beta-adrenergic antagonist) and placebo in 74 subjects, and found that phenelzine produced a 64% response rate, as compared with 30% for atenolol and 23% for placebo. They further observed that phenelzine may be more effective when social phobia is generalized to many situations, rather than restricted to specific fears, such as performance or public speaking.[84] Finally, a recent study of 65 patients compared four treatment conditions for social phobia: cognitive-behavioral therapy, alprazolam, phenelzine, and placebo. All groups improved on self-report scales, but the pharmacologic agents were superior on physician rating scales for both symptomatic and functional improvement. The phenelzine-treated group achieved the highest rating of functional improvement, although only slightly higher than for alprazolam.[41]

Conclusions

Current data suggest that MAOIs are at least as effective as heterocyclic antidepressants and benzodiazepines in the treatment of agoraphobia and social phobia, although insufficient data are available that directly compare these agents in homogeneous patient samples. Yet, if efficacy is equal, then currently available (irreversible) MAOIs must be considered quite low on the list of treatment options. Only after TCAs and benzodiazepines have failed, and only for patients with serious functional impairment, should MAOIs be prescribed, because of the difficulty of dietary compliance and the risk of hypertensive reactions.[10,78]

Moclobemide and other reversible MAOIs have not been tested for phobic disorders. These would be expected to confer equal benefit without tyramine pressor reactions, the cardiotoxic effects of TCAs, or the abuse potential of benzodiazepines. Therefore, clinical trials of reversible MAOIs for anxiety disorders are highly desirable. The phenomenologic similarity between adolescent and adult phobic disorders (agoraphobia without panic attacks and social phobia) and separation anxiety/school phobia in children suggests that reversible agents may also be effective in younger children. The relative success of the nonpharmacologic treatment of childhood anxiety disorders requires that any pharmacologic measures be of high efficacy and exceedingly low risk, criteria according to which reversible selective MAOIs may eventually become the treatment of choice, but by which current MAOIs cannot be recommended.

Attention-Deficit Hyperactivity Disorder

For a clinical description of this prominent childhood disorder, see Chapter 3. As discussed there, ADHD is most often thought of as a disorder of catecholamine underactivity. The therapeutic effects of methylphenidate and d-amphetamine provide indirect support for this concept. In addition, several studies have reported low MAO activity in children with ADHD,[123,124] and both high and low platelet MAO activity in individuals with high impulsivity,[125,136] ADHD with conduct disorder,[15] and thrill-seeking personality characteristics.[1,2,91] In at least one small study, treatment with d-amphetamine returned MAO activity to normal in hyperactive children.[124] However, it is important to note that a direct relationship between platelet MAO activity (MAO-B) and CNS MAO has not been established. Young and associates[156] have, in fact, reported poor correlation between platelet and brain MAO activity in epileptic subjects undergoing brain surgery. Therefore, it is difficult to know whether an abnormal peripheral MAO assay means that central MAO is underactive, overactive, or unrelated. Abnormal platelet MAO activity may be a manifestation rather than a biological marker of hyperactivity and impulsivity.

Whatever the significance of platelet MAO studies, preliminary clinical trials of MAOIs show promise. Zametkin and associates[158,159] at the National Institute of Mental Health (NIMH) have compared psychostimulants with several medications that alter catecholamine metabolism for the treatment of ADHD. Prompted by open trials in adults with residual ADHD symptoms[148,154] and by the hypothesis that MAOIs should have an effect on catecholamine systems comparable to that of psychostimulants, this group conducted a double-blind crossover study of MAOIs in 14 boys with ADHD. Both clorgyline (irreversible MAO-A inhibitor) and tranylcypromine were tested, and both "so closely paralleled dextroamphetamine that the treating physician could not distinguish between them."[158,159] Interestingly, a follow-up study of L-deprenyl (selegiline, an irreversible MAO-B inhibitor) suggests that it is inferior to clorgyline and tranylcypromine in the treatment of ADHD,[99] further suggesting that the effects on ADHD are also mediated by MAO-A.

The NIMH group has discouraged the use of MAOIs as a mainline treatment of ADHD, but much of this hesitancy is based on the strict dietary restrictions and potentially serious side effects of irreversible MAOIs. If reversible MAO-A inhibitors (which do not require dietary restriction) prove efficacious, they may become a viable alternative to psychostimulants. Moclobemide has, in fact, been tested in an open trial of 11 ADHD patients who had failed or were intolerant of stimulant treatment. Parent ratings of hyperactivity, as well as objective measures of attention and concentration, improved substantially.[140] Although this was an uncontrolled and nonblind study, it should prompt further research of reversible MAOIs in ADHD.

Eating Disorders

Symptoms of eating disorders occur in up to 6% of young females, but the majority of these cases are time-limited. Current estimates place the prevalence of bulimia nervosa at approximately 2% and anorexia nervosa at 0.2% of women aged 12 to 25 years (Table 6-5).[3] The prevalence of eating disorders in men is much lower, with an estimated sex ratio of 9:1. Since the peak age of onset for eating disorders is from the teens to mid-20s, these disorders are of particular interest to adolescent psychiatrists, especially in

Table 6-5
DSM-III-R Diagnostic Criteria for Eating Disorders

Anorexia nervosa	Refusal to maintan body weight over a minimal normal weight for age and height or failure to make expected weight gain during period of growth, leading to body weight 15% below that expected. Intense fear of gaining weight or becoming fat, even though underweight. Disturbance in the way in which one's body weight, size, or shape is experienced. In females, absence of at least three consecutive menstrual cycles when otherwise expected to occur.
Bulimia nervosa	Recurrent episodes of binge eating. A feeling of lack of control over eating behavior during binges. The person regularly engages in either self-induced vomiting, use of laxatives or diuretics, strict dieting or fasting, or vigorous exercise in order to prevent weight gain. A minimum average of two binge-eating episodes per week for at least three months. Persistent overconcern with body shape and weight.

Source: Reference 4.

light of potentially devastating outcomes. Although severe cases are rare, early outcome studies reported mortality rates up to 19%.[153] Of the 460 cases studied by Patton[87] between 1971 and 1981, 3.3% with anorexia and 3.1% with bulimia proved fatal. Many survivors remain underweight or amenorrheic, and psychiatric comorbidity is common. The most frequent cause of death in anorexic patients is suicide.[87]

Anorexia

Several psychotropic agents have been tried in the treatment of anorexia nervosa, but no standard pharmacologic therapy has emerged. Antidepressants have received the greatest attention, perhaps due to the strong association of eating disorders with affective disorders. Low platelet MAO activity has been reported in depressed anorectic patients, but not in nondepressed patients.[9] Although there have been no placebo-controlled studies to date, two open trials of MAOIs in anorexia have reported success. Hudson and associates[51] reported 10 cases in which a series of antidepressants were tried. MAOIs (phenelzine or tranylcypromine) were tried in five cases, and were associated with the return of body weight to acceptable levels in two.[51] Another open trial treated six anorectic and 12 bulimic women with isocarboxazid. Treatment resulted in no significant weight change, but significant improvement in depression, anxiety, and phobia.[58] Interpretation of the latter study was hampered by a high dropout rate by the bulimic subjects and initial weights above 85% of expected in five of the 14 subjects who completed the trial (115% in one subject). Therefore, weight gain may have been a weak measure of outcome in this sample.

Bulimia

The data for bulimia are somewhat more complete than for anorexia. Several placebo-controlled studies by Walsh and colleagues[145–147] suggest that MAOIs may be effective in some cases. In 1984, they studied 35 bulimic women in a single-blind design comparing phenelzine with placebo. Again, a high dropout rate was observed due to dietary noncompliance, placebo response, or intolerance of side effects, with only 20 women completing the 10-week trial. Of these, the phenelzine group showed a fourfold decrease in bingeing behavior and moderate improvement on an "eating attitudes" scale. However, long-term benefit was established in only three of the patients receiving phenelzine.[146]

More pronounced success was reported in a second study by the same group. Thirty of 53 patients completed a double-blind, placebo-controlled trial. A threefold reduction in bingeing was observed among the 14 who received phenelzine, six of whom achieved remission.[147] More recently, 50 of 82 patients completed a third trial with a design similar to that of the 1985 study. Phenelzine again produced a substantial, statistically significant reduction in bingeing and an improvement in eating attitudes.[145] In both the 1985 and 1988 studies, the effect of phenelzine on associated affective symptoms was discussed. Bulimic subjects who exhibited significant depressive or anxiety symptoms prior to treatment improved on these measures, as well as on measures of bulimia. Interestingly, the reduction in bingeing behavior was greater among nondepressed than depressed patients, although improvement in both groups was statistically significant. In all three studies, the overall effectiveness of phenelzine was limited by often intolerable side effects and the difficulty of maintaining a low-tyramine diet.

Conclusions

Eating disorders remain a possible, but by no means proven, indication for MAOIs. Only 30–40% of the subjects who completed MAOI trials in the above studies achieved long-term remission, with high relapse and dropout rates for the remaining subjects. Therefore, the treatment of anorectic and bulimic adolescents with the currently available agents cannot be recommended, since dietary noncompliance is exceptionally high in both eating disorder patients and adolescents.[115] Consideration should be given to clinical trials of moclobemide to circumvent this problem.

Borderline Personality Disorder

Personality disorders are classically resistant to both psychotherapeutic and psychopharmacologic interventions. However, borderline personality disorder (BPD) may be amenable to the treatment of associated affective and behavioral symptoms, even if the core pathology remains.[129] Although BPD is one of the personality disorders that may be diagnosed in adolescents,[4] there are no trials specific to adolescent borderline patients.

Historically, this heterogeneous syndrome has included symptoms from both neurotic and psychotic categories, including affective lability, chaotic social relationships, high interpersonal sensitivity, impulsivity, and limited psychotic episodes or perceptions. Comorbid affective disorders are common, especially atypical manifestations of depression (see description above). An interesting analysis of comorbid depression in BPD and the efficacy of MAOIs is provided by Parsons and colleagues[86] at Columbia University. They propose that the extant literature can be divided into subtypes of BPD that have different responses to pharmacologic agents. More than 300 patients with atypical major depression or atypical intermittent depressive disorder were treated in a double-blind, placebo-controlled crossover design with phenelzine and imipramine. The subjects were rated for number of borderline features and response of depressive symptoms to treatment. In patients with fewer than four borderline symptoms, the two agents were of approximately equal benefit. However, four or more features of BPD predicted a negative response to imipramine and a positive response to phenelzine. Depressed subjects with BPD showed a 91% response rate to phenelzine, 39% to imipramine, and 21% to placebo.[86] One additional controlled study reported improvement in affective symptoms on tranylcypromine, while pointing out that there was no effect on behavioral control.[23]

Hysteroid Dysphoria

Overlapping the depressive symptoms of BPD is a proposed depressive subtype, hysteroid dysphoria. Characteristic symptoms of this subtype include criteria of BPD (impulsivity, histrionic personality features, and chaotic interpersonal relationships) and atypical depression (interpersonal sensitivity and reversed neurovegetative signs).[55] The diagnostic validity and response of this syndrome to MAOIs are difficult to discern due to the overlap with BPD and atypical depression, both of which appear to respond to MAOIs. Half of patients with hysteroid dysphoria also meet the diagnostic criteria for BPD.[8,86] However, controlled studies testing the use of MAOIs for hysteroid dysphoria have demonstrated phenelzine's superiority to placebo, imipramine,[56,67,70] and amitriptyline.[56]

Conclusions

As indicated in the discussion above, there is evidence that MAOIs may be superior to heterocyclic compounds for atypical depressive disorders. Currently, hysteroid dysphoria must be considered a variant of atypical depression, and has not been validated as a separate clinical syndrome. Since BPD often coexists with atypical depression, MAOIs may also be useful in these patients. However, both MAOIs and TCAs may improve a variety of symptoms associated with BPD, independently of the effect on mood.[128] Regardless of the target symptoms, the impulsive and self-abusive symptoms inherent in BPD require extreme caution in selecting patients who are able to comply with the dietary restrictions of current agents, especially adolescents.

Contraindications

See Table 6-6.

Treatment with MAOIs is contraindicated in a variety of circumstances, most of which relate to concurrent medical illness or pharmacologic treatment. The primary contraindication for currently available agents is the inability of the patient to comply with dietary restrictions. It is advisable to test the ability to comply by reviewing a detailed log of food and beverage for two weeks prior to instituting therapy (see "Initiating and Maintaining Treatment").

Table 6-6
Contraindications to Treatment with MAOIs

- Inability to maintain dietary restrictions (see Table 6-8)
- Concurrent use of any sympathomimetic agents or other agents known to react with MAOIs (see Table 6-7)
- Concurrent use of other drugs with MAOI activity
- Concurrent use of SSUIs
- Pheochromocytoma
- Preexisting liver disease
- Preexisting cerebrovascular disease or untreated hypertension
- Impending surgery requiring general or local anesthesia (see Table 6-7)
- Asthma when sympathomimetic bronchodilators are unavoidable

Additional contraindications are given in Table 6-6. Most notable are the presence of cerebrovascular disease, which increases the risk of hypertensive consequences; preexisting hepatic disease, which has been associated with impaired tyramine clearance: pheochromocytoma, which causes high levels of endogenous sympathomimetic amines; and pending surgical procedures that will require anesthesia (Table 6-7).[92] If the patient has been treated with any serotonergic agent (including paroxetine, sertraline, buspirone, trazadone, doxepin, and TCAs), a seven- to 14-day washout period is required before starting an MAOI (see "Drug Interactions"). A 14-day washout is similarly necessary when changing from one MAOI to another.[115] Fluoxetine (Prozac) has an extended elimination half-life requiring at least a five-week washout period.[92] Sympathomimetics, either prescribed, in over-the-counter preparations, or through excessive caffeine intake, are contraindicated (Table 6-7).

Side Effects

A discussion of the side effects of MOAIs inevitably focuses on the so-called cheese effect, or the hypertensive reaction produced by dietary tyramine in patients treated with classic MAOIs. Raskin[100] reported a 3.3% incidence of this effect even when dietary restrictions were observed, but found other side effects to be quite rare. This section will discuss both the less infamous side effects of MAOIs and their interaction with tyramine and sympathomimetic amines.

Tyramine Pressor Effect

Dietary tyramine in high doses acts as a pseudotransmitter, with stimulant and pressor effects. Since tyramine is a substrate of MAO, MAOI therapy is associated with a 10- to 30-fold increase in sensitivity to these effects.[81] Tyra-

Table 6-7
Medications That Are Contraindicated with MAOI Therapy

Degree of Caution	Medication	Comments and Examples
Common agents that are absolutely contraindicated	Sympathomimetic amines	Rx—amphetamine and epinephrine analogs. OTC—ephedrine, pseudoephedrine, phenylephrine, and phenylethylamine.
	Dextromethorphan	OTC—present in Dristan, Comtrex, and many others; acts via serotonin reuptake blockade.
	SSUIs	Rx—fluoxetine, sertraline, paroxetine, etc. May produce serotonin syndrome (see text).
	Hypoglycemic agents	Rx—potentiates hypoglycemia.
	L-Dopa, methyldopa	Rx—enhances pressor effect. Dopa present in some food.
	Reserpine, tetrabenazine	Rx—similar to serotonin syndrome.
	Tryptophan	Rx—serotonin precursor.
Anesthetic agents to be avoided	Narcotic analgesics	Reserved to meperidine and other 5-HT blockers, but may also prolong action of morphine and barbiturates.
	Ketamine	Theoretical risk of cardiovascular toxicity.
	Suxamethonium	May prolong or increase neuromuscular blockade.
	Local anesthetics	Avoid epinephrine, norepinephrine, cocaine and analogues.
Agents causing adverse reactions in rare cases	Amantadine	Acts as a dopamine agonist, may produce hypertension.
	Chloral hydrate	Hypertension reported, mechanism unknown.
	Droperidol	Hypotension reported.
	Fenfluramine	Delirium reported, mechanism unknown.
	Guanethidine	May produce hypertension.
Agents to be used with caution	Tricyclic antidepressants	See guidelines in text.
	Anticholinergics	Potentiation reported in humans, hyperthermia in animals.
	Benzodiazepines	Reports of edema, probably safe.
	Caffeine	Hypertension and agitation with excessive intake.

Abbreviations: Rx—prescription drug; OTC—available without prescription.
Source: References 12, 133.

mine is a product of bacterial tyrosine metabolism, leading to high levels in aged or unfresh protein-rich foods, such as cheese. In addition, several foods (broad beans, chocolate, banana peels) have high levels of dopamine precursors and other natural pressor agents, which may produce hypertension during MAOI therapy. As little as 6–10 mg of dietary tyramine in a subject taking MAOIs can result in a significant rise in blood pressure, while 20–25 mg may induce a hypertensive crisis.[17] Normal (unmedicated) volunteers can tolerate 200–400 mg of oral tyramine before blood pressure increases.[127]

When this effect was discovered, it was felt that extreme dietary restrictions were necessary. These restrictions have moderated somewhat with experience and more detailed studies of tyramine content in foods.[36,75,137] The list in Table 6-8 represents a moderately conservative dietary guide. Violation of dietary guidelines or concurrent use of any sympathomimetic agent may result in a hypertensive crisis. Clinically, this consists of severe occipital headache, palpitations, neck stiffness, nausea, vomiting, diaphoresis, pupillary dilation, photophobia, and chest pain. Hypertension has, in rare cases, been severe enough to cause intracranial bleeding and death.[13]

The tyramine pressor effect is primarily responsible for the unpopularity of MAOIs in current clinical practice, as well as being the main impetus for the development of selective, reversible MAOIs. L-Deprenyl and other selective MAO-B inhibitors do not react significantly with dietary tyramine, but currently have no application in child and adolescent psychiatry. Irreversible, selective MAO-A inhibitors (clorgyline) react with tyramine to the same extent as phenelzine and tranylcypromine. However, reversible inhibitors of MAO-A (moclobemide) induce only a modest increase in sensitivity (Table 6-1). Because moclobemide and tyramine compete for MAO binding, much higher doses of tyramine are required to produce hypertension. For example, a 40 mg dose of tranylcypromine increases sensitivity to *intravenous* tyramine up to 162 times normal.[127] In contrast, a single dose of moclobemide increases sensitivity to IV tyramine by only two to four times normal. A study of tyramine-enriched food given to subjects taking 600 mg of moclobemide daily indicated that up to 150 mg could be ingested safely, compared with 200–400 mg in unmedicated individuals. This amount of tyramine is not found in normal meals.[160] Therefore, the availability of moclobemide and other reversible MAO-A inhibitors may eliminate the main deterrent to MAOI therapy.

The Serotonergic Syndrome

A well-established interaction has been described between fluoxetine and MAOIs, which is often referred to as the serotonergic syndrome. The reaction is not limited to this combination, however, as it has been reported

Table 6-8
Dietary Restrictions Necessary for MAOI Therapy

Dietary Guidelines	Tyramine* (mg/30 g)	Comments and Examples
Not permitted		
Cheese, aged, overripe, or spoiled	1.0–65.0	For example, blue, cheddar, Gruyere.
Smoked, pickled, or unfresh fish	0–99.0	For example, caviar, anchovies, herring.
Fermented dry sausage	3.0–45	For example, pepperoni, salami, summer sausage.
Semidry	~2.6	For example, bologna.
Beer		
Imported or import-style ale	0.05–0.4	Twelve ounces of American-style
American style	0.05–0.1	beer contains about 1 mg tyramine.
Red wine, sherry, liqueurs	0.05–0.4	Especially Chianti (0.76 mg/30 ml).
Beef or chicken liver	0–0.3	May be acceptable if very fresh.
Meat extracts	2.9–9.1	Bovril, Marmite, some dry soup bases.
Yeast extracts and supplements	2.0–68.0	Regular bakery products are permitted.
Sauerkraut	0.6–2.9	Testing done on German products.
Unfresh or overripe protein-rich foods	Varies	For example, leftover meats and expired dairy products.
Broad beans (e.g., fava beans)	NA	Contains dopa rather than tyramine.
Green banana or banana peel	0.2–2.0	Peel also contains dopamine.
Permitted in limited amounts		
Processed American cheeses	0–1.5	Up to 1.5 mg of tyramine in a single slice (1 ounce) of American cheese.
Avocado	0–0.7	Higher levels in overripe fruit and guacamole.
Bananas, fresh	0–0.2	Avoid overripe fruit and peel.
Soy sauce and variants	~0.05	Safe unless used in very large amounts.
Peanuts and other nuts	?	No documentation of tyramine content.
Raspberries, fresh or in jams	~0.3–2.9	Safe in very small servings.
White wine and distilled spirits	?	No documentation of tyramine content.
Chocolate	NA	Contains phenylethylamine.
Need not be restricted		
Yogurt, sour cream, cream cheese, cottage cheese	0–0.3	Avoid homemade or homemade styles and consume very fresh products.
Fresh fish and meats	ND	Do not allow spoilage.
Fresh fruits (except raspberries)	ND	
Figs and raisins	ND	Canned figs may contain tyramine.*
Most dried soups and bouillon	ND	

*Figures based on 1-ounce (30 g or 30 ml) portions. Up to 6 mg of tyramine may be ingested safely while taking therapeutic doses of MAOIs.
Abbreviations: ND—no detectable amount of tyramine; NA—not applicable, contains other pressor agents.
Source: References 22, 36, 75, 126, 137.

with MAOIs combined with tryptophan (serotonin precursor) and other agents that inhibit serotonin reuptake. The clinical features include mental status changes (confusion, agitation, hypomania), myoclonus, hyperreflexia, tremor, ataxia, diaphoresis, fever, and autonomic dysregulation.[134] If the patient is also being treated with an antipsychotic, this syndrome may be difficult to distinguish from neuroleptic malignant syndrome (see Chapter 7). However, the serotonergic syndrome does not commonly produce pronounced rigidity, CPK levels over 1000 units per liter, or leukocytosis.

Cardiovascular Effects

Goldman and associates[48] have reviewed and contrasted the cardiovascular side effects experienced in patients treated with heterocyclic antidepressants and MAOIs. They surmise that MAOI therapy is associated with both decreased and increased resting blood pressure (RBP). The decrease in RBP is most notable in subjects who were hypertensive at baseline.[48] Orthostatic hypotension is reportedly common, although how common it actually is has been questioned owing to methodology that fails to take into account the decrease in RBP. In either case, the symptomatic reduction of blood pressure presents a significant limitation to MAOI use.[48,83] Hypertension as a consequence of MAOI therapy is most often part of the tyramine reaction or a result of concurrent sympathomimetic use (see discussion below). In a small, but well-controlled sample, O'Brien et al.[84] found that tranylcypromine treatment had no significant effect on cardiac conduction.

Manic Symptoms

Although a well-known reaction to heterocyclic antidepressants, mania induced by MAOIs was recognized rather late. One of the first case reports was that of a 17-year-old boy who developed rapid cycling bipolar affective disorder after treatment with phenelzine.[74] Cases have also been reported of mania induced by combined MAOIs and TCAs in depressed bipolar patients.[31] The incidence of this effect has not been established, but it is probably more common in patients with bipolar depression.

General Effects

The most common side effect of MAOI use is hypotension (discussed above) and dizziness. Much less common, but established, adverse effects include insomnia, impotence, edema, weight gain, elevated hepatic enzymes, and overstimulation (jitteriness, tremors, twitching). Psychotic symptoms may emerge or be exacerbated in rare cases.[92]

Overdose

Much of the information on MAOI overdose comes not from the psychiatric literature, but from oncologic reports, where MAOI agents are used in antineoplastic regimens. The greatest concern to psychiatrists is intentional overdose. If the patient has also ingested a source of tyramine or sympathomimetics, then an overdosage is treated much like a hypertensive crisis (see below). However, death has been reported from MAOI overdose alone.[92] Gellman[42] reported the accidental overdose of phenelzine in a 14-month-old girl who became toxic despite the prompt induction of emesis with recovery of pill fragments. Periods of deep sedation alternated with unrestrainable agitation and autonomic dysregulation, although blood pressure remained stable. The child recovered after nine days of observation and IV fluid support.[42]

Toxic symptoms reported by the manufacturers include drowsiness, dizziness, mental status changes (including agitation, hyperactivity, confusion, or psychosis), headache, seizures, and coma.[92] Hypotension or hypertension may develop, along with hyperreflexia and general autonomic dysregulation (tachycardia, hyperthermia, tachypnea, pupillary dilation).[53] Toxic blood levels have not been established for humans.

Abuse/Dependence

Although one case of addiction to tranylcypromine has been reported,[16] MAOIs are not generally considered drugs of potential abuse.

Drug Interactions

In addition to the pressor effect of dietary tyramine and dopamine, the pressor effects of many medications are also increased by MAOI therapy (see Table 6-7). This includes several over-the-counter cold remedies and allergy preparations. Serotonergic agents are associated with the serotonergic syndrome, as described above. Violation of these medication guidelines may result in a hypertensive or serotonergic crisis.

Available Preparations and Cost

Three MAOIs are currently marketed for psychiatric indications in the United States: phenelzine (Nardil), tranylcypromine (Parnate), and isocarboxazid (Marplan). These are available in tablet form only, in 15-mg, 10-mg, and 10-mg sizes respectively. Isocarboxazid has not been as widely tested as the others, and is rated by the FDA as "probably" an effective treatment for refractory depression.

Current average wholesale prices per 100 tablets are as follows: phenelzine—$32.29, tranylcypromine—$38.65, and isocarboxazid—$53.97. Therefore, the approximate daily cost (wholesale) of treating an older adolescent is $0.97 for phenelzine, $1.16 for tranylcypromine, and $1.62 for isocarboxazid. Generic equivalents are not offered.[94]

Initiating and Maintaining Treatment

Education about and adherence to dietary and medication restrictions is necessary before starting MAOI therapy. Verbal discussion of restrictions is not sufficient, as the patient may remember little of what is said. It is advisable to provide well-organized and simply written handouts, which may be posted at home and referred to frequently. Since a washout period of seven to 14 days or more is required when changing from most other antidepressant agents to an MAOI (see discussion above), the authors have found it helpful to use this time to verify the patient's ability to comply with dietary restrictions. For two weeks prior to therapy, the patient and his or her parents should adhere to dietary restrictions, while keeping a detailed log of all foods and beverages ingested. The physician may then review the log for compliance, and counsel the family on any misinterpretations of the guidelines before prescribing an MAOI.

Dosage and Administration

Guidelines in child psychiatry are virtually nonexistent, since these agents are not approved for use in children younger than 16 years. Even for older children, it is recommended that the prescription start below the adult dose, with one tablet of phenelzine (15 mg) or tranylcypromine (10 mg) daily, rather than three. Dose increases should not be more frequent than every 14 days, since maximal MAO inhibition is achieved seven to 14 days after the last change. Weight-adjusted dose schedules have not been established for children, although adult studies suggest that 1.0 mg/kg/day of phenelzine is safe and effective.[109] The maximum recommended dose for adults and older adolescents is 90 mg (six tablets) of phenelzine daily or 60 mg (six tablets) of tranylcypromine daily, in divided doses. In the trial cited above[109] an average phenelzine dose of 15 mg twice daily was well tolerated by children aged 9 to 15 years.[37] Maximum doses and the general safety of MAOIs have not been established for preadolescent children.

Combining MAOIs with TCAs

The combination of MAOIs with TCAs was used in several of the adolescent cases reported by Ryan and associates,[115] and at one time was advocated as a superior treatment for refractory depression.[121] To some degree, this practice is counterintuitive, especially when one considers that SSUIs are contraindicated in the presence of MAOIs and that tricyclics inhibit both MAO and serotonin reuptake to varying degrees.[53] Nevertheless, there are reports of safe treatment in both open[36,121,132] and controlled[105,150] trials. Not all of these have been favorable, as one study found trimipramine alone to be superior to MAOIs alone and to MAOIs combined with trimipramine in mild to moderate outpatient depression.[157] Another study found ECT to be superior to a phenelzine–amitriptyline combination in severe inpatient depression.[30] In a double-blind, placebo-controlled trial on 60 patients with major depression, Razani and colleagues[105] compared amitriptyline, tranylcypromine, and the two drugs combined. They found that the combination was safe, but showed no evidence of increased effectiveness. At least one review of this approach has disapproved of combined MAOI–TCA therapy on the grounds that it has not proved more effective than single agents, has a higher incidence of adverse side effects, and increases the risk of the serotonergic syndrome with certain agents.[62] Combined treatment may or may not increase the risk of cardiotoxic effects.[62,83,84]

Although combined MAOI–TCA therapy is probably not clinically superior to single agents, tests of tyramine sensitivity show that the combination confers a relative resistance to dietary tyramine.[85] This is the basis for Ryan and colleagues'[115] recommendation that the combination be considered for adolescent (or adult) indications. If this approach is used, Kaplan and Sadock[53] recommend that imipramine and trimipramine be avoided because of their higher incidence of adverse reactions when combined with MAOIs. In addition, TCAs should not be given to a patient who is already taking MAOIs, since it is impossible to predict or control the effect of amine reuptake inhibition in the presence of greater than 80% MAO inhibition. Rather, the MAOI must be discontinued and 14 days allowed for MAO activity to return to normal. Both agents may then be started at very low doses and titrated according to response and the emergence of side effects.[53]

Management of Specific Side Effects

Hypertensive Crisis

Ryan and colleagues[115] reported several cases in which adolescents treated with MAOIs intentionally violated dietary guidelines. Even with good compliance, patients may forget about certain forbidden foods or inadvertently ingest foods that they did not realize were rich in tyramine. Extensive premedication counseling is necessary so that the symptoms of a pressor response (headache, diaphoresis, stiff neck, nausea and vomiting) will be promptly recognized and immediate medical attention will be available.[53] Patients in remote locations or without access to emergency medical services should probably not receive MAOIs. Chlorpromazine has been used as a short-term treatment measure, leading to the recommendation that several 50-mg tablets (25 mg for children) be provided for patients to take if symptoms appear, especially if they will be away temporarily from medical care.[53,115]

The manufacturers recommend the immediate discontinuation of MAOIs if a hypertensive crisis is suspected and IV phentolamine (5 mg) to treat symptomatic hypertension. Hospitalization with any indicated supportive and symptomatic measures may be necessary in such cases.[92] *Dietary and medication restrictions must be maintained for two weeks after the discontinuation of an MAOI* and during the treatment of a hypertensive reaction.

Serotonin Syndrome

A recent review has recommended several steps to be taken when the serotonin syndrome is suspected. Hospitalization and prompt discontinuation of the medications that are thought responsible are followed by an assessment of supportive needs, such as cooling blankets for fever or ventilation for respiratory depression. Myoclonus, seizures, and agitation have been reported, and may require pharmacologic treatment. Nifedipine has been used successfully in four cases where hypertension was present. Propranolol has been suggested as an adjunctive agent, since it may both provide symptomatic relief and act as a serotonin antagonist.[134]

Cardiovascular Effects

Hypotension is often tolerable or may be managed with increased fluids and salts. Decreasing the dosage may help, but may also influence the effectiveness of the drug. If the patient was hypertensive prior to treatment, any antihypertensive agents should be discontinued. Despite these interventions, a number of patients will be unable to continue MAOI therapy because of symptomatic hypotension. Hospitalization with IV fluids may be necessary in severe cases, but *pressor agents are to be avoided completely*.[92]

How to Withdraw Medication

Withdrawal symptoms have been described with MAOIs, but the mechanisms of such symptoms are difficult to conceptualize. Upon abrupt discontinuation, MAO activity returns to normal gradually over two weeks, suggesting that any withdrawal is related to non-MAOI properties of the compound itself. Nevertheless, symptoms have ranged from anxiety and agitation to frank psychosis, and have been compared to those of stimulant withdrawal.[52] Gradual discontinuation of the medication is recommended.[92]

But regardless of how the medication is discontinued, MAO activity is suppressed for up to two weeks after the last dose, necessitating full compliance with dietary and medication restrictions for that period.

References

1. Af Klinteberg, B., Levander, S.E., Oreland, L., et al. (1987). Neuropsychological correlates of platelet monoamine oxidase (MAO) activity in female and male subjects. *Biol Psychol, 24(3)*, 237–252.

2. Af Klinteberg, B., Schalling, D., Edman, G., et al. (1987). Personality correlates of platelet monoamine oxidase (MAO) activity in female and male subjects. *Neuropsychobiology, 18(2)*, 89–96.

3. Agras, S.W., Bachman, J.A. (1989). Anorexia nervosa and bulimia nervosa. In P.J. Wilner (Ed.), *Psychiatry (vol. 2)* (Chap. 102, pp. 1–12). Philadelphia: Lippincott.

4. American Psychiatric Association. (1987). *Diagnostic and Statistical Manual of Mental Disorders (3rd ed., rev.)*. Washington, D.C.: American Psychiatric Association.

5. Amrein, R., Allen, S.R., Guentert, T.W., et al. (1989). The pharmacology of reversible monoamine oxidase inhibitors. *Br J Psychiatry Suppl, 6*, 66–71.

6. Baldessarini, R.J. (1975). The basis for amine hypothesis in affective disorders. *Arch Gen Psychiatry, 32*, 1087–1093.

7. Balon, R., Rainey, J.M., Pohl, R., et al. (1987). Platelet monoamine oxidase activity in panic disorder. *Psychiatry Res, 22(1)*, 37–41.

8. Beeber, A.R., Kline. M.D., Pies, R.W., Manring, J.M., Jr. (1984). Hysteroid dysphoria in depressed inpatients. *J Clin Psychiatry, 45(4)*, 164–166.

9. Biederman, J., Rivinus, T.M., Herzog, D.B., et al. (1984). Platelet MAO activity in anorexia nervosa patients with and without a major depressive disorder. *Am J Psychiatry, 141(10)*, 1244–1247.

10. Biederman, J. (1990). The diagnosis and treatment of adolescent anxiety disorders. *J Clin Psychiatry, 51(Suppl)*, 20–26.

11. Biziere, K., Berger, M. (1990). Efficacy of a reversible monoamine oxidase-A inhibitor versus imipramine in subgroups of depressed patients. *Acta Psychiatr Scand, 360(Suppl)*, 59–60.

12. Blackwell, B. (1991). Monoamine oxidase inhibitor interactions with other drugs. *J Clin Psychopharmacol, 11(1)*, 55–59.

13. Blackwell, B., Marley, E., Price, J., Taylor, D. (1967). Hypertensive interactions between monoamine oxidase inhibitors and foodstuffs. *Br J Psychiatry, 113(497)*, 349–365.

14. Bloch, R.G., Dooneief, A.S., Buchberg, A.S., Spellman, S. (1954). The clinical effects of isoniazid and iproniazid in the treatment of pulmonary tuberculosis. *Ann Intern Med, 40*, 881–900.

15. Bowden, C.L., Deutsch, C.K., Swanson, J.M. (1988). Plasma dopamine-beta-hydroxylase and platelet monoamine oxidase in attention deficit disorder and conduct disorder. *J Am Acad Child Adolesc Psychiatry, 27(2)*, 171–174.

16. Briggs, N.C., Jefferson, J.W., Koenecke, F.H. (1990). Tranylcypromine addiction: A case report and review. *J Clin Psychiatry, 51(10)*, 426–429.

17. Brown, C., Taniguchi, G., Yip, K. (1989). The monoamine oxidase inhibitor–tyramine interaction. *J Clin Pharmacol, 29(6)*, 529–532.

18. Buigues, J., Vallejo, J. (1987). Therapeutic response to phenelzine in patients with panic disorder and agoraphobia with panic attacks. *J Clin Psychiatry, 48(2)*, 55–59.

19. Casacchia, M., Moll, E. (1990). Moclobemide (Ro 11–1163) versus imipramine in the treatment of depression. *Acta Psychiatr Scand, 360(Suppl)*, 43.

20. Casper, R.C., Redmond, D.E., Jr., Katz, M.M., et al. (1985). Somatic symptoms in primary affective disorder. *Arch Gen Psychiatry, 42*, 1098–1104.

21. Civeira, J., Cervera, S., Giner, J., et al. (1990). Moclobemide versus clomipramine in the treatment of depression: A multicentre trial in Spain. *Acta Psychiatr Scand, 360(Suppl)*, 48–49.

22. Cooper, A.J. (1989). Tyramine and irreversible monoamine oxidase inhibitors in clinical practice. *Br J Psychiatry Suppl, 6*, 38–45.

23. Cowdry, R., Gardner, D. (1988). Pharmacology of borderline personality disorder. *Arch Gen Psychiatry, 45*, 111–119.

24. Dally, P.J., Rohde, P. (1961). Comparison of antidepressant drugs in depressive illnesses. *Lancet, 1*, 18–20.

25. Davidson, J., Turnbull, C. (1984). The importance of dose in isocarboxazid therapy. *J Clin Psychiatry, 45(7 pt. 2)*, 49–52.

26. Davidson, J., McLeod, M.N., Blum, M.R. (1978). Acetylation phenotype, platelet monoamine oxidase inhibition, and the effectiveness of phenelzine in depression. *Am J Psychiatry, 135(4)*, 467–469.

27. Davidson, J., Lipper, S., Pelton, S., et al. (1988). The response of depressed inpatients to isocarboxazid. *J Clin Psychopharmacol, 8(2)*, 100–107.

28. Davidson, J.R.T., McLeod, M.N., White, H.L. (1978). Inhibition of platelet monoamine oxidase in depressed subjects treated with phenelzine. *Am J Psychiatry, 135*, 470–472.

29. Davidson, J.R., Giller, E.L., Zisook, S., Helms, M.J. (1991). Predictors of response to monoamine oxidase inhibitors: Do they exist? *Eur Arch Psychiatry Clin Neurosci, 241(3)*, 181–186.

30. Davidson, J., McLeod, M., Law-Yone, B., Linnoila, M. (1978). A comparison of electroconvulsive therapy and combined phenelzine-amitriptyline in refractory depression. *Arch Gen psychiatry, 35(5)*, 639–642.

31. De la Fuente, J.R., Berlanga, C., Leon-Andrade, C. (1986). Mania induced by tricyclic-MAOI combination therapy in bipolar treatment-resistant disorder: Case reports. *J Clin Psychiatry, 47(1)*, 40–41.

32. Delini-Stula, A., Radeke, E., Waldmeier, P.C. (1988). Basic and clinical aspects of the activity of the new monoamine oxidase inhibitors. *Psychopharmacol Ser, 5*, 147–158.

33. Demish, L., Gebhart, P., Kaczmarczyk, P., von der Muhlen, H. (1981). Low platelet MAO activity in psychiatric patients and plasma factors: No evidence for inhibitory influences on MAO in the circulating platelet population. *Biol Psychiatry, 16(1)*, 21–33.

34. Dierick, M., Cattiez, P., Franck, G., et al. (1990). Moclobemide versus clomipramine in the treatment of depression: A double-blind multicentre study in Belgium. *Acta Psychiatr Scand, 360(Suppl)*, 50–51.

35. Evans, D.A.P., Manley, K.A., McKusick, V.A. (1960). Human isoniazid metabolism—a genetically determined phenomenon. *Br Med J, 2*, 485–491.

36. (1989). Foods interacting with MAO inhibitors. *Med Lett Drugs Ther, 31(785)*, 11–12.

37. Frommer, E.A. (1967). Treatment of childhood depression with antidepressant drugs. *Br Med J, 1(542)*, 729–732.

38. Funke, H.J., Moritz, E., Hellstern, K., Malanowski, H. (1990). Moclobemide versus clomipramine in the treatment of depression: A single-centre study, Federal Republic of Germany. *Acta Psychiatr Scand, 360(Suppl)*, 46–47.

39. Gabelic, I., Moll, E. (1990). Moclobemide (Ro 11–1163) versus desipramine in the treatment of endogenous depression. *Acta Psychiatr Scand, 360(Suppl)*, 44–45.

40. Ganrot, P.O., Rossengren, E., Gottfries, C.G. (1962). Effect of iproniazid on monoamines and monoamine oxidase in human brain. *Experientia, 18*, 260–261.

41. Gelernter, C.S., Uhde, T.W., Cimbolic, P., et al. (1991). Cognitive-behavioral and pharmacological treatments of social phobia. A controlled study. *Arch Gen Psychiatry, 48(10)*, 938–945.

42. Gellman, V. (1966). Phenelzine dihydrogen sulphate (Nardil) intoxication. *Manit Med Rev, 46(2)*, 147–149.

43. Georgotas, A., McCue, R.E., Cooper, T., et al. (1987). Clinical predictors of response to antidepressants in elderly patients. *Biol Psychiatry, 22(6)*, 733–740.

44. Georgotas, A., McCue, R.E., Cooper, T.B., et al. (1989). Factors affecting the delay of antidepressant effect in responders to nortriptyline and phenelzine. *Psychiatry Res, 28(1)*, 1–9.

45. Georgotas, A., McCue, R.E., Friedman, E., Cooper, T. (1987). Prediction of response to nortriptyline and phenelzine by platelet MAO activity. *Am J Psychiatry, 144(3)*, 338–340.

46. Giller, E., Jr., Bialos, D., Harkness, L., Riddle, M. (1984). Assessing treatment response to the monoamine oxidase inhibitor isocarboxazid. *J Clin Psychiatry, 45(7 pt. 2)*, 44–48.

47. Goldberg, L.I. (1964). Monoamine oxidase inhibitors: Adverse reaction and possible mechanism. *JAMA, 190*, 132–138.

48. Goldman, L.S., Alexander, R.C., Luchins, D.J. (1986). Monoamine oxidase inhibitors and tricyclic antidepressants: Comparison of their cardiovascular effects. *J Clin Psychiatry, 47(5)*, 225–229.

49. Himmelhoch, J.M., Thase, M.E., Mallinger, A.G., Houck, P. (1991). Tranylcypromine versus imipramine in anergic bipolar depression. *Am J Psychiatry, 148(7)*, 910–916.

50. Houlihan, D.J., Gershon, S. (1994). The role of MAO inhibitors in psychiatry. In A. Lieberman, C.W. Olanow, M. Youdim, K.F. Tipton (Eds.), *Monoamine oxidase Inhibitors in Neurological Diseases* (Chapter 15, pp. 295–351). New York: Marcel Dekker.

51. Hudson, J.I., Pope, H.G., Jr., Jonas, J.M., Yurgelun-Todd, D. (1985). Treatment of anorexia nervosa with antidepressants. *J Clin Psychopharmacol, 5(1)*, 17–23.

52. Joyce, P.R., Paykel, E.S. (1989). Predictors of drug response in depression. *Arch Gen Psychiatry, 46(1)*, 89–99.

53. Kaplan, H.I., Sadock, B.J. (1991). *Synopsis of Psychiatry* (pp. 382, 656–667). Baltimore: Williams & Wilkins.

54. Kay, D.W., Garside, R.F., Fahy, T.J. (1973). A double-blind trial of phenelzine and amitriptyline in depressed out-patients. A possible differential effect of the drugs on symptoms. *Br J Psychiatry, 123(572)*, 63–67.

55. Kayser, A., Robinson, D.S., Nies, A., Howard, D. (1985). Response to phenelzine among depressed patients with features of hysteroid dysphoria. *Am J Psychiatry, 142(4)*, 486–488.

56. Kayser, A., Robinson, D.S., Yingling, K., et al. (1988). The influence of panic attacks on response to phenelzine and amitriptyline in depressed out-patients. *J Clin Psychopharmacol, 8(4)*, 246–253.

57. Kelly, D., Guirguis, W., Frommer, E., et al. (1970). Treatment of phobic states with antidepressants. *Br J Psychiatry, 116*, 387–398.

58. Kennedy, S.H., Piran, N., Garfinkel, P.E. (1985). Monoamine oxidase inhibitor therapy for anorexia nervosa and bulimia: A preliminary trial of isocarboxazid. *J Clin Psychopharmacol, 5(5)*, 279–285.

59. Kline, N.S. (1958). Clinical experience with iproniazid (Marsilid). *J Clin Exp Psychopathol, 19(Suppl 1)*, 72–78.

60. Kline, N. (1967). Drug treatment of phobic disorders. *Am J Psychiatry, 123*, 1447–1450.

61. Kramer, A.D., Feiguine, R.J. (1981). Clinical effects of amitriptyline in adolescent depression. *J Am Acad Child Adolesc Psychiatry, 20*, 636–644.

62. Lader, M. (1983). Combined use of tricyclic antidepressants and monoamine oxidase inhibitors. *J Clin Psychiatry, 44(9 pt. 2)*, 20–24.

63. Larsen, J.K. (1988). MAO inhibitors: Pharmacodynamic aspects and clinical implications. *Acta Psychiatr Scand, 345(Suppl)*, 74–80.

64. Larsen, J.K., Holm, P., Mikkelsen, P.L. (1984). Moclobemide and clomipramine in the treatment of depression. A randomized clinical trial. *Acta Psychiatr Scand, 70(3)*, 254–260.

65. Lesse, S. (1978). Tranylcypromine (Parnate)—a study of 1000 patients with severe agitated depressions. *Am J Psychother, 32(2)*, 220–242.

66. Liebowitz, M.R., Quitkin, F.M., Stewart, J.W., et al. (1988). Antidepressant specificity in atypical depression. *Arch Gen Psychiatry, 45(2)*, 129–137.

67. Liebowitz, M.R., Quitkin, F.M., Stewart, J.W., et al. (1984). Psychopharmacologic validation of atypical depression. *J Clin Psychiatry, 45(7 pt. 2)*, 22–25.

68. Liebowitz, M.R., Schneier, F., Campeas, R., et al. (1990). Phenelzine and atenolol in social phobia. *Psychopharmacol Bull, 26(1)*, 123–125.

69. Liebowitz, M.R., Fyer, A.J., Gorman, J.M., et al. (1986). Phenelzine in social phobia. *J Clin Psychopharmacol, 6(2)*, 93–98.

70. Liebowitz, M.R., Quitkin, F.M., Stewart, J.W., et al. (1984). Phenelzine v. imipramine in atypical depression. A preliminary report. *Arch Gen Psychiatry, 41(7)*, 669–677.

71. Loomer, H.P., Saunders, J.C., Kline, N.S. (1958). A clinical and pharmacodynamic evaluation of iproniazid as a psychic energizer. *Psychiatr Res Rep Am Psychiatr Assoc, 8*, 129–131.

72. Mallinger, A.G., Himmelhoch, J.M., Thase, M.E., et al. (1990). Plasma tranylcypromine: Relationship to pharmacokinetic variables and clinical antidepressant actions. *J Clin Psychopharmacol, 10(3)*, 176–183.

73. Mann, J.J., Aarons, S.F., Wilner, P.J., et al. (1989). A controlled study of the antidepressant efficacy and side effects of (-)-deprenyl. *Arch Gen Psychiatry, 46*, 45–50.

74. Mattsson, A., Seltzer, R.L. (1981). MAOI-induced rapid cycling bipolar affective disorder in an adolescent. *Am J Psychiatry, 138(5)*, 677–679.

75. McCabe, B.J. (1986). Dietary tyramine and other pressor amines in MAOI regimens: A review. *J Am Dietetic Assoc, 86(8)*, 1059–1064.

76. McDaniel, K.D. (1986). Clinical pharmacology of monoamine oxidase inhibitors. *Clin Neuropharmacol, 9(3)*, 207–234.

77. McGrath, P.J., Quitkin, F.M., Harrison, W., Stewart, J.W. (1984). Treatment of melancholia with tranylcypromine. *Am J Psychiatry, 141(2)*, 288–289.

78. Modigh, K. (1987). Antidepressant drugs in anxiety disorders. *Acta Psychiatr Scand, 335(Suppl)*, 57–74.

79. Mountjoy, C.Q., Marshall, E.F., Campbell, I.C., et al. (1980). Prediction of response to treatment with phenelzine in neurotic patients. *Prog Neuropsychopharmacol, 4(3)*, 303–308.

80. Mountjoy, C.Q., Roth, M., Garside, R.F., Leitch, I.M. (1977). A clinical trial of phenelzine in anxiety depressive and phobic neuroses. *Br J Psychiatry, 131*, 486–492.

81. Murphy, D.L., Sunderland, T., Cohen, R.M. (1984). Monoamine oxidase-inhibiting antidepressants: A clinical update. *Psychiatr Clin North Am, 7*, 549–562.

82. Murphy, D.L., Brand, E., Goldman, T., et al. (1977). Platelet and plasma amine oxidase inhibition and urinary amine excretion changes during phenelzine treatment. *J Nerv Mental Dis, 164(2)*, 129–134.

83. O'Brien, S., McKeon, P., O'Regan, M., et al. (1992). Blood pressure effects of tranylcypromine when prescribed singly and in combination with amitriptyline. *J Clin Psychopharmacol, 12(2)*, 104–109.

84. O'Brien, S., McKeon, P., O'Regan, M. (1991). A comparative study of the electrocardiographic effects of tranylcypromine and amitriptyline when prescribed singly and in combination. *Int Clin Psychopharmacol, 6(1)*, 11–17.

85. Pare, C.M.B., Kline, N., Hallstrom, C., Cooper, T.B. (1982). Will amitriptyline prevent the "cheese" reaction of monoamine oxidase inhibitors? *Lancet, 2(8291)*, 183–186.

86. Parsons, B., Quitkin, F.M., McGrath, P.J., et al. (1989). Phenelzine, imipramine, and placebo in borderline patients meeting criteria for atypical depression. *Psychopharmacol Bull, 25(4)*, 524–534.

87. Patton, G.C. (1988). Mortality in eating disorders. *Psychol Med, 18(4)*, 947–951.

88. Paykel, E.S. (1971). Classification of depressed patients: A cluster analysis derived grouping. *Br J Psychiatry, 118*, 275–288.

89. Paykel, E.S., West, P.S., Rowan, P.R., Parker, R.R. (1982). Influence of acetylator phenotype on antidepressant effects of phenelzine. *Br J Psychiat, 141*, 243–248.

90. Paykel, E.S., White, J.L. (1989). A European study of views on the use of monoamine oxidase inhibitors. *Br J Psychiatry, 6(Suppl)*, 9–17.

91. Perris, C., Jacobsson, L., von Knorring, L., et al. (1980). Enzymes related to biogenic amine metabolism and personality characteristics in depressed patients. *Acta Psychiatr Scand, 61(5)*, 477–484.

92. (1993). *Physicians' Desk Reference (47th ed.)*. Oradell, N.J.: Medical Economics.

93. Pickar, D., Cohen, R.M., Jimerson, D.C., et al. (1981). Tyramine infusions and selective monoamine oxidase inhibitor treatment II. Interrelationships among pressor sensitivity changes, platelet MAO inhibition, and plasma MHPG reduction. *Psychopharmacology, 74(1)*, 8–12.

94. (1992). *Prescription Pricing Guide*. Indianapolis: Medi-Span.

95. Puig-Antich, J., Blau, S., Marx, N., et al. (1978). Prepubertal major depressive disorder: A pilot study. *J Am Acad Child Psychiatry, 17*, 695–707.

96. Quitkin, F.M., McGrath, P., Liebowitz, M.R. et al. (1981). Monoamine oxidase inhibitors in bipolar endogenous depressives. *J Clin Psychopharmacol, 1(2)*, 70–74.

97. Quitkin, R., Rifkin, A., Klein, D.F. (1979). Monoamine oxidase inhibitors: A review of antidepressant effectiveness. *Arch Gen Psychiatry, 36*, 749–760.

98. Raft, D., Davidson, J., Wasik, J., Mattox, A. (1981). Relationship between response to phenelzine and MAO inhibition in a clinical trial of phenelzine, amitriptyline and placebo. *Neuropsychobiology, 7*, 122–126.

99. Rapoport, J.L., Zametkin, A., Donnelly, M., Ismond, D. (1985). New drug trials in attention deficit disorder. *Psychopharmacol Bull, 21(2)*, 232–236.

100. Raskin, A. (1972). Adverse reactions to phenelzine: Results of a nine-hospital depression study. *J Clin Pharmacol New Drugs, 12(1)*, 22–25.

101. Raskin, A., Schulterbrandt, J.G., Reatig, N., et al. (1974). Depression subtypes and response to phenelzine, diazepam, and a placebo. Results of a nine-hospital collaborative study. *Arch Gen Psychiatry, 30(1)*, 66–75.

102. Raskin, A., Crook, T.A. (1976). The endogenous-neurotic distinction as a predictor of response to antidepressant drugs. *Psychol Med, 6*, 59–70.

103. Ravaris, C.L., Niew, A., Robinson, D.S., et al. (1976). A multiple-dose, controlled study of phenelzine in depression-anxiety states. *Arch Gen Psychiatry, 33*, 347–352.

104. Ravaris, C.L., Robinson, D.S., Ives, J.O., et al. (1980). Phenelzine and amitriptyline in the treatment of depression. A comparison of present and past studies. *Arch Gen Psychiatry, 37(9)*, 1075–1080.

105. Razani, J., White, K.L., White, J., et al. (1983). The safety and efficacy of combined amitriptyline and tranylcypromine antidepressant treatment. A controlled trial. *Arch Gen Psychiatry, 40(6)*, 657–661.

106. Rees, L., Davies, B. (1961). Controlled trial of phenelzine (Nardil) in treatment of severe depressive illness. *J Ment Sci, 107*, 560–566.

107. Reveley, M.A., Glover, V., Sandler, M. Coppen, A. (1981). Increased platelet monoamine oxidase activity in affective disorders. *Psychopharmacology, 73(3)*, 257–260.

108. Rihmer, Z., Arato, M., Bagdy, G. (1983). Association between high platelet MAO activity and response to MAO inhibitor in depressed bipolars: Case reports. *Pharmacopsychiatria, 16(4)*, 119–120.

109. Robinson, D.S., Nies, A., Ravaris, C.L., et al. (1978). Clinical pharmacology of phenelzine. *Arch Gen Psychiatry, 35(5)*, 629–635.

110. Rose, S. (1982). The relationship of acetylation phenotype to treatment with MAOIs: A review. *J Clin Psychopharmacol, 2(3)*, 161–164.

111. Rossel, L., Moll, E. (1990). Moclobemide versus tranylcypromine in the treatment of depression. *Acta Psychiatr Scand, 360(Suppl)*, 61–62.

112. Rutter, M., Tizard, J., Yule, W., et al. (1976). Research report: Isle of Wight studies. *Psychol Med, 6*, 313–332.

113. Ryan, N.D., Puig-Antich, J., Cooper, T., et al. (1986). Imipramine in adolescent major depression. *Acta Psychiatr Scand, 73*, 275–288.

114. Ryan, N.D. (1990). New research: Pharmacologic treatment of adolescent depression. *Psychopharmacol Bull, 26(1)*, 75–79.

115. Ryan, N.D., Puig-Antich, J., Rabinovich, H., et al. V., (1988). MAOIs in adolescent major depression unresponsive to tricyclic antidepressants. *J Am Acad Child Adolesc Psychiatry, 27(6)*, 755–758.

116. Samson, J.A., Gudeman, J.E., Schatzberg, A.F., et al. (1985). Toward a biochemical classification of depressive disorders—VIII. Platelet monoamine oxidase activity in subtypes of depressions. *J Psychiatr Res, 19(4)*, 547–555.

117. Sargant, W. (1961). Drugs in the treatment of depression. *Br Med J, 1*, 225–227.

118. Sargant, W., Dally, P. (1962). Treatment of anxiety states by antidepressant drugs. *Br Med J, 6*, 6–12.

119. Sargant, W. (1962). The treatment of anxiety states and atypical depressions by the monoamine oxidase inhibitor drugs. *J Neuropsychiatry, 3(Suppl 1)*, 96–103.

120. Schoerlin, M.P., Blouin, R.A., Pfefen, J.P., Guentert, T.W. (1990). Comparison of the pharmacokinetics of moclobemide in poor and efficient metabolizers of debrisoquine. *Acta Psychiatr Scand, 360(Suppl)*, 98–100.

121. Schuckit, M., Robins, E., Feighner, J. (1971). Tricyclic antidepressants and monoamine oxidase inhibitors. *Arch Gen Psychiatry, 24(6)*, 509–514.

122. Sheehan, D.V., Ballenger, J., Jacobsen, G. (1980). Treatment of endogenous anxiety with phobic, hysterical and hypochondriacal symptoms. *Arch Gen Psychiatry, 37*, 51–59.

123. Shekim, W.O., Bylund, D.B., Alexson, J., et al. (1986). Platelet MAO and measures of attention and impulsivity in boys with attention deficit disorder and hyperactivity. *Psychiatry Res, 18(2)*, 179–188.

124. Shekim, W.O., Davis, L.G., Bylund, D.B., et al. (1982). Platelet MAO in

children with attention deficit disorder and hyperactivity: A pilot study. *Am J Psychiatry, 139(7)*, 936–938.

125. Shekim, W.O., Hodges, K., Horwitz, E., et al. (1984). Psychoeducational and impulsivity correlates of platelet MAO in normal children. *Psychiatry Res, 11(2)*, 99–106.

126. Shulman, K.I., Walker, S.E., MacKenzie, S., Knowles, S. (1989). Dietary restriction, tyramine, and the use of monoamine oxidase inhibitors. *J Clin Psychopharmacol, 9(6)*, 397–402.

127. Simpson, G.M., de Leon, J. (1989). Tyramine and new monoamine oxidase inhibitor drugs. *Br J Psychiatry Suppl, 6*, 32–37.

128. Singer, T.P. (1987). Perspectives in MAO: Past, present, and future. A review. *J Neural Transm, 23(Suppl)*, 1–23.

129. Soloff, P.H., Cornelius, J., Foglia, J., et al. (1991). Platelet MAO in borderline personality disorder. *Biol Psychiatry, 29(5)*, 499–502.

130. Solyom, C., Solyom, L., LaPierre, Y., et al. (1981). Phenelzine and exposure in the treatment of phobias. *Biol Psychiatry, 16(3)*, 239–247.

131. Solyom, L., Kenny, F., Ledwidge, B. (1969). Evaluation of a new treatment paradigm for phobias. *Can Psychiatr Assoc J, 14*, 3–9.

132. Spiker, D.G., Pugh, D.D. (1976). Combining tricyclic and monoamine oxidase inhibitor antidepressants. *Arch Gen Psychiatry, 33(7)*, 828–830.

133. Stack, C.G., Rogers, P., Linter, S.P.K. (1988). Monoamine oxidase inhibitors and anaesthesia. *Br J Anaesth, 60*, 222–227.

134. Sternbach, H. (1991). The serotonin syndrome. *Am J Psychiatry, 148(6)*, 705–713.

135. Stewart, J.W., McGrath, P.J., Quitkin, F.M., et al. (1989). Relevance of DSM-III depressive subtype and chronicity of antidepressant efficacy in atypical depression. Differential response to phenelzine, imipramine, and placebo. *Arch Gen Psychiatry, 46(12)*, 1080–1087.

136. Stoff, D.M., Friedman, E., Pollock, L., et al. (1989). Elevated platelet MAO is related to impulsivity in disruptive behavior disorders. *J Am Acad Child Adolesc Psychiatry, 28(5)*, 754–760.

137. Sullivan, E.A., Shulman, K.I. (1984). Diet and monoamine oxidase inhibitors: A re-examination. *Can J Psychiatry, 29*, 707–711.

138. Sullivan, J.L., Dackis, C., Stanfield, C. (1977). In vivo inhibition of platelet MAO activity by tricyclic antidepressants. *Am J Psychiatry, 134*, 188–190.

139. Thase, M.E., Mallinger, A.G., McKnight, D., Himmelhoch, J.M. (1992). Treatment of imipramine-resistant recurrent depression, IV: A double-blind crossover study of tranylcypromine for anergic bipolar depression. *Am J Psychiatry, 149(2)*, 195–198.

140. Trott, G.E., Friese, H.J., Menzel, M., Nissen, G. (1992). Use of moclobemide in children with attention deficit hyperactivity disorder. *Psychopharmacology, 106(Suppl)*, 134–136.

141. Ucha Udabe, R., Marquez, C.A., Traballi, C.A., Portes, N. (1990). Double-blind comparison of moclobemide, imipramine and placebo in depressive patients. *Acta Psychiatr Scand, 360(Suppl)*, 54–56.

142. Vallejo, J., Gasto, C., Catalan, R., Salamero, M. (1987). Double-blind study of imipramine versus phenelzine in melancholias and dysthymic disorders. *Br J Psychiatry, 151*, 639–642.

143. Versiani, M., Mundim, F.D., Nardi, A.E., Liebowitz, M.R. (1988). Tranylcypromine in social phobia. *J Clin Psychopharmacol, 8(4)*, 279–283.

144. Versiani, M., Oggero, U., Alterwain, P., et al. (1989). A double-blind comparative trial of moclobemide v. imipramine and placebo in major depressive episodes. *Br J Psychiatry Suppl, 6*, 72–77.

145. Walsh, B.T., Gladis, M., Roose, S.P., et al. (1988). Phenelzine vs placebo in 50 patients with bulimia. *Arch Gen Psychiatry, 45(5)*, 471–475.

146. Walsh, B.T., Stewart, J.W., Roose, S.P., et al. (1984). Treatment of bulimia with phenelzine. A double-blind, placebo-controlled study. *Arch Gen Psychiatry, 41(11)*, 1105–1109.

147. Walsh, B.T., Stewart, J.W., Roose, S.P., et al. (1985). A double-blind trial of phenelzine in bulimia. *J Psychiatr Res, 19(2–3)*, 485–489.

148. Wender, P., Wood, D., Reimherr, F., Word, M. (1983). An open trial of pargyline in the treatment of attention deficit disorder—residual type. *Psychiatry Res, 9*, 329–336.

149. West, E.D., Dally, P.J. (1959). Effect of iproniazid in depressive syndrome. *Br Med J, 1*, 1491–1494.

150. White, K., Pistole, T., Boyd, J.L. (1980). Combined monoamine oxidase inhibitor–tricyclic antidepressant treatment: A pilot study. *Am J Psychiatry, 137(11)*, 1422–1425.

151. White, K., Razani, J., Cadow, B., et al. (1984). Tranylcypromine vs nortriptyline vs placebo in depressed outpatients: A controlled trial. *Psychopharmacology, 82(3)*, 258–262.

152. Wiesel, F.A., Raaflaub, J., Kettler, R. (1985). Pharmacokinetics of oral moclobemide in healthy human subjects and effects on MAO-activity in platelets and excretion of urine monoamine metabolites. *Eur J Clin Pharmacol, 28(1)*, 89–95.

153. Williams, E. (1958). Anorexia nervosa—a somatic disorder. *Br Med J, 2*, 190–195.

154. Wood, D., Reimherr, F., Wender, P. (1983). The use of L-deprenyl in the treatment of attention deficit disorder, residual type. *Psychopharmacol Bull, 19*, 627–629.

155. Youdim, M.B. (1975). Monoamine oxidase. Its inhibition. *Mod Prob Pharmacopsychiatry, 10*, 65–88.

156. Young, W.F., Jr., Laws, E.R., Jr., Sharbrough, F.W., Weinshilboum, R.M. (1986). Human monoamine oxidase. Lack of brain and platelet correlation. *Arch Gen Psychiatry, 43(6)*, 604–609.

157. Young, J.P., Lader, M.H., Hughes, W.C. (1979). Controlled trial of trimipramine, monoamine oxidase inhibitors, and combined treatment in depressed outpatients. *Br Med J, 2(6201)*, 1315–1317.

158. Zametkin, A., Rapoport, J.L., Murphy, D.L., et al. (1985). Treatment of hyperactive children with monoamine oxidase inhibitors. II. Plasma and urinary monoamine findings after treatment. *Arch Gen Psychiatry, 42(10)*, 969–973.

159. Zametkin, A., Rapoport, J.L., Murphy, D.L., et al. (1985). Treatment of hyperactive children with monoamine oxidase inhibitors. I. Clinical efficacy. *Arch Gen Psychiatry, 42(10)*, 962–966.

160. Zimmer, R., Puech, A.J., Philipp, F., Korn, A. (1990). Interaction between orally administered tyramine and moclobemide. *Acta Psychiatr Scan, 360(Suppl)*, 78–80.

161. Zisook, S., Braff, D.L., Click, M.A. (1985). Monoamine oxidase inhibitors in the treatment of atypical depression. *J Clin Psychopharmacol, 5(3)*, 131–137.

C h a p t e r   7

Antipsychotic Agents

Although a mainstay of chemotherapy in adults, antipsychotic agents (also called neuroleptics or major tranquilizers) are far less commonly used in child and adolescent psychiatry. Only seven agents have FDA approval for psychiatric indications in children younger than 12 years. The main causes for controversy are the potentially severe neurologic and developmental sequelae of long-term use and the risks of unpleasant short-term side effects that may hamper learning, socialization, and affect. Therefore, their use is appropriately limited to debilitating psychiatric illness and a duration of treatment that is as short as possible.

Chemical Properties

The prototype antipsychotic is the phenothiazine chlorpromazine (thorazine), discovered over 50 years ago during the synthesis of potential antihistaminic compounds. Since that time, many agents have been developed in an effort to improve efficacy and minimize unwanted effects (Figure 7-1). Neuroleptics may be classified by either chemical structure or relative potency at target receptors (Table 7-1). Antipsychotic agents bind to a number of receptor sites, including dopaminergic, muscarinic cholinergic, serotonergic, alpha-adrenergic,

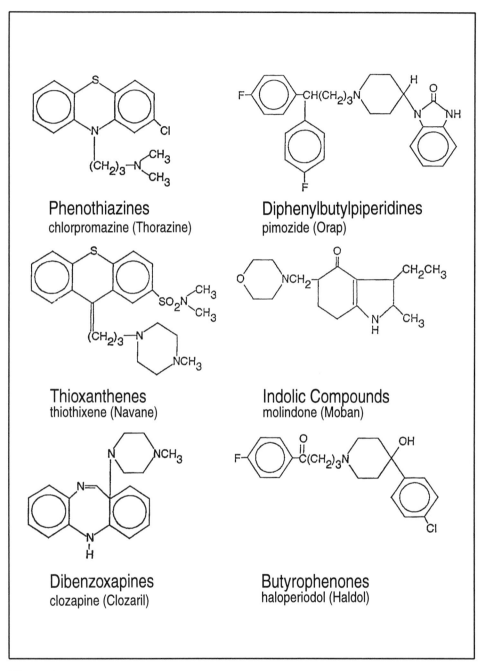

Phenothiazines
chlorpromazine (Thorazine)

Diphenylbutylpiperidines
pimozide (Orap)

Thioxanthenes
thiothixene (Navane)

Indolic Compounds
molindone (Moban)

Dibenzoxapines
clozapine (Clozaril)

Butyrophenones
haloperiodol (Haldol)

Figure 7-1
Sample of Chemical Structures from Major Neuroleptic Classes

Table 7-1
Relative Potencies of Neuroleptics in Clinical Use and at Dopaminergic and Muscarinic Cholinergic Neuroreceptors

Compound	Trade Name	Clinical Potency*	D_2 Affinity*	mACh Affinity†	Dose Range—Adult (mg/day)
Phenothiazines					
Chlorpromazine	Thorazine	1	1.0	330	400–1000
Thioridazine	Mellaril	1	0.72	1300	200–800
Mesoridazine	Serentil	2	1.0	330	100–400
Trifluoperazine	Stelazine	30	7.2	35	15–40
Fluphenazine	Prolixin	50–100	24	13	2.5–10.0
Perphenazine	Trilafon	10	13	16	16–64
Prochlorperazine	Compazine	7	2.6	43	30–150
Thioxanthenes					
Chlorprothixene	Taractan	1	2.5	—	100–600
Thiothixene	Navane	25	42	8.1	20–60
Indolic compounds					
Molindone	Moban	10	0.16	0.062	50–225
Diphenylbutylipiperdines					
Pimozide	Orap	≈50‡	≈5.3	—	1–10
Butyrophenones					
Haloperidol	Haldol	50	4.7	1.0	1–15
Droperidol		—	≈6.2	—	≈8
Dibenzoxapines					
Loxapine	Loxitane	7	0.26	52	60–250
Clozapine	Clozaril	≈1	0.11	2000	300–900

*Clinical potency and affinity for dopamine type 2 receptors expressed as ratios to chlorpromazine.[101,114]
†Affinity for muscarinic cholinergic receptors expressed as ratios to haloperidol.[101,114]
‡Reference 106.

and histaminic.[101] Most are lipophilic and achieve high CNS-to-plasma concentration ratios. Although clinical potency correlates best with the affinity for dopaminergic receptors, these agents often bind to other receptor populations with equal or greater affinity, accounting for common side effects.[33,123] For example, the sedative property of antipsychotics is likely mediated by adrenergic blockade, and the most potent alpha-adrenergic inhibitors (thioridazine, chlorpromazine, clozapine, droperidol) are also the most sedating neuroleptics (Table 7-2).[102] Nearly all antipsychotics are antagonists at serotonin receptors, particularly the newer agent, clozapine.[32]

Central-nervous-system dopamine receptors vary in both form and function. Traditionally, clinical potency has been thought to correlate directly with a neuroleptic's antagonist potency at the type 2 dopamine receptor (D_2). Recent data suggest that this concept is oversimplified. Clozapine has emerged as one of the more effective antipsychotics available in adult schizophrenia, and yet possesses an in vitro affinity for D_2 that is only 11% that of chlorpromazine and 0.5% that of fluphenazine (Table 7-1). Two recent studies using positron emission tomography (PET) and single photon emission computerized tomography (SPECT) to measure in vivo D_2 binding showed that traditional neuroleptics occupy 70–89% of D_2 receptors, while clozapine occupies only 38–63%. Extrapyramidal side effects were more strongly correlated with D_2 occupancy than were clinical effects.[45] Despite lower D_2 occupancy in vivo, clozapine appears to be clinically superior to traditional

Table 7-2
Relative Potency of Neuroleptics for Common Side Effects

Compound	Sedative	Anticholinergic	Extrapyramidal
Phenothiazines			
Chlorpromazine	High	High	Low
Thioridazine	High	High	Low
Trifluoperazine	Medium	Medium	High
Fluphenazine	Medium	Medium	High
Thioxanthenes			
Thiothixene	Low	Low	High
Diphenylbutylpiperidines			
Pimozide	Low	Low	High
Butyrophenones			
Haloperidol	Low	Low	High
Dibenzoxapines			
Clozapine	High	High	Low

Adapted from Keks, N.A., Kulkarni, J., Copolov, D.L.[71]

neuroleptics, while conferring a much lower risk of extrapyramidal side effects.[105]

Currently, at least five subpopulations of dopamine receptor have been isolated in the human CNS (D_1–D_5), with additional genetic variants identified.[53,141] Of these, clozapine has the greatest affinity for D_4.[32] Taken together, these new data suggest that an antipsychotic response in schizophrenic adults is only indirectly related to D_2 receptor blockade, and that selective pharmacologic agents may be able to reduce psychotic symptoms without substantial extrapyramidal side effects.

Absorption and Metabolism

Although the absorption and metabolism of neuroleptics have been widely studied in adults, scant data are available in children. Therefore, the general principles of developmental pharmacology outlined in Chapter 2 bear additional importance. Where data on children are not available, the practitioner must allow for a higher rate of absorption for oral medications, a lower rate of plasma protein binding, a lower percentage of body fat (for lipophilic drugs), and more rapid enzymatic metabolism in prepubescent children. Therefore, higher mg/kg doses are required in children than in adults to achieve comparable plasma levels.[109] Based on these metabolic differences alone, one would suspect that children should receive higher mg/kg doses than equivalent adult doses before declaring the therapeutic failure of an agent. However, Teicher and Glod[138] correctly point out that in the few pharmacokinetic studies available, individual variability in metabolism is far greater than the developmental variability seen across age groups. Therefore, doses in prepubescent children should begin at the equivalent of 0.01–0.05 mg/kg/day of haloperidol and titrated slowly on the basis of individual clinical response and the emergence of side effects.

The metabolism of antipsychotics is hepatic, yielding a substantial first-pass effect for oral preparations and wide variability in plasma level for a given mg/kg dose. Oral doses of phenothiazines, thioxanthenes, and butyrophenones reach a peak plasma level two to three hours after ingestion; IM injections reach peak levels in 30–60 minutes.[35] Metabolites of neuroleptics are excreted primarily through the urine and, to a lesser extent, in bile. Steady-state levels of chlorpromazine have been shown to be two to three and one-half times lower in children than in adults for mass-equivalent doses. In adults, the elimination half-lives of most neuroleptics are in the 10–30-hour range. A marked exception is pimozide, the half-life of which has been shown to vary from 24 to 142 hours in preadolescent children and from 50 to 200 hours in adults.[119] Clozapine, a dibenzodiazepine derivative, recently was tried in psychotic adolescents.[14] Although its metabolism is unstudied in children, the half-life of clozapine in adults is 10–16 hours.[28]

The relationship of plasma level to clinical response is unclear, and is currently rendered academic by the lack of readily available and affordable clinical assays. Smith et al.[130] demonstrated that when compliance was insured, peak and steady-state levels of butaperazine, thioridazine, and haloperidol were significantly lower in chronic nonresponding schizophrenic adults than in treatment responders. This suggests that some treatment failures are due to increased rates of drug clearance and inadequate plasma levels. A simple dose–response relationship has not been described for most neuroleptics, but available data do suggest basic dosing guidelines. In the treatment of schizophrenic adults, Van Putten et al.[142] found that there was little benefit to plasma chlorpromazine levels above 100 ng/ml, and that higher levels increased the incidence of adverse reactions. Within the broad "therapeutic" window of 30–100 ng/ml, plasma level and clinical response were poorly correlated. The findings are similar to those for most other antipsychotic agents, although many studies have found no relationship between plasma level and clinical response. Estimated therapeutic and toxic doses for adult chronic psychosis derived from such studies appear in Table 7-3. The degree to which this experience may be generalized to children and adolescents is unclear.

General Indications

Antipsychotics are, of course, indicated primarily for the treatment of psychosis, and their use for childhood psychosis parallels that in adults. Other

Table 7-3
Suggested Therapeutic and Toxic Plasma Levels of Neuroleptic Drugs (ng/ml), Measured Eight to 12 Hours After Oral Dose

Compound	Therapeutic Range	Toxic Range
Chlorpromazine	>30	>100–150
Fluphenazine	>0.2	>2.0
Haloperidol	>5.0	>20–30
Perphenazine	>0.8	>2.4
Thiothixene	>2.0	>15

Adapted with permission from Dahl, S.G., Hals, P.A.[36]

definite indications include Tourette's syndrome and the short-term symptomatic treatment of severe self-injurious behavior or aggression. Probable indications include severe, treatment-resistant ADHD, pervasive developmental disorders (PDD), and a variety of uses in pediatric medicine (Tables 7-4 and 7-5). Despite these fairly narrow indications, neuroleptics have been tried for most psychiatric diagnoses. Some are approved, but not recommended according to current practice standards, for generalized anxiety and nonspecific behavioral problems. Antipsychotic use in anxiety disorders is limited to cases that have defied standard treatment and have severe functional consequences. In adults, antipsychotics have seen use in personality

Table 7-4

**Psychiatric Indications and Approved Age Ranges
for Neuroleptic Agents***

Compound	Age Range	Approved Indications	Recommended Pediatric Doses
Chlorpromazine	≥6 months	Psychosis, SBD, ADHD, mania[†]	0.25 mg/kg PO q4–h6 or IM q6–8h. Maximum IM dose is 45 mg/day («5 years) or 75 mg/day (15–12 years)
Thioridazine	≥2 years	Psychosis, SBD, ADHD	0.5 mg/kg/day divided b.i.d. or t.i.d. to maximum of 3.0 mg/kg/day in ages 2–12 years
Trifluoperazine	≥6 years	Psychosis, NPA	1–15 mg/day given b.i.d. or t.i.d.
Prochlorperazine	≥2 years	Psychosis, NPA	2.5 mg PO/PR, b.i.d. or t.i.d. to maximum of 20 mg/day (2–5 years) or 25 mg/day (6–12 years)
Chlorprothixene	≥6 years	Psychosis	10–25 mg PO t.i.d. or q.i.d. IM route not recommended for under 12 years
Pimozide	≥2 years[‡]	Tourette's disorder	1–2 mg/day in divided doses. Maximum is lesser of 0.2 mg/kg/day or 10 mg/day
Haloperidol	≥3 years	Psychosis, ADHD, Tourette's, SBD	0.05–0.15 mg/kg/day divided b.i.d. or t.i.d. for psychosis or 0.05–0.075 for others

*Neuroleptic drugs not listed are not recommended for use under 12 years of age. Loxapine and clozapine are not recommended under 16 years. Pediatric doses are not established for these agents.
[†]Abbreviations are as follows: SBD—severe behavioral disorders; MR—mental retardation; ADHD—attention-deficit hyperactivity disorder; NPA—nonpsychotic anxiety.
[‡]Safety of pimozide in children under 12 years of age is not well established.

Table 7-5
Nonpsychiatric Pediatric Indications for Neuroleptic Drugs

Compound	Trade Name(s)	Approved Ages	Approved Indications
Prochlorperazine	Compazine	≥2 years	Nausea/vomiting
Thiethylperazine	Norzine Torcan	≥2 years	Nausea/vomiting
Metoclopramide	Reglan	Any	Nausea/vomiting
Chlorpromazine	Thorazine	≥6 months	Nausea/vomiting Intractable hiccups Preoperative restlessness or anxiety
Trimethobenzamide	Tigan	Any	Nausea/vomiting
Perphenazine	Trilafon	≥12 years	Nausea/vomiting
Promethazine	Phenergan	≥2 years	Nausea/vomiting Motion sickness Allergic reactions Preoperative, postoperative, and obstetric sedation Sedation and sleep
Promethazine + meperidine (narcotic)	Mepergan	Any	Preanesthetic sedation Adjunct to general or local anesthesia

disorders, but both the diagnosis and treatment of personality disorders in children remain controversial. Some agents have been used, but not systematically studied, for child and adolescent OCD.

Schizophrenia

The term childhood schizophrenia has undergone several changes since its first use in the early 1900s. The first descriptions were based on adult symptomatology, altered only to account for developmental stage.[65] Bender[13] initiated a trend to include child cases that did not exhibit what are now termed Schneiderian first-rank symptoms of schizophrenia. Such child cases are now largely subsumed within the diagnoses of PDD and schizoid or schizotypal personality disorders.[8,13,46] These early criteria produced an estimated prevalence for childhood schizophrenia of 1.4 to 4.5 per 10,000 (aged under 13 years).[15,78] The diagnosis of schizophrenia in children is now reserved for patients who meet adult criteria.[8] Based on this definition, Burd and Kerbeshian[19] recently reported the existence of only two cases of schizophrenia in North Dakotan children aged 2 to 12 years (approximately 0.19 per 10,000).

Despite the current application of adult criteria, phenomenologic differences between child- and adult-onset schizophrenia do exist. The distinction is pertinent to the interpretation of early medication trials, the persisting diagnostic confusion between schizophrenia and PDD, and the differential response of these entities to antipsychotic medication. When it appears after puberty, schizophrenia is comparable to the adult syndrome. However, in prepubescent children, the diagnosis is more complicated. The frequency of visual hallucinations appears to be higher in child than in adult schizophrenia,[76] while hallucinatory experiences in general may be less frequent in schizophrenic children younger than 8 years old.[64] Most writers have emphasized developmentally inappropriate formal thought disorder, poorly organized delusional systems, ideas of reference, poor affective regulation, and impaired social functioning as the most selective clinical signs.[12] A single sign in this constellation does not seem to predict an eventual diagnosis of schizophrenia, as many normal developmental phenomena may be construed as psychotic by adult standards, such as imaginary friends, irrational concern about parental safety, and illogical beliefs. Kotsopoulos and colleagues[77] have reported a high frequency of hallucinations (1.1% of psychiatric consults) in children served in a large pediatric outpatient department, none of whom had schizophrenia and all of whom were effectively treated without antipsychotic medication.

Once the diagnosis of schizophrenia is established in a child or adolescent, treatment guidelines parallel those for adult schizophrenia. This is due more to the lack of controlled studies in children than to proven strategies. In the acute phase of adult schizophrenia, all commonly prescribed antipsychotics are superior to placebo in treating psychosis.[75,89,90,114] Maintenance treatment with neuroleptics is likewise superior to placebo in the prevention of relapse, and is influenced by the preservation of social supports and lowered emotional demands.[61]

In one of the few placebo-controlled trials in children, Campbell and associates[24] compared chlorpromazine with lithium in 10 "severely disturbed" children, six of whom were diagnosed with schizophrenia. All of the children with schizophrenia improved when treated with chlorpromazine, based on an examination by a nonblind psychiatrist, and one showed marked improvement.[24] These changes did not reach statistical significance in blind measurements, but analysis included all 10 subjects and was not separately reported for the six with schizophrenia. Spencer et al.[134] have presented the preliminary results of a double-blind, placebo-controlled study of haloperidol in seven schizophrenic children, and these showed marked benefit.

The manifestations of schizophrenia have classically been divided into positive symptoms (hallucinations, delusions, ideas of reference, and formal thought disorder) and negative symptoms (withdrawal, flattening of affect, amotivation, and apathy). While antipsychotic agents are unequivocally effective against the former, the question of whether they treat, aggravate, or have any effect on negative symptoms remains undecided. Meltzer[91] reviewed this issue in adults with emphasis on the confounding factors of psychosocial environment, and determined that antipsychotics probably have a mild beneficial effect on negative symptoms. The contribution of specific antipsychotic side effects to negative symptoms of schizophrenia will be discussed below.

Case History

R., a 13-year-old postpubertal girl, had exhibited a six-month deterioration in functioning that initially consisted of avoidance of group activities, deterioration in school performance, and refusal to complete school assignments. Later she began to refuse to prepare herself for school, and for six weeks she had exhibited even more unusual behavior. She would sit, laughing for no apparent reason, and appear to be listening to something. She felt that people watched her and laughed at her. She believed she smelled and took numerous showers. Within the family, she became increasingly hostile, particularly toward her younger sister. Her handwriting deteriorated. She wrote notes to her friends remarking on her persecution and torment. A few days prior to admission to a psychiatric hospital, she suddenly refused to enter the bathroom, believing that she was being spied on from outside. She gradually became increasingly upset and tearful, talked of God and the Devil speaking to her, and wished to die to end her persecution.

R. was the product of a liaison her mother had had outside of marriage while separated from her husband. She was, therefore, a half-sister to three of her siblings (30-year-old brother, 28-year-old sister, 26-year-old brother), and had a full sister one year younger than herself. R.'s mother later reconciled with her husband. The mother was a high school graduate. She was overtalkative, bossy, and irritable with R. The maternal grandmother had received psychiatric treatment. The natural father was a convert to a fundamentalist religion who lived with his own family in another state. He was not in contact with R. The stepfather was a railroad foreman who seemed calm and appropriate in managing the family situation.

Although the birth history was unremarkable, R. had respiratory problems at 2 weeks of age, which almost led to a crib death. She was cyanotic and required resuscitation. In a nonspecific way, she had always been considered "weak" and sensitive. For example, she had to be walked to sleep throughout her toddler years. She had been placed on tranquilizers for hyperactivity from 18 months to 4 years of age. There were no reported delays in development, and R. was a competent student prior to her illness. However, she had appeared less mature and "sillier" compared with her peers. Psychological testing (after her illness began) revealed a WISC-R full-scale IQ of 90, with verbal and performance scales identical at 91.

Examination of her physical and mental state showed a tall, heavy 13-year-old girl with slow, rigid gait and an air of confusion. Affect was mostly flat, but she had bouts of inappropriate giggling. Her thought patterns showed marked blocking, but other than a slow and deliberate speech, she did not exhibit other thought disorders. She described numerous psychotic symptoms. She felt controlled by God and the Devil, and believed she was being watched. She had auditory, olfactory, tactile, and possibly visual hallucinations. She believed thoughts were inserted into her head and that others would read her mind. The only significant physical findings were orthopedic abnormalities (thoracic kyphosis, lumbar lordosis, spina bifida occulta).

Pharmacologic therapy with haloperidol significantly reduced the psychotic phenomena, and behavioral management techniques were used to address continuing unusual behaviors secondary to her delusional ideas. Because of extrapyramidal side effects, pharmacotherapy was changed to trifluoperazine. On discharge from the hospital, R. continued to have a flat affect and occasional psychotic experiences. In addition, family stresses were apparent. She was referred to a therapist who focused on these family problems and withdrew the medication. R. rapidly returned to her earlier psychotic state and did not respond at the time of follow-up to reinstitution of neuroleptic therapy. (Pomeroy, J.C. (1990). Infantile autism and childhood psychosis. In B.D. Garfinkel, G.A. Carlson, E.B. Welles (Eds.), *Psychiatric Disorders in Childhood and Adolescence* (pp. 288–289). Philadelphia: W.B. Saunders.)

Transient Psychoses

Transient psychotic symptoms are associated with affective disorders such as major depression and bipolar disorder (Chapters 4 and 8), psychoactive drug overdose (Chapter 14), nonschizophreniform paranoid disorders, and organic mental disorders. Paranoid disorders are rarely diagnosed in children, largely because of the difficulty in differentiating transient psychotic symptoms from normal developmental phenomena. However, drug abuse and organic mental disorders are encountered. Although the use of neuroleptics in such cases has not been systematically studied, case studies and clinical practice have demonstrated their effectiveness under certain conditions.

Drug Overdose

Neuroleptics are useful during acute intoxication with psychoactive drugs, especially hallucinogens and phencyclidine (PCP). High-potency agents (haloperidol) in low doses are preferable. However, neuroleptics are contraindicated for sedative overdose and during withdrawal states, as they may further depress consciousness or mask life-threatening withdrawal symptoms. Low-potency agents are not generally useful due to their anticholinergic properties, especially in cases of delirium in which anticholinergic agents may be a suspected cause.[41]

Delirium

Delirium is distinguished from other psychiatric diagnoses by a relatively rapid onset, the presence of a fluctuating level of consciousness, and a known or inferred medical or neurologic cause. Thought is disorganized and the ability to maintain attention is impaired. Sleep/wake cycles are nearly always disrupted, and psychotic symptoms such as hallucinations, formal thought disorder, illusions, and delusions are often present. Diffuse background slowing on an EEG may help to distinguish delirium from other mental syndromes, especially if a previous EEG is available for comparison. Pediatric causes include direct brain injury, CNS neoplasms, Addison's disease, Wilson's disease, hyper- or hypothyroidism, and other metabolic disorders.[67] There are no controlled studies of neuroleptics for these disorders in children, but their use in adult causes of delirium is well documented. Low-dose haloperidol is favored due to its minimal anticholinergic activity.[89] Intravenous haloperidol combined with a benzodiazepine has been advocated for hospitalized, medically ill adults with delirium on the basis that it provides superior response with fewer extrapyramidal side effects (see Chapter 13).[1,92]

Tourette's Syndrome

Gilles de la Tourette described this syndrome of chronic motor and vocal tics in 1885. Current standards define a tic as: "An involuntary, sudden, rapid, recurrent, nonrhythmic, stereotyped motor movement or vocalization. It is experienced as irresistible, but can be suppressed for varying lengths of time."[8]

Although several tic disorders are recognized, only Tourette's syndrome is an approved indication for treatment with neuroleptic agents. Therefore, care must be taken to distinguish Tourette's from other chronic or transient

203

tic disorders. A diagnosis depends on the presence of multiple motor tics (involving more than one muscle group) *and* at least one phonic tic, onset before age 21, and persistence of symptoms beyond one year.[8] More stringent diagnostic criteria have been suggested and are often used in clinical trials, narrowing the age of onset to between 2 and 15 years and requiring the presence of more than one phonic tic.[81] Both motor and phonic tics may take virtually any form. Simple motor tics usually appear early in the disorder, and may include eye blinking, facial grimacing or twitching, shoulder shrugging, or head turning. A simple phonic tic is any respiratory movement that produces a sound, such as grunting, coughing, sighing, sniffing, throat clearing, or unintelligible vocalizations. Complex tics typically arise later in the syndrome, and may include complex motor movements and intelligible words. The most recognized symptom of Tourette's syndrome is coprolalia, or the involuntary utterance of obscenities. Despite its infamy, coprolalia appears in only 20–40% of cases.[81]

Other disorders may mimic Tourette's and must be ruled out before initiating a trial of neuroleptics. If the tics emerged during treatment with psychostimulants for ADHD (see Chapter 3) or with sympathomimetics for asthma, these agents should be discontinued to ensure that the syndrome is not pharmacologically induced. A portion of such cases will have persistent symptoms, but whether psychostimulants can cause Tourette's or they simply speed its emergence in susceptible individuals is unknown (Chapter 3). If the repetitive movements are complex, they may be indistinguishable from the behavioral symptoms of OCD, and this diagnosis must be considered[63] (see Chapter 4). The possibility of partial complex seizures should be ruled out with serial EEGs. However, nonspecific EEG abnormalities are not contrary to the diagnosis, since they occur in as many as half of Tourette's cases.[81]

Two antipsychotic agents are approved for use in Tourette's syndrome: haloperidol (Haldol) and pimozide (Orap). The effectiveness of each has been well demonstrated in a number of placebo-controlled studies,[20,50,72,126,128] but the two agents have not been compared with each other in a double-blind, placebo-controlled design. Sandor et al.[120] reported long-term experience with a retrospective cohort of Tourette's cases treated with haloperidol, pimozide, or no medication over a period of one to 15 years. The pimozide group had significantly fewer adverse side effects and the haloperidol group showed a higher rate of noncompliance, suggesting that pimozide may be more clinically effective despite equal efficacy at symptom reduction.

The most important clinical question, however, is not whether haloperidol or pimozide will reduce the symptoms of Tourette's disorder, as they seem to do this quite reliably, but whether the reduction of symptoms is necessary.

Erenberg[43] estimates that, with appropriate support and education, as many as 50% of patients can tolerate tics without significant functional compromise, and without incurring the risks associated with neuroleptic therapy.

Tourette's is associated with a number of nonspecific behavioral symptoms, such as increased impulsivity, low frustration tolerance, poor concentration and academic performance, impaired social development, and motoric hyperactivity.[81] A concurrent diagnosis of ADHD is common. For patients in whom behavioral symptoms predominate, clonidine should be considered as an alternative to pimozide or haloperidol (see Chapter 11). Stimulants (methylphenidate, *d*-amphetamine, pemoline) are contraindicated in Tourette's, as they greatly increase the severity of tics (Chapter 3).

Pervasive Developmental Disorder

Autism was initially thought by Kanner to be a distinctive manifestation of schizophrenia in childhood,[66] but he later abandoned this idea in favor of a separate classification.[65] The issue was actively debated until the late 1970s when clinical, epidemiologic, and neurophysiologic evidence made a conclusive case for autism as a unique clinical entity.[94] The DSM-III-R now includes autistic disorder as the primary diagnosis in the category of Pervasive Developmental Disorder.[8] Because of the early diagnostic confusion and greater prevalence, more clinical trials of neuroleptics have been conducted on autism than on childhood schizophrenia. Subjects studied in early schizophrenia trials must be considered a mixed diagnostic group of developmental disorders and psychosis, limiting the usefulness of those studies.

A diagnosis of autistic disorder is based on a clinical triad of abnormal development. The child must demonstrate marked impairment in reciprocal social interaction, characteristic abnormalities in verbal and nonverbal communication, and a restricted range of spontaneous interests. After 50 years of research, this definition remains difficult to operationalize. Recent attempts to standardize the diagnosis of autism across research sites have led to the development of structured diagnostic instruments, such as the Autism Diagnostic Interview (ADI)[80] and the Autism Diagnostic Observation Schedule (ADOS).[86] More clinically based instruments, such as the Childhood Autism Rating Scale (CARS), may aid in diagnosis.[121] However, most medication trials on autistic subjects lack standardized methods and their results should be interpreted in the light of probable diagnostic heterogeneity.[129]

Before reviewing the efficacy of neuroleptics in the treatment of autism, it is important to determine what aspects of the disorder are targeted. Autistic children display a broad range of developmental and behavioral pathology, little of which can be expected to respond to pharmacologic intervention.[55] Of the core symptoms, treatment has focused on increasing spontaneous social interaction and communication skills. Associated symptoms that may respond to medication include behavioral impulsivity, hyperactivity, self-injury, and stereotypy. In all cases, the goal of treatment is to ameliorate or compensate for individual symptoms rather than to cure autism.[129]

Magda Campbell and colleagues have been most active in evaluating neuroleptics for this disorder. In the study cited above, only one of the 10 "severely disturbed" children was diagnosed with autism. That child was judged to have improved slightly on chlorpromazine.[24] Subsequent studies from this group evaluated the effects of haloperidol on an exclusively autistic sample. In a comparison of haloperidol and two levels of a response-contingent behavioral paradigm in 40 autistic children, the medication conditions yielded significantly more improvement in stereotypy, withdrawal, and word learning than did the nonmedication conditions. Behavioral treatment was effective in improving imitative speech and compliance.[26] In 1982, Campbell and associates[27] studied a group of 33 subjects treated with haloperidol in a double-blind, placebo-controlled crossover design. Modest, but statistically significant, improvement was noted in withdrawal, stereotypy, abnormal object relations, and performance on a discrimination learning task, while hyperactivity improved markedly. Finally, a more recent study of 45 autistics confirmed the behavioral findings, but failed to demonstrate improved performance on discrimination learning.[9] A recent secondary analysis of these data indicated that within a cumulative sample of 125 autistic children treated with haloperidol, the fraction of subjects who improved varied from 28% to 84%, depending on the outcome measure, and a number of patients worsened.[85] Between 15% and 34% of subjects improved on placebo, although haloperidol was superior to placebo on all measures. Age and higher IQ predicted a better response to haloperidol. Therefore, haloperidol may be relatively less effective in younger autistic children or those with lower IQs. A 1990 presentation by Campbell and associates[21] indicated a similar reduction in behavior problems in three autistic boys treated with pimozide.

It should be noted that these studies are probably not appropriate to address the effect of neuroleptics on learning and socialization. Since severely disruptive behavior precludes normal learning and social interaction, a medication that treats the behavioral symptoms will appear to increase learning and socialization. To evaluate a specific effect on the core symptoms of autism, trials must be conducted on high-functioning, nonretarded individuals who exhibit few associated behavioral symptoms.

In summary, neuroleptics are not indicated as a primary treatment of autistic disorder. Available clinical trials suggest they may be useful in the treatment of associated behavioral symptoms, such as self-injurious behavior, stereotypy, and hyperactivity. However, the data neither support nor refute an effect on the core symptoms of autism.

Attention-Deficit Hyperactivity Disorder

A clinical description of ADHD, as well as of the standard treatment of the disorder, appears in Chapter 3. Neuroleptics are generally not considered for the treatment of ADHD unless standard measures (behavioral therapy, psychostimulants, antidepressants, clonidine) have either failed or are contraindicated. Nevertheless, most reviews of child psychopharmacology mention their use. As with autistic disorder, case reports in ADHD indicate that antipsychotics are most useful for the short-term management of disruptive behavior. Several placebo-controlled studies have reported improvement when neuroleptics were used alone or in combination with stimulants.[51,54,143] Werry and colleagues[146] reported that very low doses of haloperidol were comparable to methylphenidate in treating both hyperactivity and attention in ADHD, but that haloperidol produced more unwanted side effects. In contrast to psychostimulants, neuroleptics have more often been shown to hamper cognitive performance in hyperactive children.[60,135] The positive trials have been criticized on the grounds that they failed adequately to measure cognitive parameters, including attention.[56] In general, the relative success of nonpharmacologic treatment, the cognitive side effects of antipsychotics, and the liability of long-term risks limit the usefulness of neuroleptics, and interest in them, for treating ADHD.

Personality Disorders

Due to the lack of available studies and diagnostic uncertainty regarding severe personality disorders in children, a clinical description of this diverse class of diagnoses will not be included here. However, the benefit of neuroleptics in the treatment of severe character pathology in adults, especially BPD, has long been recognized,[17,42] and recently was subjected to stringent clinical trials.[132,133] Although there is mounting evidence that BPD exists in children and adolescents,[104] there have been no controlled trials of neuroleptics in this population, and their use is not currently recommended.

Nonspecific Behavioral Problems

Behavioral disorders account for the bulk of child psychiatric referrals. Neuroleptics have been used in the treatment of those behaviors that are seen as dangerous or severely disruptive to the child's development, and have failed to respond to behavioral or other pharmacologic measures.

207

Self-Injurious Behavior

Self-injurious behavior (SIB) is a common problem in mental retardation, pervasive developmental disorder, Lesch-Nyhan syndrome, and other genetic syndromes. It has been estimated that 10% of institutionalized mentally retarded individuals exhibit such behaviors.[122] It was also one of the first clinical indications for neuroleptics, with controlled trials dating back to 1958.[2] Pharmacologic intervention should be considered when the behavior is chronic, is severe enough to produce injury, and has failed behavioral treatment and other pharmacologic trials (stimulants, antidepressants, anticonvulsants). Common manifestations include head banging, biting, scratching, picking, and self-mutilation. Severe cases have resulted in subdural hematoma, detached retina, fracture, infection, deformity, and even death.[44,122] Farber[44] has reviewed the available controlled studies, and concludes that although nearly all trials of neuroleptics have reported success in decreasing SIB, it remains uncertain whether the effect is due to dopaminergic blockade or to general sedation.

Severe Aggression

Severe aggression is also associated with many child psychiatric diagnoses, particularly developmental disorders, conduct disorder, and ADHD. Pharmacologic treatment alone is not sufficient in any case, but may be used in a limited fashion to augment a broader treatment program.[136] Neuroleptics have been shown to be helpful in aggression appearing specifically in conduct disorder,[22,145] in ADHD,[6] and in mixed diagnostic groups.[24,34] Several agents have FDA approval for severe behavioral disruption in children (Table 7-4).

Nonspecific Agitation

Nonspecific agitation, such as is often encountered in severely retarded children, anxiety disorders, and situational reactions, has resulted in the use of sedating neuroleptics on a short-term basis. Specific behavior may include restlessness, pacing, verbal disruption, or property destruction. Several agents are approved for episodes of severe agitation, subsumed under the terms "severe behavioral disruption" and "nonpsychotic anxiety" (Table 7-4). However, neuroleptics should not be considered first in such situations, and may produce side effects (akathisia) that exacerbate the symptoms.

Especially in institutionalized children and adults, the chronic prescription of neuroleptics without clear diagnostic indications has been deemed an epidemic problem in mental health care, accounting for 30–55% of neuroleptic prescriptions in *reporting* institutions.[62,83,147] There is some evidence that such use is declining.[69,112] The current availability of diagnostically specific treatments, the sequelae of chronic neuroleptic exposure, and the existence of sedative agents with vastly superior benefit-to-risk profiles (such as benzo-diazepines) render the long-term use of neuroleptics inappropriate as a non-specific behavioral sedative.

Uses in Pediatric Medicine

Nausea and Vomiting

Nausea and vomiting are ameliorated by low-potency neuroleptics, especially the phenothiazines. Seven neuroleptics are approved for this use, not all of which are approved for psychiatric indications (Table 7-5). The most appropriate indication for neuroleptics as antiemetic agents is in the treatment of severely medically ill children, such as cancer patients undergoing chemotherapy, when vomiting places them at serious risk. Their use for emesis during pregnancy should be limited due to potential damage to a fetus, although specific malformations and substantially increased risk with in utero exposure have not been demonstrated (see "Contraindications"). It should be noted that in several of the case reports of severe dystonia or neuroleptic malignant syndrome appearing in the pediatric literature, the condition arose after only a brief exposure to antiemetics.[74,139]

Sedation

Sedation prior to surgery or office procedures is a common, but controversial indication for neuroleptics. In particular, the DPT cocktail, an injected combination of the narcotic analgesic Demerol (meperidine) and the phenothiazines Phenergan (promethazine) and Thorazine (chlorpromazine), has come under criticism. This combination is used in children's emergency rooms and clinics for surgical and orthopedic procedures and has been associated with the full spectrum of neuroleptic side effects.[131] If neuroleptics must be used, close monitoring for dystonia, akathisia, and extrapyramidal symptoms is necessary. Alternative means of sedation are vastly preferable.

Intractable Hiccups and Motion Sickness

These are infrequent applications for which some neuroleptics have been approved, but they cannot be recommended for such purposes (Table 7-5).

Contraindications

See Table 7-6.

The only absolute contraindications to neuroleptics are type IV hypersensitivity, acute agranulocytosis, and current episodes of neuroleptic malignant syndrome (NMS). However, probable contraindications include comatose or obtunded patients, patients who have received high doses of CNS depres-

Table 7-6
Contraindications to Neuroleptic Therapy

Definite
• Hypersensitivity to neuroleptics
• Agranulocytosis associated with neuroleptics
• Neuroleptic malignant syndrome (acute)
Probable
• Comatose or obtunded patients
• Patients receiving high-dose CNS depressants
• Preexisting bone marrow suppression
• Subcortical temperature
Relative
• History of neuroleptic malignant syndrome
• Pregnancy

sants (such as narcotics or barbiturates), patients with a history of blood dyscrasias or bone marrow suppression (especially if related to neuroleptic use), and the presence of subcortical brain injury with temperature dysregulation. Relative contraindications include pregnancy and previous NMS, both of which bear further discussion.

Past Episode of NMS

This rare, potentially fatal reaction to dopamine antagonists is described below (see "Adverse Reactions"). When a nonpsychotic patient has a history of NMS, retreatment with antipsychotic agents is contraindicated. However, many victims of NMS require continuation of treatment for chronic psychosis. Recent studies on schizophrenic adults suggest that the risk of recurrent NMS upon restarting neuroleptic therapy may be lower than predicted.

Addonizio and colleagues[3] reviewed 115 case studies and found that the authors reported reinstitution of therapy in 26 cases, 10 of which saw a recurrence of NMS. Pelonero and associates[100] reviewed the cases in which neuroleptics were reinstituted, and recommended that an agent from a different chemical class be chosen, one of lower potency and at the lowest possible dose. Both groups of authors recommended intensive monitoring for fever and laboratory markers of NMS with rechallenge. However, retrospective reviews of NMS recurrence are confounded by trends in clinical practice over the past two decades, most significantly that maintenance doses are lower now than in the past. Recently, Rosebush and associates[115] successfully reinitiated neuroleptic therapy in 13 of 15 cases of NMS with no apparent relationship to neuroleptic dose or potency. Similarly, Pope and colleagues[108] rechallenged 11 of 20 consecutive cases of NMS and found no recurrences of NMS even with long-term neuroleptic treatment. However, the risk of recurrent NMS has not been assessed in children. Retreatment should be attempted only when neuroleptic therapy is clearly necessary and alternative treatments have failed.

Pregnancy

Animal studies have shown an increase in congenital anomalies, a decrease in viability, and abnormal neuronal growth with prolonged, high-dose exposure to antipsychotic agents in utero.[40] Human studies, however, consist largely of psychiatrically normal populations who received short-term, low-dose neuroleptics for emesis. Therefore, it is difficult to differentiate the risk of neuroleptic exposure from that of the multiple causes of severe emesis. In these populations, there have been reports of a slightly increased, but statistically insignificant, risk of birth defects, especially for exposure during the first trimester.[39,93,118] Interestingly, one of the few controlled studies found that a retrospective cohort of children exposed to neuroleptics for at least two months in utero had significantly increased height and weight, as compared with controls.[107]

A recent survey in France found no increased risk of malformation in children of schizophrenic mothers who were exposed to neuroleptics in utero.[52] Therefore, although psychotropic medication should always be avoided in pregnancy when possible, current experience does not indicate a significantly higher risk of birth defects at therapeutic doses of antipsychotics. Their use may be warranted when the symptoms of psychosis are judged to be a health risk to the mother and fetus.

Side Effects and Adverse Reactions

See Table 7-7.

The term neuroleptic literally means "agent that causes neurologic dysfunction." As such, it highlights the potential toxicity of this category of medication and the reason for controversy surrounding the use of these agents in children.

Anticholinergic Effects

Anticholinergic side effects are those common to atropine-like agents, including blurred vision, exacerbation of narrow-angle glaucoma, constipation, agitation, and delirium. Table 7-1 indicates the relative anticholinergic potency of common antipsychotic agents, as well as their affinity for other neuro-receptors. Highly anticholinergic agents should be avoided when these side effects are of concern, such as in the presence of delirium, other anticholiner-

Table 7-7

Side Effects and Adverse Reactions to Neuroleptics

Short Term	Long Term	Idiosyncratic
Extrapyramidal symptoms Acute dystonia Cardiac arrythmias Anticholinergic symptoms Akathisia Sedation Affective blunting Cognitive dulling Social withdrawal	Tardive dyskinesia Hyperprolactinemia Hepatic toxicity Ocular pigmentation	Neuroleptic malignant syndrome Agranulocytosis Sudden death

gic agents (antidepressants), glaucoma, encopresis, or neurologic illness in which the level of consciousness must be monitored.

Extrapyramidal Symptoms

Extrapyramidal symptoms (EPS) are common effects of antipsychotic therapy and their severity is proportional to the degree of dopaminergic blockade. The usual presentation is of a parkinsonian-like syndrome including muscular rigidity with or without cogwheeling, tremor, bradykinesia, masked facies, shuffling or festinating gait, and drooling. These effects are most common with high-potency neuroleptics possessing little or no anticholinergic and antihistaminic properties, but can be produced with higher doses of low-potency agents.

The proposed mechanism of EPS is the interruption of inhibitory dopaminergic input to the caudate nucleus by D_2 receptor blockers. As discussed under "Chemical Properties," the severity of EPS is most closely correlated with the percent of D_2 receptor blockade, and is greatly reduced with clozapine. When dopaminergic inhibition of the caudate is interrupted, the net effects are increased excitatory cholinergic activity in the caudate and parkinsonian abnormalities of movement.[68] The two main pharmacologic approaches to treating EPS are based on this mechanism: anticholinergic agents that reduce cholinergic activity in the caudate, and dopaminergic agonists that increase nigrostriatal inhibition of the caudate.

Anticholinergic drugs used to treat EPS include both specific and nonspecific agents, many with significant antihistaminic activity as well. These include benztropine (Cogentin, Tremin), biperiden (Akineton), and trihexyphenidyl (Artane). Diphenhydramine (Benadryl) is primarily antihistaminic, but has significant anticholinergic activity and is more sedating than the other agents. Specific treatment guidelines are given below.

Dopamine agonists (L-dopa, bromocriptine, amantadine) have been used in adults to treat EPS by enhancing dopamine transmission in the nigro-striatal tract. As one might predict, a significant side effect of this approach is increased psychosis, mania, or agitation. Most adults appear to tolerate the cautious use of dopamine agonists, and often report fewer unpleasant side effects than with anticholinergics. Amantadine is well studied, and probably has the lowest risk of increasing psychosis.[7] In contrast, L-dopa has been ineffective in open trials, and may have a higher incidence of side effects.[58]

Although amantadine has been used as an antiviral agent in children and has seen limited (unsuccessful) testing for ADHD, its safety has not been established. One single-blind crossover trial exists that compared amantadine with benztropine for the treatment of EPS in children with Tourette's syndrome. Of seven patients, six developed akathisia, four experienced dystonic reactions, and four developed parkinsonian symptoms upon treatment with haloperidol. Amantadine and benztropine were equally effective in reducing parkinsonian symptoms, but amantadine appeared to be superior against dystonia and akathisia.[16] Despite this finding, dopamine agonists must be considered an experimental treatment for EPS in children an adolescents until safety and efficacy are more firmly established.

Acute Dystonia

Dystonia is also more common with high-potency agents. This effect is characterized by the sudden development of cramping and pain, usually involving head, neck, and back musculature, and can be severe enough to compromise respiration or cause skeletal injury. Oculogyric or opisthotonic crises may occur, and, untreated, can be life-threatening. Subacute cases may present with dysarthria, jaw or tongue cramping, or dysphagia.

Treatment
The treatment of dystonic reactions is based on the rapid introduction of antiparkinsonian agents. Intramuscular or IV injection of diphenhydramine (50 mg) or benztropine (2 mg) is often sufficient for large children and adolescents, although intermittent dosing may be necessary. Initial doses may be reduced for smaller children, although dystonic reactions are less common in preadolescents.[23] If dystonia fails to resolve within 15 to 20 minutes after the first injection, the dose is repeated, followed by either a third dose or augmentation with a rapid-acting benzodiazepine (lorazepam, 1 mg IM or IV), if needed. Long-term management includes a decrease or discontinuation of the antipsychotic agent, changing to a lower-potency agent, or the addition of regular doses of antiparkinsonian agents (Table 7-8). As noted above, recurrent dystonia may respond to amantadine.

Table 7-8
Acute Management of Adverse Reactions

Reaction	Management*
Anticholinergic symptoms	Decrease dose. Eliminate concurrent anticholinergic drugs. Change to higher-potency agent.
Extrapyramidal symptoms	Decrease dose. Add antiparkinsonian agent (e.g., benztropine or biperiden).
Acute dystonia	Airway management. Diphenhydramine 50 mg IM or IV. *or* Benztropine 2 mg IM (may repeat dose every 15–20 minutes). Lorazepam 1–2 mg IM or IV.
Akathisia	Decrease dose. Antiparkinsonian agents may be ineffective. Propranolol 10–30 mg t.i.d. *or* Clonazepam 0.5–1.0 mg b.i.d.
Neuroleptic malignant syndrome	Discontinue neuroleptics. Cardiorespiratory support. Hydration. May use bromocriptine 2.5–10 mg t.i.d. *or* Dantrolene 1–3 mg/kg/day, divided. Benzodiazepines may alleviate agitation and rigidity.
Hyperprolactinemia	Reduce or discontinue medication. Amantadine 100–300 mg/day, divided, may be effective.

*Doses and safety of pharmacologic approaches are not established in preadolescents.

Akathisia

Akathisia is the frequent subjective complaint of a need for constant movement. This may or may not be observed on exam as restlessness, agitation, or motoric hyperactivity. In fact, although exceedingly unpleasant for patients, it may yield no observable change in behavior, and may be indistinguishable from anxiety. The mechanism underlying this side effect of antipsychotics is unknown, but is thought to be mediated by extrapyramidal D_2 blockade, and is reduced or absent with agents that show low D_2 occupancy (clozapine). Again, decreasing the antipsychotic dose may be effective. Antiparkinsonian agents may provide some relief, but are often less effective at reducing akathisia than parkinsonian EPS. In adults, beta-adrenergic blocking agents are best studied, and appear to be the current medication of choice for neuroleptic-induced akathisia. Propranolol, a nonselective, lipophilic beta-adrenergic antagonist, has been used most widely at doses of 20–40 mg t.i.d. However, selective beta-1 (betaxolol and metoprolol) and beta-2 (ICI 118,551) antagonists have been equally effective in double-blind trials.[5,38,73] Interestingly, nadolol, a nonlipophilic beta-blocker, appears to be ineffective at reducing akathisia, suggesting that central rather than peripheral beta-adrenergic receptor blockade is required.[144] Whether beta-adrenergic agents are safe or effective for children with akathisia remains unclear, and safety must be better demonstrated before this approach can be recommended (see Chapter 11).

Trials of benzodiazepines suggest that these agents may be equal in efficacy, but controlled and long-term studies are few. Both diazepam[37] and clonazepam[79] have been shown to be beneficial for adults with akathisia, but neither has been compared with propranolol in a controlled fashion.

Clonidine has been tried for akathisia with mixed results and is untested in children for this indication.

Movement Disorders

Abnormal involuntary movements are the most common long-term side effect of neuroleptic use, but may also be seen with other medications and disorders (Table 7-9). There are several manifestations, mostly involving involuntary, often unconscious, movements of the tongue, face, and neck. Muscle groups with the densest motor innervation are the most severely affected, so that dyskinesias of the hands and feet are next most common, followed by limb and trunk movements. Specific movements may appear choreoathetoid, ticlike, or even as mimicking voluntary habits.[137] Movements that appear after lowering or discontinuing medication are termed withdrawal dyskinesia, while those that appear during chronic administration are called tardive dyskinesia. The latter manifestation is rare in patients exposed to neuroleptic treatment for less than six months. Although long thought to be irreversible, there are cases of tardive dyskinesia that resolve over time, or with dopamine agonist treatment (L-dopa or amantadine).[10,87] There are reports of dyskinesia appearing after as little as one dose of a low-potency neuroleptic. However, in general, risk increases with the age of the patient (particularly over 50 years), the length of exposure, and the potency of dopamine blockade.

Since there is no proved treatment for neuroleptic-induced dyskinesia, proper management involves thorough pretreatment counseling, minimiza-

Table 7-9
Nonneuroleptic Causes of Tardive Dyskinesia

Medications
• L-dopa
• Amphetamines
• Anticholinergics
• Antidepressants
• Lithium
• Phenytoin
Psychiatric conditions
• Stereotypes of schizophrenia or autism
• Spontaneous oral dyskinesia of old age or senility
• Oral dyskinesias secondary to dentures or dental conditions
• Idiopathic torsion dystonia
• Tourette's disorder and simple tics
Medical/neurologic conditions
• Wilson's disease
• Huntingdon's disease
• Fahr's syndrome
• Postanoxic and encephalitic EPS
• Sydenham's chorea
• CNS manifestation of systemic metabolic disorder
• CNS neoplasm

Adapted from Task Force on Late Neurological Effects of Antipsychotic Drugs. (1980). Tardive dyskinesia: Summary of a Task Force Report of the American Psychiatric Association. *Am J Psychiatry, 137(10)*, 1163–1172.

tion of neuroleptic dose and exposure, and periodic standardized examination for involuntary movements. The Abnormal Involuntary Movement Scale (AIMS) is useful for this purpose (Figures 7-2A and 7-2B).[97]

Neuroleptic Malignant Syndrome

A potentially life-threatening adverse reaction to neuroleptics, NMS is characterized by hyperthermia, "lead pipe" muscular rigidity, altered mental status, hyper- or hypotension, tachycardia, diaphoresis, and pallor. Laboratory findings include myoglobinuria and elevated white blood cell count and muscle and hepatic enzymes. The clinical picture may be mistaken for psychosis, catatonia, EPS, infection, or fever of unknown origin.[59] Levenson[82] has suggested diagnostic criteria for NMS. In a review of 53 cases, he found fever, rigidity, and elevated creatinine phosphokinase (CPK) to be major manifestations, and tachycardia, abnormal blood pressure, tachypnea, altered consciousness, diaphoresis, and leukocytosis to be minor manifestations. The

		(Circle One)				

PATIENT'S NAME

RATER

DATE

ABNORMAL INVOLUNTARY MOVEMENT SCALE (AIMS)

INSTRUCTIONS: Complete Examination Procedure (reverse side) before making ratings.
MOVEMENT RATINGS: Rate highest severity observed.

Code: 0 = None
1 = Minimal, may be extreme normal
2 = Mild
3 = Moderate
4 = Severe

		(Circle One)
FACIAL AND ORAL MOVEMENTS:	1. Muscles of Facial Expression e.g., movements of forehead, eyebrows, periorbital area, cheeks; including frowning, blinking, smiling, grimacing	0 1 2 3 4
	2. Lips and Perioral Area e.g., puckering, pouting, smacking	0 1 2 3 4
	3. Jaw e.g., biting, clenching, mouth opening, lateral movement	0 1 2 3 4
	4. Tongue Rate only increase in movement both in and out of mouth NOT inability to sustain movement	0 1 2 3 4
EXTREMITY MOVEMENTS:	5. Upper *(arms, wrists, hands, fingers)* Include choreic movements (i.e. rapid, objectively purposeless, irregular, spontaneous), athenoid movements (i.e., slow, irregular complex, serpentine) Do NOT include tremor (i.e., repetitive, regular, rhythmic)	0 1 2 3 4
	6. Lower *(legs, knees, ankles, toes)* e.g., lateral knee movement, foot tapping, heel dropping, foot squirming, inversion and eversion of foot	0 1 2 3 4
TRUNK MOVEMENTS:	7. Neck, shoulders, hips e.g., rocking, twisting, squirming, pelvic gyrations	0 1 2 3 4
GLOBAL JUDGMENTS:	8. Severity of abnormal movements	None, normal 0 Minimal 1 Mild 2 Moderate 3 Severe 4
	9. Incapacitation due to abnormal movements	None, normal 0 Minimal 1 Mild 2 Moderate 3 Severe 4
	10. Patient's awareness of abnormal movements Rate only patient's report	No awareness 0 Aware, no distress 1 Aware, mild distress 2 Aware, moderate distress 3 Aware, severe distress 4
DENTAL STATUS:	11. Current problems with teeth and/or dentures	No 0 Yes 1
	12. Does patient usually wear dentures?	No 0 Yes 1

Source: NIMH. AIMS (Abnormal Involuntary Movement Scale). *Psychopharmacology Bulletin*, 21:1077-1080.

Figure 7-2A
Abnormal Involuntary Movement Scale (AIMS)

Either before or after completing the Examination Procedure, observe the patient unobtrusively, at rest (e.g., in waiting room).

The chair to be used in this examination should be a hard, firm one without arms.

1. Ask patient whether there is anything in his/her mouth (i.e., gum, candy, etc.), and if there is, to remove it.

2. Ask patient about the *current* condition of his/her teeth. Ask patient if he/she wears dentures. Do teeth or dentures bother patient *now*?

3. Ask patient whether he/she notices any movements in mouth, face, hands, or feet. If yes, ask to describe and to what extent they *currently* bother patient or interfere with his/her activities.

4. Have patient sit in chair with hands on knees, legs slightly apart, and feet flat on the floor. (Look at entire body for movements while in this position.)

5. Ask patient to sit with hands hanging unsupported. If male, between legs; if female and wearing a dress, hanging over knees. (Observe hands and other body areas.)

6. Ask patient to open mouth. (Observe tongue at rest within mouth.) Do this twice.

7. Ask patient to protrude tongue. (Observe abnormalities of tongue in movement.) Do this twice.

* 8. Ask patient to tap thumb, with each finger, as rapidly as possible for 10-15 seconds; separately with right hand, then with left hand. (Observe facial and leg movements.)

9. Flex and extend patient's left and right arms (one at a time). (Note any rigidity and rate on DOTES.)

10. Ask patient to stand up. (Observe in profile. Observe all body areas again, hips included.)

*11. Ask patient to extend both arms outstretched in front with palms down. (Observe trunk, legs, and mouth.)

*12. Have patient walk a few paces, turn, and walk back to chair. (Observe hands and gait.) Do this twice.

*Activated movements

Examiner's Comments _____

_____

_____

_____

_____

_____

Figure 7-2B

presence of all three major, or two major plus four minor, manifestations is diagnostic of NMS, if the clinical history supports this.[82]

Adityanjee[4] has cautioned against overdependence on CPK levels to diagnose NMS, since mild elevations in CPK are common in agitated patients, in those receiving IM injections, and in active children. Therefore, levels below 1000 U/L may not be a manifestation of NMS. Specific diagnostic criteria are still debated, but most descriptions emphasize the presence of four main features: fever, muscular rigidity, altered level of consciousness, and autonomic dysregulation.[98] Although specific risk factors are not known, high-potency agents, multiple antipsychotics, and polypharmacy have been implicated. Keck et al.[70] compared 18 cases of NMS with controls, and found significantly higher neuroleptic doses, rates of dosage increase, and number of IM doses among the NMS cases.

Occurrence

Occurrence rates have been estimated at between 0.5% and 1.4%, based on the number of reported cases and estimates of the number of patients exposed to neuroleptics.[116] However, since cases have been reported for even brief or accidental exposure to neuroleptics,[18,74,95,139] the number of patients at risk is probably underestimated in these studies. Keck et al.[69] prospectively tracked 2695 patients treated with neuroleptics and saw only four cases of NMS, or 0.15%. A number of cases have been reported in children as young as 11 months of age,[99] although differential risk factors and treatment methods for children have been virtually unexplored.

Treatment

The treatment of mild cases may require only supportive measures and cessation of all antidopaminergic and anticholinergic medication. However, treatment with the dopamine agonist bromocriptine or the peripheral muscle relaxant dantrolene has been advocated.[116] Close monitoring of cardiac and renal status is required to avoid arrhythmias and myonecrotic kidney failure respectively. Fever may reach 41°C or higher, requiring hydration and cooling. Bromocriptine mesylate, at (adult) doses of 2.5 to 10 mg t.i.d., appears to improve rigidity and mental status through central dopaminergic stimulation, while sodium dantrolene, in four divided doses of 1–3 mg/kg/day, decreases rigidity, tachycardia, and myonecrosis through direct action on musculature. Both agents may be used simultaneously.[57,59,82] Rosenberg and Green[116] reviewed available case reports and compared the speed of recovery for patients treated with supportive measures alone with that for patients treated with bromocriptine or dantrolene. They found that the mean response and recovery times for either pharmacologic treatment were significantly shorter than for supportive treatment alone. This observation, combined with the low incidence of adverse reactions to dantrolene or bromo-criptine, strongly supports pharmacologic treatment of NMS. Other authors have argued that improvements in supportive care techniques may account for these results,[99] and one prospective study of 24 cases found no advantage of medication over supportive care alone.[117]

Mortality

Mortality has been estimated from reviews of adult NMS case reports at 11–22%.[3,82,124,125] Shalev and colleagues[124] reviewed 202 cases of NMS and concluded that mortality has significantly decreased from 25% before 1984 to 11.6% currently, independent of the use of dantrolene or bromocriptine. The strongest predictors of poor outcome in their analysis were myoglobinu-ria and renal failure. Mortality in the presence of these two factors was esti-mated at 50%.

Reinstitution

The reinstitution of neuroleptics in a patient who has recovered from NMS is discussed under "Contraindications."

Sudden Death

Several case reports exist describing sudden, unexplainable demise during treatment with high-potency neuroleptics. In particular, haloperidol and droperidol have been associated with death during the administration of high, but clinically acceptable, injected doses. The mechanisms and relative risk of this rare reaction are unknown.

Other Side Effects

Secondary receptor mechanisms underlie a variety of neuroleptic side ef-fects. Low-potency agents commonly produce postural hypotension and/or syncope, presumably through adrenergic blockade, and may produce quini-dine-like effects on cardiac conduction. Cases of heart block and ventricular tachycardia have been reported, especially in overdose. Pimozide and thiorid-azine are notable for higher incidences of QT prolongation and reports of ar-rhythmias even at therapeutic doses.

Agranulocytosis

Reported hematologic effects include leukopenia, thrombocytopenia, and lym-phopenia. However, the most serious of these is rare, idiosyncratic agranulo-cytosis. Prior to the introduction of clozapine, agranulocytosis occurred in less than 1:2000 cases of, mainly, phenothiazine use. With the recent intro-duction of clozapine, this adverse effect has become of greater concern. As of

December 1989, the manufacturer reported agranulocytosis in 1.3% of patients receiving clozapine, with 32% proving fatal. However, since implementation of mandatory weekly blood monitoring with the prescription of clozapine, the mortality rate has dropped substantially. Since January 1991, 68 cases of agranulocytosis were reported, with one fatality. The manufacturer continues to require that each treatment center assess hematologic and cardiac effects weekly in patients receiving clozapine.

Hyperprolactinemia

Prolonged dopaminergic blockade may produce hyperprolactinemia by interfering with dopamine's role in inhibiting prolactin secretion via tuberoinfundibular projections to the anterior pituitary. Possible clinical effects include galactorrhea (both females and males), amenorrhea, and impotence. Neuroleptic-induced hyperprolactinemia has been successfully treated in adults with dopamine agonists (bromocriptine and amantadine),[30,31,88,128] although these agents bear the risk of producing or exacerbating psychosis and mania in some cases.[113,140] Dopaminergic agonists have not been tested for neuroleptic-induced side effects in children, and the emergence of endocrine abnormalities should prompt the reduction or cessation of neuroleptics whenever possible.

Other Adverse Effects

Other adverse effects include increased risk of seizure, hepatic toxicity (especially with chlorpromazine), photosensitivity, and ocular pigmentation.

Overdose

The therapeutic index of most neuroleptics is high with regard to lethal toxicity (Table 7-3). Severe side effects of dopamine blockade usually ensue, and constitute a medical emergency, before lethal plasma levels are reached (see "Acute Dystonia"). With pimozide or thioridazine, cardiac arrhythmias may appear sooner rather than later in the progression of toxic symptoms. Signs and symptoms of toxicity include severe forms of the side effects noted above, CNS and cardiovascular depression, severe hypotension, and respiratory depression. Hypertension has been reported with childhood overdoses of haloperidol. An overdose of agents with potent anticholinergic properties may present as delirium.

The treatment of neuroleptic overdose is supportive and symptomatic, as there are no antidotes. Extrapyramidal symptoms and NMS are treated as described in those sections. Cardiac monitoring and respiratory support are needed. There are few reports of death from an overdose of neuroleptics.

Abuse/Dependence

Because of their unpleasant side effects and nonreinforcing primary effects, these medications are not generally abused. Tolerance is not described in the classic sense, although receptor up-regulation, decreased tissue sensitivity, and withdrawal syndromes are described. Abrupt withdrawal is most often associated with transient dyskinesia and psychosis. The emergence of psychotic symptoms after withdrawal of a long-term neuroleptic is sometimes termed supersensitivity psychosis, and is thought to be a result of dopamine receptor up-regulation and subsequent overstimulation upon removal of the drug.

Available Preparations

See Table 7-10.

For most applications in children and adolescents, antipsychotics are administered orally. Intramuscular preparations are available for conditions in which rapid absorption is desirable, such as for sedation. Most neuroleptics are highly lipophilic, allowing for oil-based depot preparations that may be used to extend normal half-lives. This is desirable only when the chronic use of high-potency neuroleptics is clearly indicated, but extremely long half-lives are needed for convenience or compliance—conditions that are rarely, if ever, met in the treatment of children. Currently, haloperidol ($t_{1/2}$ = approximately 21 days) and fluphenazine ($t_{1/2}$ = 7–10 days) decanoates are available for monthly or twice-monthly injections respectively.

Initiating and Maintaining Treatment

It is advisable to complete diagnostic procedures prior to neuroleptic treatment, when possible. Antipsychotic agents have been shown to produce abnormalities on EEG, psychometric testing, and neurologic examination. Baseline CBCs with differential and hepatic enzymes are needed for comparison if abnormalities arise during treatment. If therapy is likely to be long term, an initial CPK and an ECG are likewise advisable. Prior to treatment, patients and their parents should be informed of the risks both of side effects and of adverse reactions, as noted above, and of the risk of nontreatment. A screen for abnormal involuntary movements (AIMS) is usually included in the initial neurologic examination to rule out preexisting movement disorders. Although no specific teratogenic effects have been described with these agents, a negative pregnancy test and adequate contraceptive use are preferred (see "Contraindications").

Since dystonia, akathisia, and anticholinergic and hematologic effects generally appear within the first two months of starting or increasing medication, it is advisable to monitor these closely after initiating treatment with anti-psychotics. Particularly with long-acting agents, blood levels may require up to 50 days to reach steady state, so that continual adjustment of EPS treatment may be required. Neuroleptic malignant syndrome, dyskinesia, and idiosyncratic agranulocytosis may appear at any time during therapy. The AIMS exam, a CBC with differential, transaminases, and CPK should be repeated at six-month intervals. Electrocardiograms should follow any dose change of pimozide or thioridazine, in particular. Clozapine requires taking a CBC, as well as blood pressure and pulse, weekly during treatment.

Management of Specific Side Effects

See Table 7-8.

Clinical Practice

Starting and maintenance doses, where established, are listed in Table 7-4. Clinical trials comparing doses of neuroleptics are even scarcer than those proving their efficacy in children. Maintenance doses are determined on an individual basis by starting at the minimal recommended dose and titrating upward to clinical response or unacceptable side effects. As extrapyramidal symptoms emerge, they may be managed by the addition of antiparkinsonian agents, as described above, but should first prompt a reduction of dose where possible. In adults, the incidence of acute dystonia is reduced by the prophylactic use of anticholinergic agents,[11] but this may be unnecessary in many cases.

Selecting a Specific Agent

Two main functional spectra influence the choice of a specific antipsychotic: potency for dopaminergic receptor blockade and potency for anticholinergic side effects (Table 7-1). In general, the former correlates with antipsychotic potency and the risk of precipitating extrapyramidal side effects, although clozapine is a highly potent antipsychotic that produces minimal EPS. The latter correlates with the risks of hypotension, sedation, and peripheral and central anticholinergic effects, as well as the ability of the agent to inhibit its own EPS. In general, a lower-potency agent is chosen when nonspecific sedation is desirable, such as in presurgical sedation, the short-term treatment of severe aggression and impulsivity, or agitated psychoses. Higher-potency agents are preferable (in equivalent doses) for schizophrenia, Tourette's syndrome, organic psychoses, and longer-term behavior disorders, due to their milder effect on cognition and socialization.

Table 7-10

Available Preparations and Average Costs of Neuroleptic Drugs

Compound	Trade Name	Non-parenteral Preparations	INJ	GEN	Average Dose/Day	Average Cost/Day
Chlorpromazine	Thorazine	Liquid: 30, 100 mg/ml Tablet: 10, 25, 50, 100, 200 Sup: 25, 100 SR: 30, 75, 150, 200	Yes	No	200 mg	$1.38
Thioridazine	Mellaril	Liquid: 25, 30, 100 mg/ml Tablet: 10, 15, 25, 50, 100, 150, 200	Yes	Yes	200 mg	$1.00 ($0.21)
Mesoridazine	Serentil	Liquid: 25 mg/ml Tablet: 10, 25, 50, 100	Yes	No	100 mg	$1.33
Trifluoperazine	Stelazine	Tablet: 1, 2, 5, 10	Yes	No	10 mg	$1.93
Fluphenazine	Prolixin	Liquid: 5 mg/ml Tablet: 1, 2.5, 5, 10	Yes	No	5 mg	$2.26
Perphenazine	Trilafon	Tablet: 2, 4, 8, 16	Yes	No	16 mg	$1.68
Prochlorperazine	Compazine	Liquid: 1 mg/ml Tablet: 5, 10, 25 Sup: 2.5, 5, 25 SR: 10, 15, 30	Yes	No	50 mg	$1.93

Chlorprothixene	Taractan	Tablet: 10, 25, 50, 100	Yes	No	100 mg	$1.37
Thiothixene	Navane	Liquid: 5 mg/ml Cap: 1, 2, 5, 10, 20	Yes	Yes	20 mg	$1.96 ($0.50)
Molindone	Moban	Liquid: 20 mg/ml Tablet: 5, 10, 25, 50, 100	No	No	100 mg	$2.51
Pimozide	Orap	Tablet: 2	No	No	2 mg*	$0.60
Haloperidol	Haldol	Liquid: 2 mg/ml Tablet: 0.5, 1, 2, 5, 10, 20	Yes	Yes	6 mg†	$2.17 ($0.09)
Droperidol	Inapsine	Inj: 2.5 mg/ml	No	No	2.5 mg‡	Not Available
Loxapine	Loxitane	Liquid: 25 mg/ml Cap: 5, 10, 25, 50	Yes	Yes	50 mg	$2.94 ($1.56)
Clozapine	Clozaril	Tablet: 25, 100	No	No	300 mg†	$10.26

For comparison, all average doses are the lowest effective *adult* maintenance dose reported by the manufacturer for hospitalized psychotic patients. Cost is based on b.i.d. dosing (unless otherwise indicated) at the average wholesale price and availability reported by Medi-Span for June 1992.[110] Cost of generic equivalent given in parentheses, where applicable.
*For Tourette's disorder—not approved for psychosis.
†Based on t.i.d. dosing.
‡For sedation—not approved for psychiatric indications.

Schizophrenia

As noted above, there are few controlled trials of neuroleptics in diagnostically homogeneous childhood schizophrenia. Agents that have been reported as efficacious include chlorpromazine, loxapine, thioridazine, thiothixene, trifluoperazine, and haloperidol. However, children and adolescents are exceedingly sensitive to the sedative and cognitive dulling effects of neuroleptics. Therefore, high-potency agents should be considered first-line therapy.[47,111] In all reports, doses were individualized. Haloperidol is started at 0.01–0.05 mg/kg/day in two or three divided doses for small children, or 0.5 mg b.i.d. for older children and adolescents. Although the manufacturer does not declare a maximum dose, maintenance doses above 15 mg/day are usually prohibited by their side effects, and add little to clinical response. If clinical response is not achieved within this range after two weeks of uninterrupted therapy, consideration should be given to other neuroleptics or to augmentation with lithium (Chapter 8), anticonvulsants (Chapter 9), or benzodiazepines (Chapter 10). Fish and colleagues[48] reported similar experience with trifluoperazine in autistic schizophrenic children. Children in that study tolerated maintenance doses at from 2 to 6 mg/day in the least impaired group and from 4 to 20 mg/day in the most impaired group, with decreased response rates noted in children requiring higher doses.

Tourette's Syndrome

In Tourette's syndrome, haloperidol is initiated in the same manner as for schizophrenic children. However, the maintenance doses are much lower. The recommended range is 0.05–0.075 mg/kg/day or up to 3 mg/day, although doses as high as 10 mg/day are occasionally necessary.[43] Since the smallest available haloperidol tablet is 0.5 mg, these may be cut to allow for 0.25-mg increments.

Pimozide is available in 2-mg tablets, which also may be cut to allow for smaller dose increments. The dose is then titrated to 0.2 mg/kg/day or 10 mg/day, whichever is smaller. At higher doses, QT prolongation is evident on an ECG, and sudden death has occurred at doses above 20 mg/day. Therefore, serial ECGs must be performed during dose titration, and periodic follow-up ECGs are recommended during maintenance therapy.

Pervasive Developmental Disorder and Behavioral Disorders

Since there are no studies demonstrating that neuroleptics relieve the core symptoms of autism, it is not a first-line treatment here. Neither have these agents been proven in the treatment of nonbehavioral symptoms of ADHD. Therefore, before using neuroleptics in these disorders, the practitioner must counsel the patient and family on both the realistic benefits to be gained and the potentially severe liability. Clear clinical guidelines are not available for any behavioral indication, but the best data come from studies of behaviorally disturbed autistic children.

Perry and associates[103] showed that haloperidol (0.25–4.0 mg/day) was beneficial in irritable, oppositional, autistic children, and that cumulative neuroleptic exposure could be limited by a discontinuous administration schedule without decreasing overall response. Therefore, intermittent treatment may be sufficient and prudent. Campbell and colleagues[27] have reported success with 0.5–3.0 mg/day (0.02–0.23 mg/kg/day) of haloperidol. Pimozide has been effective in a range of 1–9 mg/day.[96]

Monitoring for neuroleptic-associated movement disorders is particularly important in this population, as it may be difficult to distinguish drug side effects from the stereotypies of autism.[25]

How to Withdraw Medication

Withdrawal symptoms associated with the abrupt cessation of long-term neuroleptic use include cholinergic rebound (nausea, vomiting, diaphoresis, restlessness, insomnia); withdrawal dyskinesia (including oral dyskinesia, ataxia, or choreiform movements); and psychosis.[49] The last is rarely, if ever, seen in patients who did not have psychosis prior to neuroleptic treatment, but it has been suggested that withdrawal of neuroleptics in schizophrenic patients may induce a supersensitivity psychosis that differs from a simple relapse.[29]

Prior to lowering or discontinuing neuroleptic dosage, the patient and family must be cautioned about the possibility of withdrawal symptoms. Withdrawal of the drug should be gradual if treatment has been lengthy or a low-potency agent was used. Close follow-up is needed to monitor for signs of relapse or withdrawal.

References

1. Adams, F. (1988). Emergency intravenous sedation of the delirious, medically ill patient. *J Clin Psychiatry, 49(suppl.)*, 22–27.

2. Adamson, W.C., Nellis, B.P., Runge, G., et al. (1958). Use of tranquilizers for mentally deficient patients. *Am J Dis Child, 96*, 159–164.

3. Addonizio, G., Susman, V.L., Roth, S.D. (1987). Neuroleptic malignant syndrome: Review and analysis of 115 cases. *Biol Psychiatry, 22(8)*, 1004–1020.

4. Adityanjee, P.D. (1992). The myth of elevated creatine phosphokinase level and neuroleptic malignant syndrome. *Br J Psychiatry, 158*, 706–707.

5. Adler, L.A., Duncan, E., Kim, A., et al. (1989). Akathisia: Selective beta-blockers and rating instruments. *Psychopharmacol Bull, 25(3)*, 451–456.

6. Alderton, H.R., Hoddinott, B.A. (1964). A controlled study of the use of thioridazine in the treatment of hyperactive and aggressive children in a children's psychiatric hospital. *Can Psychiatr Assoc J, 9*, 239–247.

7. Allen, R. (1983). Role of amantadine in the management of neuroleptic-induced extrapyramidal syndromes: Overview and pharmacology. *Clin Neuropharmacol, 6(suppl.)*, 64–73.

8. American Psychiatric Association. (1987). *Diagnostic and Statistical Manual of Mental Disorders* (3rd ed., rev.). Washington D.C.: American Psychiatric Association.

9. Anderson, L.T., Campbell, M., Adams, P., et al. (1989). The effects of haloperidol on discrimination learning and behavioral symptoms in autistic children. *J Autism Dev Disord, 19(2)*, 227–239.

10. Ankenman, R. (1989). The combination of amantadine and neuroleptics plus time may cure tardive dyskinesia (Letter). *J Neuropsychiatry Clin Neurosci, 1(1)*, 96–97.

11. Arana, G.W., Goff, D.C., Baldessarini, R.J., Keepers, G.A. (1988). Efficacy of anticholinergic prophylaxis for neuroleptic-induced acute dystonia. *Am J Psychiatry, 145(8)*, 993–996.

12. Beitchman, J.H. (1985). Childhood schizophrenia. A review and comparison with adult-onset schizophrenia. *Psychiatr Clin North Am, 8(4)*, 793–814.

13. Bender, L. (1947). Childhood schizophrenia. *Am J Orthopsychiatry, 17*, 40–56.

14. Birmaher, B., Baker, R., Kapur, S., et al. (1992). Clozapine for the treatment of adolescents with schizophrenia. *J Am Acad Child Adolesc Psychiatry, 31(1)*, 160–164.

15. Bomberg, D., Szurek, S.A., Etemad, J.G. (1973). A statistical study of a group of psychiatric children. In S.A. Szurek, I.N. Berlin (Eds.), *Clinical Studies in Childhood Psychosis* (pp. 330–347). New York, Brunner/Mazel.

16. Borison, R.L., Davis, J.M. (1983). Amantadine in Tourette syndrome. *Curr Psychiatr Ther, 20*, 127–130.

17. Brinkley, J.R., Beitman, B.D., Friedel, R.O. (1979). Low-dose neuroleptic regimens in the treatment of borderline patients. *Arch Gen Psychiatry, 36(3)*, 319–326.

18. Brown, F.E., Nierenberg, D.W., Nordgren, R.E., et al. (1991). Neuroleptic malignant syndrome: Occurrence in a child after reconstructive surgery. *Plastic Reconstr Surg, 87(5)*, 961–964.

19. Burd, L., Kerbeshian, J. (1987). A North Dakota prevalence study of schizophrenia presenting in childhood. *J Am Acad Child Adolesc Psychiatry, 26(3)*, 347–350.

20. Caine, E.D. (1985). Gilles de la Tourette's syndrome. A review of clinical and research studies and consideration of future directions for investigation. *Arch Neurol, 42(4)*, 393–397.

21. Campbell, M., Magee, H., Lynch, N., Locascio, J.J. (1990). A pilot study of pimozide in autistic children. Paper presented at the 37th Annual Meeting of the American Academy of Child and Adolescent Psychiatry, Chicago.

22. Campbell, M., Small, A.M., Green, W.H., et al. (1984). Behavioral efficacy of haloperidol and lithium carbonate: A comparison in hospitalized aggressive children with conduct disorder. *Arch Gen Psychiatry, 41(7)*, 650–656.

23. Campbell, M. (1985). Schizophrenic disorders and pervasive developmental disorders/infantile autism. In J.M. Wiener (Ed.), *Diagnosis and Psychopharmacology of Childhood and Adolescent Disorders*. New York: Wiley.

24. Campbell, M., Fish, B., Korein, J., et al. (1972). Lithium and chlorpromazine: A controlled crossover study of hyperactive severely disturbed young children. *J Autism Child Schizophr, 2(3)*, 234–263.

25. Campbell, M., Locascio, J.J., Choroco, M.C., et al. (1990). Stereotypies and tardive dyskinesia: Abnormal movements in autistic children. *Psychopharmacol Bull, 26(2)*, 260–266.

26. Campbell, M., Anderson, L.T., Meier, M., et al. (1979). A comparison of haloperidol, behavior therapy, and their interaction in autistic children. *Psychopharmacol Bull, 15(2)*, 84–86.

27. Campbell, M., Anderson, L.T., Small, A.M., et al. (1982). The effects of haloperidol on learning and behavior in autistic children. *J Autism Child Schizophr, 12(2)*, 167–175.

28. Cheng, Y.F., Lundberg, T., Bondesson, U., et al. (1988). Clinical pharmacokinetics of clozapine in chronic schizophrenic patients. *Eur J Clin Pharmacol, 34(5)*, 445–449.

29. Chouinard, G., Jones, B.D. (1980). Neuroleptic-induced supersensitivity psychosis: Clinical and pharmacologic characteristics. *Am J Psychiatry, 137(1)*, 16–21.

30. Cohn, J.B., Brust, J., DiSerio, F., Singer, J. (1985). Effect of bromocriptine mesylate on induced hyperprolactinemia in stabilized psychiatric outpatients undergoing neuroleptic treatment. *Neuropsychobiology, 13(4)*, 173–179.

31. Correa, N., Opler, L.A., Kay, S.R., Birmaher, B. (1987). Amantadine in the treatment of neuroendocrine side effects of neuroleptics. *J Clin Psychopharmacol, 7(2)*, 91–95.

32. Coward, D.M. (1992). General pharmacology of clozapine. *Br J Psychiatry, 17*, 5–11.

33. Creese, I., Burt, D.R., Snyder, S.H. (1976). Dopamine receptor binding predicts clinical and pharmacological potencies of antischizophrenic drugs. *Science, 192*, 481–483.

34. Cunningham, M.A., Pillai, V., Blanchford-Rogers, W.J. (1968). Haloperidol in the treatment of children with severe behavior disorders. *Br J Psychiatry, 114*, 845–854.

35. Dahl, S.G. (1990). Pharmacokinetics of antipsychotic drugs in man. *Acta Psychiatr Scand, 358(suppl.)*, 37–40.

36. Dahl, S.G., Hals, P.A. (1987). Pharmacokinetic and pharmacodynamic factors causing variability in response to neuroleptic drugs. In S.G. Dahl, L.F. Gram, S.M. Paul, W.Z. Potter (Eds.), *Clinical Pharmacology in Psychiatry*, (pp. 266–275). Berlin: Springer-Verlag.

37. Donlan, P.T. (1973). The therapeutic use of diazepam for akathisia. *Psychosomatics, 14*, 222–225.

38. Dumon, J.P., Catteau, J., Lanvin, F., Dupuis, B.A. (1992). Randomized, double-blind, crossover, placebo-controlled comparison of propranolol and betaxolol in the treatment of neuroleptic-induced akathisia. *Am J Psychiatry, 149 (5)*, 647–650.

39. Edlund, M.J., Craig, T.J. (1984). Antipsychotic drug use and birth defects: An epidemiologic reassessment. *Compr Psychiatry, 25*, 32–37.

40. Elia, J., Katz, I.R., Simpson, G.M. (1987). Teratogenicity of psychotherapeutic medications. *Psychopharmacol Bull, 23(4)*, 531–586.

41. Elinwood, E.H., Woody, G., Krishnan, R.R. (1990). Treatment for drug abuse. In R. Michels et al. (Eds.), *Psychiatry, Revised Edition 1990* (vol. 2, chap. 90). Philadelphia: Lippincott.

42. Ellison, J.M., Adler, D.A. (1984). Psychopharmacologic approaches to borderline syndromes. *Compr Psychiatry, 25(3)*, 255–262.

43. Erenberg, G. (1988). Pharmacologic therapy of tics in childhood. *Pediatr Ann, 17(6)*, 395–404.

44. Farber, J.M. (1987). Psychopharmacology of self-injurious behavior in the mentally retarded. *J Am Acad Child Adol Psychiat, 26(3)*, 296–302.

45. Farde, L., Nordstrom, A.L., Wiesel, F.A., et al. (1992). Positron emission tomographic analysis of central D1 and D2 dopamine receptor occupancy in patients treated with classical neuroleptics and clozapine. Relation to extrapyramidal side effects. *Arch Gen Psychiatry, 49(7)*, 538–544.

46. Faretra, G. (1979). Lauretta Bender on autism: A review. *Child Psychiatry Hum Dev, 10(2)*, 118–129.

47. Fish, B., Campbell, M., Shapiro, T., Floyd, A., Jr. (1969). Comparison of trifluperidol, trifluoperazine and chlorpromazine in preschool schizophrenic children: The value of less sedative antipsychotic agents. *Curr Ther Res Clin Exp, 11(10)*, 589–595.

48. Fish, B., Shapiro, T., Campbell, M. (1966). Long-term prognosis and the response of schizophrenic children to drug therapy: A controlled study of trifluoperazine. *Am J Psychiatry, 123(1)*, 32–39.

49. Gardos, G., Cole, J.O., Tarsy, D. (1978). Withdrawal syndromes associated with antipsychotic drugs. *Am J Psychiatry, 135(11)*, 1321–1324.

50. Gillies, D.R., Forsythe, W.I. (1984). Treatment of multiple tics and the Tourette syndrome. *Dev Med Child Neurol, 26(6)*, 830–833.

51. Gittelman-Klein, R., Klein, D.F., Katz, S., et al. (1976). Comparative effects of methylphenidate and thioridazine in hyperactive children. I. Clinical results. *Arch Gen Psychiatry, 33*, 1217–1231.

52. Godet, P.F., Marie-Cardine, M. (1991). Neuroleptiques, schizophrenie et gossesse. Etude epidemiologique et teratologique. *Encephale, 17(6)*, 543–547.

53. Grandy, D.K., Zhang, Y.A., Bouvier, C., et al. (1991). Multiple human D5 dopamine receptor genes: A functional receptor and two pseuodogenes. *Proc Natl Acad Sci USA, 88(20)*, 9175–9179.

54. Greenberg, L.M., Deem, M.A., McMahon, S. (1972). Effects of dextroamphetamine, chlorpromazine, and hydroxyzine on behavior and performance in hyperactive children. *Am J Psychiatry, 129*, 532–539.

55. Gualtieri, C.T., Randall, E.W., Patterson, D.R. (1987). The medical treatment of autistic people. In E. Schopler, G.B. Mesibov (Eds.), *Neurobiological Issues in Autism* (pp. 373–388). New York: Plenum.

56. Gualtieri, C.T., Hicks, R.E. (1985). Stimulants and neuroleptics in hyperactive children (Letter). *J Am Acad Child Psychiatry, 24(3),* 363–364.

57. Guze, B.H., Baxter, L.R. (1985). Neuroleptic malignant syndrome. *N Engl J Med, 313,* 163–166.

58. Hardie, R.J., Lees, A.J. (1988). Neuroleptic-induced Parkinson's syndrome: Clinical features and results of treatment with levodopa. *J Neurol, Neurosurg Psychiatry, 51(6),* 850–854.

59. Harpe, C., Stoudemire, A. (1987). Etiology and treatment of neuroleptic malignant syndrome. *Med Toxicol, 2(3),* 166–176.

60. Helper, M.M., Wilcott, R.C., Garfield, S.L. (1963). Effects of chlorpromazine on learning and related processes in emotionally disturbed children. *J Consult Psychol, 27,* 1–9.

61. Hogarty, G.E., Goldberg, S.C., Schooler, N.R., et al. (1974). Drug and sociotherapy in the aftercare of schizophrenic patients: Two-year relapse rates. *Arch Gen Psychiatry, 31,* 603.

62. Hughes, P.S. (1977). Survey of medication in a subnormality hospital. *Br J Ment Subnormality, 23,* 88–94.

63. Jagger, J., Prusoff, B.A., Cohen, D.J., et al. (1982). The epidemiology of Tourette's syndrome: A pilot study. *Schizophr Bull, 8,* 267.

64. Jordan, K., Prugh, D.G. (1971). Schizophreniform psychosis of childhood. *Am J Psychiatry, 128,* 323–331.

65. Kanner, L. (1971). Childhood psychosis: A historical overview. *J Autism Child Schizophr, 1(1),* 14–19.

66. Kanner, L. (1943). Autistic disturbances of affective contact. *Nerv Child, 3(2).*

67. Kaplan, H.I., Sadock, B.J. (1991). *Synopsis of Psychiatry* (pp. 241–245). Baltimore: Williams & Wilkins.

68. Kaufman, D.M. (1990). *Clinical Neurology for Psychiatrists (3rd ed.)* (pp. 358–370). Philadelphia: W.B. Saunders.

69. Keck, P.E., Jr., Pope, H.G., Jr., McElroy, S.L. (1991). Declining frequency of neuroleptic malignant syndrome in a hospital population. *Am J Psychiatry, 148(7),* 880–882.

70. Keck, P.E., Jr., Pope, H.G., Jr., Cohen, B.M., et al. (1989). Risk factors for neuroleptic malignant syndrome. A case-control study. *Arch Gen Psychiatry, 46(10),* 914–918.

71. Keks, N.A., Kulkarni, J., Copolov, D.L. (1989). Treatment of schizophrenia. *Med J Aust, 151(8)*, 462–467.

72. Kerbeshian, J., Burd, L. (1988). A clinical pharmacological approach to treating Tourette syndrome in children and adolescents. *Neurosci Biobehav Rev, 12(3–4)*, 241–245.

73. Kim, A., Adler, L., Angrist, B., Rotrosen, J. (1989). Efficacy of low-dose metoprolol in neuroleptic-induced akathisia. *J Clin Psychopharmacol, 9(4)*, 294–296.

74. Klein, S.K., Levinsohn, M.W., Blumer, J.L. (1985). Accidental chlorpromazine ingestion as a cause of neuroleptic malignant syndrome in children. *J Pediatr, 107*, 970–973.

75. Klein, D.F., Gittelman, R., Quitkin, F., Rifkin, A. (1980). *Diagnosis and Drug Treatment of Psychiatric Disorders: Adult and Children (2nd ed.)* (pp. 88–144). Baltimore: Williams & Wilkins.

76. Kolvin, I., Ounsted, C., Humphrey, M., et al. (1971). The phenomenology of childhood psychoses. *Br J Psychiatry, 118*, 385–395.

77. Kotsopoulos, S., Kanigsberg, J., Cote, A. Fiedorowicz, C. (1987). Hallucinatory experiences in nonpsychotic children. *J Am Acad Child Adolesc Psychiatry, 26(3)*, 375–380.

78. Kramer, M. (1978). Population changes and schizophrenia, 1970–1985. In L.C. Wynne, R.L. Cromwell, and S. Matthysse (Eds.), *The Nature of Schizophrenia: New Approaches to Research and Treatment* (pp. 545–571). New York: Wiley.

79. Kutcher, S., Williamson, P., MacKenzie, S., et al. (1989). Successful clonazepam treatment of neuroleptic-induced akathisia in older adolescents and young adults: A double-blind, placebo-controlled study. *J Clin Psychopharmacol, 9(6)*, 403–406.

80. Le Couteur, A., Rutter, M., Lord, C., et al. (1989). Autism diagnostic interview: A standardized investigator-based instrument. *J Autism Dev Disord, 19(3)*, 363–387.

81. Leckman, J.F., Cohen, D.J. (1990). Tourette's disorder and other stereotyped movement disorders. In R. Michels et al. (Eds.), *Psychiatry, Revised Edition 1990* (vol. 2, chap. 38). Philadelphia: Lippincott.

82. Levenson, J.L. (1985). Neuroleptic malignant syndrome. *Am J Psychiatry, 142(10)*, 1137–1145.

83. Linaker, O.M. (1990). Frequency of and determinants for psychotropic

drug use in an institution for the mentally retarded. *Br J Psychiatry, 156,* 525–530.

84. Lipowski, Z.J. (1992). Update on delirium. *Psychiatr Clin North Am, 15(2),* 335–346.

85. Locascio, J.J., Malone, R.P., Small, A.M., et al. (1991). Factors related to haloperidol response and dyskinesias in autistic children. *Psychopharmacol Bull, 27(2),* 119–126.

86. Lord, C., Rutter, M., Goode, S., et al. (1989). Autism diagnostic observation schedule: A standardized observation of communicative and social behavior. *J Autism Dev Disord, 19(2),* 185–212.

87. Ludatscher, J.I. (1989). Stable remission of tardive dyskinesia by L-dopa. *J Clin Psychopharmacol, 9(1),* 39–41.

88. Matsuoka, I., Nakai, T., Miyake, M., et al. (1986). Effects of bromocriptine on neuroleptic-induced amenorrhea, galactorrhea and impotence. *Jpn J Psychiatry Neurol, 40(4),* 639–646.

89. May, P.R.A., Tuma, H., Dixon, W.J. (1976). Schizophrenia—a follow-up study of results of treatment: I Design and other problems. *Arch Gen Psychiatry, 33,* 474–478.

90. May, P.R.A., Tuma, H., Yale, C., et al. (1976). Schizophrenia—a follow-up study of results of treatment: II. Hospital stay over two to five years. *Arch Gen Psychiatry, 33,* 481–486.

91. Meltzer, H.Y. (1987). Effect of neuroleptics on the schizophrenic syndrome. In S.G. Dahl, L.F. Gram, S.M. Paul, W.Z. Potter (Eds.), *Clinical Pharmacology in Psychiatry.* Berlin: Springer-Verlag.

92. Menza, M.A., Murray, G.B., Holmes, V.F., Rafuls, W.A. (1988). Controlled study of extrapyramidal reactions in the management of delirious, medically ill patients: Intravenous haloperidol versus intravenous haloperidol plus benzodiazepines. *Heart Lung, 17(3),* 238–241.

93. Milkovich, L., Van Den Berg, B.J. (1976). An evaluation of teratogenicity of certain anti-nauseant drugs. *Am J Obstet Gynecol, 125,* 244–248.

94. Minshew, N.J., Payton, J.B. (1988). New perspectives in autism. Part II: The differential diagnosis and neurobiology of autism. *Curr Prob Pediatr, 18(11),* 615–694.

95. Moore, A., O'Donohoe, N.V., Monaghan, H. (1986). Neuroleptic malignant syndrome. *Arch Dis Child, 61(8),* 793–795.

96. Naruse, H., Nagahata, M., Nakane, Y., et al. (1982). A multicenter double-blind trial of pimozide (Orap), haloperidol and placebo in children with behavioral disorders, using crossover design. *Acta Paedopsychiatr, 48,* 173–184.

97. National Institute of Mental Health. (1985). AIMS (abnormal involuntary movement scale). *Psychopharmacol Bull, 21,* 1077–1080.

98. Nierenberg, D., Disch, M., Manheimer, E., et al. (1991). Facilitating prompt diagnosis and treatment of the neuroleptic malignant syndrome. *Clin Pharmacol Ther, 50(5 Pt. 1),* 580–586.

99. Numa, A. (1991). Neuroleptic malignant syndrome in children. *Med J Aust, 155(6),* 417–419.

100. Pelonero, A.L., Levenson, J.L., Silvermann, J.J. (1985). Neuroleptic therapy following neuroleptic malignant syndrome. *Psychosomatics, 26,* 946–948.

101. Peroutka, S.J., Synder, S.H. (1980). Relationship of neuroleptic drug effects at brain dopamine, serotonin, alpha-adrenergic, and histamine receptors to clinical potency. *Am J Psychiatry, 137(12),* 1518–1522.

102. Peroutka, S.J., U'Prichard, D.C., Greenberg, D.A., et al. (1977). Neuroleptic drug interactions with norepinephrine alpha-receptor binding sites in rat brain. *Neuropharmacology, 16,* 549–556.

103. Perry, R., Campbell, M., Adams, P., et al. (1989). Long-term efficacy of haloperidol in autistic children: Continuous versus discontinuous drug administration. *J Am Acad Child Adolesc Psychiat, 28(1),* 87–92.

104. Petti, T.A., Vela, R.M. (1990). Borderline disorders of childhood: An overview. *J Am Acad Child Adolesc Psychiat, 29(3),* 327–337.

105. Pilowsky, L.S., Costa, D.C., Ell, P.J., et al. (1992). Clozapine, single photon emission tomography, and the D2 dopamine receptor blockade hypothesis of schizophrenia. *Lancet, 340(8813),* 199–202.

106. Pinder, R.M., Brogden, R.N., Swayer, R., et al. (1976). Pimozide: A review of its pharmacological properties and therapeutic uses in psychiatry. *Drugs, 12(1),* 1–40.

107. Platt, J.E., Friedhoff, A.J., Broman, S.H., et al. (1988). Effects of prenatal exposure to neuroleptic drugs on children's growth. *Neuropsychopharmacology, 1(3),* 205–212.

108. Pope, H.G., Harlyn, G.A., Keck, P.E., McElroy, S.L. (1991). Neuroleptic malignant syndrome: Long-term follow-up of 20 cases. *J Clin Psychiatry, 52(5),* 208–212.

109. Popper, C.W. (1990). Child and adolescent psychopharmacology. In Michels et al. (Eds.), *Psychiatry, Revised Edition 1990* (vol. 2, chap. 59). Philadelphia: Lippincott.

110. *Prescription Pricing Guide*. (1992). Indianapolis: Medi-Span, Inc.

111. Realmuto, G.M., Erickson, W.D., Yellin, A.M., et al. (1984). Clinical comparison of thiothixene and thioridazine in schizophrenic adolescents. *Am J Psychiatry, 141*, 440–442.

112. Reardon, G.T., Rifkin, A., Schwartz, A., et al. (1989). Changing patterns of neuroleptic dosage over a decade. *Am J Psychiatry, 146(6)*, 726–729.

113. Rego, M.D., Giller, E.L., Jr. (1989). Mania secondary to amantadine treatment of neuroleptic-induced hyperprolactinemia. *J Clin Psychiatry, 50(4)*, 143–144.

114. Richelson, E. (1990). Schizophrenia: Treatment. In Michels et al. (Eds.), *Psychiatry, Revised Edition* (vol. 1, chap. 55). Philadelphia: Lippincott.

115. Rosebush, P.I., Stewart, T.D. (1989). A prospective analysis of 24 episodes of neuroleptic malignant syndrome. *Am J Psychiatry, 146*, 717–725.

116. Rosenberg, M.R., Green, M. (1989). Neuroleptic malignant syndrome. Review of response to therapy. *Arch Intern Med, 149(9)*, 1927–1931.

117. Rosebush, P.I., Stewart, T.D. (1989). A prospective analysis of 24 episodes of neuroleptic malignant syndrome. *Am J Psychiatry, 146*, 717–725.

118. Rumeau-Rouquette, C., Goujard, J., Huel, G. (1976). Possible teratogenic effects of phenothiazines in human beings. *Teratology, 15*, 57–64.

119. Sallee, F.R., Pollock, B.G., Stiller, R.L., et al. (1987). Pharmacokinetics of pimozide in adults and children with Tourette's syndrome. *J Clin Pharmacol, 27(10)*, 776–781.

120. Sandor, P., Musisi, S., Moldofsky, H., Lang, A. (1990). Tourette syndrome: A follow-up study. *J Clin Psychopharmacol, 10(3)*, 197–199.

121. Schopler, E., Reichler, R., Renner, B.R. (1988). The childhood autism rating scale. Los Angeles: Western Psychological Services.

122. Schroeder, S., Schroeder, C., Smith, B., et al. (1978). Prevalence of self-injurious behaviors in a large state facility for the retarded: A three-year follow-up study. *J Autism Child Schizophr, 8*, 261–269.

123. Seeman, P., Lee, T., Chau-Wong, M., et al. (1976). Antipsychotic drug doses and neuroleptic/dopamine receptors. *Nature, 261*, 717–719.

124. Shalev, A., Hermesh, H., Munitz, H. (1989). Mortality from neuroleptic malignant syndrome. *J Clin Psychiatry, 50(1)*, 18–25.

125. Shalev, A., Munitz, H. (1986). The neuroleptic malignant syndrome: Agent and host interaction. *Acta Psychiatr Scand, 73(4)*, 337–347.

126. Shapiro, A.K., Shapiro, E. Fulop, G. (1987). Pimozide treatment of tic and Tourette disorders. *Pediatrics, 79(6)*, 1032–1039.

127. Shapiro, E., Shapiro, A.K., Fulop, G., et al. (1989). Controlled study of haloperidol, pimozide and placebo for the treatment of Gilles de la Tourette's syndrome. *Arch Gen Psychiatry, 46(8)*, 722–730.

128. Siever, L.J. (1981). The effect of amantadine on prolactin levels and galactorrhea on neuroleptic-treated patients. *J Clin Psychopharmacol, 1(1)*, 2–7.

129. Sloman, L. (1991). Use of medication in pervasive developmental disorders. *Psychiatr Clin North Am, 14(1)*, 165–182.

130. Smith, R.C., Crayton, J., Dekirmenjian, H., et al. (1979). Blood levels of neuroleptic drugs in nonresponding chronic schizophrenic patients. *Arch Gen Psychiatry, 36(5)*, 579–584.

131. Snodgrass, W.R., Dodge, W.F. (1989). Lytic/"DPT" cocktail: Time for rational and safe alternatives. *Pediatr Clin North Am, 36(5)*, 1285–1291.

132. Soloff, P.H., George, A., Nathan, S., et al. (1989). Amitriptyline versus haloperidol in borderlines: Final outcomes and predictors of response. *J Clin Psychopharmacol, 9(4)*, 238–246.

133. Soloff, P.H., George, A., Nathan, S., et al. (1986). Progress in pharmacotherapy of borderline disorders. A double-blind study of amitriptyline, haloperidol, and placebo. *Arch Gen Psychiatry, 43(7)*, 691–697.

134. Spencer, E., Padron-Gayol, M., Kafantaris, V., et al. (1990). Haloperidol in schizophrenic children. Poster presented at the 37th Annual meeting of the American Academy of Child and Adolescent Psychiatry, Chicago.

135. Sprague, R.L., Barnes, K.R., Werry, J.S. (1970). Methylphenidate and thioridazine: Learning, reaction time, activity and classroom behavior in disturbed children. *Am J Orthopsychiatry, 40*, 615–628.

136. Stewart, J.T., Myers, W.C., Burket, R.C., Lyles, W.B. (1990). A review of the pharmacology of aggression in children and adolescents. *J Am Acad Child Adolesc Psychiatry, 29(2)*, 269–277.

137. Task Force on Late Neurological Effects of Antipsychotic Drugs. (1980). Tardive dyskinesia: Summary of a task force report of the American Psychiatric Association. *Am J Psychiatry, 137(10),* 1163–1172.

138. Teicher, M.H., Glod, C.A. (1990). Neuroleptic drugs: Indications and guidelines for their rational use in children and adolescents. *J Child Adolesc Psychopharmacol, 1(1),* 33–56.

139. Thacker, A.K., Radhakrishnan, K., Maloo, J.C., Bohlaga, N.H. (1990). Neuroleptic malignant syndrome in a girl without psychosis. *Br J Clin Psychiatry, 44(8),* 425–427.

140. Turner, T.H., Cookson, J.C., Wass, J.A., et al. (1984). Psychotic reactions during treatment of pituitary tumours with dopamine agonists. *Br Med J—Clin Res, 289(6452),* 1101–1103.

141. Van Tol, H.H., Wu, C.M., Guan, H.C., et al. (1992). Multiple dopamine D4 receptor variants in the human population. *Nature, 358(6382),* 149–152.

142. VanPutten, T., May, P.R.A., Jenden, D.J. (1981). Does a plasma level of chlorpromazine help? *Psychol Med, 11,* 729–734.

143. Weizman, A., Weitz, R., Szekely, G.A., et al. (1984). Combination of neuroleptic and stimulant treatment in attention deficit disorder with hyperactivity. *J Am Acad Child Psychiatry, 23(3),* 295–298.

144. Wells, B.G., Cold, J.A., Marken, P.A., et al. (1991). A placebo-controlled trial of nadolol in the treatment of neuroleptic-induced akathisia. *J Clin Psychiatry, 52(6),* 255–260.

145. Werry, J., Aman, M.G. (1975). Methylphenidate and haloperidol in children: Effects on attention, memory and activity. *Arch Gen Psychiatry, 32,* 790–795.

146. Werry, J., Aman, M., Lampen, E. (1976). Haloperidol and methylphenidate in hyperactive children. *Acta Paedopsychiatr, 42,* 26–40.

147. Wressell, S.E., Tyrer, S.P., Berney, T.P. (1990). Reduction in antipsychotic drug dosage in mentally handicapped patients. A hospital study (see comments). *Br J Psychiatry, 157,* 101–106.

C h a p t e r   8

Lithium

Lithium is the drug of choice for the treatment of adults with bipolar disorder.[1] While there are no extensive lithium versus placebo-controlled, double-blind studies assessing its efficacy in treating bipolar disorder in children and adolescents, open-label studies have revealed that it can be helpful in this population.[3,4] Lithium's only FDA-established indication, however, is for the acute and maintenance treatment of bipolar disorders in patients at least 12 years old. Nonetheless, active investigation into lithium's usefulness in treating a wide variety of psychiatric disorders in both adolescents and children younger than 12 years of age continues. Currently, these studies are exploring lithium's utility in the treatment of children and adolescents with bipolar disorder, in augmenting antidepressants in the treatment of depression and aggressive behavior, and in treating children and adolescents with behavior control problems whose parents have responded to lithium therapy.

Chemical Properties

See Table 8-1.

Lithium carbonate (Li_2CO_3) is a very soluble cation salt that is rapidly absorbed after oral administration by the GI tract. A citrate form of lithium is also available as a syrup that contains 8 mEq lith-

Table 8-1
Pharmacokinetic Properties of Lithium

Absorption	Peak Serum Levels (hours)	Serum Half-Life (hours)	Principal Route of Excretion
Gastrointestinal	2–4	20–24	Renal

ium/5 ml. Peak blood levels are achieved within approximately two hours for standard preparations of lithium, while peak levels for the sustained-release form are generally achieved within four and one-half hours.[1] Baldessarini and Stephens[5] demonstrated that complete absorption of lithium usually occurs within eight hours of its administration. Lithium circulates in the bloodstream unbound to protein, and penetrates the blood–brain barrier within about one day of administration.[1] It is excreted predominantly by the kidney, with approximately 80% being reabsorbed in the proximal renal tubules.

The proximal reabsorption of lithium competes with the proximal reabsorption of sodium. This becomes important when a patient is receiving a thiazide diuretic that decreases the proximal reabsorption of sodium, leading to increased lithium reabsorption and consequently increased lithium serum levels. In other words, the greater the sodium reabsorption in the proximal tubules, the lesser is the lithium reabsorption and hence lithium serum level, and vice versa. In adults, the elimination half-life of lithium is approximately 24 hours, and over 60% of an acute dose is excreted within 12 hours. Children generally have a shorter elimination half-life of lithium because of their increased ratio of kidney to whole-body size as compared with adults. As a consequence, steady-state levels of lithium are reached sooner in children than in adults.

Indications

See Table 8-2.

Bipolar Disorder

Acute Mania
There have not been any large-scale double-blind, placebo-controlled studies of lithium in children and adolescents. In clinical practice, however, the guidelines that apply to lithium's use in adults are commonly used for these younger patients.[6,7] Because of their increased renal clearance as compared with adults, children and adolescents treated with lithium often are able to tolerate higher oral doses.[8,9] In a survey of the literature, Youngerman and

Table 8-2
Indications for Lithium in Child and Adolescent Psychiatry

FDA established:
- Bipolar disorder—acute mania in patients >12 years
- Prophylaxis for bipolar disorder in patients >12 years

Possible indications:
- Bipolar disorder—acute mania in children <12 years
- Bipolar disorder—acute depression
- Unipolar depression
- Augmentation of tricyclic-refractory depression
- Prophylaxis for unipolar depression
- Cyclothymia
- Psychosis
- Aggression and violent behavior
- ADHD
- Alcohol abuse/dependence
- Bulimia
- Personality disorders
- Functional encopresis

Canino[10] found that in open trials of lithium in children with bipolar disorder, the positive response rate was 66%, which is similar to that seen in adults treated with lithium.

Varanka and colleagues[3] treated 10 prepubertal children diagnosed with bipolar disorder with psychotic features with lithium carbonate doses of up to 1800 mg/day. Significant improvement, including amelioration of mood and psychotic symptoms, occurred, an average of 11 days after the lithium was begun. No antipsychotic medication was utilized. The lithium was well tolerated by these children and with minimal side effects. This is contrary to what is usually done in bipolar adults with and without psychosis. Because lithium may take seven to 10 days before exerting its effect, many have advocated starting a neuroleptic agent such as haloperidol concomitantly with the lithium to acutely control agitation. Although standard clinical practice in many settings, this treatment regimen has been called into question since lithium and haloperidol can have synergistic effects on each other, and because of haloperidol's (and the other neuroleptics') side-effect profile. Child psychiatrists must be particularly cautious in using an antipsychotic with lithium in view of the increased risk of such side effects as tardive dyskinesia and dystonia. Some clinicians are opting to try lithium first, and to add an antipsychotic only after a therapeutic trial of lithium fails. This is obviously more feasible for small children and younger adolescents where the disruptive and often dangerous behavior that can be associated with mania is likely to have less severe consequences.

McKnew and colleagues[13] studied six prepubescent children and found that two of the children with mixed bipolar disorder had good responses to lithium therapy. Brumback and Weinberg[14] reported that two of six prepubescent children with mania or hypomania experienced sustained improvement after being treated with lithium.

Case History

A 16-year-old girl with no past psychiatric history but whose parents claimed that she "always ran a little higher than the rest of us" was admitted for inpatient psychiatric evaluation after having run away from home and having a police officer apprehend her when, while nude, she tried to direct traffic at a busy intersection at 2 a.m. When she arrived in the emergency room, she alternately would yell at the emergency room staff that she had to get back to work downtown at the station, and then would spontaneously burst into singing the national anthem. She refused to let the emergency room staff examine her physically, saying she was a special agent of the President and carried dangerous and priceless material that could not be "contaminated." Her speech was pressured and she had racing thoughts. She reported that she had been unable to sleep for the past seven days, and had begun to work feverishly. She had completed all of her homework in every course for the remainder of the year. She had made several long-distance phone calls after midnight to various acquaintances. She had also recently charged $5000 to her father's credit card. Indeed, her father found out about the charge on the evening of admission and confronted his daughter about it. Although initially jovial during the encounter, she suddenly became upset, threw a knife at her father's head, and ran out the door.

There was no history of drug or alcohol use, no prior depressive episodes, and no recent psychosocial stressor. Her parents did admit to a family history of mood disorder. The patient's mother was on nortriptyline for depression. An older sister had been diagnosed as having bipolar disorder and was currently receiving lithium, to which she had experienced a remarkable response. Medication-free observation for three days revealed the patient to be clearly manic, and she was diagnosed with bipolar disorder. A trial of lithium was initiated after TFTs, BUN/creatinine, U/A, electrolytes, CBC, a urine pregnancy test, and a urine drug screen were assayed and found to be normal. Lithium 300 mg t.i.d., was started. After five days on this dose, a plasma lithium level was drawn and found to be 0.6 mEq/L. Since she was still exhibiting prominent manic symptoms, her lithium dose was increased by 300 mg every five days to an ultimate dose of 1800 mg/day (lithium level 1.2 mEq/L). She tolerated this dose well without side effects. TFTs and BUN/creatinine were also checked and found to be normal.

It has been reported that good responders to lithium therapy include those patients with an onset of bipolar disorder in late adolescence and a positive family history of good response to lithium.[11] Poor responders to lithium include younger prepubescent children with a rapid cycling type of bipolar disorder. It should be noted, however, that Strober and colleagues[12] observed that 15 adolescent-onset bipolar disorder patients who all came from families with high rates of mood disorder responded poorly to lithium therapy. These adolescents had a history of behavior problems beginning in early childhood. Therefore, certain questions regarding the diagnostic purity of this sample are raised. Of those who showed some response to lithium, it appeared much later (six to eight weeks after the initiation of therapy) and was of lesser degree than the response reported in adolescents without prepubescent behavior problems.

The difficulty in distinguishing bipolar disorder from ADHD and conduct disorders in children is often difficult. It is believed that they can coexist, but identifying a particular population most likely to respond to lithium for the most part has been unsuccessful. This should not be entirely surprising, since in adults, age, sex, age at onset, rate of mood attacks, family history of mood disorder, and the nature of the prior episode have absolutely no predictive value regarding the success or failure of lithium treatment.[16]

Carlson and colleagues[17] studied the effect of lithium treatment in 11 hospitalized children at four and eight weeks using weekly ratings of mood, behavior, and cognitive effects. These children were chosen for the study because, based on literature review, their condition at the time of hospitalization, diagnoses, and family history, it was suggested that they would be positive responders to lithium therapy. The children improved most significantly by week 8 and less so by week 4 in areas of self-control, aggression, and irritability. It should be noted, however, that seven of the children were studied by conducting a double-blind placebo crossover, and behavioral and cognitive improvements were observed on placebo. Only three of the 11 children (27%) improved enough to be discharged on lithium.[17] These authors concluded that lithium should be tried in children with bipolar disorder and refractory behavior disturbances, since some may show positive responses.[17] It is also their assertion, from a review of the literature, that antimanic responses are different from antiaggressive responses. In bipolar disorder, a longer time is generally needed to produce a positive response to lithium therapy, and when successful, it may be more complete.

Carlson[18] has also speculated on the implications of comorbid diagnoses of ADHD and conduct disorder with bipolar disorder in children. One possibility is that disruptive behavior disorders may be the antecedent of full-blown mania, which takes on its characteristic form in adolescence. Another theory is that ADHD/conduct disorder and bipolar disorder together make up a very severe and often refractory type of bipolar disorder due to its early onset.[18] Other authors have theorized that the mania may actually be secondary to the ADHD or conduct disorder.[19,20] Black and colleagues[21] report that such "complicated mania" has a poorer response to lithium. Rancurello[22] posed a particularly intriguing possibility that the manic symptoms are "epiphenomena" without predictive validity when occurring with ADHD and/or conduct disorder in prepubescent children. Moreover, Rancurello hypothesized that response to an antidepressant such as desipramine would suggest a primary depression and/or ADHD diagnosis.

Clearly, further study is required. Longitudinal studies are necessary accurately to delineate what happens to these children diagnosed with bipolar disorder—that is, do they become bipolar adults?

Acute Depression

Lithium is not effective as often as antidepressants (see Chapter 4) in the treatment of acute depressive episodes in adult patients with bipolar disorder.[23] Therefore, in adults, it is most common to add an antidepressant to the medical regimen of a patient being treated with lithium for bipolar disorder, depressed type. There are no data on children and adolescents. This poses something of a dilemma, since the antidepressants have not been shown to be effective in child and adolescent unipolar depression (see Chapter 4). Further study is clearly warranted. The clinician should always make sure to check thyroid function tests when a child or adolescent on lithium becomes depressed, since lithium can cause hypothyroidism, sometimes resulting in decreased energy levels and other depressive signs and symptoms. Further study assessing the treatment and management of bipolar children and adolescents with an acute depressive episode is necessary.

Prophylaxis of Bipolar Disorder

As in adults, lithium is thought to be indicated for the prophylactic treatment of bipolar disorder.[24] Since the majority of patients with bipolar disorder experience recurrent episodes of illness, prophylaxis is advised as well-conducted studies in adults have shown that bipolar prophylaxis with lithium decreases the frequency and intensity of manic episodes in up to 80% of bipolar patients.[24–27] Lithium appears to be less effective in decreasing depressive recurrences than manic recurrences. There are no data on children and adolescents. Generally, if a child or adolescent has responded well to lithium, it is advisable to keep him or her on a maintenance dose for a minimum of six to nine months. Careful monitoring for efficacy versus toxicity is also advocated. Compliance may be a major issue in adolescence, and communication with the patient and family about the medication and what taking the medication means is often crucial.

Unipolar Depression

Lithium often has a mood-stabilizing effect when it is effective in treating psychiatric disorders. It is not, however, believed to be as effective as antidepressants in the treatment of unipolar depression in adults.[28] There are no data on children and adolescents on the use of lithium alone in the treatment of an acute unipolar depression. It should be noted, however, that with the lack of success of this modality in adults and its many side effects, lithium's future use for children and adolescents with acute unipolar depression is probably limited.

Interest is being generated in using lithium to augment the effects of antidepressants such as the TCAs and SSUIs to treat refractory depression in children and adolescents. This interest is attributable in large part to the fact that antidepressants have not yet proved effective for child and adolescent depression. In consequence, clinicians are looking for alternatives.

In adults, several well-conducted studies have demonstrated clinical improvement when lithium was added to the medical regimen of unipolar depressed patients who had not responded to TCA drug therapy alone.[29-37] There are no controlled studies of lithium augmentation of TCAs in the treatment of nonbipolar depression in children and adolescents. Ryan and colleagues[37] conducted a retrospective chart review of 14 adolescent patients diagnosed with unipolar depression who were subsequently treated openly with a TCA (desipramine, nortriptyline, amitriptyline)–lithium combination after an inadequate response to a TCA alone. Six of the 14 patients (over 40%) had a good response on the lithium augmentation of the TCA. Moreover, all of the adolescents tolerated the combination well without toxicity. Obviously, conclusions from this report are premature at this time, since it was an open trial with only 14 patients in the sample. Nonetheless, with the poor results obtained with TCA treatment in children and adolescents, these results are intriguing and suggestive that there may be a population of adolescents who respond to the TCA–lithium combination. Ryan and colleagues[37] observed that the duration of treatment with the TCA before the lithium was added was six to eight weeks, which was longer than the average of three weeks in the adult studies. Quitkin and colleagues[38] have written a great deal about the duration of antidepressant treatment and what constitutes a "good" trial. According to their criteria, since the improvement occurred after the eighth week of the tricyclic trial, it is unlikely that the positive response to lithium was due to the late effects of the antidepressant alone.[37,38] The authors also note that the duration of lithium augmentation required to produce a significant clinical response was longer than that reported in the adult literature.[37] In fact, seven adolescents continued to show improvement in their symptoms as long as six weeks after the lithium augmentation. Nonetheless, this was not a placebo-controlled crossover trial, so the possibility that the patients improved with time as opposed to medication cannot be discounted.[37] Further studies are warranted.

Prophylaxis for Unipolar Depression

In contrast to bipolar prophylaxis where lithium is considered to be the drug of choice, most psychiatrists do not use lithium as a first-line agent for the prophylaxis of unipolar depression in adults. Prien and colleagues[39] in a large multicenter study observed that lithium was effective in prophylaxis for unipolar depression only when the most recent depressive episode had been mild, and that lithium was not significantly better than placebo in prophylaxis against unipolar depression when the prior episode had been severe. There are no data on children and adolescents. It should be noted, however, that lithium's role in prophylaxis against childhood and adolescent depression appears rather limited due to the lack of efficacy in adults.

Cyclothymia

Cyclothymia is characterized by periods of hypomania alternating with periods of depression not severe enough to meet the criteria for a major depressive episode or mania.[2] In children and adolescents, only a one-year period of alternating moods (i.e., depression and hypomania) is required, as opposed to the two years required for diagnosis in adults. There are no data on children and adolescents. Since cyclothymic patients often have a family history of mood disorders and may look similar to rapid-cycling bipolar disorder patients, a lithium trial is probably worthwhile as long as there are no confounding factors affecting the diagnosis.

Psychosis

As mentioned previously, Varanka and colleagues[3] used lithium successfully to treat 10 prepubertal children 6 to 12 years of age with manic episodes, family psychiatric histories, and psychotic symptoms. All of the children improved when treated with lithium alone. Manic and psychotic symptoms were noted to be improved an average of 11 days after lithium was started. Because of the unfavorable side-effect profile of the antipsychotic drugs, which can cause lifelong disability (such as tardive dyskinesia) in some syndromes where psychosis may occur, it is probably best to start with lithium alone. Careful monitoring can determine whether or not the lithium is sufficient to control the mood and psychotic symptoms. If it is insufficient, the use of another agent, such as carbamazepine or valproic acid, either alone or in combination with the lithium can be considered (see Chapter 9). Antipsychotics should be reserved for use as a last resort when other medications that have more favorable side-effect profiles have failed.

Since lithium often takes seven to 10 days to take effect, antipsychotics such as haloperidol were often given concomitantly over the short term until the lithium began to exert its effect. Now, however, there is a move away from polydrug therapy toward monotherapy whenever possible. Neuroleptics are often used only when the patient becomes so agitated that he or she threatens his or her own or other lives. This is especially true for children and adolescents where it is often possible to implement behavior techniques such as time-outs and physical restraint without resorting to chemical "restraint."

Schizoaffective disorder is seen in patients who have discrete periods of psychosis without afffective symptoms and mood syndromes without psychosis.[2] In psychotic adults, lithium is often used as an adjunct to a neuroleptic.[70] Lithium can also be the drug of choice to treat associated mania. It is rare for lithium to be the sole medication in schizoaffective disorder in adults. There are no data on children and adolescents, and the very diagnosis is somewhat controversial. Further research into the validity of the diagnosis, as well as into its therapy, is required.

Schizophrenic patients often suffer mood symptoms. Psychosis of sudden onset, especially if the family history is positive for mood disorder, may warrant a trial of lithium, depending on the mood symptoms.[23] It has been reported that nearly all children and adolescents with major depression with psychotic features go on to develop bipolar disorder. This does not necessarily mean that lithium is the first drug of choice when a patient presents as depressed and psychotic, but that careful monitoring for mania should take place. This is especially true if an antidepressant is started. Antidepressants can produce mania, particularly in a biologically vulnerable patient (see Chapter 4).

In summary, when mood symptoms are observed during a psychotic process, lithium therapy should be considered. In fact, lithium's mood-stabilizing properties may be particularly beneficial in psychotic patients prone to disconcerting shifts in their moods. Lithium is not infrequently added to schizophrenic adult patient regimens. There are no data on this in children and adolescents, but it remains an interesting consideration. Adding lithium to a neuroleptic not only may enhance mood, but may result in lower requirements for the neuroleptic.[1,43,44,48,49] Further study is needed in this area as well.

Severe Aggression and Explosive Behavior

Schiff and colleagues[40] observed lithium to be effective in decreasing episodic and explosive behavior in patients with antisocial personality disorder,
particularly in those with a family history positive for mood disorders. Its potential role in the treatment of children and adolescents with severe aggression and explosive behavior is currently being evaluated.

Greenhill and colleagues[41] used lithium to treat nine children 9 to 14 years
of age with hyperactivity, aggression, and "giddy" behavior, and noted clinical improvement in only two of the children. These two children got worse
when the lithium was removed. The other children got worse on the lithium
or showed no improvement. The authors did note that the two children who
responded had more mood "lability, euphoria, and depression" symptoms
than those children who did not respond to lithium therapy. DeLong and
Nieman[42] used lithium to treat 16 children and adolescents 6 to 13 years of
age who had significant behavior problems beginning by 5 years, and who
also exhibited manic-type symptoms. The patients had all proved refractory
to stimulant medication, and had family histories positive for mood disorder.
Eleven of the patients exhibited clinical improvement on lithium in an open
trial and were subsequently given placebo in a double-blind manner (i.e.,
three weeks of lithium treatment, three weeks of placebo). These patients
did significantly better on lithium than on placebo.

Campbell and colleagues[43] conducted a double-blind, placebo-controlled
study of 61 inpatient children with DSM-III diagnoses of conduct disorder
undersocialized aggression, and found that haloperidol and lithium were
more effective than placebo in improving behavior. Lithium was noted to be
especially helpful in decreasing explosive behavior. Moreover, it caused
fewer and less toxic side effects than haloperidol. The lithium was relatively
well tolerated. Its use was found to result in decreased performance of the
children on the Porteus maze test, but did not impair short-term memory
and performance on other cognitive tests.[44]

DeLong and Aldershof[45] used lithium to treat children with behavioral disorders who had a variety of concomitant neurologic disorders, including mental retardation, and noted a significant decrease in aggression, explosive
outbursts, and encopresis in these children. The decrease in encopresis was
not an anticipated finding, but since it is often associated with disruptive behavior disorders, perhaps the amelioration of the behavioral symptoms resulted in the secondary decrease in encopresis.

Finally, Vetro and colleagues[46] used lithium to treat 17 very aggressive children 3 to 12 years of age who had severe social maladjustment difficulties.
Ten of the 17 children had proved refractory to haloperidol combined with

various psychological interventions. At mean serum lithium levels of 0.68 mEq/L, Vetro and his associates observed that 13 of the 17 children improved, with decreased aggressiveness and better social adjustment to the environment. The children needed continuous treatment with lithium for periods greater than six months for maximal efficacy. The authors also pointed out that three of the four patients who did not demonstrate clinical improvement had been noncompliant with the medication regimen. Further research into lithium's role in the treatment of severe aggression problems and explosive, violent behavior is required.

Attention-Deficit Hyperactivity Disorder

Lithium is a last-line treatment option for children and adolescents with ADHD. Stimulants are the pharmacologic treatment of choice (see Chapter 3), followed by the antidepressants, such as desipramine (Chapter 4), and clonidine (see Chapter 11). It is only when these more standard and more efficacious treatments of ADHD are unsuccessful that alternative medications such as lithium, carbamazepine, and such antipsychotics as haloperidol are considered. Some advocate trying lithium in treatment-refractory children and adolescents with ADHD who have a family history of mood disorder or who are exhibiting mood-type symptoms along with their ADHD. As mentioned previously, the differential diagnosis between ADHD and bipolar disorder, especially the rapid cycling type, can be difficult. Moreover, the two entities can coexist. Investigation to date, however, has shown that lithium has been ineffective when used to treat children diagnosed with ADHD.[41,45] Further study is necessary, but lithium's usefulness in treating ADHD appears limited to that of being utilized only when all else has failed.

Alcohol Abuse

See Chapter 14.

Bulimia

Hsu[71] conducted a study in which 14 bulimic patients were treated with lithium. While 12 of the 14 patients showed moderate to marked improvement on lithium, 10 had a coexistent mood disorder. Coexistent mood disorders are not, however, uncommon in patients with eating disorders.

In addition, the antidepressant fluoxetine recently generated attention for its effectiveness in ameliorating bulimic symptoms (see Chapter 4). Moreover, upon comparing the side-effect profiles of lithium and fluoxetine, fluoxetine is seen to be preferable. Patients with eating disorders often abuse laxatives and diuretics, which can result in lithium toxicity in those receiving lithium, while it is not a risk when fluoxetine is used. Perhaps in those

249

patients for whom fluoxetine is ineffective or only marginally effective, lithium can be cautiously added to the antidepressant. This may be an area for future research.

Personality Disorders (Borderline Personality Disorder)

The use of lithium in personality disorder patients is controversial. This is complicated by the fact that coexistent mood disorders are not uncommon in patients with personality disorders, so that it is often difficult to delineate specific medication effects on the personality disorder. In general, personality disorders are not indications for lithium's use. If there is a coexistent mood disorder (i.e., bipolar disorder), then the mood disorder should be treated. Obviously, an Axis I mood disorder can have a negative impact on an Axis II personality disorder, and vice versa, so that ameliorating symptoms of the mood disorder may result in improvement in some personality symptoms.

There are no data on children and adolescents. Moreover, many practicing clinicians are reluctant to diagnose this population with personality disorders. As with adults, until more is known it is probably best to treat mood disturbances as indicated, but not directly to target personality/character pathology with lithium.

Contraindications

See Table 8-3.

Pregnancy

Lithium is contraindicated in pregnancy unless there are urgent circumstances requiring its use, such as danger to self or others. Lithium use, particularly in the first trimester of pregnancy, significantly increases the risk of cardiac deformities and malformations. Ebstein's anomaly, the downward

Table 8-3
Contraindications to Lithium Use in Child and Adolescent Psychiatry

Absolute:
• Allergic drug reaction (rare)
Relative:
• Pregnancy
• Renal disease
• Cardiovascular disease
• Thyroid disease
• Severe dehydration/sodium depletion

displacement of the tricuspid valve, is the best-known and most common anomaly seen. Kallen and Tandberg[47] also observed that 7% of infants of women who took lithium in early pregnancy suffered severe heart defects other than Ebstein's anomaly. Thus it is crucial to emphasize to the adolescent and family the importance of informing the treating physician if the adolescent intends to or might accidentally become pregnant. Because of the high risk for side effects, we strongly urge avoiding this medication, particularly during the first trimester, in pregnant adolescents unless urgent circumstances dictate otherwise. These circumstances are likely to be less common in children and younger adolescents than in adults.

Renal Disease

Lithium is relatively contraindicated for children and adolescents with renal disease as it is primarily excreted by the kidneys.

Cardiovascular Disease

Lithium is relatively contraindicated for children and adolescents with cardiovascular disease as it has been associated with AV block and other cardiovascular side effects. Its use in such patients can significantly raise the likelihood that lithium toxicity will develop.[51]

Thyroid Disease

Thyroid disease no longer is felt to be an absolute contraindication to lithium's use. Carefully monitoring thyroid function and using supplemental thyroxine (Synthroid) when necessary obviate not using the medication. The risks/benefits must be assessed, and if the child or adolescent's condition is harmful to his or her well-being, the potential benefits with careful monitoring may outweigh the risks. If the patient had previously been on lithium and shown a poor response, or if the symptoms were not too severe, use of this medication may be deferred in favor of other medications that do not affect thyroid function.

Severe Dehydration/Sodium Depletion

Severe dehydration and sodium depletion are relative contraindications to lithium's use in children and adolescents because of the very high risk of toxicity.

History of Hypersensitivity/Allergy

A child or adolescent who has experienced an allergic reaction to lithium should not receive lithium again. Such reactions are, however, uncommon.

Patients on Thiazides

Lithium is not contraindicated for patients taking thiazides. An alternative dosing strategy is necessary for these patients (see below).

Electroconvulsive Therapy

Concurrent administration of lithium with ECT may prolong the muscular blockade of succinyl choline.[69] Therefore, prior to initiating ECT, lithium should be discontinued.

Side Effects

See Table 8-4.

Gastrointestinal Discomfort

General GI distress is a frequently encountered early side effect of lithium therapy.[51] Signs and symptoms include nausea, vomiting, loose stools, abdominal discomfort, and irritation and feelings of malaise. These effects are usually short-lived and may be related to peak plasma lithium levels. Having the patient take lithium with meals may help ameliorate GI symptoms. Starting with a low dose and increasing the dose gradually so that the patient becomes tolerant to the medication may be helpful. Certain lithium preparations (e.g., Lithobid) may be tolerated better. Cessation of lithium

Table 8-4
Side Effects of Lithium

Common:
• GI (nausea/vomiting, diarrhea)
• Tremor
• Leukocytosis
• Malaise
Uncommon:
• Renal (polydipsia/polyuria)
• Ocular irritation/stomatitis
• Hypothyroidism/nontoxic goiter
• Dermatologic
• Cardiovascular
• Weight gain/edema
• NMS/encephalopathic syndrome
• Diabetes
• Hair loss
• Growth and development

therapy should be considered if its use results in significant electolyte and volume depletion via emesis and/or diarrhea.

Tremor

A fine tremor is often seen early during lithium treatment, and usually signifies that lithium is at therapeutic levels in the bloodstream.[51] This is in contrast to the gross tremor seen with lithium toxicity.

Renal Dysfunction

Polyuria and polydipsia may occur at any time during lithium therapy due to its direct effect on the kidney,[24] and can result in a nephrogenic diabetes insipidus–like syndrome. This side effect may necessitate decreasing the dose, discontinuing the lithium, or, more rarely, treating the condition with chlorthiazide. Patients who suffer from severe polyuria secondary to lithium have been reported to excrete several liters of urine per day. It is, therefore, essential that kidney function be monitored since lithium has been rarely reported to result in a decreased glomerular filtration rate as a result of glomerular sclerosis and tubular atrophy.[48]

Ocular Irritation/Contact Stomatitis

Ocular irritation and/or contact stomatitis may result when lithium is secreted into body fluids.[24]

Hypothyroidism/Nontoxic Goiter

Lithium can produce hormonal side effects, including hypothyroidism and nontoxic goiter.[50] Decreased circulating thyroid hormones T3 and T4 and elevated TSH may result. Vetro and colleagues[46] observed that two of the children in their sample developed nontoxic goiter after being on lithium for one and one-half to two years. Hyperthyroidism has been reported with lithium use in adults, but occurs far less frequently than does hypothyroidism.

Dermatologic Effects

Dermatologic side effects can be particularly problematic for adolescent patients. The most common of these side effects are increase in acne vulgaris and maculopapular eruptions.[52] Less commonly, exacerbation and/or aggravation of psoriasis may occur.

Weight Gain and Edema

Weight gain and edema are common side effects associated with lithium's use.[51]

Leukocytosis

Lithium not infrequently causes a clinically insignificant increase in the white blood cell count of between 10,000 and 15,000 cells/mm^3, with increased polymorphonuclear leukocytes, lymphocytopenia, and platelet count.[53]

Malaise and Fatigue

Fatigue and malaise are not uncommonly seen in patients receiving lithium. This does not always imply toxicity (see "Overdose/Toxicity"). Children and adolescents may complain of feeling sluggish, tired, and uncomfortable. Sometimes, this goes away with time as the child adjusts to the medication. In other cases, decreasing the dose is helpful. Starting with a low dose and increasing the dose gradually may also help to avert some of these side effects.

Neuroleptic Malignant Syndrome

The neuroleptic malignant syndrome has been seen in patients treated with a combination of lithium and antipsychotic medications.[55] In a few such patients, a full-blown encephalopathic syndrome has developed, which is characterized by weakness, lethargy, fever, confusion, extrapyramidal side effects, increased white blood cell count, increased BUN, increased serum enzymes, and increased fasting blood sugar. It is, therefore, essential to monitor patients receiving both lithium and neuroleptics extremely closely for the presence of neurotoxicity, since some patients who developed this syndrome have died. As this usually occurs at toxic plasma lithium levels, careful monitoring of lithium plasma blood levels is essential when haloperidol and lithium are administered simultaneously. If such symptoms are seen, lowering the dose of lithium or discontinuing the medication is often necessary. Some clinicians view the encephalopathic syndrome and NMS in these instances as being very similar or the same.

Diabetes

Lithium's associated hormonal side effects may occasionally accelerate the development of diabetes.[50]

Hair Loss

Hair loss is a rare side effect of lithium.[51]

Growth and Development

It is known that lithium can interfere with calcium metabolism by mobilizing calcium from immature bones. It is, therefore, recommended that regular physical examinations looking specifically at the growth and development of children on lithium be done. Moreover, some investigators believe that calcium, phosphorus, and alkaline phosphatase need to be monitored in children who are still growing.[50,54]

Overdose/Toxicity

Lithium toxicity is very closely related to serum lithium levels, and in fact, can be seen at doses close to therapeutic levels.[55] Moreover, lithium has a low therapeutic index and can be lethal after overdose. It is important to remember, however, that although lithium overdose may result in lithium toxicity, the most common cause of toxicity in compliant patients is a change in sodium balance leading to sodium depletion,[23] which elevates lithium levels. In fact, the clinician must monitor the patient closely to determine any condition that can alter the sodium balance, such as dehydration or change in diet. It is important that the patient and family be advised that the child or adolescent on lithium must get sufficient amounts of table salt and liquids. Some have wondered if patients on lithium should be counseled either to reduce their exercising or stop it altogether, particularly in hot weather. Jefferson and colleagues[1] assessed four athletes in good health who were placed on stable doses of lithium for one month before they were to compete in a 20-km race. After the race, the four patients were found to be dehydrated, but instead of having increased serum lithium levels, these levels had decreased by 20%. Interestingly, the sweat-to-serum ratio for the lithium cation was four times greater than that for the sodium ion.[1] It was concluded that vigorous exercise that resulted in large amounts of perspiration was more likely to necessitate an increase or no change in the lithium dose, since serum lithium levels after strenuous exercise appeared to be more likely to decrease than to increase. Nonetheless, Jefferson and his associates still recommend careful monitoring of the fluid–electrolyte status in patients on lithium who engage in strenuous exercise.

There are different degrees of lithium toxicity: mild, moderate, and severe.[23] Mild intoxication can be manifested by subtle symptoms, such as GI distress or dizziness. In these cases, the lithium should be withheld until the level returns to the therapeutic range.[23] It is important to search for the cause of the increased level (noncompliance, accidental overingestion, etc.). If no obvious cause for the increased level and toxicity is found, a renal workup is indicated, which should include a urinalysis, electrolytes, BUN/creatinine, creatinine clearance, urinary sodium, and 24-hour protein. With moderate or severe lithium toxicity, the patient needs to be admitted to the hospital so that sodium can be administered while frequent monitoring of lithium levels is carried out.[23]

Acute Lithium Intoxication

Lithium levels above 3 mmol/L can be life-threatening and represent a medical emergency.[23] It is important to emphasize that the reversibility of lithium intoxication is directly related to the serum level of lithium and the length of time it remains elevated. Thus it is important that measures to reduce the toxic level be commenced with haste. It also is important to note that even with very high lithium serum levels and after a significant overdose, symptoms may be quite mild and subtle.[23] The physician must not be lulled into a false sense of security. Severe symptoms can arise suddenly and without warning, resulting in the death of the patient. Therefore, it is important to counsel patients and their families on the importance of looking for any early-warning signs of lithium toxicity, and of the need to tell the physician immediately if they should appear. Signs of serious lithium intoxication include ataxia, dysarthria, gross tremor, delirium, hallucinations, seizure, coma, renal failure, diarrhea, and neuromuscular irritability or flaccidity.[23] Patients who survive severe lithium toxicity may suffer permanent impairment to memory, gait, and other functions.[56]

There is no specific antidote to lithium poisoning, that is, after an overdose.[23] It is, however, believed that treatment should be aggressive in attempting to remove the excess lithium from the body. As with any overdose/overingestion, the clinician should obtain a toxicologic screen to see if the patient has taken any other drugs. Treatment is very similar to that for barbiturate overdoses. Gastric lavage should be undertaken in acute overdose patients.[23] Lithium levels are often quite high in gastric secretions, so gastric aspiration is very important.[23] It is also essential that correction of the fluid and electrolyte imbalance be initiated promptly. When lithium levels are less than 3 mmol/L and the signs of intoxication are mild, this fluid and electrolyte imbalance can be corrected by administering IV normal saline at rates of 150–200 ml/hr as long as the patient is producing adequate urine.[23] At lithium levels greater than 3 mmol/L and with evidence of severe toxicity (i.e., if there is minimal urine output and/or renal failure), dialysis is necessary. Hemodialysis is the preferred treatment, as it rapidly removes lithium ions from the toxic patient. Urea, mannitol, and aminophylline are capable of significantly increasing the excretion of lithium.[55] It is very important to monitor lithium levels frequently during dialysis, as lithium will reequilibrate from the tissues after hemodialysis treatment.[23] Targeted lithium levels are 1 mmol/L or less six hours after dialysis. When such levels are reached, the dialysis can be stopped. As with any overdose, it is also important to monitor the patient's airway, breathing, and circulation.

Abuse

There appears to be virtually no risk for recreational abuse of lithium.

Drug Interactions

See Table 8-5.

Available Preparations

See Table 8-6.

Initiating and Maintaining Treatment

Before treatment with lithium is begun in children and adolescents, a premedication workup is required that is similar to that performed on adults. Children and adolescents must have a complete history taken and physical examination performed by their primary medical physician. Laboratory assessment includes a pregnancy test on every female patient, because lithium crosses the placenta and is associated with an increased risk of congenital heart disease in infants born to mothers using lithium during pregnancy. The period of greatest risk appears to be the first trimester. The most common cardiac malformation is Ebstein's anomaly, but other cardiac disturbances can occur in these infants, and there is also an increased risk for cyanosis, hypotonia, and lethargy.[57] It is essential that the patient and family be counseled about the importance of informing the psychiatrist if there is any chance that the patient might be pregnant. Screening for the use of and knowledge about birth control is necessary. If, during treatment with lithium, the adolescent admits to having missed menstrual periods and/or to having had unprotected sex, the lithium should be withheld until a preg-

Table 8-5
Lithium Drug Interactions

Increase serum lithium levels: • Antibiotics • Carbamazepine • Diuretics • Nonsteroidal anti-inflammatory agents
Decrease serum lithium levels: • Acetazolamide • Caffeine • Osmotic diuretics • Theophylline
Interact with lithium to produce sedation and/or confusional states: • Alcohol • Antihypertensives • Antipsychotics (especially haloperidol)

Table 8-6
Available Preparations of Lithium

Generic	Proprietary	Strength
Lithium carbonate	Eskalith	300 mg
Lithium carbonate	Lithium carbonate	300 mg
Lithium carbonate	Lithonate	300 mg
Lithium carbonate	Lithotabs	300 mg
Lithium carbonate, slow release	Eskalith CR	450 mg
Lithium carbonate, slow release	Lithobid	300 mg
Lithium citrate syrup	Cibalith	8 mEq/5 ml (equal to one 300-mg tablet)

nancy test is performed that documents that the patient is not pregnant. The clinician should not rely on the patient or her family to guarantee this, as certain situations might force the adolescent to deny her pregnancy. Most important, however, is establishing a good relationship with the adolescent and caregivers and emphasizing that, due to the risk of congenital heart malformations, she should not become pregnant while on lithium. If she does decide to become pregnant, she must immediately inform the physician and/or stop taking the medication. Counseling and further assessment can then be conducted.

It is important to assess all children and adolescents for evidence of kidney and thyroid disease before lithium is started, in order to ascertain the patient's baseline function. In healthy patients, this merely requires checking a urinalysis for BUN and creatinine.[58] If renal anomaly is noted prior to initiating lithium therapy, it is probably best to avoid lithium and to try an alternative medication such as carbamazepine. If all other alternatives have been exhausted and the clinician believes that lithium is essential to the patient's functioning (i.e., a very strong positive family history of response to lithium or the patient has responded well to lithium in the past), then consultation with a nephrologist is recommended. If it is decided to initiate lithium therapy, very careful monitoring, with frequent checks of kidney function, is required.

When a stable dose has been achieved, checking kidney function one week later is recommended. If kidney function is normal, assessing it every six months is sufficient. If an anomaly occurs, consultation with a medical specialist is recommended. Laboratory tests to be checked include a urinalysis, paying particular attention to specific gravity, BUN and creatinine, creatinine clearance, 24-hour urine protein, and urinary sodium. While the patient is on lithium, the patient and family should be active participants in monitoring how the patient is doing. If any anomaly is noted, such as the child's going to the bathroom more frequently than usual, drinking more fluids than usual, or complaining of increased thirst, the parents should be instructed to call the psychiatrist immediately, and to hold the lithium until they speak with the doctor and/or have the child assessed.

Jefferson and colleagues[1] found that as many as 15% of patients receiving lithium therapy will show increased TSH levels. Lithium causes these thyroid anomalies by reducing thyroid hormone release, leading to decreased levels of T3, T4, and protein-bound thyroid hormone, and to increased TSH and I_{131} levels. Therefore, it is essential to determine baseline thyroid function prior to initiating lithium therapy by checking T4, T3, T3RU, and TSH levels. Some investigators recommend checking antithyroid antibodies, since hypothyroidism secondary to lithium may be related to a preexisting Hashimoto's thyroiditis.[59] Anomalies do not necessarily preclude treatment with lithium. Elevated TSH levels are felt to be the most sensitive index for hypothyroidism. If this occurs, it is best to repeat the level and consult an endocrinologist. If the level remains elevated, the clinician can use another medication and/or, upon consultation with the endocrinologist, consider treating the hypothyroidism with thyroxine (Synthroid) while the lithium is administered. Frequent monitoring of lithium blood levels and thyroid function is necessary. The patient should also be monitored for signs of hypothyroidism, such as thinning hair, dry skin, heat/cold intolerance, and decreased energy.

Other anomalies of thyroid function, such as alterations in T4, T3, or T3RU, are less sensitive than the TSH index. Therefore, if there is an anomaly of one or more of these factors with a normal TSH, it is best to repeat the whole battery. If repeat testing is normal, lithium therapy can be commenced with monitoring as described above. If anomalies persist, a TRH stimulation test that is very sensitive to picking up thyroid pathology can be conducted. Consultation with an endocrinologist is advised. It should be noted, however, that transiently abnormal TFTs without coexisting thyroid pathology have been observed in up to 33% of patients in psychiatry.[60] Thus a number of thyroid anomalies detected on routine testing spontaneously resolve, so that lithium therapy may not be precluded. Checking thyroid function tests after each increase of the lithium dose in this situation, and then after a stable dose has been achieved, every three months instead of every six months is recommended. If the thyroid function test anomaly subsequently resolves, switching to routine monitoring is recommended, as long as the patient is asymptomatic.

If thyroid function is normal at baseline, it should be checked one week after the maintenance dose of lithium has been achieved. If it is normal, thyroid function tests need to be checked every six months. The patient should also be monitored clinically, and if he or she shows clinical signs suspicious of thyroid illness, such as cold intolerance, apathy, and decreased energy, thyroid function tests should be checked at that time.

If at any time during the lithium therapy thyroid anomaly is noted, consultation with an endocrinologist is recommended. First of all, it is important to determine whether or not the condition requires medical treatment. Second, sometimes lowering the dose of lithium instead of simply discontinuing it will reverse the thyroid anomaly. Discontinuation of lithium in some cases can reverse the hypothyroid or, more rarely, hyperthyroid condition. Lithium therapy not uncommonly can result in the patient's developing a nontoxic goiter. Again, medical consultation is necessary, but discontinuation of the drug is not always required. If the patient is doing well on the medication, and it is determined, after assessing the risks versus benefits, that it should be continued, this can be done safely with careful monitoring of the patient. Fortunately, some conditions, such as hypothyroidism, can be treated very effectively with thyroid hormone. This is often not a major inconvenience for the family as the thyroid hormone usually can be taken once per day, for example, with the morning lithium dose.

All children and adolescents to be started on lithium should receive a baseline ECG, since conduction abnormalities, bradycardia, and reversible ECG anomalies have been observed occasionally in adults on lithium.[58] Therefore, although some might argue that a baseline ECG is not necessary for healthy children and adolescents, we advocate performing this relatively simple and noninvasive test so that, if problems occur, it can be compared with the premedication ECG. If cardiac anomalies develop, cardiology consultation is recommended prior to starting or continuing lithium therapy.

Children and adolescents treated with lithium should have a CBC and differential and platelet count, since lithium is known to cause a leukocytosis with neutrophilia, lymphocytopenia, and increased platelet counts in some patients.[53] This leukocytosis is benign, and can often be distinguished from leukocytosis caused by true infection, since during lithium therapy the neutrophils are in a more mature form, while infection affects the younger forms of neutrophils. It is essential that the patient and family be told to inform all medical professionals that the child is on lithium. They should be given a handout listing lithium's side effects so that they know that lithium can cause leukocytosis. This may be important if the child sees a medical physician and is found to have an unexplained leukocytosis. Moreover, some medical personnel may not know that lithium causes this side effect. That is why it is best that it be explained to the patient and/or his or her family that it is a side effect with lithium therapy so that they can inform their medical doctor. It is also important that the patient, family, and other clinicians understand that lithium does not have to be discontinued when a leukocytosis develops.

It is very important to check electrolytes prior to initiating lithium therapy. Particular attention needs to be paid to sodium to ensure that it is not low, since decreased sodium results in reduced excretion of lithium and can lead to lithium toxicity. It is probably a good idea to check electrolytes with kidney function tests, since they are often checked together with the BUN and creatinine. The patient and family must be counseled to make sure that the child receives adequate quantities of table salt. Moreover, if the child is participating in any kind of strenuous exercise in which he or she perspires a great deal, the psychiatrist must be consulted and lithium levels monitored more frequently (see "Side Effects"). The patient and family should be advised particularly of the risks involved if the patient becomes dehydrated, since dehydration can result in sodium imbalance and consequent lithium toxicity.

There is some debate as to whether baseline EEGs should be performed on children and adolescents being started on lithium. Children with conduct disorders on lithium have been observed to have increased EEG abnormalities, including focal and paroxysmal changes, as compared with EEGs done prior to treatment.[60] The EEG anomalies do not, however, correlate with lithium toxicity, and behavioral improvement was noted in more of the children on lithium than on placebo. Therefore, we do not recommend EEG as a baseline workup measure for healthy children and adolescents. If, however, the child has a history of EEG disturbance (seizures and/or family history of seizure disorder), we endorse getting a baseline EEG, and then monitoring the EEG periodically thereafter. Lithium levels should be checked on the same morning that the EEG is performed to correlate the levels with the EEG.

Clinical Practice

Dosage and Administration

See Table 8-7.

In children older than 12 years of age, the dosing of lithium is started low and gradually increased, with repeated monitoring of lithium level.

Starting with an initial dose of 150–300 mg of lithium carbonate per day and gradually increasing the dose by 150- to 300 mg increments every five to seven days is advisable. It has been reported that many of the aversive side effects of lithium that occur early during treatment—including GI irrita-

261

Table 8-7

Dosing and Administration of Lithium for Children and Adolescents

Children <12 years:	Children >12 years:
Not FDA approved.	FDA approved (see Table 8-2).
Guidelines from Weller and colleagues:	Start with dose 150–300 mg/day. Check serum levels
> 25 kg initial dose on t.i.d. schedule: 150/150/300	five days after dose. Increase gradually by 150–300
25–40kg—300/300/300	mg every five to seven days. For acute mania, doses
40–50kg—300/300/600	of 1800 mg/day (level 1–1.5 mEq/L) usually
50–60kg—600/300/600	required. For long-term maintenance, doses of
	900–1200 mg/day are usually required, yielding
	serum levels of 0.6–1.2.
• Targeted therapeutic serum levels 0.6–1.2 mEq/L.	
• Should not exceed level 1.4 mEq/L.	
• Increase dose gradually, monitoring efficacy versus toxicity.	
• Keep on specific dose five to seven days.	
• Draw lithium levels 12 hours after giving medication.	

Adapted from: Weller, E.B., Weller, R.A., Fristad, M.A. (1986). Lithium dosage guide for prepubertal children. *J Am Acad Child Psychiatry, 25,* 92–95.

tion, such as nausea/vomiting and diarrhea; dizziness and confusion; muscle aches; weakness; polyuria and polydipsia; and hand tremor—take place when the dose of lithium is increased too rapidly, so that serum lithium levels rise too quickly for the body to adjust.[63] Moreover, the lithium cation directly irritates the gastric mucosa, so that making sure that the lithium is taken after eating (i.e., after breakfast, lunch, and dinner) will often decrease or eliminate the GI irritation, since this dose regimen slows lithium's absorption. The combination of gradually increasing the lithium dose and taking the medication after meals often is successful in ameliorating the GI symptoms. If the symptoms persist, switching to enteric-coated lithium such as Lithobid capsules might be helpful. In addition, the slow-release form of lithium, which can be administered twice a day, is often better tolerated by patients. If lithium is to be given four times per day, having the patient have a bedtime snack before taking the lithium is recommended.

Lithium blood levels should be checked five days after the dose is increased. Because of their increased renal clearance, it is not uncommon for children and adolescents to require higher doses of lithium than adults—1800 mg/day or higher.[11,61] This dosage often results in lithium levels of 1–1.5 mEq/L, which are necessary to control an acute mania. It is believed that acutely manic patients require such high doses of lithium because while they are manic, they metabolize lithium more rapidly than when they are euthymic. This necessitates dosage adjustment when the manic phase abates (i.e., low ering the dose). Long-term maintenance therapy usually involves the administration of 900–1200 mg of lithium carbonate daily in three or four divided doses, which usually produces levels of 0.6–1.2 mEq/L.[55] Occasionally, children and adolescents will require higher maintenance doses to maintain adequate lithium levels. Berg and colleagues[63] described one 14-year-old girl with bipolar disorder who required lithium doses of 2400 mg per day to reach therapeutic levels.

Because of lithium's pharmacokinetics, it is necessary to administer it in three to four divided doses when the immediate-release form is given. When the sustained-release form is utilized, it should be given twice daily. It is not advisable to give the entire dose of lithium at one time. In other words, if a patient is receiving a total daily lithium dose of 900 mg, it is better to give this as 300 mg three times per day instead of all 900 mg at bedtime. This minimizes the risk of serum lithium level toxicity and resultant patient discomfort.

Lithium levels must be checked twice a week when the patient is acutely manic. When the mania abates and the patient is more stable, the levels may be checked less frequently. After it has been determined that the patient is euthymic and in remission, maintenance therapy is necessary for at least six to nine months. During this period, lithium levels should be checked at least once every three months. We recommend checking the lithium on a monthly basis for at least the first three months of the maintenance period, because child and adolescent pharmacokinetics can be so variable and because lithium has been less studied in this population. Kidney and thyroid function, as mentioned, can be checked twice a year. It is important to emphasize that, in contrast with adults, the National Institute of Mental Health/National Institute of Health Consensus Development Panel specifically states that there are no set standards for the prophylactic use of lithium in children and adolescents.[63] The decision to maintain a patient on preventative lithium therapy chronically is a clinical decision that must be made by the individual clinician in consultation with the patient and family.

Although children under 12 years of age are generally treated with therapeutic doses of lithium similar to those used for older adolescents, Weller and colleagues[61,66] have written a guide for calculating the initial total lithium dose that differs significantly from the initial dose given to adolescents and young adults. The guide's goal is to help the clinician achieve therapeutic lithium levels of 0.6–1.2 mEq/L as rapidly as possible, thus maximizing the efficacy of the medication and minimizing its toxicity. Weller and colleagues[61] devised this strategy after studying the effects of lithium on 10 children with bipolar disorder, manic type, and five children with conduct disorders. What was most remarkable about their study was that 13 of the 15 children achieved therapeutic lithium levels within five days of initiating treatment and suffered very minimal side effects, which were mostly short-term effects and none of which required discontinuation of the medication.

Weller and colleagues divided prepubertal children according to their weight and determined specific initial doses for these children. In children weighing less than 25 kg, the initial recommended dose is 600 mg/day in divided doses, 150 mg after breakfast, 150 mg after lunch, and 300 mg after dinner. This dosage schedule should be maintained for five days. Lithium levels should be drawn every other day 12 hours after the last lithium dose during this period, until two consecutive lithium levels between 0.6 and 1.2 mEq/L are obtained. It is then recommended that doses be adjusted gradually according to clinical efficacy versus side effects and serum lithium level. The authors do not recommend exceeding lithium levels of 1.4 mEq/L.

For children weighing between 25 and 40 kg, initial doses of lithium recommended by the authors are 300 mg after breakfast, lunch, and dinner, for a total of 900 mg/day.[61] Children weighing 40–50 kg should be started with a total daily lithium dose of 1200 mg in divided doses of 300 mg after breakfast, 300 mg after lunch, and 600 mg after dinner. Finally, children weighing between 50 and 60 kg should be given an initial lithium dose of 1500 mg/day in three divided doses of 600 mg after breakfast, 300 mg after lunch, and 600 mg after dinner.

Further study in this area is clearly necessary. The sample studied by Weller and colleagues was small, and larger, placebo-controlled trials in which various doses of lithium are used to treat these children are required. Nonetheless, Weller's guide is an important first step, and may prove to be quite useful.

It behooves the clinician to be aware of the fact that a liquid lithium preparation—lithium citrate—is available (see Table 8-6). This may be particularly helpful for younger children, who often have difficulty in swallowing pills.

One final point regarding the dosing and administration of lithium that needs to be addressed is whether or not it is acceptable to monitor lithium by checking saliva levels as opposed to blood levels. While the authors prefer serum blood levels, we recognize that drawing repeated lithium serum blood levels can be traumatic for children, and thus saliva tests must be considered, particularly for children and adolescents who become especially upset by repeated blood draws. Several authors have reported that saliva lithium levels are higher than serum lithium levels, ranging from 1.0 to 3.99 times higher.[65–68] Moreover, these saliva/serum ratios show marked interindividual variability. Nonetheless, the saliva/serum ratio is fairly constant for a specific patient.[67,68] Obviously, this area requires further study. Clinicians are urged to consider getting an initial saliva lithium level. This does not preclude drawing an initial blood level, as the ratio will be important when checking future saliva levels. We recommend assessing the patient and family first. If the patient is not unduly upset at having his or her blood drawn, then this is to be preferred. If, on the other hand, venipuncture is especially disconcerting and traumatic for the youngster, checking saliva lithium levels may be preferable.

References

1. Jefferson, J.W., Greist, J.H., Ackerman, D.L. (1987). *Lithium Encyclopedia for Clinical Practice*. Washington, D.C.: American Psychiatric Press.

2. *Diagnostic and Statistical Manual of Mental Disorders (3rd rev.)*. (1987). Washington, D.C.: American Psychiatric Association.

3. Varanka, T.M., Weller, R.A., Weller, E.B., Fristad, M.A. (1988). Lithium treatment of manic episodes with psychotic features in prepubertal children. *Am J Psychiatry, 145*, 1557–1559.

4. Sylvester, C.E., Burke, P.M., McCanky, E.A., Clark, C.J. (1984). Manic psychosis in childhood: Report of two cases. *J Nerv Men Dis, 172*, 12–15.

5. Baldessarini, R.J., Stephens, J.H. (1970). Clinical pharmacology and toxicology of lithium salts. *Arch Gen Psychiatry, 22*, 72–77.

6. Delong, G.R., Aldershof, A.L. (1987). Long-term experience with lithium treatment in childhood: Correlation with clinical diagnosis. *J Am Acad Child Adolesc Psychiatry, 26*, 389–394.

7. McDaniel, K.D. (1986). Pharmacologic treatment of psychiatric and neurodevelopmental disorders in children and adolescents (part 3). *Clin Pediatr, 25*, 198–204.

8. Gualtieri, C.T., Golden, R.N., Fahs, J.J. (1983). New developments in pediatric psychopharmacology. *Dev Behav Pediatr, 4*, 202–209.

9. Ryan, N.D., Puig-Antich, J. (1987). Pharmacological treatment of adolescent psychiatric disorders. *J Adolesc Health Care, 8*, 137–142.

10. Youngerman, J., Canino, I.A. (1978). Lithium carbonate use in children and adolescents: A survey of the literature. *Arch Gen Psychiatry, 35*, 216–224.

11. Jefferson, J.W. (1982). The use of lithium in childhood and adolescence: An overview. *J Clin Psychiatry, 43*, 174–177.

12. Strober, M., Morrell, W., Burroughs, J., et al. (1988). A family study of bipolar I in adolescence. *J Affective Disords, 15*, 255, 268.

13. McKnew, D.H., Cytryn, L., Buchsbaum, M.D., et al., (1981). Lithium in children of lithium responding parents. *Psychiatry Res, 4*, 171–180.

14. Brumback, R.A., Weinberg, W.A. (1977). Mania in childhood II: Therapeutic trail of lithium carbonate and further description of manic-depressive illness in children. *Am J Dis Child, 131*, 1122–1126.

15. Varanka, T.M., Weller, R.A., Weller, E.B., Fristad, M.A. (1988). Lithium treatment of manic episodes with psychotic features in prepubertal children. *Am J Psychiatry, 145*, 1557–1559.

16. Dunner, D.L., Fleiss, J.L., Fieve, R.R. (1976). Lithium carbonate prophylaxis failure. *Br J Psychiatry, 129*, 40–44.

17. Carlson, G.A., Rapport, M.D., Pataki, C.S., Kelly, K.L. (1992). Lithium in hospitalized children at 4 and 8 weeks: Mood, behavioral, and cognitive effect. *J Child Psychol Psychiatry, 33(2)*, 411–425.

18. Carlson, G.A. (1990) Annotation: Child and adolescent mania—diagnostic considerations. *J Child Psychol Psychiatry, 31*, 331–341.

19. Krauthammer, C., Klerman, G.L. (1978). Secondary mania. *Arch Gen Psychiatry, 35*, 1333–1339.

20. Woodruff, R.A., Murphy, G.E., Herjanic, M. (1967). The natural history of affective disorders I: Symptoms of 72 patients at the time of index admission. *J Psychiat Res, 5*, 225–263.

21. Black, D.W., Winokur, G., Bell, S., et al. (1988). Complicated mania—comorbidity and immediate outcome in the treatment of mania. *Arch Gen Psychiatry, 45*, 232–236.

22. Rancurello, M.D. (1986). Antidepressants in children: Indicating benefits and limitations. *Am J Psychother, 40*, 377–392.

23. Arana, G.W., Hyman, S.E. (1991). *Handbook of Psychiatric Drug Therapy (2nd ed.)* (pp. 162–170.). Boston: Little Brown.

24. Lapierre, Y.D., Raval, K.J. (1989). Pharmacotherapy of affective disorders in children and adolescents. *Psychiat Clin North Am, 12(4)*.

25. Baastrup, P.C., Poulson, J.C., Schou, M., et al. (1970). Prophylactic lithium: Double-blind discontinuation in manic-depressive and recurrent disorders. *Lancet, 2*, 326.

26. Fieve, R.R., Kumbarachi, T., Dunner, D.L. (1976). Lithium prophylaxis

of depression in bipolar I, bipolar II, and unipolar patients. *Am J Psychiatry, 133*, 925.

27. Prien, R.F., Kupfer, D.J., Mansky, P.A., et al. (1984). Drug therapy in the prevention of recurrences in unipolar and bipolar affective disorders. *Arch Gen Psychiatry, 41*, 1096.

28. Mendels, J., Ramsey, A., Dyson, W.L., Frazer, A. (1979). Lithium as an antidepressant. *Arch Gen Psychiatry, 36*, 845.

29. Neubauer, H., Bermingham, P. (1976). A depressive syndrome responsive to lithium. *J Nerv Ment Dis, 163*, 276–281.

30. DeMontigny, C., Cournoyer, G., Morissette, R., et al. (1983). Lithium carbonate addition to tricyclic antidepressant-resistant unipolar depression. *Arch Gen Psychiatry, 40*, 1327–1334.

31. DeMontigny, C., Grunberg, F., Mayer, A., Deschenes, J.P. (1981). Lithium induces rapid relief of depression in tricyclic antidepressant drug nonresponders. *Br J Psychiatry, 138*, 252–256.

32. Heninger, G.R., Charney, D.S., Sternberg, D.E. (1983). Lithium carbonate augmentation of antidepressant treatment. *Arch Gen Psychiatry, 40*, 1336–1342.

33. Garbutt, J.C., Mayo, J.P., Gilette, G., et al. (1986). Lithium potentiation of tricyclic antidepressants following lack of T_3 potentiation. *Am J Psychiatry, 143*, 1038–1039.

34. Louie, A.K., Meltzer, H.Y. (1984). Lithium potentiation of antidepressant treatment. *J Clin Psychopharmacol, 4*, 316–321.

35. Price, L.H., Charney, D.S., Heninger, G.R. (1984). Variability of response to lithium augmentation in refractory depression. *Am J Psychiatry, 143*, 1387–1392.

36. Schrader, G.D., Levien, H.E.M. (1985). Response to sequential administration of clomipramine and lithium carbonate in treatment resistant depression. *Br J Psychiatry, 147*, 573–575.

37. Ryan, N.D., Meyer, V., Dachille, S., et al. (1988). Lithium antidepressant augmentation in TCA-refractory depression. *J Am Acad Child Adolesc Psychiatry, 27(3)*, 371–376.

38. Quitkin, F.M., Rabkin, J.G., Ross, D., McGrath, P.J. (1984). Duration of antidepressant drug treatment: What is a good trial? *Arch Gen Psychiatry, 41*, 238–245.

39. Prien, R.F., Kupfer, D.J., Mansky, P.A., et al. (1984). Drug therapy in the prevention of recurrences in unipolar and bipolar affective disorders. *Arch Gen Psychiatry, 41*, 1096.

40. Schiff, H.B., Sabin, T.D., Geller, A., et al. (1982). Lithium in agressive behavior. *Am J Psychiatry, 139*, 1346.

41. Greenhill, L.L., Reider, R.O., Wender, P.H., et al. (1973). Lithium carbonate in the treatment of hyperactive children. *Arch Gen Psychiatry, 28*, 636–640.

42. DeLong, G.R., Nieman, G.W. (1983). Lithium-induced behavior changes in children with symptoms suggesting manic-depressive illness. *Psychopharmacol Bull, 19*, 258–265.

43. Campbell, M., Small, A.M., Green, W.H., et al. (1984). Behavioral efficacy of haloperidol and lithium carbonate—Comparison in hospitalized aggressive children with conduct disorder. *Arch Gen Psychiatry, 41*, 650–656.

44. Platt, J.E., Campbell, M., Green, W.H., Grega, D.M. (1984). Cognitive effects of lithium carbonate and haloperidol in treatment of resistant aggressive children. *Arch Gen Psychiatry, 41*, 657–662.

45. DeLong, G.R., Aldershof, A.L. (1987). Long-term experience with lithium treatment in childhood: Correlation with clinical diagnosis. *J Am Acad Child Adolesc Psychiatry, 26*, 389–394.

46. Vetro, A., Szentistvangi, I., Pallag, L., et al. J. (1985). Therapeutic experience with lithium in childhood aggressivity. *Pharmacopsychiatry, 14*, 121–127.

47. Källèn, B., Tandberg, A. (1983). Lithium and pregnancy. *Acta Psychiatr Scand, 68*, 134–139.

48. Vestergaard, P. (1980). Renal side effects of lithium. In F.N. Johnson (Ed.), *Handbook of Lithium Therapy* (pp. 354–357). Baltimore: University Park Press.

49. Lena, B., Surtees, S.J., Maggs, R. (1978). The efficacy of lithium in the treatment of emotional disturbances in children and adolescents. In F.N. Johnson & S. Johnson (Eds.), *Lithium in Medical Practice* (pp. 79–83). Baltimore: University Park Press.

50. Herskowitz, J. (1987). Developmental neurotoxicology. In C. Popper (Ed.), *Psychiatric Pharmacoscience of Children and Adolescents* (pp. 81–123). Washington, D.C.: American Psychiatric Press.

51. Jefferson, J.W., Greist, J.H. (1991). Lithium therapy. In H.I. Kaplan, B.J. Sadock (Eds.), *Comprehensive Textbook of Psychiatry (5th ed.)* (p. 1661). Baltimore: Williams & Wilkins.

52. McDaniel, K.D. (1985). Pharmacologic treatment of psychiatric and neurodevelopmental disorders in children and adolescents. *Can J Psychiatry, 30*, 119–129.

53. Reisberg, B., Gershon, S. (1979). Side effects associated with lithium therapy. *Arch Gen Psychiatry, 36*, 879–887.

54. Joyce, P.R. (1984). Age of onset in bipolar affective disorder and misdiagnosis as schizophrenia. *Psychol Med, 14*, 145–149.

55. *Physicians Desk Reference* (45th ed.). (1991). Oradell, NJ: Medical Economics.

56. Schou, M. (1984). Long-lasting neurological sequelae after lithium intoxication. *Acta Psychiatr Scand, 70*, 594.

57. *United States Pharmacoperal Dispensing Information: Drug Information for the Health Care Professional.* (1990). Rockville, Md.: United States Pharmacopeial Convention.

58. Rosse, R.B., Geise, A.A., Deutsch, S.I., Morihisa, J.M. (1989). *Laboratory Diagnostic Testing in Psychiatry.* Washington, D.C.: American Psychiatric Press.

59. Spratt, D.L., Pont, A., Miller, M.B., et al. (1982). Thyroxinaemia in patients with acute psychiatric disorders. *Am J Med, 73*, 41–47.

60. Bennett, W.G., Korein, J., Kalmyn, M., et al. (1983). Electroencephalogram and treatment of hospitalized agressive children with haloperidol or lithium. *Biol Psychiatry, 12*, 1427–1440.

61. Weller, E.B., Weller, R.A., Fristad, M.A. (1986). Lithium dosage guide for prepubertal children. *J Am Acad Child Psychiatry, 25*, 92–95.

62. National Institute of Mental Health/National Institutes of Health Consensus Development Panel. (1985). Mood disorders: Pharmacologic prevention of reoccurrences. *Am J Psychiatry, 142*, 469–476.

63. Berg, I., Hullin, R., Allsopp, M., et al. (1974). Bipolar manic-depressive psychosis in early adolescence: A case report. *Br J Psychiatry, 125*, 416–417.

64. Campbell, M., Perry, R., Green, W.H., (1984). The use of lithium in children and adolescents. *Psychosomatics, 25*, 95–106.

65. Perry, R., Campbell, M., Grega, D.M., Anderson, L. (1984). Saliva lithium levels in children: Their use in monitoring serum lithium levels and lithium side effects. *J Clin Psychopharmacol, 4*, 199–202.

66. Weller, E.B., Weller, R.A., Fristad, M.A., et al. (1987). Saliva lithium monitoring in prepubertal children. *J Am Acad Child Psychiatry, 26*, 173–175.

67. Vitiello, B., Behar, D., Malone, R., et al. (1988). Pharmacokinetics of lithium carbonate in children. *J Clin Psychopharmacol, 8,* 355, 359.

68. Bernstein, J.G. (1988). *Handbook of Drug Therapy in Psychiatry (2nd ed.).* Littleton, Mass.: PSG Publishing.

69. Fink, M. (1988). A manual of practice. In A.J. Frances, R.E. Hales (Eds.), *Review of Psychiatry* (p. 482). Washington, D.C.: American Psychiatric Press.

70. Procci, W.R. (1991). Schizoaffective disorder and brief reactive psychosis. In H.I. Kaplan, B.J. Sadock (Eds.), *Comprehensive Textbook of Psychiatry (5th ed.)* (pp. 839–840). Baltimore: Williams & Wilkins.

71. Hsu, L. (1984). Treatment of bulimia with lithium. *Am J Psychiatry, 141,* 1260–1262.

Chapter 9

Anticonvulsants

Anticonvulsants are the mainstay in the treatment of epileptic disorders, but intense investigation has also revealed that they have established efficacy in the treatment of psychiatric behavior disorders.[1] Interest in their application to child and adolescent psychiatry is now emerging as a consequence of their increasing use, with documented efficacy, in adult populations. Anticonvulsants have shown great promise in many psychiatric disorders, particularly mood disorders and aggression and impulse control disorders, but there has been a significant shift in the choice of drugs used in such applications. In past years, phenobarbital and phenytoin were frequently the first tried anticonvulsants in treating behavior disorders. Now clinicians are more commonly utilizing carbamazepine and valproic acid as the first-line agents, particularly in mood disorders. However, despite the fact that anticonvulsants are being used more frequently for both adults and children, there is much yet to be learned, and further investigation into their role in child and adolescent psychiatry is needed.

Chemical Properties

See Figures 9-1, 9-2, and 9-3, and Table 9-1.

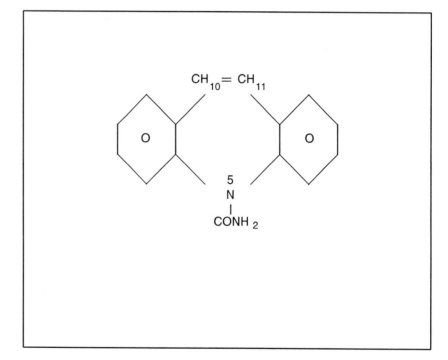

Figure 9-1
Carbamazepine

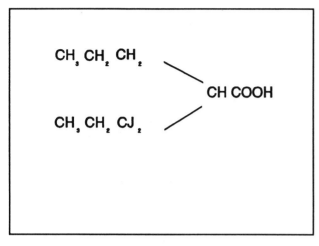

Figure 9-2
Valproic Acid

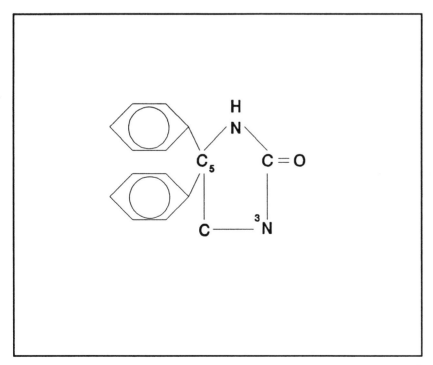

Figure 9-3
Phenytoin (Dilantin)

Table 9-1
Pharmacokinetic Properties of Anticonvulsants

Drug	Elimination	Protein Binding (%)	Half Life (hours)	Desired Serum Level (μg/ml)
Carbamazepine	Hepatic	40–90	12	8–12
Valproic acid	Renal	95	8–20	50–100
Phenytoin	Hepatic	90	10–34	10–20
Phenobarbital	Hepatic	50	46–136	20–40
Primidone	Hepatic	80	3–19	8–12
Ethosuximide	Hepatic	0	50–70	80–100

The chemical structures of the individual anticonvulsants are relatively unique. Carbamazepine, for example, has a structure similar to that of the TCAs.[1] Valproic acid's structure resembles that of fatty acids, and phenytoin has qualities similar to those of barbiturates.

When prescribing anticonvulsants, it is particularly important to keep in mind the pharmacokinetics of the agent being employed. Carbamazepine is relatively easy to dose since, as it has linear kinetics, a dose increase will result in a predicted increase in serum blood levels.[1] Valproic acid, on the other hand, has a much longer duration of action since its effects on the brain last longer than the drug remains in the blood, making monitoring of serum levels less helpful in predicting responsiveness to the medication.[1] Phenytoin follows zero-order kinetics, and so there is a nonlinear relationship between dose and serum level.[1]

Carbamazepine, valproic acid, and phenytoin are highly bound to protein (over 90%).[1] When protein binding capacity is altered, marked changes in the free fractions of these agents can penetrate the blood–brain barrier and enter the brain.

Indications

See Table 9-2.

Bipolar Disorder

Carbamazepine has demonstrated efficacy in adults with bipolar disorder, and is often used in patients who fail to respond to lithium.[7] Numerous open and controlled, double-blind medication versus placebo trials have shown it to have antimanic and antidepressive effects in the acute stage of bipolar

Table 9-2
Psychiatric Indications for Anticonvulsants

Established indications:
• Bipolar disorder in adults
• Alcohol withdrawal
• Chronic pain/pain associated with nerve injury
Possible indications:
• Bipolar disorder in children and adolescents
• Major depression
• Episodic dyscontrol syndrome
• ADHD
• Conduct disorders
• Psychotic disorders as adjunct
• Functional enuresis
• Sleep terror disorder

disorder and during prophylaxis.[8–14] Increased severity of mania and depression, rapid cycling between mania and depression, and poor response to lithium often predict an improved response to carbamazepine.[8–14] It has also been found useful when added to lithium treatment for patients who have only partially responded to lithium.[14–17] There are no data on children and adolescents. This is an important area for investigation, and placebo-controlled studies are much needed as many practicing child psychiatrists are empirically prescribing carbamazepine to bipolar children and adolescents.

Valproic acid has been reported to have antimanic properties and to be an effective mood-stabilizing agent. There are some who believe it to be as effective as, or even more effective than, carbamazepine. In adults, there have been reports of refractory patients being treated with lithium, carbamazepine, and valproic acid combinations. Thus far, these properties have not been definitively established by controlled clinical trials, and the literature to date is mostly preliminary and/or anecdotal. There are no data on children; however, this is an area in which further study is needed on both adults and children to determine its efficacy for the treatment of this disorder.

Major Depressive Disorder

Because carbamazepine has a tricyclic moiety similar to the TCAs, investigators were optimistic that it would prove useful in the treatment of major depressive disorder. Nonetheless, its antidepressant effects have been found to be weaker and less rapid than its antimanic effects, and it improves depression in only a minority of patients.[13,14,16] Carbamazepine is, therefore, a treatment of last resort in adult patients with major depression. On the

275

other hand, in an open study, Groh[18] studied 62 children with abnormal behaviors who did not have epilepsy and found that of the 27 patients who showed improvement, the majority had what the author described as a "dysphoric or dysthymic syndrome" characterized by irritability and mood lability. In addition, one literature review determined that positive results were seen in children treated with carbamazepine for the target symptoms of dysphoria.[24] Since the TCAs have been ineffective in the treatment of child and adolescent depression, and since there is no established efficacious treatment of this disorder in children and adolescents, further study of the use of carbamazepine for certain depressive subtypes is warranted. These depressive subtypes may include CNS anomalies, EEG irregularities, and/or behavioral disturbances coexistent with depressive symptoms.

Valproic acid is not believed to be effective in the treatment of pure unipolar major depressive disorder.[19]

Alcohol Withdrawal

Using anticonvulsants, which are not addictive, to treat alcohol withdrawal has obvious advantages. Concern has been raised, however, that to protect adequately against withdrawal, agents that are cross-tolerant to alcohol should be used. Nonetheless, at least theoretically, the anticonvulsants may be useful alternatives since these agents are antiepileptic and are used to treat one of the most serious complications of alcohol withdrawal, namely, seizures. Malcolm and colleagues[20] conducted a controlled, randomized double-blind study of 86 male adults with severe alcohol withdrawal. Carbamazepine 800 mg/day was found to be as effective as oxazepam 120 mg/day in the treatment of these patients. There have been other open trials in which carbamazepine successfully detoxified patients from benzodiazepines, including diazepam and alprazolam, which are often quite difficult to taper in addicted patients.[21]

There are no data on children and adolescents. Further study of carbamazepine's efficacy in alcohol withdrawal in adults is also necessary before definitive conclusions can be made. Nevertheless, carbamazepine, which is not addictive, may offer certain advantages for those children and adolescents who are having some difficulty while they are being detoxified, even if they are not actually suffering a severe, life-threatening withdrawal reaction. The other anticonvulsants are believed to have very limited use in the treatment of alcohol withdrawal.[1]

Intermittent Explosive Disorder

Anomalies of the CNS, including EEG abnormalities and seizures, are more common in patients with intermittent explosive disorder.[22] Kuhn-Gebhart[23]

studied a large sample of children with behavioral disorders and without seizure disorders and found that approximately 80% improved on carbamazepine, 20% showed no change in behavior, and only one patient out of 50
worsened. Those children with abnormal EEGs responded better to carbamazepine than did those with normal EEGs. It should be noted, however, that
many of the children who showed favorable responses to carbamazepine
came from homes with a strong parental coalition, whereas poor responders
were wont to come from more chaotic home environments. Remschmidt,[24] in
a rather comprehensive review of the literature in 1976, found that clinical
improvement resulted for the target symptom of aggressive/hyperaroused behavior disorders. Puente[25] treated 46 aggressive children with carbamazepine (average dose, 300 mg/day with a range of 100–600 mg/day for a mean
duration of three months) and observed significant improvement in 70% of
the children. Further study is clearly warranted to define more clearly carbamazepine's role in treating aggressiveness in child and adolescent psychiatry.

Phenytoin has also been reported to be of therapeutic value in the treatment
of intermittent explosive disorder.[1] Its use in children and adolescents has
been markedly curtailed because of its wide variability of absorption and its
high incidence of side effects.[2] It is rarely, if ever, indicated in child and adolescent psychiatry since other anticonvulsants such as carbamazepine and
valproic acid are now available.

Recently, some practitioners have begun to use valproic acid both for adults
and for children and adolescents with aggressive behavior disorders. Some
have claimed success with this agent. There is, however, a need for systematic, controlled studies, and at the present time the reported efficacy of valproic acid remains anecdotal and unsubstantiated.

Chronic Pain

In adults, carbamazepine has been found effective in the treatment of
chronic pain due to trigeminal neuralgia and is the drug of choice for treating this condition.[19] Phenytoin has also been found to be effective in the
treatment of this disorder, although less so than carbamazepine. Trigeminal
neuralgia is an uncommon condition in children, and there are no data on
its use for children with this disorder.

Carbamazepine has been found to be helpful in the treatment of pain associated with specific nerve damage or injury.[1] Neuropathies secondary to diabetes, multiple sclerosis, herpes, and physical injury or surgical trauma to
peripheral neurons have also been found to be responsive to anticonvulsants
such as carbamazepine and phenytoin.[1,19] After a specific neuronal insult,
carbamazepine can be used acutely during the first few weeks after the injury to help ameliorate the pain. Nontraumatic pain, such as that due to dia-

betic neuropathy, can also be treated long-term with carbamazepine. It is usually started at a dose of 100 mg twice a day and increased gradually until relief of pain occurs.[19] Plasma levels should be monitored for evidence of toxicity, but have not, as of yet, been found to correlate with symptom improvement. Patients who do not respond to carbamazepine or phenytoin are often then treated with a TCA such as amitriptyline, which has been found to be effective in the treatment of some forms of chronic pain (see Chapter 4). Clonazepam, a high-potency benzodiazepine, may also be effective in treating some forms of chronic pain. There are no data on children and adolescents. Further study of these agents in this population is necessary before definitive recommendations can be given.

Attention-Deficit Hyperactivity Disorder

In a review of carbamazepine's efficacy in the treatment of over 800 nonepileptic children and adolescents, positive results were noted in patients with symptoms of hyperactivity.[24] This agent is used rather commonly in Europe for the treatment of children with ADHD, but is not often used for this disorder in the United States.[1] When it is used, it is often as a last resort after all other behavioral and pharmacologic treatments have failed. Evans and colleagues[26] report that carbamazepine can reduce ADHD symptoms, with variable ultimate dosages required for different children. Doses of only 50 mg/day have reportedly improved symptoms in some children, while doses of 1 gram per day have been required for other children. It is important to monitor carbamazepine plasma levels and CBC and differential in these children, regardless of the dose. Plasma levels have not, however, been found to correlate with clinical improvement. Carbamazepine appears to be particularly efficacious in the amelioration of the target symptoms of aggression, hyperactivity, distractibility, impulsivity, and poor frustration tolerance.[26] There are no data on adolescents or adults with ADHD. Moreover, carbamazepine has not been directly compared with stimulants, antidepressants, or clonidine in the treatment of ADHD in children.[1] Still, it may prove to be helpful, and merits further study in children and adolescents refractory to standard therapy.

There are no data on valproic acid's efficacy for children and adolescents. Anecdotal reports of its efficacy in treating behavior disorders both in adults and in children and adolescents warrant investigation.

In contrast to carbamazepine, and possibly valproic acid, phenobarbital and the high-potency benzodiazepine clonazepam should be avoided in children and adolescents with disruptive behavior disorders such as ADHD, since their use in this population has been associated with paradoxical behavioral rebound with a precipitation or exacerbation of hyperactive behavior.[27]

Conduct Disorders in Children and Adolescents

Children with conduct disorders have responded favorably to carbamazepine treatment. Twenty children and adolescents with conduct disorders were found to exhibit significant improvement when treated with carbamazepine in a double-blind, placebo-controlled crossover trial.[18] Trimble and Corbett[28] found that higher serum levels of carbamazepine (i.e., 8–12 μg/ml) were associated with decreased behavior problems. They also noted that phenobarbital use was associated with paradoxical worsening of behavior. There are no current data on treatment with valproic acid, phenytoin, or the other anticonvulsants. The data at present must be regarded as preliminary and further study is needed.

Psychosis

With regard to psychotic adults with affective symptomatology, there is evidence to suggest that carbamazepine may be helpful in the treatment of some of these patients.[9,16] It appears to be most effective as an adjunct to an antipsychotic medication in these patients. Carbamazepine itself is not effective in the treatment of psychosis, but may ameliorate some affective symptoms, as in patients with schizoaffective disorder.[9] This agent might be indicated particularly for those patients with a psychotic disorder with affective components who had failed a trial of lithium. Valproic acid might also be considered for similar reasons, although it has received even less study than carbamazepine. Clonazepam, a high-potency benzodiazepine (see Chapter 10), has also been found useful as an adjunct in bipolar disorder, and may have some benefit for psychotic patients with affective symptomatology. There are no data on children and adolescents with psychotic disorders, and so further investigation into the potential role of anticonvulsants in the treatment of psychosis is warranted.

Functional Enuresis

Puente[3] observed that carbamazepine at mean daily doses of 300 mg decreased enuresis in eight of nine children with severe behavioral disorders but no neurologic impairment. However, carbamazepine cannot be endorsed at this time for the routine treatment of enuretic children due to the paucity of available data.

Sleep Terror Disorder

Puente[3] reported that all six children with night terrors (pavor nocturnus) responded favorably to carbamazepine therapy. Moreover, 16 of 17 children with other sleep disturbances also responded positively to carbamazepine treatment. Most often, medication is not required for sleep disorders in children and adolescents, and behavioral interventions are preferred. When pharmacotherapy is indicated, benzodiazepines are the drugs of choice (see Chapter 10). If these are unsuccessful, TCAs (i.e., imipramine) have been utilized effectively. Carbamazepine, therefore, cannot be endorsed for routine use in children and adolescents suffering from sleep disorders.

Contraindications to Carbamazepine

See Table 9-3.

History of Hypersensitivity to Carbamazepine and/or Antidepressants

A known history of allergic reaction to carbamazepine and/or TCAs is an absolute contraindication to the use of carbamazepine. It is important to remember that carbamazepine has a tricyclic moiety similar to that of the antidepressants.[1]

A history of bone marrow depression also is an absolute contraindication to the use of carbamazepine.

Patients on an MAOI

The *Physicians' Desk Reference* recommends that carbamazepine not be used for any patient who has received an MAOI within the past two weeks.[4]

Pregnancy

Since carbamazepine crosses the placenta, there is virtually no psychiatric indication for its use during pregnancy.

Table 9-3
Contraindications to Carbamazepine Use

Absolute:
• Known hypersensitivity to carbamazepine or TCAs
• History of bone marrow depression
• On MAOI within past two weeks
• Pregnancy
Relative:
• Liver disease
• Kidney disease

Liver Disease

Since carbamazepine is metabolized by the liver, its use is relatively contra-indicated for children and adolescents with liver disease. Consultation with the patient's medical physician is essential, and the risks versus potential benefits of carbamazepine's use must be considered.

Renal Disease

Renal disease in children and adolescents is a relative contraindication to the use of carbamazepine. The patient's physician should be consulted if carbamazepine is felt to be important to the mental health of the child or adolescent.

Contraindications to Valproic Acid

See Table 9-4.

Known Hypersensitivity to Valproic Acid or a Related Drug

Hypersensitivity to valproic acid or a related drug is an absolute contraindication to its use.

Previous bone marrow depression is also an absolute contraindication to the use of valproic acid.

Pregnancy

There is virtually no psychiatric indication for valproic acid's use during pregnancy since it crosses the placenta.

Patients on Clonazepam

Coadministration of valproic acid and clonazepam can result in status epilepticus.[30] Therefore, valproic acid is absolutely contraindicated for patients receiving clonazepam.

Table 9-4
Contraindications to Valproic Acid Use

Absolute:
• Known hypersensitivity to valproic acid or related drug
• History of bone marrow depression
• Pregnancy
Relative:
• Liver disease
• Kidney disease

Children Under 3 Years of Age

Because children under 3 years of age have an increased risk for liver toxicity (see "Side Effects"), valproic acid is absolutely contraindicated for this population.

Liver Disease

Valproic acid is relatively contraindicated for children and adolescents with liver disease (see "Side Effects").

Renal Disease

Since valproic acid is cleared mostly by renal mechanisms, it should be avoided in children and adolescents with renal disease.

Contraindications to Phenytoin

See Table 9-5.

Known Hypersensitivity to Phenytoin or a Related Drug

Hypersensitivity to phenytoin is an absolute contraindication to its use.

Pregnancy

Phenytoin is absolutely contraindicated for pregnant women.

Cardiac Disorders

Phenytoin is relatively contraindicated in certain cardiac disorders.

Liver Disease

Phenytoin is relatively contraindicated for patients with liver disease.

Table 9-5
Contraindications to Phenytoin Use

Absolute:
• Known hypersensitivity to phenytoin or a related drug
• Pregnancy
Relative:
• Alcohol use/dependence
• Cardiac disorders
• Diabetes
• Liver disease
• Renal disease

Renal Disease

Phenytoin is relatively contraindicated for children and adolescents with renal disease.

Diabetes

It is best to avoid using phenytoin for children and adolescents with diabetes, and to choose another anticonvulsant instead.

Alcohol Abuse/Dependence

Phenytoin is relatively contraindicated for patients who abuse alcohol, because of the synergistic neurotoxic effects these two agents can have when used simultaneously.[1]

Contraindications to Other Anticonvulsants

Since the foregoing anticonvulsants are the primary agents used in the treatment of psychiatric disorders, the contraindications to the use of the other anticonvulsants, such as phenobarbital, will not be discussed. In fact, the other anticonvulsants are themselves felt by most authorities to be *contraindicated* in the treatment of psychiatric disorders owing to their exacerbation or precipitation of certain behavior problems in children and adolescents and their unfavorable side-effect profiles. The reader is referred to any comprehensive neurology textbook for more information on these agents.

Since all of the anticonvulsants can be associated with significant psychiatric side effects that the practicing clinician who uses the medications will inevitably encounter, these side effects will be discussed in the next section.

Side Effects of Carbamazepine

See Table 9-6.

Table 9-6
Side Effects of Carbamazepine

Common:	Uncommon:
• Diplopia	• Agranulocytosis and aplastic anemia
• Drowsiness	• Hyponatremia and water intoxications
• Incoordination	• Liver toxicity
• Nystagmus	• Neurotoxicity
• Nausea	• Mania
• Leukopenia	• Exacerbation/precipitation of behavior
• Skin rashes	problems
	• Hypocalcemia

Diplopia

Diplopia is the most common side effect seen with the use of carbamazepine, and often remits spontaneously or after the dose is decreased.[30] There does not appear to be any relationship between carbamazepine blood level and this side effect, however.[32]

Drowsiness, Incoordination, Vertigo, Nystagmus, Mild Nausea

These are common, usually transient side effects that usually are seen at the beginning of therapy or when the dose is increased too quickly.[1,30]

Leukopenia

Leukopenia is a very common side effect of carbamazepine treatment and should not be confused with the far less common but potentially life-threatening ogranulocytosis and aplastic anemia.[1] Pellock[29] found that a stable, nonprogressive leukopenia is not an uncommon side effect of carbamazepine use, Pellock observing a leukopenia of less than 4000/mm³ in approximately 13% of the children studied and of less than 3000 in only 2.3%. Drug discontinuation was not required, and the leukopenia was not progressive, with spontaneous reversal of the blood counts in 75% of the children. A viral illness can result in a decrease in the number of white blood cells in some of these patients.[30] Rarely, this progresses to agranulocytosis or aplastic anemia, which is a medical emergency; careful monitoring of blood counts is indicated (see below).

Agranulocytosis and Aplastic Anemia

Agranulocytosis and aplastic anemia are uncommon, but potentially very serious, life-threatening side effects of carbamazepine therapy. The clinician should monitor for bruising, bleeding, sore throat, fever, lethargy, and mouth ulcers, with a precipitous drop in white blood cell count.[1] A decrease in white blood cell count necessitates prompt medical attention and consultation with a hematologic specialist. A drop in the granulocyte count to less than 1000 necessitates the gradual tapering and then discontinuation of the medication.[1] These effects are usually reversible, but since death has been reported in one in 50,000 cases, caution is advised.[1]

It does appear that agranulocytosis and aplastic anemia are more commonly encountered in older patients. In fact, one noted authority believes that routine blood tests are unnecessary in youngsters receiving carbamazepine.[30] But because carbamazepine remains an experimental medication in child and adolescent psychiatry with no established FDA indications for its use in this population, we recommend that blood counts be monitored during treatment with this drug (see "Initiating and Maintaining Treatment").

Skin Rashes

Rashes are relatively common when carbamazepine is used.[29] Pellock observed rashes in 5% of children treated with carbamazepine. Severe skin rashes appear to be relatively uncommon, however.[1] Nevertheless, the occasional occurrence of the Stevens-Johnson syndrome or a systemic lupus erythematosus (SLE)–like syndrome has been reported, sometimes requiring emergency treatment. When a rash develops, we advise discontinuing the medication and seeking medical consultation.

Hyponatremia and Water Intoxication

Since carbamazepine has a direct CNS effect of stimulating the release of antidiuretic hormone (ADH), its use can result in the development of a syndrome of inappropriate ADH characterized by hyponatremia, water intoxication, lethargy, headache, nausea/vomiting, increased urination, edema, seizures, and, very rarely, acute renal failure.[1] These effects may be more likely to result when lithium and carbamazepine are used concomitantly, since lithium can alter fluid balance as well.[1] If this side effect occurs, the carbamazepine should be discontinued and another anticonvulsant used instead.

Liver Toxicity

Liver toxicity is a very rare side effect of carbamazepine therapy.[1] Mild and nonprogressive increases in LFTs are not uncommon, however. Camfield and colleagues[33] found that 9% of children on carbamazepine had mildly elevated aspartate aminotransferase.

Neurotoxicity

When carbamazepine is administered in therapeutic doses to children with atypical absence or other minor motor seizures, it can exacerbate the seizure disorder or precipitate status epilepticus.[30] Pleak and colleagues[31] observed that two 11-year-old boys who were treated with carbamazepine developed sharp waves and spike abnormalities on their EEGs. Very infrequently, a continuous, nonepileptic myoclonus can be seen.[34,35] Slurred speech, nystagmus, dystonic reactions, muscle rigidity, and tinnitus occasionally are seen.[1] When carbamazepine is given with other drugs, such as diltiazem, verapamil, erythromycin, isoniazid (INH), propoxyphene (Demerol), or alcohol, neurotoxicity can be induced.[36] Caution should be exerised in giving these drugs to children and adolescents.

Mania

Despite the fact that carbamazepine is used to treat bipolar disorder, carbamazepine-induced mania has been reported as an occasional side effect.[1] Antidepressant-induced mania has been well documented (see Chapter 4), and since carbamazepine has a tricyclic moiety similar to that of the antidepressants, perhaps it is not surprising that it occasionally induces a manic episode. Pleak and colleagues[31] observed the precipitation of a severe mania in a 16-year-old treated with carbamazepine, and a 10-year-old child treated with carbamazepine developed what the authors referred to as a hypomania. Other investigators have reported cases of carbamazepine-induced mania in children.[37,38]

Exacerbation/Precipitation of Problem Behaviors

Evans and colleagues[26] report that in their extensive use of carbamazepine in the treatment of children and adolescents with conduct disorders and hyperactivity, side effects of the medications, including aggression, increased irritability and mood lability, tantrums, and the disruption of normal sleep patterns with insomnia, are not uncommon. These symptoms often resemble the target symptoms, and close monitoring is essential so that the carbamazepine dose is not increased to treat symptoms that are, in fact, being caused or aggravated by the medication itself. This differential can be even more difficult to detect in children who have not yet achieved adequate communication skills. It is clear that children and adolescents who receive carbamazepine must be carefully monitored for adverse behavioral side effects. Comparing the patient's behavior on and off carbamazepine may help in elucidating whether the drug is helping or hindering therapy.

Hypocalcemia

Hypocalcemia is a rare side effect of carbamazepine therapy.[1] Very occasionally, muscle cramps and decreased control of seizures are seen.

Side Effects of Valproic Acid

See Table 9-7.

Gastrointestinal Upset

Gastrointestinal upset such as nausea and vomiting is the most common side effect encountered in patients receiving valproic acid.[39] The medication should be taken with food/formula to minimize stomach upset. The use of the enteric-coated preparation Depakote may also minimize this side effect.

Table 9-7
Side Effects of Valproic Acid

Common:	Uncommon:
• GI upset	• Liver toxicity
• Increased appetite/weight gain	• Hyperammonemia
• Sedation	• Blood dyscrasias
• Tremor	• Alopecia
	• Decreased serum carnitine
	• Neural tube defects
	• Pancreatitis
	• Hyperglycinemia
	• Menstrual irregularity

Increased Appetite/Weight Gain

The Collaborative Study Group[40] found increased appetite to be a significant side effect of valproic acid use, particularly in those receiving enteric-coated medication. Interestingly enough, Menkes[30] reports that, in his experience, significant weight gain is frequently seen in those patients who respond particularly well to the medication.

Sedation

Sedation is considered a common side effect of valproic acid, but its incidence can be reduced by avoiding polydrug therapy.[1] The Collaborative Study Group[40] found that sedation due to valproic acid occurred in approximately 10% of the patients, but that when it did, it tended to be self-limited and often attributable to another anticonvulsant that was also being administered. Stupor is a very uncommon side effect of valproic acid treatment, and is most likely to occur in patients on more than one anticonvulsant, especially when valproic acid is coadministered with benzodiazepines or barbiturates. In fact, the coadministration of valproic acid and the high-potency benzodiazepine clonazepam can have extremely powerful hypnotic effects, and can precipitate status epilepticus.[1]

Tremor

Tremor is a common side effect of valproic acid therapy,[1] and is observed most commonly in patients receiving doses greater than 40–50 mg/kg/day.[41] A family history of essential tremor is not uncommon in these children. Asterixis is very rarely seen in children, and is most commonly associated with polydrug therapy.[42]

Liver Toxicity

Valproic acid causes dose-related increases in LFTs in as many as 44% of patients being treated with this agent alone.[30] Most commonly, these elevations are transient and nonprogressive. Dose reduction also often results in liver enzymes' returning to baseline. Hepatitis, liver failure, and death have been reported, but appear to be limited almost exclusively to children under 3 years of age who are receiving polydrug therapy.[1] This effect usually is seen during the first six months of therapy and is unrelated to drug dosage.[30,43] Young children with mental retardation receiving anticonvulsant polydrug therapy appear to be at greatest risk. The incidence of liver toxicity in children over 2 years of age is far less than in children less than 2 years old.

Hyperammonemia

Hyperammonemia is commonly seen in patients treated with valproic acid.[30] Laub[44] has reported that elevated fasting ammonia levels were seen in asymptomatic patients receiving therapeutic dosages of valproic acid, and that ammonia levels rose even higher following protein loading. High blood ammonia levels in the absence of other clinical symptoms do not necessitate the discontinuation of valproic acid since there is no correlation between increased ammonia levels and liver failure.[44] It is not clear as to whether or not hyperammonemia plays a role in the development of stupor.[45]

Blood Dyscrasias

Neutropenia and thrombocytopenia are uncommon side effects of valproic acid therapy.[1] When a fall in platelet count occurs, it is most often transient, and is believed to have an autoimmune basis.[30] This alteration is dose related, but does not usually necessitate the reduction or discontinuation of valproic acid. It should be noted, however, that infection can aggravate the thrombocytopenia, resulting in bruising and minor bleeding.[46]

Alopecia

Hair loss is an uncommon side effect of valproic acid therapy, and is reversible and possibly dose related.[1]

Lowered Serum Carnitine Levels

Valproic acid decreases free serum carnitine levels,[30] but there is no correlation between the dose and the decrease in carnitine. As children with low carnitine levels are generally asymptomatic, dietary supplementation with carnitine is not felt to be indicated.[47]

Neural Tube Defects

Valproic acid use during pregnancy has been associated with the development of neural tube defects.[48,49] We recommend avoiding valproic acid for the treatment of psychiatric disorders in pregnant adolescent girls (see "Contraindications"). However, when consulted on a case involving a pregnant woman who has taken valproic acid during her pregnancy, to determine whether or not a neural tube defect is present, the drawing of alpha-fetoprotein levels is warranted.[1,48,49]

Pancreatitis/Hyperglycemia/Menstrual Irregularity

These are rare side effects of valpric acid therapy.[1,40,48]

Side Effects of Phenytoin

See Table 9-8.

Hirsutism

Seventy-five percent of patients receiving phenytoin develop hirsutism.[30] Menkes reports that this complication does not usually lead to his discontinuing the medication.

Gum Hypertrophy

Gingival hyperplasia is a common complication of phenytoin therapy, and usually occurs two to three months after the medication is started.[30] This side effect is seen at therapeutic levels of phenytoin.[50] Adolescents may find it particularly troubling and embarrassing. Good oral hygiene, daily gum massage, and surgical excision of hyperplastic tissue are helpful.[30]

Table 9-8
Side Effects of Phenytoin

Common:	**Uncommon:**
• Hirsutism	• Encephalopathy ("Dilantin dementia")
• Gum hypertrophy	• Altered vitamin D/calcium metabolism
• Folate deficiency	• Biotin deficiency
• Psychomotor retardation	• Vitamin E deficiency
	• Liver toxicity
	• Neurotoxicity
	• Hypersensitivity reaction
	• Coarsening of facial features
	• Headache
	• Gynecomastia
	• Hyperglycemia

Folate Deficiency

Megaloblastic anemia and decreased serum folate concentrations are common side effects of chronic phenytoin therapy.[30] Reynolds and Wales[51] observed that dementia and psychotic-like states were associated with the prolonged phenytoin therapy of epileptics, and occurred more commonly in patients treated with polydrug therapy. Folic acid therapy can raise serum folate levels, but has no effect on the behavior or mental impairment of chronic epileptic patients.[52]

Psychomotor Retardation

Phenytoin commonly causes cognitive impairment, with disturbances in memory, attention, and concentration, that does not appear to be due to sedation and can be dose related or idiosyncratic.[1] Decreased motor efficiency may be particularly problematic in the adolescent population and may result in behavior problems. Moreover, phenytoin, like phenobarbital, has been reported to aggravate underlying behavior disorders.[53]

Encephalopathy

Phenytoin encephalopathy is usually observed at toxic blood levels.[30] Mentally retarded patients may be especially vulnerable to this side effect.[54] This encephalopathy is commonly referred to as "Dilantin dementia."[53]

Vitamin D and Calcium Metabolism Changes

Disturbed vitamin D metabolism resulting in rickets, decreased serum calcium and phosphorus, and increased alkaline phosphatase is seen in some patients after long-term treatment with phenytoin, primidone, or phenobarbital.[55] Therefore, children who are on long-term anticonvulsant therapy with any of these agents should be given vitamin D supplementation and allowed to get sufficient exposure to sunlight.[56]

Biotin deficiency

Plasma biotin levels are decreased in patients on long-term phenytoin therapy.[57]

Vitamin E Deficiency

In epileptic patients, decreased vitamin E is frequently observed, so that vitamin E is frequently added to the anticonvulsant regimen to improve seizure control.[58] Whether there is any association with behavioral disorders with or without EEG abnormalities is not known.

Liver Toxicity

Liver toxicity is a rare side effect of phenytoin therapy that is generally seen only in adults.[1]

Neurotoxicity

Nystagmus, ataxia, confusion, muscle weakness, and slurred speech are occasional adverse effects of phenytoin therapy, most often seen with toxic blood levels.[1] Peripheral neuropathy has also been observed in patients receiving long-term phenytoin therapy.[30] In fact, deep tendon reflexes are found to be absent in approximately 50% of patients on phenytoin for longer than 15 years.[59]

Hypersensitivity Reaction

Up to 5% of patients receiving phenytoin develop fever, a rash, and lymphadenopathy within two weeks of initiating treatment.[30] This reaction is generally found at therapeutic blood levels for the drug,[60] and the symptoms resolve once the drug is discontinued. The drug should not be restarted due to the risk for developing severe hypersensitivity reactions such as the Stevens-Johnson syndrome or an SLE-like syndrome.[61] Moreover, the incidence of malignant lymphomas and Hodgkin's disease in patients receiving long-term phenytoin therapy is as much as 10 times greater than expected, which suggests that phenytoin-induced lymphadenopathy may not necessarily be a benign condition.[62]

Coarsening of Facial Features

Thickened lips and eyebrow prominence are occasional adverse effects of phenytoin seen in patients receiving this drug for many years.[1]

Headache

Headache is an uncommon side effect of phenytoin therapy.[1]

Gynecomastia in Males

Male patients and their families must be warned that gynecomastia is an occasional adverse effect of phenytoin therapy.[1]

Hyperglycemia

Over the short term, phenytoin appears to impair glucose-induced insulin release.[2] This effect generally resolves spontaneously, and in clinical practice, hyperglycemia is only encountered at drug levels that produce neurotoxicity.

Side Effects of Ethosuximide

Ethosuximide is not used for psychiatric indications, but as it has significant psychiatric side effects, it will be discussed here briefly.

Psychosis

Very occasionally, ethosuximide use can result in psychosis, especially in children with abnormal spikes on their EEGs.[63]

Side Effects of Phenobarbital

See Table 9-9.

Phenobarbital has no indication for the treatment of psychiatric disorders, but its use is associated with significant psychiatric side effects, and so it will be discussed here.

Dysphoria/Depression

Corbett and colleagues[64] originally reported the high occurrence of depressive symptomatology in children treated with phenobarbital. Robertson and his colleagues[65] found that patients with major depression and epilepsy on phenobarbital recorded higher depression scores than did patients on carbamazepine. Brent and colleagues[6] compared 15 children treated with phenobarbital with 24 children treated with carbamazepine, and found that 40% of those treated with phenobarbital had a major depressive disorder versus only 4% of those receiving carbamazepine. Moreover, 47% on phenobarbital had suicidal ideation, as compared with only 4% on carbamazepine. Brent[5] evaluated 131 consecutive suicide attempts made by 126 children and adolescents at a children's hospital over a five-year period, and discovered that nine of the patients (which corresponded to an incidence 15 times higher than expected) had epilepsy and that eight of the nine were being treated with phenobarbital.

Table 9-9
Side Effects of Phenobarbital

- Depression
- Mood changes
- Suicidal ideation
- Paradoxical behavior rebound/worsening
- Hyperactivity
- Cognitive impairment
- Drowsiness

Case History

A 13-year-old epileptic child who had recently made a serious suicide attempt by overdose was referred to the child psychiatry service for evaluation of depression. Evaluation revealed that the child had a history of major depressive disorder that required his hospitalization at the age of 10 years. He had been in good health until one week prior to psychiatric evaluation, at which time his parents reported he had become more depressed. They were perplexed because he had not had a seizure in over one year. Nonetheless, he had been having increased difficulty falling asleep, and was reporting decreased appetite and decreased energy level. Moreover, usual activities that he found pleasurable, such as going to baseball games, failed to improve his mood. The night prior to his admission, he had become despondent and swallowed an entire bottle of his mother's fluoxetine. One hour after ingestion, he told his mother what he had done. He was taken by ambulance to the emergency room. After being medically cleared, he was found to be significantly depressed with active suicidal ideation. He claimed he was sorry he had told his mother and wished, "I'd just ended it." He was noted to be frequently tearful. There was no history of drug or alcohol use: He gave no evidence of psychotic or manic symptoms. Family history was significant for an older brother with major depression, which had been treated with cognitive and behavioral therapy; an older sister with bipolar disorder, who had made several suicide attempts; and his mother who carried the diagnosis of major depression, and who was currently being treated with fluoxetine. The patient was on no medications other than the anticonvulsant phenobarbital, 100 mg t.i.d. The phenobarbital level was therapeutic at 75 µg/ml.

Because of the patient's mental history of depression and the significant family history of depression in his first-degree relatives, the treating psychiatrist sought consultation with the patient's family and neurologist. They discussed phenobarbital's increased association with suicidal behavior in children. The psychiatrist advocated switching from phenobarbital to another anticonvulsant. The anticonvulsant carbamazepine was recommended because of its lower risk of inducing affective symptoms and because it is often effective in treating affective symptoms and disorders. The parents were initially reluctant because of phenobarbital's success in treating their child's seizure disorder. The neurologist informed the parents that carbamazepine had been shown to be effective in the treatment of their child's type of epilepsy (temporal lobe). The psychiatrist and neurologist agreed that, because of the potential lethality of the patient's suicide attempt and his continued depression and suicidal ideation, the risk/benefit ratio did not favor phenobarbital's continued use in spite of its effectiveness in suppressing seizure activity. The patient's parents agreed to a trial of carbamazepine. The patient was gradually tapered off his phenobarbital and carbamazepine therapy initiated, with the neurologist monitoring and titrating the dose for epileptic effect and the psychiatrist monitoring mood symptoms. At 200 mg t.i.d, the patient experienced symptom remission and remained seizure-free. The carbamazepine level was 9.4 mg/ml. His CBCs with differential and platelet counts were all within normal limits. Subsequently, the patient admitted to feeling less depressed and denied suicidal ideation. Milieu reports confirmed that his depression had decreased. He did, however, continue to have periods when he was described as feeling "blue" and, according to his parents, was still "not his usual self" despite denying suicidal ideation. Since no antidepressant therapy has been demonstrated to be effective in treating child and adolescent depression, and because of their potential for lowering the seizure threshold, the psychiatrist was reluctant to initiate such a trial. Cognitive and behavioral therapy and family therapy were recommended. The patient and family were told that if this psychosocial approach failed, medication could then be considered. As long as the patient was maintained on a stable anticonvulsant regimen, the risk of altering the seizure threshold with an antidepressant would be relatively low. Nonetheless, the parents agreed that they would rather try family therapy and cognitive/behavioral therapy first.

Drowsiness

Drowsiness is a common side effect of phenobarbital.[30]

Hyperactivity

Phenobarbital use can precipitate and/or exacerbate behavior problems, leading to paradoxical behavior rebound and hyperactivity.[30]

Cognitive Impairment

Position emission tomography scanning done before and after the withdrawal of therapeutic doses of phenobarbital reveals that phenobarbital produces a 37% reduction in local cerebral glucose metabolism.[66] Thompson and Trimble[67] showed that the substitution of carbamazepine for phenobarbital or phenytoin resulted in improved memory, concentration, and mental and motor speed.

Side Effects of Primidone

Primidone is metabolized to phenobarbital, and is likely to cause the same side effects as phenobarbital.[1] It is not indicated for the treatment of any psychiatric disorder.

Overdose/Toxicity

Carbamazepine

Carbamazepine toxicity is manifest by drowsiness, nausea/vomiting, gait disturbance, nystagmus, confusion, neuromuscular excitability, and seizures.[1] It is important to remember that when carbamazepine is taken in overdose, peak levels may not occur until the second or third day postingestion because of its slow absorption.[19] Since it has a tricyclic structure, overdose with carbamazepine can be lethal. Nonetheless, it appears to be less lethal in overdose than the standard TCAs such as imipramine.[19] Overdose is, however, a medical emergency requiring close monitoring.

Cardiac monitoring is required since overdose with carbamazepine can result in AV block.[2,19] There is also the risk of aspiration pneumonia, and when large quantities of carbamazepine are taken, respiratory depression can occur, although it is usually mild. Stupor and coma can also occur. The management of carbamazepine overdose is primarily supportive; since the drug is so highly protein-bound, hemodialysis is of no help.[19]

Valproic Acid

Valproic acid toxicity is manifest by drowsiness, weakness, incoordination, and confusion.[1] Valproic acid is generally not very dangerous in overdose, except when it is taken in combination with other drugs.

Phenytoin

Phenytoin toxicity is manifest by diplopia, ataxia, nystagmus, dysarthria, confusion, vertigo, drowsiness, nausea, tremor, and slurred speech.[1] Phenytoin is generally not very dangerous in overdose, except when it is taken in combination with other drugs.

Barbiturates

The barbiturates are quite dangerous when taken in overdose, and this is considered a medical emergency. These agents are particularly harmful when taken in combination with other drugs, such as alcohol.[1] Epileptic patients most frequently use barbiturates to commit suicide.

Abuse

With the exception of the barbiturates, there is little potential for abuse of these agents.

Drug Interactions

See Tables 9-10 through 9-13.

Available Preparations and Costs of Anticonvulsants

See Table 9-14.

Initiating and Maintaining Treatment

Choosing an anticonvulsant to use in the treatment regimen of children and adolescents can be difficult since there are no current FDA-established indications for such use in psychiatric disorders. None of these agents can be considered first-line treatments. Their use is indicated in child and adolescent psychiatry when other, more standard treatments have proved unsuccessful. Carbamazepine is the best-studied agent of its class with reported efficacy in specific behavioral syndromes (see "Indications"), and should be the first anticonvulsant tried in children and adolescents. Because of valproic acid's reported effectiveness in adults and some preliminary data on children and adolescents, its use is warranted if the child or adolescent proves refractory to carbamazepine. The other anticonvulsants are not generally felt to be of much use in the treatment of psychiatric disorders, and because of their rather significant side effects, we recommend avoiding them. Phenytoin has been reported to be effective in certain behavioral conditions and in the treatment of chronic pain syndromes, but we believe that its

Table 9-10
Anticonvulsant Drug Interactions

Anticonvulsant effects increased by:	Anticonvulsant effects decreased by:
• Cimetidine	• Birth control pills
• Chloramphenicol	• Cortisol
• Chlorpheniramine	• Coumarin
• Disulfiram	• Dexamethasone
• Erythromycin	• Diazepam
• Isoniazid	• Digoxin
• Methylphenidate	• Neuroleptics
• Phenothiazine	• Phenylbutazone
• Propoxyphene	• Prednisolone
• Sulthiame	• TCAs
• TCAs	• Warfarin

Table 9-11
Carbamazepine Drug Interactions

Decreases serum half-life of:
• Haloperidol
• Phenytoin
• Theophylline

Increases serum concentrations of lithium

Serum levels decreased by simultaneous administration of:
• Phenobarbital
• Phenytoin
• Primidone

side-effect profile is so unfavorable that it is best avoided and alternative medications considered. Phenobarbital should never be given for psychiatric disorders since its use has been associated with the aggravation and/or precipitation of behavioral problems, including hyperactivity, depression, and suicidal ideation.[5]

The consultation-liaison psychiatrist may be consulted on a child or adolescent with epilepsy who is experiencing mood symptoms (see Chapter 13). Children and/or adolescents with epilepsy and a mood disorder such as major depression who are receiving sedative anticonvulsants such as phenobarbital and primidone should have these drugs removed from their regimen and started on anticonvulsant monotherapy with either carbamazepine or valproic acid.[68] In addition, children and adolescents with epilepsy and a coexistent mood disorder being treated with phenytoin are probably best treated by removing the phenytoin and switching to carbamazepine or valproic acid.[68] The mood stabilizing effects of carbamazepine have been documented, and although not as well documented as with valproic acid, clinical reports continue to advocate its efficacy. Therefore, in this section, we will focus our discussion on the initiation, dosing, and maintenance of anticonvulsant therapy with carbamazepine and valproic acid. Phenytoin administration will be discussed very briefly, since the authors believe that its prescription is not warranted for child and adolescent psychiatric disorders. Nonetheless, some clinicians still believe it to be of limited use as a

Table 9-12
Valproic Acid Interactions

Decreases effect of:	**Increases effect of:**
• Hepatically metabolized drugs	• Carbamazepine
	• Phenytoin

Table 9-13
Phenytoin Drug Interactions

Drugs increasing phenytoin levels	Drugs decreasing phenytoin levels:
• Alcohol (acutely) • Benzodiazepines • Methylphenidate • Phenothiazine • Salicylates	• Alcohol (chronically) • Benzodiazepines • Carbamazepine • Molindone

Table 9-14
Available Preparations and Costs of Anticonvulsants

Drug	Available Preparations	Average Cost/Day
Carbamazepine	**Generic:** 200 mg scored tablets 100 scored tablets, chewable **Tegretol:** 200 mg scored tablets 100 mg scored tablets, chewable 100 mg/5 ml oral suspensions	$0.90
Valproic Acid	**Generic:** 250 mg capsules 250 mg 5/ml oral syrup **Depakene:** 250 mg capsules 250 mg/5 ml oral syrup	$0.84
Divalproex (enteric coated)	**Generic:** 125, 250, 500 mg unscored tablets **Depakote:** 125, 250, 500 mg unscored tablets "Sprinkles," can be put directly on food	$1.14
Phenytoin	**Generic:** 100 mg tablets Extended 100 mg capsules **Dilantin:** 30, 50, 100 mg scored, chewable tablets 30 mg/5 ml and 125 mg/5 mg oral suspension Extended 30, 50, 100 mg scored, chewable capsules Extended 30 mg/5 ml and 125 mg/5 ml oral suspension Parenteral formulations	$0.10

Source: Red Book Annual Pharmacist Reference, 1989–1990. Oradell, NJ: Medical Economics.

last resort in patients with certain behavior disorders. The other anticonvulsants—namely, phenobarbital, primidone, and ethosuximide—are generally agreed upon by most authorities to have no utility in the treatment of psychiatric disorders and will not be discussed here. For more information, the reader is referred to any comprehensive textbook on child neurology.

It is important that the child or adolescent undergo the taking of a complete history and a physical examination by his or her pediatrician or medical doctor prior to the initiation of anticonvulsant therapy. In addition, a complete blood count with differential and platelet count should be obtained, and LFTs, including bilirubin, SGPT, SGOT, and alkaline phosphatase, should be checked. An assessment of kidney function should be performed (i.e., BUN and creatinine). It is important to inform the patient and family about possible side effects, especially the rare anticonvulsant-induced agranulocytosis or liver failure, as these side effects are not dose or blood level related, and can appear suddenly despite careful monitoring.[1] The patient and parents should be advised to inform the physician if there is any unexplained bruising or bleeding. It is important to tell adolescent female patients that anticonvulsants cross the placenta, and that if they decide to or inadvertently become pregnant, they should notify their physician. At each visit, the clinician should do a sexual history so as to be alert to a possible pregnancy.

Parents should be advised to use acetaminophen instead of aspirin when their child develops a fever or cold.[4] In addition, cough/cold preparations often contain over 5% alcohol and may increase the sedative effects of anticonvulsants. It is important that parents and/or adolescents check the labels of over-the counter medications and get advice from their nurse or physician. Adolescents should be further warned of the danger of using alcohol while on anticonvulsants.

It is important to inform the patient and family that anticonvulsants can be taken with food or formula to decrease GI upset. If a single dose is missed, the dose may be given one to two hours later, and then the regular dosing schedule continued. If a dose is vomited within one half hour of its administration, it may be given again. It should be emphasized to the patient and parents that anticonvulsants need to be taken regularly, since it takes several days to get to a steady-state blood level. Once steady state is achieved, there is little variability in blood levels from day to day in compliant patients.

It is also important to remember that the anticonvulsants have been known to interfere with and alter standard diagnostic laboratory tests. Patients on carbamazepine may have false-negative pregnancy tests if the human chorionic gonadotropin (HCG) is being assayed.[1] Thyroid function tests may also be altered, and false-positive results may be obtained on the dexamethasone suppression test in children and adolescents on carbamazepine.[1] Valproic acid has been known to alter thyroid function tests, such as decreasing free T4 and free T3. Tests for urinary ketones may be falsely positive. Finally, phenytoin use can lower free T4, elevate blood glucose, and also result in a false-positive dexamethasone suppression test.[1]

The monitoring of serum anticonvulsants is advised, but this is not necessary at every visit. Getting an anticonvulsant blood level is most valuable after a recent change in medication dose or if the prescribing clinician believes that the patient either is not taking his or her medication or is taking more than the prescribed amount.[1] White blood cell counts with differential and platelet counts and LFTs are warranted if there is clinical suspicion, such as unexplained bruising or bleeding.

Monitoring Carbamazepine

After the patient is on a stable dose and provided there were no sources of concern during initial screening, a CBC, differential and platelet counts and BUN, creatinine, serum iron, and liver function tests should be drawn one month after beginning treatment, and then once every three to six months.[1] The platelet count may signal the first apparent change in bone marrow suppression, although this often comes on suddenly and without warning. Serum iron may also increase if this condition arises.[1]

Monitoring Valproic Acid

Liver function tests should be obtained every month for children less than 10 years of age.[1] For older children and adolescents, LFTs and CBCs should be done every week for the first month of therapy, and then every four to six months.[1]

Maintenance on Phenytoin

A CBC and differential should be taken every six months.[1]

Treatment Duration

There are no firm guidelines regarding the duration of treatment with anticonvulsants in children and adolescents with psychiatric disorders. Epileptic children and adolescents, of course, generally receive long-term treatment for control of their seizures. When these agents are used to treat psychiatric conditions, it is probably best to adopt the standard guidelines for other psychotropic agents used in the treatment of psychopathology.[1] The anticonvulsants usually should be given for nine to 12 months. Gradual tapering of the medication can be considered at the end of this period if symptom reduction has been achieved.[1] As with other psychiatric medications, this is often a judgment call.

There are now data to support maintenance medication of certain psychiatric disorders, such as recurrent major depression in adults (see Chapter 4). If the patient's behavior has shown marked improvement and he or she is experiencing no side effects, the patient and family may decide that it is not worth discontinuing the medication. In that case, following the child closely and maintaining him or her on the medication may be warranted. On the other hand, as many parents dislike having their children take medication, a trial off of the anticonvulsant may be warranted. The family should be warned of the risk that the symptom will recur. Nonetheless, if a child or adolescent has responded well to a particular medication, his or her likelihood of responding to the medication again if it is restarted is good. Obviously, however, with some problems, such as severe self and other-directed physical aggression, continued therapy may be necessary. It is advisable to get input from as many sources as possible, including the family, teachers, and school principal.

Withdrawal Seizures

Withdrawal seizures can occur in patients without a history of seizure disorder.[1] They are very rare with carbamazepine, valproic acid, and phenytoin,[69] and are seen primarily with barbiturates and benzodiazepines.

Clinical Practice

Dosage and Administration

There are no FDA-established guidelines for administering anticonvulsants to children and adolescents with psychiatric disorders. Generally, standard pharmacokinetics in children and adolescents and the guidelines established in treating epilepsy are utilized. For instance, prepubertal children savagely metabolize anticonvulsants, so they are eliminated rather rapidly.[1] In fact, adult metabolic states are often not achieved until very late adolescence. Liver and kidney metabolisms are significantly faster in children than in adolescents, and faster in adolescents than in adults. Therefore, children, and to a lesser extent adolescents, require higher doses.[1] Children also generally do better with more frequent and divided doses than when given large single doses. It is always advisable to start with low doses and to increase them gradually, as children appear to be very susceptible to anticonvulsant side effects.

Carbamazepine
See Table 9-15.

Children should be started at a dose of 100 mg/day.[1] For children under 4 years of age, the dose should be even lower (50 mg or half of a tablet). If the initial dose is well tolerated, it should be increased by 100 mg per week to a maximum daily dose of 1000 mg for children younger than 15 years. In children 15 years old and older, the dose can be increased to a maximum of 1200 mg/day to control symptoms.[1] This generally corresponds to a range of 10–50 mg/kg/day. Carbamazepine should be given three to four times daily to children and adolescents. Serum levels of 4–12 µg/ml are therapeutic.[1]

Valproic Acid
See Table 9-16.

Valproic acid (or sodium divalproex—Depakote) is initiated at a dose of 15 mg/kg day and increased every week to a maximum of 30–60 mg/kg/day.[70] Some investigators advocate giving the drug as a single bedtime dose to enhance patient compliance.[1] We agree that although this may be attempted initially, if problems such as GI upset occur, standard pediatric pharmacologic dosing should be employed. Generally, the dose is determined by tolerance to medication side effects and blood level.[1] Children and adolescents appear to respond best at valproic acid levels of 80–100 µg/ml with 50–100 µg/ml being considered the therapeutic range. The enteric-coated equivalent—divalproex generic or Depakote—can be given if the child experiences GI distress on regular valproic acid.

Phenytoin
See Table 9-17.

Phenytoin is started at a low dose in children or adolesents (50–100 mg/ day), and increased gradually every two weeks by 50 mg, until therapeutic serum levels approach the upper limit of 20 µg/ml. The standard dose range for phenytoin is 4–7 mg/kg/day.[71] Doses are usually closer to 4 mg/kg/day for older children and 7 mg/kg/day for younger children. This dosing strategy is used to treat seizure and behavioral disorders.[1]

Table 9-15
Dosage Scheduled for Treating Children and Adolescents with Carbamazepine

• Children under 6 years: Not recommended.
• Children over 6 years and adolescents: Dose initiated at 100 mg/day and increased by 100 mg/week to a maximum of 1000 mg/day (<15 years) or 1200 mg/day (>15 years).

Table 9-16
**Dosage Schedule for Treating Children and Adolescents
with Valproic Acid**

- Not recommended for children less than 3 years of age due to increased liver toxicity.
- Use with caution in mentally retarded children due to increased sensitivity to liver failure.
- Children >3 years: Dose initiated at 15 mg/kg/day and increased at weekly intervals to a maximum of 60 mg/kg/day.

Table 9-17
**Dosage Schedule for Treating Children and Adolescents
with Phenytoin**

- No age limit.
- Children under 6 years: Dose initiated at 50–100 mg/day and increased by 50 mg/day every two weeks to a maximum dose of 8 mg/kg/day.
- Children 6 years and older: Dose initiated at 50–100 mg/day and increased by 50 mg/day every two weeks to a maximum of 300 mg/day.

References

1. Trimble, M.R. (1990). Anticonvulsants in children and adolescents. *J Child Adolesc Psychopharmacol, 1(2)*.

2. Dodson, W.E. (1982). Nonlinear kinetics of phenytoin in children. *Neurology, 32,* 42.

3. Puente, R.M. (1976). The use of carbamazepine in the treatment of behavioral disorders in children. In W. Birkmayer (Ed.), *Epileptic Seizures—Behavior—Pain* (pp. 243–252). Bern: Hans Huber.

4. *Physicians' Desk Reference (45th ed.)* (1991). Oradell, N.J.: Medical Economics.

5. Brent, D.A. (1986). Overrepresentation of epileptics in a consecutive series of suicide attempters seen at a children's hospital. *J Am Acad Child Psychiatry, 25,* 242–246.

6. Brent, D.A., Crumrine, P.K., Varma, R.R., et al. (1987). Phenobarbital treatment and major depressive disorder in children with epilepsy. *Pediatrics, 80,* 909–917.

7. Stuppaeck, C., Barnas, C., Miller, C., et al. (1990). Carbamazepine in the prophylaxis of mood disorders. *J Clin Psychopharmacol, 10,* 39–42.

8. Post, R.M. (1987). Mechanisms of action of carbamazepine and related anticonvulsants in affective illness. In H.Y. Meltzer (Ed.), *Psychopharmacol-*

ogy: *The Third Generation of Progress* (pp. 567–576). New York: Raven Press.

9. Takezaki, H., Hanaoka, M. (1971). The use of carbamazepine (Tegretol) in the control of manic-depressive psychosis and other manic-depressive states. *Seishinigaku, 13*, 173–183.

10. Okuma, T., Kishimoto, A., Inove, K., et al. (1973). Antimanic and prophylactic effects of carbamazepine (Tegretol) on manic-depressive psychosis: A preliminary report. *Folia Psychiat Neurol Jpn, 27*, 283–297.

11. Ballenger, J.C., Post, R.M. (1978). Therapeutic effects of carbamazepine in affective illness: A preliminary report. *Commun in Psychopharmacol, 2*, 159–175.

12. Kishimoto, A., Ogura, C., Hazama, H. Inove, K. (1983). Long-term prophylactic effects of carbamazepine in affective disorder. *Br J Psychiatry, 143*, 327–331.

13. Okuma, T., Ianagu, K., Otsuki, S., et al. (1981). A preliminary double-blind study on the efficacy of carbamazepine in prophylaxis of manic-depressive illness. *Psychopharmacology, 73*, 95–96.

14. Post, R.M., Uhde, T.W. (1985). Carbamazepine in bipolar illness. *Psychopharmacol Bull, 21*, 10–17.

15. Inove, K., Arima, S., Tanaka, K., et al. (1981). A lithium and carbamazepine combination in the treatment of bipolar disorder: A preliminary report. *Folia Psychiat Neurol Jpn, 35*, 465–475.

16. Schaffer, C.B., Mungas, D., Rockwell, E. (1985). Successful treatment of psychotic depression with carbamazepine. *J Clin Psychopharmacol, 5*, 233.

17. Watkins, S.E., Callender, K., Thomas, D.R., et al. (1987). The effect of carbamazepine and lithium on remission from affective illness. *Br J Psychiatry, 150*, 180.

18. Groh, C. (1976). The psychotropic effect of Tegretol in non-epileptic children with particular reference to the drug's indications. In W. Birkmayer (Ed.), *Epileptic Seizures—Behavior—Pain* (pp. 259–263). Bern: Hans Huber.

19. Arana, G.W., Hyman, S.E. (1991). *Handbook of Psychiatric Drug Therapy* (2nd ed.). Boston: Little Brown.

20. Malcolm, R., Ballenger, J.C., Sturgis, E.T., Anton, R. (1989). Double-blind controlled trial comparing carbamazepine to oxazepam treatment of alcohol withdrawal. *Am J Psychiatry, 146*, 617.

21. Ries, R.K., Roy-Byrne, P.P., Ward, N.G., et al. (1989). Carbamazepine treatment for benzodiapazine withdrawal. *Am J Psychiatry, 145*, 536.

22. Monroe, R.R. (1970). *Episodic Behavioral Disorders: A Psychodynamic and Neurophysiologic Analysis*. Cambridge, Mass.: Harvard University Press.

23. Kuhn-Gebhardt, V. (1976). Behavioral disorders in non-epileptic children and their treatment with carbamazepine. In W. Birkmayer (Ed.), *Epileptic Seizures—Behavior—Pain* (pp. 264–267). Bern: Hans Huber.

24. Remschmidt, H. (1976). The psychotropic effect of carbamazepine in non-epileptic patients, with particular reference to problems posed by clinical studies in children with behavioral disorders. In W. Birkmayer (Ed.), *Epileptic Seizures—Behavior—Pain*. Bern: Hans Huber.

25. Puente, R.M. (1976). The use of carbamazepine in the treatment of behavioral disorders in children. In W. Birkmayer (Ed.), *Epileptic Seizures—Behavior—Pain*. Bern: Hans Huber.

26. Evans, R.W., Clary, T.H., Gualtieri, C.T. (1987). Carbamazepine in pediatric psychiatry. *J Am Acad Child Psychiatry, 26*, 2–8.

27. Wolf, S.M., Forsyth, A. (1955). Behavior disturbance, phenobarbital and febrile seizures. *Pediatrics, 61*, 728–731.

28. Trimble, M.R., Corbett, J. (1980). Behavioral and cognitive disturbances in epileptic children. *Irish Med J, Suppl. 73*, 21–28.

29. Pellock, J.M. (1987). Carbamazepine side effects in children and adults. *Epilepsia, 28(suppl. 3)*, 564.

30. Menkes, J.H. (1990). *Textbook of Child Neurology* (4th ed.) (pp. 641–642). Philadelphia: Lea & Febiger.

31. Pleak, R.R., Birmahr, B., Gaurilescu, A., et al. (1988). Mania and neuropsychiatric excitation following carbamazepine. *J Am Acad Child Adolesc Psychiatry, 27*, 500–503.

32. Lesser, R.P., et al. (1978). High-dose monotherapy in the treatment of epilepsy. *J Neurol Neurosurg Psychiatry, 41*, 907.

33. Camfield, C., et al. (1986). Asymptomatic children with epilepsy: Little benefit from screening for anticonvulsant-induced liver, blood, or renal damage. *Neurology, 36*, 838.

34. Snead, O.C., Hosey, L.C. (1985). Exacerbation of seizures in children by carbamazepine. *N Engl J Med, 313*, 916.

35. Agulgia, U., Zappin, M., Quattrone, A. (1987). Carbamazepine-induced nonepileptic myoclonus in a child with benign epilepsy. *Epilepsia, 28*, 515.

36. Macphee, G.J., et al. (1986). Verapamil potentiates carbamazepine neurotoxicity: A clinically important inhibitory interaction. *Lancet, 1*, 700.

37. Myers, W.C., Carrera, F. III. (1989). Carbamazepine-induced mania with hypersexuality in a 9-year-old boy. *Am J Psychiatry, 146,* 400.

38. Reiss, A.L., O'Donnell, D.J. (1984). Carbamazepine-induced mania in two children: Case report. *J Clin Psychiatry, 45,* 272–274.

39. Wilder, B.J., et al. (1983). Gastrointestinal tolerance of divalprorex sodium. *Neurology, 33,* 808.

40. Collaborative Study Group: Bourgeois, B., et al. (1987). Monotherapy with valproate in primary generalized epilepsies. *Epilepsion, 28(suppl. 2),* 58.

41. Hyman, N.M., Dennis, P.D., Sinclair, K. (1979). Tremor due to sodium valproate. *Neurology, 29,* 1177.

42. Bodensteiner, J.B., Morris, H.H., Golden, G.S. (1981). Asterixis associated with sodium valproate. *Neurology, 31,* 186.

43. Dreifuss, F.E., Langer, D.H. (1987). Hepatic considerations in the use of antiepileptic drugs. *Epilepsia, 28(suppl. 2),* 523.

44. Laub, M.C. (1986). Nutritional influence on serum ammonia in young patients receiving sodium valproate. *Epilepsia, 27,* 55.

45. Coulter, D.L., Allen, R.J. (1980). Secondary hyper-ammonaemia: A possible mechanism for valproate encephalopathy. *Lancet, 1,* 1310.

46. Barr, R.D., et al. (1982). Valproic acid and immune thrombocytopenia. *Arch Dis Child, 57,* 681.

47. Laub, M.C., et al. (1986). Serum carnitine during valproic acid therapy. *Epilepsia, 27,* 559.

48. Gram, L., Bensten, K.D. (1985). Valproate: An updated review. *Acta Neurol Scand, 72,* 129.

49. Robert, E., Guibaud, P. (1982). Maternal valproic acid and congenital neural tube defects. *Lancet, 2,* 937.

50. Kapur, R.N., et al. (1973). Diphenylhydantoin-induced gingival hyperlasia: Its relationship to dose and serum level. *Dev Med Child Neurol, 15,* 483.

51. Reynolds, E.H., Wales, M.B. (1967). Effects of folic acid on the mental state and fit-frequency of drug-treated epileptic patients. *Lancet, 1,* 1086–1088.

52. Reynolds, E.H. (1973). Anticonvulsants, folic acid, and epilepsy. *Lancet, 1,* 1376.

53. Trimble, M.R., Reynolds, E.H. (1976). Anticonvulsant drugs and mental symptoms: A review. *Psychol Med, 6*, 169.

54. Ambrosetto, G., et al. (1977). Phenytoin encephalopathy as probably idiosyncratic reaction: Case report. *Epilepsia, 18*, 405.

55. Crosley, C.J., Chee, C., Berman, P.H. (1975). Rickets associated with long-term anticonvulsant therapy in a pediatric out-patient population. *Pediatrics, 56*, 52.

56. Morijiri, Y., Sato, T. (1981). Factors causing rickets in institutionalized handicapped children on anticonvulsant therapy. *Arch Dis Child, 56*, 446.

57. Krause, K.H., et al. (1985). Biotin status of epileptics. *Ann NY Acad Sci, 447*, 297.

58. Ogunmekan, A.O., Huang, P.A. (1989). A randomized, double-blind, placebo-controlled, clinical trial of D-tocopheryl acetate (vitamin E) as add-on therapy, for epilepsy in children. *Epilepsia, 30*, 84.

59. Lovelace, R.E., Horwitz, S.J. (1968). Peripheral neuropathy in long-term diphenylhydantoin therapy. *Arch Neurol, 18*, 69.

60. Dawson, K.P. (1973). Severe cutaneous reactions to phenytoin. *Arch Dis Child, 48*, 239.

61. Beernink, D.H., Miller, J.J. (1973). Anticonvulsant-induced antinuclear antibodies and lupus-like disease in children. *J Pediatr, 82*, 113.

62. Li, F.P., et al. (1975). Malignant lymphoma after diphenylhydantoin (dilantin) therapy. *Cancer, 36*, 1359.

63. Sherwin, A.L. (1983). How to use ethosuximide. In P.L. Morselli, C.E. Pippenger, J.K. Penry (Eds.), *Antiepileptic Drug Therapy in Pediatrics* (pp. 229–236). New York: Raven Press.

64. Corbett, J.A., Trimble, M.R., Nichol, T.C. (1985). Behavioral and cognitive impairment in children with epilepsy: The long-term effects of anticonvulsant therapy. *J Am Acad Child Psychiatry, 24*, 17–23.

65. Robertson, M.M., Trimble, M.R., Townsend, H.R.A. (1987). The phenomenology of depression in epilepsy. *Epilepsia, 28(4)*, 364–372.

66. Theodore, W.H., et al. (1986). Barbiturates reduce human cerebral glucose metabolism. *Neurology, 36*, 60.

67. Thompson, P.J., Trimble, M.R. (1982). Anticonvulsant drugs and cognitive functions. *Epilepsia, 23*, 531.

68. Blumer, D. (1991). Epilepsy and disorders of mood. In D. Smith, D. Trei-

man, M. Trimble (Eds.), *Advances in Neurology (vol. 55)*. New York: Raven Press.

69. Duncan, M.R., Shorvon, S., Trimble, M.R. (1989). Withdrawal symptoms from phenytoin, carbamazepine, and sodium valproate. *J Neurol Neurosurg Neuropsychiatry, 51*, 924–928.

70. Dreifuss, F.E. (1983). How to use valproic acid. In I.L. Morselli, C.E. Pippenger, J.K. Penry (Eds.), *Antiepileptic Drug Therapy in Pediatrics* (pp. 219–228). New York: Raven Press.

71. Albani, M. (1983). How to use phenytoin. In I.L. Morselli, C.E. Pippenger, J.K. Penry (Eds.), *Antiepileptic Drug Therapy in Pediatrics* (pp. 253–262). New York: Raven Press.

Chapter 10

Anxiolytics

Anxiolytic and sedative agents are among the most frequently prescribed drugs in medicine. However, "anxiolytic" is a deceiving term
for this category. Antidepressants are the long-term treatment of
choice for most anxiety disorders in children and adolescents, and are
discussed separately (see Chapters 4 and 6). Similarly, antipsychotics
and beta-adrenergic antagonists, which are often used for their sedative and anxiolytic properties, are reviewed in Chapters 7 and 11.
Therefore, although the medications discussed in this chapter are
commonly known as anxiolytics, they do not necessarily represent
the current standards of treatment for childhood anxiety disorders.
The distinction is an important one, since most anxiolytics are actually of limited use for children and adolescents.

Thirty years ago, this category could have been defined as those medications that produce prompt sedation, rapid tolerance, and possible
drug dependence. They included the barbiturates, which were widely
prescribed as hypnotics and anxiolytics; the newly developed benzodiazepines, which offered improved efficacy with less risk of toxicity;
and the sedating antihistamines. Since barbiturates are now all but
absent from the psychiatrist's armamentarium, the term anxiolytic
has become nearly synonymous with benzodiazepine. However, antihistamines continue to see frequent use as hypnotics, and recently a

new category of nonsedating, nonaddictive anxiolytic (azapirones) was introduced. Therefore, this chapter will focus on the current use of benzodiazepines, antihistamines, and azapirones (buspirone) in child and
adolescent psychiatry.

Chemical Properties

Benzodiazepines

Since their introduction in the early 1960s, benzodiazepines (BZPs) have become the most widely prescribed psychoactive agents in the world, owing
mainly to their ease of use, relatively low toxicity, and tremendous effectiveness in alleviating anxiety. Although specific agents have undergone wide
swings in popularity, the overall market for BZPs has remained rich. Over
17 million prescriptions for these agents were filled in 1989 in the United
States.[51] The BZPs are so effective at relieving anxiety that they have also
become one of the most widely abused prescription drugs, prompting New
York State to institute mandatory triplicate prescription regulation for all
BZPs.[131] However, it is clear that the majority of prescriptions are not
abused and BZPs are likely to remain useful for specific conditions.[125]

Absorption and Metabolism

Chlordiazepoxide (Librium) was introduced in 1960 for the treatment of anxiety, followed closely by diazepam (Valium). Many agents are now available
and can be classified by chemical structure (Figure 10-1) or metabolic pathways (Figure 10-2). Kaplan and Sadock[61] categorize the compounds as 2-
keto-, 3-hydroxy-, or triazolo-benzodiazepines, corresponding to their structures and metabolic pathways. All are rapidly absorbed via oral or parenteral routes. The 2-keto-BZPs (diazepam, chlordiazepoxide) undergo a
complex sequence of hepatic biotransformations, the end product of which is
the active metabolite, desmethyldiazepam. The elimination half-life of this
metabolite is approximately 72 hours and it accounts for the long duration
of action seen with 2-keto-BZPs (Table 10-1). The 3-hydroxy BZPs (temazepam, oxazepam) are the metabolic products of desmethyldiazepam and do
not give rise to further active metabolites. These compounds and their derivatives (lorazepam) are glucuronidated and then excreted, yielding intermediate half-lives of 8–24 hours. Triazolo-BZPs (alprazolam, triazolam) undergo
hydroxylation followed by glucuronidation and have intermediate or short
half-lives with no active metabolites.[69] Although flurazepam is considered a
2-keto-BZP, its metabolic pathway differs. For both flurazepam and quazepam, the rate-limiting active metabolite is desalkylflurazepam, which has
a half-life of 48–120 hours.[52] Clonazepam follows a unique metabolic pathway, but its half-life in adults is comparable to those of chlordiazepoxide
and diazepam.

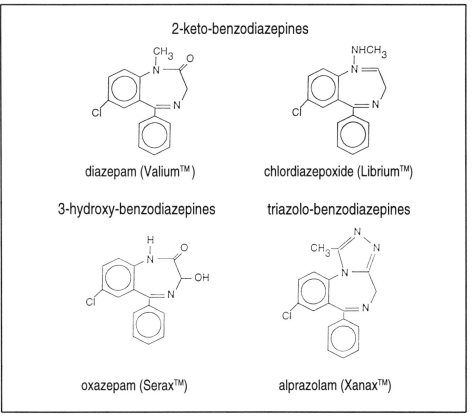

2-keto-benzodiazepines

diazepam (Valium™)

chlordiazepoxide (Librium™)

3-hydroxy-benzodiazepines

triazolo-benzodiazepines

oxazepam (Serax™)

alprazolam (Xanax™)

Figure 10-1
Chemical Structures of Common Benzodiazepines

The metabolism of BZPs in newborns is better understood than in older children. Infants gain the limited ability to metabolize diazepam at around 13 weeks of gestation and reach maximum capacity in early childhood.[28] Thereafter, the general principles of preadolescent pharmacodynamics probably hold true: faster hepatic metabolism necessitates more frequent and higher (weight-corrected) doses for children than for adults. This is supported by studies of midazolam and diazepam, which have half-lives in children of 1.2–2.4 and 18 hours respectively.[90,94,111] The BZPs that do not undergo hepatic transformation are less affected by increased metabolic rates in children. Metabolic rates in adolescents resemble those in adults.[28]

Mechanism of Action
Several hypotheses have been proposed to explain the clinical effects of BZPs. The most prominent followed the discovery that these drugs bind to specific neuroreceptors, for which an endogenous ligand has not yet been found.[54,76] This receptor (BZP-R) apparently mediates the anxiolytic proper-

311

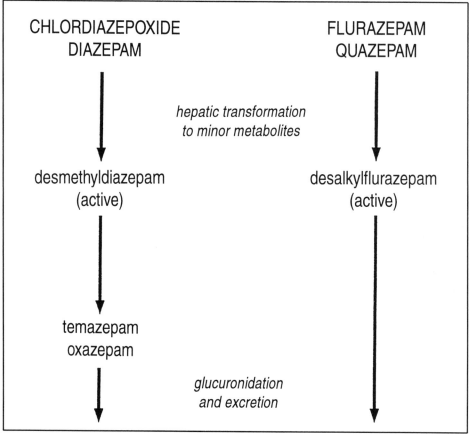

CHLORDIAZEPOXIDE
DIAZEPAM

FLURAZEPAM
QUAZEPAM

*hepatic transformation
to minor metabolites*

desmethyldiazepam
(active)

desalkylflurazepam
(active)

temazepam
oxazepam

*glucuronidation
and excretion*

Figure 10-2
Major Metabolic Pathways of Benzodiazepines

ties of BZPs, since affinity for BZP-R is highly correlated with clinical potency.[87] The BZP-R function is also closely linked with the gamma-aminobutyric acid (GABA) system and the GABA receptor. The BZP-R agonists increase GABA transmission, while GABA agonists enhance the binding of BZPs to their receptor.[142]

Tolerance develops quickly to the sedative and muscle-relaxant properties of BZPs, but less obviously to their anxiolytic properties. Most BZPs maintain anxiolytic efficacy during long-term treatment, but withdrawal does produce anxiety symptoms, and this suggests some degree of tolerance.[91,103] Although BZP-R does not undergo clear down-regulation in response to chronic BZP exposure, there are reports of both down-regulation[85] and up-regulation.[37] Biochemical studies also suggest multiple subtypes of BZP-R.[76,158] Some BZPs possess other receptor affinities that account for additional properties, such as the antidepressant effect of alprazolam, which is presumed to be related to activity at catecholamine receptors.

Those BZPs marketed exclusively as hypnotics have shorter elimination half-lives and are preferred for their relative freedom from daytime sedation after a bedtime dose. There is evidence that the quality of sleep induced by BZPs differs among specific drugs. For example, alprazolam and diazepam reduce sleep latency and awakenings with equal efficacy, but alprazolam is a more potent REM suppressant.[17] In addition to promoting sleep, BZPs slow reaction time and impair general cognitive abilities.[12,154] Therefore, academic function may be affected in children when long-acting agents or daytime doses are used.

Buspirone

Recently, a novel anxiolytic agent was introduced that cannot be classified with other common agents. Buspirone has no approved clinical indications for patients younger than 18 years, and few controlled pediatric studies have been conducted. However, it is marketed for adults as an anxiolytic agent with minimal sedation and abuse potential,[70] making it of great potential interest to pediatricians and child psychiatrists.

Absorption and Metabolism

Buspirone is the first azapirone anxiolytic to be marketed in the United States, and it is distinct from the BZPs in both structure and function (Figure 10-3). It is rapidly absorbed and reaches peak plasma level in 60–90 minutes in adults. Clinical anxiolytic effects require two to four weeks of chronic administration. The mean half-life of the parent compound is two to three hours,[44] but the primary metabolite (1-[2-pyrimidinyl]-piperazine) is pharmacologically active and has a mean half-life of 6.1 hours.[58] No pharmacokinetic studies have been conducted on children.

Mechanism of Action

The most prominent pharmacologic action of buspirone is agonist binding to postsynaptic serotonin receptors (5-HT1A), and this probably represents the anxiolytic mechanism of action.[80,146] The drug binds to a lesser degree to 5-HT2 and dopamine (D2) receptors, but the relevance of these affinities to the clinical effects is unknown. One of the postulated advantages of buspirone over BZPs is that it does not interact with the BZP–GABA receptor complex, thereby avoiding the addictive properties of BZPs.[146] Accordingly, buspirone possesses no anticonvulsant or muscle-relaxant properties,[58] nor does it cause the cognitive impairment seen with BZPs and antihistamines.[12,148] Buspirone produces minimal initial sedation and is, therefore, ineffective as a hypnotic.[37,79] Antidepressant qualities are hypothesized for buspirone, but have not been adequately evaluated.[39]

Table 10-1
Sample of Available Benzodiazepines, Usual Adult Doses, and Costs

Compound (Brand Name)	How Available	Age Range	Adult Half-Life (hours)	Usual Adult Daily Dose	Approximate Daily Cost*
Lorazepam (Ativan)	INJ—2, 4 mg/ml Tab—0.5, 1.0, 2.0 mg	⩾12 years	12	2–6 mg/day divided	$2.58
Prazepam (Centrax)	Tab—5, 10, 20 mg	⩾18 years	30–200	20–60 mg/day divided	$2.81
Chlordiazepoxide (Librium)	INJ—100/2 ml Tab—5, 10, 25 mg Cap—5, 10, 25 mg	⩾12 years	24–48	5–25 mg b.i.d. or t.i.d.	$1.55†
Oxazepam (Serax)	Tab—15 Cap—10, 15, 30 mg	⩾6 years	6–11	10–30 mg t.i.d. to q.i.d.	$2.08
Clorazepate (Tranxene)	Tab—3.75, 7.5, 15 mg SR—11.25, 22.5 mg	⩾9 years	30–200	15–60 mg/day divided	$4.81†
Diazepam (Valium)	INJ—5/ml Tab—2, 5, 10 mg SR—15 mg	⩾6 months	20–100	2–10 mg t.i.d. to q.i.d.	$1.60†

Alprazolam (Xanax)	Tab—0.25, 0.5, 1.0, 2.0 mg	≥18 years	6–27	5–6 mg/day divided (for panic disorder)	$4.33
Temazepam (Restoril)	Cap—15, 30 mg	≥18 years	9–12	15 or 30 mg q.h.s.	$0.84†
Midazolam (Versed)	INJ—1, 5 mg/ml	≥18 years	1–12	No approved psychiatric indication	NA
Flurazepam (Dalmane)	Cap—15, 30 mg	≥15 years	40–100	15 or 30 mg q.h.s.	$0.74†
Quazepam (Doral)	Tab—7.5, 15 mg	≥18 years	40–100	7.5 or 15 mg q.h.s.	$0.88
Triazolam (Halcion)	Tab—0.125, 0.25 mg	≥18 years	2–6	0.25 or 0.125 mg q.h.s.	$0.89
Estazolam (Prosom)	Tab—1, 2 mg	≥18 years	10–24	1 or 2 mg q.h.s.	$1.05

*Cost estimates based on median effective adult dose for primary psychiatric indication and average wholesale price as published in *Prescription Pricing Guide*, Medi-Span, Inc., June 1992.
†Generic available.
Abbreviations: INJ—injectable; TAB—tablet; CAP—capsule; SR—sustained release.

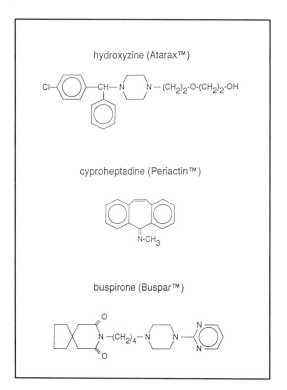

hydroxyzine (Atarax™)

cyproheptadine (Periactin™)

buspirone (Buspar™)

Figure 10-3
**Chemical Structures of Common Nonbenzodiazepine Anxiolytic
Drugs**

Antihistamines

Antihistamines have a wide variety of uses in psychiatry and medicine, from
the treatment of allergic rhinitis to preanesthetic sedation. Of those used in
psychiatry (Table 10-2), the most common is diphenhydramine (Benadryl).
This drug has both antihistaminic and anticholinergic properties, and is commonly used as a hypnotic or to treat extrapyramidal symptoms induced by
antipsychotic drugs (see Chapter 7). One antihistamine (hydroxyzine) has
been approved by the FDA for the short-term treatment of anxiety, although
its efficacy has not been well demonstrated. Several others are used for
sleep induction or the acute management of agitated states.

Absorption and Metabolism
Antihistamines are rapidly absorbed after oral administration and undergo
hepatic metabolism. Intramuscular and IV routes are available for diphenhydramine and promethazine, but are usually reserved for the treatment of ex-

trapyramidal symptoms or severe allergic reactions, or for immediate sedation. Sedative effects reach their peak one to three hours after an oral dose and average four to six hours in duration.[97] All antihistamines used for psychiatric indications have short elimination half-lives (Table 10-2). The manufacturers report half-lives of less than five hours for all commonly used agents. However, in practice, the half-life of diphenhydramine varies from three to 13 hours.[139] Estimates for hydroxyzine likewise vary, from three to 29 hours.[138] As with the BZPs, children metabolize antihistamines more rapidly than do adults. The half-life of diphenhydramine in children is 40% that in elderly adults and 60% that in young adults.[139] Children metabolize hydroxyzine approximately three times faster than do adults.[137]

Mechanism of Action
The antihistamines used in psychiatry produce sedation through central histamine H_1 receptor blockade, but their chemical structures are diverse (Figure 10-3). Several newer antihistamines were specifically designed *not* to produce sedation, and they accomplish this by reducing CNS penetration. No anxiolytic mechanism has been postulated for antihistamines apart from that of general sedation, making these agents of limited use in the long-term treatment of anxiety disorders.

Other properties pertinent to psychiatry are based on nonhistaminic mechanisms. Antiparkinsonian effects are strongly related to anticholinergic properties, making diphenhydramine the most effective agent for this application. Cyproheptadine has antiserotonergic properties and has been used in adults to treat sexual dysfunction induced by SSUIs (e.g., fluoxetine).[61] One sedating antihistamine (promethazine) is a phenothiazine derivative. Although it is a weak dopamine antagonist (one tenth the potency of chlorpromazine), it can produce the side effects common to other antipsychotic drugs (see Chapter 7).

Indications

Despite the approval of some BZPs for pediatric use, controlled studies of their efficacy in children and adolescents are scarce. Waters[161] has suggested that their clinical use far exceeds that supported by research. In one large Canadian study, BZP prescriptions were more common than all other pediatric psychotropics combined.[106] Likewise, antihistamines have long been used as sedatives and hypnotics despite a lack of evidence to prove their effectiveness for specific indications. Buspirone is still relatively new and unstudied, but has several promising applications in child and adolescent psychiatry.

Table 10-2
Sample of Available Antihistamine Agents, Usual Adult Doses, and Costs

Agent (Brand Name)	Available Forms	Adult Half-Life (hours)	Dose Range	Psychiatric Indications	Approximate Daily Cost*
Diphenhydramine (Benadryl)	CAP—25, 50 mg INJ—1, 5, 50 mg/ml	3–14	≤5 mg/kg/day, div q.i.d. Max. 300 mg/day 50–100 mg as hypnotic	EPS Hypnotic	$0.37†
Hydroxyzine (Atarax, Vistaril)	TAB—10, 25, 50, 100 mg LIQ—2 mg/5 ml	3–29	50–100 mg/day, divided 0.6 mg/kg as sedative	Anxiety Sedation	$0.89†
Cyproheptadine (Periactin)	TAB—4 mg LIQ—2 mg/5 ml	<5	0.25 mg/kg/day, divided Max. 16 mg/day	None	NA
Promethazine (Phenergan)	TAB—12.5, 25, 50 mg SUP—12.5, 25, 50 mg LIQ—6.25, 25 mg/5 ml INJ—25, 50 mg/ml	<5	1.1 mg/kg single dose Usual dose ≤50 mg	Hypnotic Sedation	$0.31†

*Cost estimates based on median effective sedation dose for adults and average wholesale price as published in *Prescription Pricing Guide*, Medi-Span, Inc., June 1992.
†Generic available.
Abbreviations: CAP—capsule; TAB—tablet; INJ—injectable; LIQ—liquid; SUP—suppository.

Anxiety Disorders

A recent review has judged anxiety disorders to have the highest point prevalence of any category of child and adolescent psychiatric illness. Between 9% and 17% of children meet the DSM-III-R criteria for at least one disorder.[14] These include syndromes that are diagnosed in adults (panic disorder, OCD, PTSD) and those that are exclusive to children (separation anxiety, overanxious disorder, avoidant disorder). Despite the high prevalence of anxiety, the majority of pharmacologic trials in children are single case reports or small open trials. This may be partly attributed to the success of nonpharmacologic therapies. For example, simple phobia has never been subjected to systematic pharmacologic trial in children, but has been shown to respond well to a variety of behavioral and psychotherapeutic interventions.[14] However, many anxiety disorders are not as amenable to psychotherapy, and the lack of complementary pharmacologic trials represents a serious deficit in child and adolescent research.

Panic Disorder

Though panic attacks were at one time considered an adult problem, they most certainly occur in children. A recent Australian survey found that 43% of adolescents reported at least one episode during their lives.[63] Estimates of the number of children experiencing at least one moderate to severe panic attack vary from 0.6% to 13.3%, but the rate of panic disorder based on full DSM-III-R criteria has not been established.[94]

Although there are no controlled pharmacologic trials for child and adolescent panic disorder, the short-term efficacy of BZPs in adult panic disorder is well documented,[2,5,29,78,126,140] and alprazolam has received FDA approval for the treatment of panic disorder in patients 18 years of age or older. Experience with BZPs in childhood panic disorder is limited to case reports of success with clonazepam[15,68] and the combination of alprazolam with imipramine.[10] Therefore, although it seems likely that the short-term efficacy of BZPs in youngsters will prove similar to that in adults, the long-term efficacy and adverse effects have not been established.

Antidepressants are currently the pharmacologic treatment of choice for panic disorder in children (see Chapter 4), but the conservative use of alprazolam as reported by Ballenger and colleagues[10] is a reasonable extension of its use in adults. They reported two cases in which children (aged 8 and 13 years) were treated with alprazolam plus imipramine, showed rapid resolution of symptoms, and then underwent an alprazolam taper without complications. Since the anxiolytic response to alprazolam is rapid and imipramine may require two or more weeks, this combination provides prompt treatment with a minimal risk of dependence on or withdrawal from the BZP.

However, this approach is not without problems. Woods and colleagues[157] compared imipramine with combined imipramine and alprazolam in adults and found that although the combined treatment produced a more rapid response, it was also associated with intolerance of the alprazolam taper. The study used alprazolam for up to six weeks before attempting a taper, suggesting that if combined treatment is used, it should be limited to the first two weeks of therapy.

Buspirone was recently tested for adult panic disorder, but the results do not support its efficacy. Controlled trials have reported failed[134] or modestly successful[102] treatment of panic attacks. One case series suggested that it may be an effective adjunct to BZP treatment,[45] but this requires replication. Unless further controlled trials support its use, buspirone cannot be recommended for child and adolescent panic disorder.

Antihistamines have no application in child and adolescent panic disorder.

Separation Anxiety/School Refusal

Separation anxiety and the symptoms of school refusal are closely related, since they often coexist and they overlap with the older term "school phobia." Separation anxiety accounts for up to half of anxiety-related treatment referrals in children and adolescents and has a lifetime prevalence of up to 84% in children diagnosed with any anxiety disorder.[71] Although school refusal is not a separate diagnosis in the DSM-III-R, it is a common manifestation of separation anxiety, as implied by the earlier diagnostic entity, school phobia. Up to 80% of children with school refusal meet the criteria for separation anxiety.[14]

Accordingly, the treatment of separation anxiety has been somewhat better studied than other childhood anxiety disorders, and several studies report success with BZPs. In 1962, D'Amato[33] conducted an open trial of chlordiazepoxide on nine children with school phobia, eight of whom showed excellent results. A few years later, Kraft and colleagues[65] conducted an open trial of chlordiazepoxide with 130 diagnostically heterogeneous children ranging in age from 2 to 17 years. Of the 18 children with school phobia, 10 were considered "excellent" responders and four were considered "good" responders (78%). Two children (11%) became worse. In contrast, 38% of children with a primary behavioral disorder responded and 22% became worse. More recently, a double-blind controlled study of alprazolam by Bernstein and associates[13] found a trend toward improvement, but no statistically significant benefit, in 24 children and adolescents with school refusal. These children also had no significant improvement on imipramine.

These data are inconclusive. The open trials showing a good response to BZPs were conducted using diagnostic criteria that differ from the current definition of separation anxiety and probably represented a mixed sample of children with school refusal and anxiety. The one controlled study may have been less sensitive to a positive effect because the sample was selected for school refusal rather than for separation anxiety, and included children with depressive disorders.[14] Further controlled trials are necessary before the short-term efficacy of BZPs can be established for separation anxiety. The long-term efficacy is unknown.

There have been, as yet, no controlled trials of buspirone for the treatment of separation anxiety, although a single case study reported success in a young boy[66] Buspirone would seem a viable treatment for this disorder and should be tested in clinical trials.

As with most anxiety disorders, antihistamines have no proved or postulated role in the treatment of separation anxiety.

Overanxious Disorder and Nonspecific Childhood Anxiety

There is one study of BZPs for overanxious disorder diagnosed according to current DSM-III-R criteria. Simeon and Ferguson[136] conducted a single-blind trial of alprazolam in 12 overanxious children, yielding at least moderate improvement in seven. Virtually all other trials of BZPs in general childhood anxiety are diagnostically nonspecific (Table 10-3). Benzodiazepines have been reported to improve, worsen, or produce no change in nonspecific anxiety symptoms.

The most practical application that may be gleaned from these studies is the pretreatment of anticipatory anxiety prior to a painful procedure, as reported by Pfefferbaum and colleagues.[99] Single doses of BZPs are likely to reduce the psychologic trauma of such procedures and are unlikely to produce untoward effects. This practice should probably be reserved for developmentally normal children, since two studies have noted that a minority of children exhibit behavioral disinhibition when treated with BZPs, and that this effect appears more frequently in children with mental retardation or "brain damage."[4,96] Behavioral disinhibition is the most significant risk of using these agents for anticipatory anxiety or as p.r.n. sedatives (see "Adverse Reactions").

Buspirone has not been evaluated for overanxious disorder or nonspecific anxiety in children. However, it was found effective for generalized anxiety in adults in double-blind comparisons with diazepam, alprazolam, and lorazepam.[30,40,92] A single case study reported success in a young boy with overanxious disorder and separation anxiety.[66] Adult generalized anxiety is currently the only FDA-approved indication for buspirone, but it seems a likely candidate for the future treatment of overanxious disorder.

Table 10-3
Trials of Benzodiazepines for Nonspecific Childhood Anxiety Symptoms

Citation	Design*	No. of Subjects	Symptoms	Treatment	Outcome
Gleser et al., 1965[47]	P-C	46	Severe behavioral disorders	Chlordiazepoxide	Improved anxiety and hostility
Kraft et al., 1965[65]	Open	130	Behavior disorders (50) School phobia (18) Adjustment reaction (17) Other (45)	Chlordiazepoxide	Best response—school phobia Worst response—brain damage 13 developed disinhibition
Lucas and Pasley, 1969[77]	P-C	10	"Psychoneurotic" with anxiety	Diazepam	No benefit
Aman and Werry,1982[4]	P-C	15	General anxiety and developmental reading delay	Diazepam	Slight exacerbation of anxiety compared with placebo
Petti et al., 1982[96]	Open	9	"Severely disturbed"	Chlordiazepoxide	Improved depression and anxiety; worsened impulsivity and psychosis
Pfefferbaum et al., 1987[99]	Open	13	Anticipatory anxiety prior to bone marrow or spinal tap	Alprazolam	Improved anxiety before procedures
Biederman, 1987[15]	Open	3	Paniclike symptoms	Clonazepam	Improved with follow-up of 5–36 months
Simeon and Ferguson, 1987[136]	P-C	12	Overanxious or avoidant disorder	Alprazolam	Significant improvement in anxiety

*P-C—Placebo controlled.

Hydroxyzine, diphenhydramine, and promethazine have been used for non-specific anxiety symptoms in both children and adults, but have not been systematically studied. One early controlled trial measured decreased physiologic and psychological signs of anxiety in a mixed group of adult psychiatric patients after a single IM dose of hydroxyzine,[101] but no data are available on children. Although anxiety is an approved indication for hydroxyzine, there is no evidence supporting the long-term benefit of antihistamines in the treatment of anxiety disorders. They are often used and may be effective for anticipatory or situational anxiety, such as a child might experience prior to an office procedure, but this, too, is unstudied.

Posttraumatic Stress Disorder

Most research on PTSD has been conducted on adult war veterans. However, this disorder may also affect children exposed to single or repeated traumatic events, such as sexual abuse or a natural disaster.[49,82,143] Antidepressants are the pharmacologic treatment of choice for adults (see Chapter 4), but BZPs and buspirone have also been evaluated, with mixed results.

The scant data on BZPs are not favorable. Clonazepam fails to inhibit the hyperactive startle reflex in adults with PTSD,[133] and a double-blind, placebo-controlled study of alprazolam in 16 adults found no benefit.[22] Six of the patients (three of whom were receiving alprazolam) dropped out of the study because of the drug's ineffectiveness, and those who completed the trial showed a trend toward improvement of anxiety symptoms, but no effect on the major symptoms of PTSD. Furthermore, withdrawal effects exacerbated anxiety in subjects receiving alprazolam.[22] Similar problems with withdrawal were observed in eight combat veterans who had received long-term alprazolam treatment, including severe sleep and anxiety problems, as well as an increase in the major symptoms of PTSD.[116] The only favorable report is a letter by Feldman,[41] who saw improvement in 16 of 20 war veterans on alprazolam, but increased aggressive outbursts in the remaining four. Based on this limited experience, BZPs cannot be recommended for use in children with PTSD. In fact, these studies suggest that they should be avoided.

In contrast, a single open trial of buspirone in three PTSD patients reported improvement in anxiety, insomnia, depression, and flashbacks on 35–60 mg/day.[153] Controlled trials of buspirone for PTSD are warranted, but have not been conducted, and there are no controlled trials of any agent for childhood PTSD.

No studies of antihistamines in the treatment of PTSD have been conducted, nor are they warranted.

Obsessive-Compulsive Disorder

General clinical opinion does not favor the use of BZPs as a primary treatment for OCD.[53] However, they are used as adjuncts to antidepressants. Much recent research has focused on the antiobsessive properties of SSUIs, in both children and adults (see Chapter 4). Animal studies have demonstrated that clonazepam, in particular, has an indirect effect on serotonergic transmission that is not mediated by reuptake inhibition or receptor binding.[55] This effect provides a theoretical basis for clinical trials of clonazepam in OCD, but only one open trial is available to test the theory. Good symptomatic improvement was observed in three adults with OCD, and it persisted up to one year in two subjects. However, one subject was terminated when she began using alcohol in conjunction with the medication.[55] No controlled trials are available, and there is no evidence supporting the use of BZPs in childhood OCD.

Since buspirone is an agonist at postsynaptic serotonergic receptors, one might predict that it would be useful in treating OCD. Although one open trial did not support the efficacy of buspirone as a single agent,[59] a more recent double-blind, controlled trial in adults found that 60 mg of buspirone daily was as effective as clomipramine.[93] There has also been some success in using buspirone in combination with other serotonergic agents, including a recent case report of buspirone augmenting the response to fluoxetine in an 11-year-old girl with OCD and depression.[3] Markovitz and associates[80] found the combination of buspirone and fluoxetine to be superior to fluoxetine alone in an open trial for young adults with treatment-resistant OCD. In contrast to the favorable reports, a recent placebo-controlled trial of patients who responded incompletely to clomipramine treatment found no group effect from adding buspirone, despite a 25% reduction of symptoms in four of the 14 patients. The authors suggested that these results may indicate a subgroup of OCD patients who are responsive to buspirone. An alternative interpretation is that selecting clomipramine-resistant patients represents a sampling bias and yields a subgroup of OCD patients with poor response to serotonergic agents.[100] Although further controlled trials of buspirone in nonrefractory OCD patients are needed, the drug has a low incidence of side effects and would be a reasonable adjunctive agent in patients who appear to respond to serotonergic agents, but are intolerant of clomipramine's side effects. No studies of buspirone in childhood OCD are available.

Conclusions

Controlled pharmacologic studies on child and adolescent anxiety disorders are very scarce, so that recommendations for treatment must be drawn from open trials and the adult literature. When pharmacologic treatment is necessary, antidepressants are the first-line treatment for panic disorder, separation anxiety, PTSD, and OCD (see Chapter 4). Benzodiazepines may be useful for the treatment of anticipatory anxiety and for the first two weeks of panic disorder therapy in children, but are of questionable benefit in separation anxiety. There is little support for their use for OCD or the long-term treatment of overanxious disorder. They should be avoided in the treatment of PTSD based on the lack of demonstrable benefit in adult studies and the possible exacerbation of symptoms upon withdrawal. Many questions remain about optimal agents, dosage schedules, and duration of treatment for any child or adolescent anxiety disorder. Controlled trials of BZPs are most clearly needed for the treatment of separation anxiety and panic disorder, where their efficacy and the risks of long-term therapy in children must be established.

Buspirone has been most promising as a nonaddictive alternative to BZPs for the long-term treatment of generalized anxiety in adults. There is almost no research experience with children, but the low risk of dependence and its favorable side-effect profile make this agent more attractive than BZPs for early clinical use. While there are no established indications, possible uses include overanxious disorder, OCD, and PTSD. There are no studies of buspirone for separation anxiety, although this would seem a likely application. Buspirone may be less effective than standard agents for panic disorder, but this requires further study in both adults and children.

Finally, hydroxyzine has gained FDA approval for the treatment of anxiety, despite a lack of academic support for this indication. Sedating antihistamines are commonly used for anticipatory or situational anxiety in children and may be appropriate for these indications, but are by no means proven. Antihistamines cannot be recommended as the primary treatment for any chronic child or adolescent anxiety disorder.

Insomnia

Insomnia is estimated to afflict 30–35% of the population each year,[83] and is the most common problem for which sedatives and anxiolytics are prescribed. Academic debate concerning the most appropriate use of anxiolytic drugs for insomnia by no means has been concluded, but it seems clear that only a fraction of the prescriptions written for hypnotic drugs are justified. As used here, the term "hypnotic" will refer to those sedatives and anxiolytics that are commonly prescribed for sleep induction, including primarily antihistamines and the short-acting BZPs.

Insomnia is most often secondary to a treatable problem such as concurrent affective illness, pain, or substance use (including caffeine, alcohol, nicotine, and illicit drugs), and in such cases should be addressed through treatment of the primary disorder. Secondary insomnia is not a usual indication for hypnotic drugs. Primary insomnia (also called psychophysiologic insomnia) is an approved indication for hypnotic drugs, but since tolerance develops to the sedative properties of both BZPs and antihistamines, they are only effective for a limited time.[56] Chronic primary insomnia is not an indication for long-term hypnotic drugs.[152] Therefore, hypnotics are most appropriate for *transient primary insomnia*, loosely defined as cases that last fewer than 30 days. Transient primary insomnia accounts for 15% of cases in adults[31] and is at least as common in children.[34]

Transient insomnia usually follows an acute stressor such as psychosocial problems or circadian phase shifts.[56] If sleep does not normalize within one to two weeks, then a diagnosis of chronic insomnia or concurrent affective disorder should be considered. Because the disorder is self-limited, pharmacologic treatment is often unnecessary and behavioral techniques (structured sleep schedules, improved sleep hygiene, and supportive measures) are usually effective.[19,46] In young children, learning to self-initiate and maintain sleep may represent a developmental and behavioral milestone, making nonpharmacologic techniques the clear treatment of choice.[34,38,43] But despite the success of nonpharmacologic treatments, hypnotic agents are occasionally indicated, and are quite often prescribed.

Benzodiazepines

At their introduction to the medical community BZPs represented a welcome departure from barbiturates, which had been the primary hypnotic agents of the past. As indicated in Table 10-4, most short-acting BZPs are approved for the short-term treatment of adult insomnia when nonpharmacologic measures are ineffective. Virtually all BZP hypnotics reduce sleep latency, arousals, and partial arousals under laboratory conditions. Placebo-controlled trials of up to five days' treatment have demonstrated this for specific agents, including alprazolam,[17] quazepam,[145,147] triazolam,[121,115] temazepam[118] and others. The study by Uhthoff and associates[147] illustrates the effect. Subjects treated with quazepam showed a significant improvement in sleep quality and latency during the first four days of treatment, but were similar to controls by the fifth day (Figure 10-4).

Beyond five days of treatment, the effectiveness of BZPs is less certain. Rebound insomnia occurs even after very limited use of hypnotics and may predispose to drug dependence.[60] Roehrs and colleagues[117] found that significant rebound insomnia occurred in both insomniac subjects and noninsomniac controls after six nightly doses of triazolam, 0.5 mg. The degree of rebound was similar for subjects and controls, but was more severe after abrupt discontinuation. When rebound takes place, the probability that a patient will continue self-administering hypnotics increases with the severity of the initial sleep problem, regardless of whether the subject received active

Table 10-4
Approved Indications for Benzodiazepine Drugs

Compound	Anxiety Disorder	Insomnia	Procedural Sedation	Alcohol Withdrawal	Other
Lorazepam	Yes	No	Yes	No	
Prazepam	Yes	No	No	No	
Chlordiazepoxide	Yes	No	No	Yes	
Oxazepam	Yes	No	No	Yes	
Clorazepate	Yes	No	No	Yes	
Diazepam	Yes	No	Yes	Yes	Muscle spasm
Alprazolam	Yes	No	No	No	Panic disorder
Temazepam	No	Yes	No	No	
Midazolam	No	No	Yes	No	
Flurazepam	No	Yes	No	No	
Quazepam	No	Yes	No	No	
Triazolam	No	Yes	No	No	
Estazolam	No	Yes	No	No	

drug or placebo.[119] This would suggest that *rebound and dependence are of significant concern in insomniac patients treated with BZPs*, although the propensity to self-medicate may be a characteristic of the sleep disorder, as well as of the reinforcing properties of the medication. In addition to these concerns, a reduction in next-day performance and alertness may be experienced after a bedtime dose of a BZP, especially with long-acting agents (see "Adverse Reactions"). Therefore, BZP hypnotics should be used only if the immediate benefits of improved sleep outweigh both the immediate risk of residual daytime effects and the eventual risk of rebound insomnia or drug dependence.

When a patient experiences chronic primary insomnia, short courses of BZPs may be helpful while nonpharmacologic measures are being instituted, although the risk of dependence may be greater than with situational insomnia. Hishikawa[56] reviewed the use of BZP hypnotics for adult insomnia and recommended that hypnotics be added only in severe cases and that treatment not exceed three weeks. The American Psychiatric Association has concluded that there is little evidence supporting the effectiveness of BZP hypnotics past 30 days of treatment.[125]

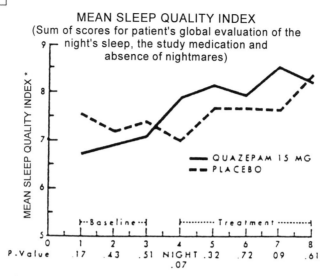

MEAN SLEEP QUALITY INDEX
(Sum of scores for patient's global evaluation of the night's sleep, the study medication and absence of nightmares)

* A higher score indicating better sleep (possible score 3.11)

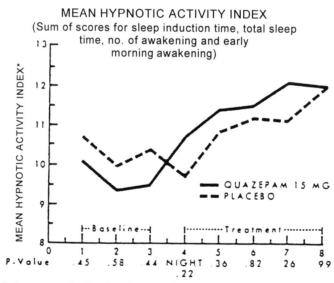

MEAN HYPNOTIC ACTIVITY INDEX
(Sum of scores for sleep induction time, total sleep time, no. of awakening and early morning awakening)

* A higher score indicating better sleep (possible score 4.17)

(Reprinted with permission from Uhthoff, H.K., Brunet, J.A., Aggerwal, A., Varin, R. (1981). A clinical study of quazepam in hospitalized patients with insomnia. *J Int Med Res, 9,* 288-291.)

Figure 10-4
Sleep Response to Quazepam

The above data are exclusively based on experience with adults. Benzodiazepine hypnotics have not been well studied in children. They are, however, widely prescribed despite the apparent clinical consensus that BZPs are inferior to behavioral measures and low-dose antidepressants.[34,106,112] The extant literature does not clearly answer the question of when to use BZP hypnotics, but suggests that they will be most helpful for severe transient insomnia that is related to time-limited stressors. Appropriate situations for children and adolescents might include insomnia following psychosocial or physical trauma, travel to a different time zone, or changing from one work shift to another. Since even single doses may produce rebound insomnia and this effect is worse with abrupt discontinuation, the most appropriate strategy may be to provide two or three therapeutic doses of a short-acting hypnotic followed by tapering the doses over several days. Admittedly, this appears to be the least common prescribing practice. A recent chart review found that 88% of hypnotic prescriptions written by outpatient primary physicians not only failed to diagnose the type of sleep disturbance, but failed to document sleep symptoms at all. Furthermore, 30% of prescriptions were for 180 or more doses.[135] This is clearly unacceptable for children and adolescents, since chronic BZP prescription may encourage dependence, create iatrogenic sleep and anxiety symptoms, and affect school performance.

Case History

A 14-year-old girl hospitalized for an appendectomy was observed to have insomnia and anxiety. The child psychiatry service was called in to evaluate the patient. The patient had no prior psychiatric history. She denied neurovegetative symptoms of depression and was not suicidal. She had no history of anxiety, insomnia, panic attacks, or the like. According to her parents, she had always been a confident, rather calm child. This was, however, her first hospitalization, and she admitted to being scared even though her mother or father was with her throughout the day and night. She had no history of drug or alcohol use or abuse. The family history was negative for anxiety disorders, panic disorder, phobia, and psychiatric disorders such as depression or bipolar disorder. Significantly, there was no history of substance abuse disorders in the family. A trial of relaxation training exercises, including having the patient listen to relaxing tapes and being instructed in breathing techniques to relieve anxiety, was initiated. This was quite effective in reducing the child's anxiety, but not effective in ameliorating her sleep disturbance. In view of the patient's continued insomnia, and since she had no personal or family history of substance-abuse disorders, a short-term trial of triazolam 0.125 mg q.H.S for insomnia was initiated. The patient tolerated this dose well the first night it was prescribed and slept eight hours of uninterrupted sleep. The next two nights, she again requested triazolam 0.125 mg. Each night her insomnia was relieved. By her third and final night in the hospital, she was feeling much happier and looking forward to returning home. The operation had been successful and she was observed to be joking with the nursing staff. She did not request triazolam for insomnia on this night. She subsequently slept soundly for the entire night and was discharged home. Subsequent follow-up revealed that she was doing quite well medically and psychologically. She showed no evidence of anxiety or insomnia and was not requesting medication to calm her nerves or to sleep.

Buspirone

The absence of prominent sedative properties predicts that buspirone would be ineffective for primary insomnia. This was confirmed by Manfredi and colleagues,[79] who tested the hypnotic effectiveness of buspirone in a manner similar to that for BZP hypnotic trials: four nights of placebo—baseline, seven nights of buspirone 10 mg, and five nights of placebo—withdrawal. The six adults with chronic insomnia showed a significant *decrease* in total sleep, which was most prominent during the first three nights. Similarly, a three-week course of buspirone was tested by De Roeck and associates[35] in adult patients with anxiety and insomnia, and also yielded no hypnotic effect.

Antihistamines

Antihistamines have been used for over three decades for mild, rapid sedation. Diphenhydramine is now available without a prescription, so its use as a hypnotic agent undoubtedly exceeds physician prescriptions for that purpose. There are fewer controlled trials of antihistamines than of BZPs, but those that are available support their short-term use for transient primary insomnia.

A 50-mg dose of diphenhydramine produces sedation roughly equivalent to that afforded by 100 mg of pentobarbital.[24,144] In controlled clinical trials, diphenhydramine was found superior to placebo in improving sleep latency, number of arousals, and total sleep time,[67,114,141] while having few effects on the sleep of normal subjects.[20] Interestingly, Meulman and associates[84] found that 50 mg of diphenhydramine was modestly superior to 15 mg of temazepam in improving total sleep time after five days of treatment ($p <$ 0.05). The only placebo-controlled comparison of an antihistamine and a BZP, this trial was conducted on a small sample of elderly nursing home residents and is difficult to generalize to children. Promethazine is also superior to placebo in adult insomniacs.[1] Hydroxyzine has not been subjected to controlled trial, but is probably effective.[130]

Like BZP hypnotics, residual morning effects and a reduction in daytime performance tasks are reported and are discussed below (see "Adverse Effects"). Although tolerance to the sedative effects of diphenhydramine has been described,[67] dependence and rebound insomnia have not.

Conclusions

Psychophysiologic or primary insomnia accounts for an impressive number of hypnotic prescriptions for both adults and children. The majority of these prescriptions are not justified, and an unknown number may produce iatrogenic sleep, anxiety, or drug-dependence problems. However, when transient insomnia is severe and is related to time-limited stressors, both short-acting BZPs and sedating antihistamines effectively improve sleep for at least one week. After that time, tolerance develops to both types of medication. If BZPs are used, the treatment must be short and the medications must be tapered upon discontinuation to minimize rebound insomnia. Because of this additional liability, antihistamines or low-dose, sedating antidepressants are preferable to BZPs for children. However, nonpharmacologic measures should be used instead of hypnotic drugs whenever possible, and should replace hypnotic drugs within the first two weeks of treatment in all cases.

Parasomnias

Parasomnias are defined as abnormal behaviors during sleep, including arousal disorders (sleepwalking, night terrors), sleep–wake transition disorders (sleep talking, leg movements), and REM-associated disorders (nightmares, REM behavior disorder).[48] Two common and one unusual parasomnia have been successfully treated with BZPs, although studies on children are limited. No studies have tested buspirone for parasomnias, and antihistamines have been reported to exacerbate some cases.

Sleepwalking

Sleepwalking, or somnambulism, occurs in up to 15% of children and adolescents, but is rare in adults.[48] The phenomenon is more common among children with a family history of sleepwalking. Several medications have been reported to exacerbate the syndrome, including neuroleptics, BZP and non-BZP hypnotics, and TCAs.[48,72,160] Case studies have reported both success[110] and failure[32] with diazepam, but no BZP has been systematically studied.

Even if the efficacy of hypnotics were supported in clinical trials, pharmacologic treatment is seldom necessary for somnambulism in children. The goal of treatment is to ensure the safety of the child, and this almost always can be achieved by environmental controls, such as locking doors and windows, removing or padding dangerous objects in the child's room, and placing the

bed on the ground floor.[75] Given that any benefit from hypnotics is likely to
be short lived and bears the risks of rebound insomnia, decreased daytime
performance, and possible exacerbation of the syndrome, hypnotics are not
recommended for sleepwalking in children.

Night Terrors

Night terrors, or pavor nocturnus, consist of the sudden onset of intense fear
and autonomic discharge, usually taking place during slow-wave sleep. The
child screams, is confused and inconsolable, and may cause injury by bolting
from his or her bed. The incidence is less than that of somnambulism (3–4%
of preadolescents) and the manifestations are more distressing to both parents and children.[48] Environmental measures, supportive psychotherapy,
and improved sleep habits are usually sufficient treatment, but short-term
hypnotic therapy may be used in severe cases. This use of BZPs has been
somewhat better studied than other sleep disorders in children. Diazepam
was noted to be successful in one early study.[42] More recently, midazolam
was evaluated in a single-blind, placebo-controlled study of 15 children with
nightly sleep terrors. Midazolam, 15 mg at the hour of sleep, eliminated terrors in all but one patient and significantly decreased sleep latency and increased total sleep.[104] However, medication was administered for only two
nights and its longer-term efficacy is unknown. It is likely that tolerance
would occur, and that hypnotic therapy of night terrors should be limited to
short-term, intermittent courses. More studies with longer follow-ups are required before this can be considered a standard treatment.

REM Behavior Disorder

A rare and unusual syndrome that generally appears in adults,[127,128] REM
behavior disorder has also been reported in children.[129] The syndrome is
characterized by the maintenance of muscle tone during REM sleep, causing
elaborate, seemingly purposeful, behavior during sleep. Specific behaviors
may include the acting out of dreams, self-injury, or violence. The majority
of pharmacologic trials are uncontrolled adult case series from a single research center, where the syndrome has been successfully managed with clonazepam.[162] Tricyclic antidepressants and SSUIs may exacerbate or produce
the disorder.[163] There is no consensus regarding treatment of its rare occurrence in children.

Aggression

One of the most common uses of sedatives is also one of the least studied.
Benzodiazepines, antihistamines, and antipsychotics are all commonly used
as "chemical restraints" on an as-needed basis in inpatient psychiatric populations.[150] Although this is a logical application for sedative agents, it has

been poorly tested and is not an approved indication for BZPs or antihistamines. Some antipsychotics are approved for this purpose, and these are reviewed in Chapter 7. Buspirone is not used on a p.r.n. basis, but has been tested for the chronic management of aggression.

Acute Violence

Several open trials have reported success using BZPs for the acute management of aggression in adults,[8,88] while others have reported the exacerbation of hostility.[9,36] There are no controlled studies. Bond and colleagues[16] reported success with midazolam in two mentally retarded and aggressive adolescents (aged 14 and 17 years). The medication was given via IM injection in 5 or 10 mg doses and produced rapid calming within 15 to 20 minutes where other sedative agents (hydroxyzine, amobarbital, and triflupromazine) had failed. Because of the frequency of disinhibitory reactions to BZPs (see "Adverse Reactions"), children are thought to be at higher risk for the exacerbation of agitated states by BZPs.[149] However, BZPs do possess some important advantages over antipsychotics as acute sedatives—the incidence of severe adverse reactions is far lower with BZPs than with antipsychotics, the sedative effects are time-limited with short-acting agents, and the therapeutic index of BZPs is superior. Therefore, for children it is preferable to try BZPs before resorting to sedating antipsychotics for the acute pharmacologic management of aggression. Furthermore, it is conceivable that disinhibitory reactions occur at lower doses than effective sedation, suggesting that a multidose, placebo-controlled trial of p.r.n. BZPs would be valuable.

After decades of use, diphenhydramine was recently tested in a small controlled trial for acute agitation in child psychiatric inpatients. Interestingly, Vitiello and associates[151] found that administering an IM agent to agitated children had a significant calming effect, but that it did not matter whether this agent was diphenhydramine or placebo. These results further support the need for placebo-controlled trials of acute sedative agents, and the prominent placebo effect suggests that only agents with a very low risk of toxicity should be used. Diphenhydramine will probably cause the least harm, although large doses may produce toxicity. The main risk of using BZPs is the possibility of a disinhibitory reaction. Both are preferable to antipsychotics for children (see Chapter 7).

Chronic Aggression

While p.r.n. medication is often necessary for acute management, it would be preferable to prevent aggressive outbursts. Lithium, beta-adrenergic blockers, antipsychotics, and anticonvulsant medications, which are all commonly used for the chronic management of aggression, are reviewed in their respective chapters. The development of tolerance to BZPs suggests that they would not be effective over the long term, but neither BZPs nor antihistamines have been systematically tested in the management of chronic aggression. Recently, Ratey and associates[107,108] published promising data on the use of buspirone for aggression in mentally retarded and schizophrenic adults. An open trial reported that low-dose buspirone (15 mg/day) was effective in reducing aggressive and self-abusive behavior in nine of 14 developmentally disabled adults. Similar effects have been noted in aggressive children with ADHD[105] and autism.[109] Although controlled trials are needed to verify these findings, it is reasonable to try buspirone in aggressive children when lithium and beta-adrenergic agents have failed. The risks and side-effect profile of buspirone are probably superior to those of anticonvulsants and antipsychotics.

Depression

Several trials of triazolo-BZPs (alprazolam and adinazolam) have suggested that these agents possess an independent antidepressant property, presumably through noradrenergic and serotonergic receptor activity.[51,62] However, concerns about tolerance and abuse have limited their acceptance for this application. No studies are available that evaluate their use in childhood depression, and they are not currently recommended for that purpose.

Buspirone performed favorably in one controlled study of major depression, showing a 70% response rate.[113] Its serotonergic activity makes it a good candidate for further research in this area, although it is currently unproven as an antidepressant.

Bipolar Affective Disorder

Clonazepam has emerged as a probable antimanic agent in adult studies of bipolar affective disorder, used either as an adjunct to lithium or as a single agent.[25,81,122,123] However, there is one contrary open trial that was terminated when the first five subjects on clonazepam suffered relapse.[7] Lorazepam has also been used successfully,[73,86] and in one double-blind study it was superior to clonazepam.[21] However, no comparable studies have been performed on children, and their long-term efficacy must be established in this population before BZPs see widespread use for mania.

Contraindications

Benzodiazepines

Benzodiazepines are absolutely contraindicated only for patients with known hypersensitivity. Most agents are also contraindicated in narrow-angle glaucoma. Relative contraindications include patients with a history of disinhibitory reactions, BZP dependence or abuse, abuse of alcohol or other substances, or hepatic dysfunction (for agents that undergo hepatic metabolism); debilitated patients or patients at risk for aspiration; and patients with the autoimmune deficiency syndrome (AIDS) who are receiving zidovudine.[27,97] Due to the muscle-relaxant properties of most BZPs, these drugs also should be avoided for patients with symptomatic sleep apnea. Patients must be cautioned against driving or performing dangerous tasks while taking BZPs, especially early in therapy.

Buspirone

Buspirone is contraindicated for patients with known hypersensitivity to the drug. Because of the risk of hypertension and the so-called central excitatory syndrome, it should not be given concurrently with MAOIs. Buspirone is relatively contraindicated for patients with hepatic or renal dysfunction.[97]

Antihistamines

Antihistamines are contraindicated in a variety of situations, depending on their degree of anticholinergic activity. Narrow-angle glaucoma, GI or urinary obstructions, and mental-status changes that may be due to anticholinergic toxicity are contraindications to diphenhydramine and cyproheptadine. Most antihistamines potentiate other CNS depressants and analgesics, necessitating caution with these agents. Like BZPs, these agents may cause impairment of driving or work performance and patients must be cautioned against using antihistamines in these situations.

Adverse Effects

Benzodiazepines

Sedation
Sedation is the most frequent side effect of BZP use. Patients must be cautioned against undertaking any activity in which drowsiness may place them at risk. Tolerance to sedation develops rapidly with long-term administration. In children and adolescents, drowsiness may affect school performance.

Decreased Psychomotor and Cognitive Performance
Johnson and Chernik[159] provided a comprehensive review of performance testing following a single nighttime dose of BZP hypnotic in both insomniac patients and normal volunteers. They concluded that all BZPs decrease next-day performance on a broad range of cognitive and psychomotor tests, depending on the dose and pharmacokinetics of the specific agent. Psychomotor performance may be persistently suboptimal, even throughout long-

term BZP treatment.[124] In school-age children, cognitive performance is of obvious importance and represents a significant risk of BZP prescription.

Disinhibitory Reactions

A case series by Kraft and associates[65] reported a paradoxical reaction to chlordiazepoxide in 13 of 130 children treated for diverse psychiatric disorders, with most of these reactions in children with neurologic impairment. According to Werry,[154] there is nothing paradoxical about the reaction, since it may be considered the amplification of behaviors normally held in check by social inhibition. Therefore, a more accurate term for this frequent reaction to BZPs is behavioral disinhibition. Beyond the 10% incidence noted by Kraft and colleagues, there are very little data in the psychiatric literature on the incidence or risk factors of disinhibitory reactions to BZPs. However, Van der Bijl and Roelofse[149] have reviewed the substantial surgical literature on the phenomenon. They define behavioral disinhibition as an "abolishment of the restraining influence of the cortex [which] has been associated with talkativeness and excitement, depression, agitated toxic psychosis, increased anxiety, hostility and rage." Anesthesia studies have reported frequencies as high as 23% in children and adolescents undergoing presurgical sedation.[74,120]

Rare Side Effects

Withdrawal seizures occur with unknown frequency, but are more common after the abrupt cessation of BZPs with short elimination half-lives. Hallucinations have been reported in rare instances and recurrent psychosis in response to BZP treatment has been reported in children.[98,99] Mania has been described with alprazolam.[6] Blood dyscrasias, including leukopenia, thrombocytopenia, and agranulocytosis, have been described in adults.[27]

Teratogenicity

There are no prospective studies of in utero exposure to BZPs. Several early studies suggested a relationship between diazepam and birth defects, but these have not been substantiated. A retrospective study of maternal drug history failed to find an increased incidence of birth defects among children born to mothers who received BZPs during the first trimester.[50] Nevertheless, because detailed prospective data are not available, BZPs must be considered potential teratogens and appropriate contraception should be ensured in women of childbearing age.

Buspirone

Buspirone induces less sedation than BZP anxiolytics, but this still remains a possible side effect. Other effects include dizziness, insomnia, GI upset, headache, fatigue, anxiety, and irritability or excitement. Disinhibition has not been described as such, but excitement might be considered a disinhibitory reaction. There is no known effect on the seizure threshold, nor has there been any report of withdrawal seizures. Teratogenicity has not been established, making prevention of pregnancy necessary.

Antihistamines

These medications generally have few serious side effects, although minor side effects can be quite unpleasant. Sedation and dizziness are most common. Anticholinergic side effects (dry mouth, constipation, urinary retention, blurred vision, confusion) are observed, especially with diphenhydramine and cyproheptadine. Rare, but important, side effects include lowered seizure threshold, hypotension and tachycardia, blood dyscrasias, and GI disturbances. Involuntary-movement disorders have been reported at high doses. There is evidence from animal studies that antihistamines may induce fetal abnormalities, and thus although there are no human studies that confirm this, antihistamines should be avoided in pregnancy.[97]

Overdose

Benzodiazepines

The symptoms of BZP toxicity include drowsiness, ataxia, confusion, slurred speech, tremor, and diplopia. Respiratory depression can occur, but is rare. In extreme cases, bradycardia and coma may result. Pfefferbaum and colleagues[98] reported two cases of toxicity in children that were characterized by visual and tactile hallucinations and insomnia.

Buspirone

Buspirone toxicity consists of more severe forms of common side effects, especially gastric distress. Miosis is common. No deaths have been reported from buspirone overdose.

Antihistamine

Antihistamine overdose is associated with sedation and hypotension. Diphenhydramine and cyproheptadine, in particular, may cause anticholinergic toxicity and delirium characterized by flushing, dry mouth, fixed and dilated pupils, and confusion. The manufacturers of these agents report that children are more susceptible to hyperarousal with overdose. One large German study examined the clinical symptoms in 136 suicide attempts by diphenhydramine overdose and found that impaired consciousness, catatonic-like stupor, hallucinations, mydriasis, and tachycardia were the most common symptoms.[64] The anticholinesterase physostigmine may be used as an antidote to anticholinergic toxicity in severe cases.

Abuse/Dependence

Benzodiazepines

A German study estimated that 7% of psychiatric inpatients had abused prescribed medication when not hospitalized, and that 80% of these abused BZPs.[156] Most such abuse took place in a therapeutic situation, with increased incidences among middle-aged women and young men. Alcoholics appear to be at greater risk for BZP abuse,[26] and short-acting BZPs are more likely to be abused than are the long-acting forms.[156]

Little data are available on the abuse potential in children, but a large epidemiologic study from Norway estimated the one-year prevalence of nonprescription BZP use in adolescents to be 10% (ages 13–18).[95] Of those who had used BZPs, 87% of boys and 80% of girls reported taking the drugs for therapeutic reasons. Thirteen percent of boys and 20% of girls reported taking BZPs for intoxication. Equivalent data for the United States are not available.

The American Psychiatric Association has determined that although most BZP abuse is by individuals with a history of opiate, sedative, or alcohol abuse, the prolonged prescription of BZPs increases the risk of dependence in all patients.[125] For these reasons, patients with a history of substance abuse should not be prescribed BZPs, and all prescriptions should be monitored for escalation of dose. Their appropriate use in child and adolescent psychiatric disorders is almost always short-term, as discussed above.

Buspirone

Buspirone was initially marketed as an anxiolytic without significant sedation or abuse potential, based on animal studies. Clinical experience thus far is consistent with that claim. No significant withdrawal syndrome has been described, even after abrupt cessation, and no cases of abuse have been reported.[11]

Antihistamines

Tolerance to the sedative effects of antihistamines has been described, and with tolerance comes the concern about potential dependence and abuse. However, antihistamines have few reinforcing effects and several unpleasant side effects. Diphenhydramine is available without a prescription and is not considered a drug of abuse. There is one study that reported that sedative abusers rated 600 mg of diphenhydramine as pleasurable, but only five of the 10 subjects could tolerate that dose.[155] Therefore, the abuse potential of antihistamines may be considered low.

Drug Interactions

See Table 10-5.

Table 10-5
Drug Interactions with Anxiolytics and Sedatives

Benzodiazepines	Drugs whose activity or blood levels may increase: • alcohol • sedatives (narcotic, analgesic, recreational) • TCAs • phenytoin • zidovudine Drugs that may increase the activity of benzodiazepines: • antimicrobials (erythromycin, isoniazid) • oral contraceptives • cimetidine • alcohol • sedatives • neuroleptics • MAOIs Drugs whose activity may be impaired: • carbamazepine Drugs that may decrease the activity of benzodiazepines: • antacids Drugs that may produce adverse reactions: • MAOIs (central excitatory syndrome)
Buspirone	Drugs whose activity or blood levels may increase: • neuroleptics (theoretical and one report of increased haloperidol levels) Drugs that may produce adverse reactions: • trazodone (one report of hepatic toxicity) • MAOIs (theoretical risk of central excitatory syndrome) • neuroleptics (theoretical risk of increased effects of dopamine antagonism)
Antihistamines	Drugs whose activity or blood levels may increase: • alcohol • sedatives (narcotic, analgesic, recreational) Drugs that may produce adverse reactions: • potentiation of anticholinergic side effects and possible toxicity with any anticholinergic agent)

Available Preparations and Cost

See Tables 10-1 and 10-2.

Initiating and Maintaining Treatment

Benzodiazepines

Since the efficacy of BZPs in children and adolescents has not been established, neither have precise clinical guidelines for their use. No specific premedication laboratory evaluation is recommended. As with most medications, preadolescent children generally require more frequent doses than adolescents or adults because of their higher rates of hepatic metabolism. Coffey[27] has published dosing guidelines for benzodiazepines based on clinical experience, and the recommendations in Table 10-6 are based on these guidelines, as well as on the studies cited above. The 0.25-mg tablet of alprazolam is scored, allowing for a starting dose for preadolescent children of 0.125 mg b.i.d. for panic disorder. For sleep induction, a reasonable dose of short-acting hypnotics is one half the adult starting dose for preadolescent children and the lower limit of the adult dose for adolescents. Long-term efficacy has not been demonstrated in children for either indication, so the course of treatment should be short—less than 30 days for panic disorder and less than two weeks for insomnia.

Buspirone

Buspirone is likewise without guidelines for children and is not approved for use under the age of 18. Coffey[27] suggests titrating up to 20 mg/day in divided doses for adolescents and 5–10 mg/day in divided doses for preadolescents for the treatment of overanxious disorder. The 5-mg tablet may be cut to allow for increments of 2.5 mg. Ratey and colleagues[107,108] have suggested that the optimal daily dose of buspirone for the treatment of aggression may be lower than for anxiety. They found 15 mg/day to be optimal in aggressive adults, with some loss of effect on higher doses, as compared with 30–60 mg/day commonly reported for adult anxiety disorders. Therefore, the optimal dose for the treatment of chronic aggression in children may also be low.

Antihistamines

There is little or no evidence supporting the use of antihistamines in the treatment of anxiety disorders. The two most appropriate indications are insomnia and situational or anticipatory anxiety. These situations require single doses or very brief courses of treatment, the dosing guidelines for which appear in Table 10-6.

Table 10-6
Suggested Agents and Dosing Guidelines for the Use of Anxiolytic Agents in Children and Adolescents

Indication	Suggested Agents	Starting Doses		Maximum Daily Dose	
		Preadolescent	Adolescent	Preadolescent	Adolescent
Panic disorder	Alprazolam	0.125 mg b.i.d. or t.i.d.	0.25 mg b.i.d. or t.i.d.	1–4 mg	8–10 mg
	Clonazepam	0.25 mg q.d.	0.5 mg q.d.	0.1–0.2 mg/kg*	0.1–0.2 mg/kg*
Anticipatory anxiety	Alprazolam	0.125–0.25 mg	0.25–0.5 mg	NA	NA
	Diphenhydramine	25–50 mg	50–100 mg	5 mg/kg	5 mg/kg
	Hydroxyzine	0.6 mg/kg	0.6 mg/kg	NA	NA
Overanxious disorder	Buspirone	2.5 mg b.i.d.	5 mg b.i.d.	20 mg/day	60 mg/day
Insomnia	Diphenhydramine	25–50 mg	50–100 mg	5 mg/kg	5 mg/kg
	Any short-acting BZP hypnotic	50% of adult starting dose	Lower limit of adult dose	50% of adult maximum	Adult maximum

*Dose is the maximum recommended for seizure disorders; maximum for psychiatric indications is not established.

341

Management of Specific Side Effects

Benzodiazepines

Behavioral Disinhibition and Overdose

There is no specific treatment strategy for BZP-induced behavioral disinhibition. Supportive and behavioral management may be sufficient while the symptoms abate. In an emergency setting, a drug history and laboratory screen should be performed to rule out concurrent alcohol or other substance use's adding to the syndrome.[27] Physostigmine has been used by anesthesiologists to treat BZP-induced delirium, as has the BZP antagonist flumazenil. However, these are by no means established treatments and should not be used to treat behavioral disinhibition.[149] In massive overdose or when other CNS depressants are present in the system, respiratory and cardiac support may be required.

Sedation and Decreased Cognitive Performance

These effects of BZPs are of great importance in children and adolescents and require careful and ongoing assessment. Tolerance may develop to sedation, but not to cognitive and psychomotor deficits. Since there is no specific treatment, minimizing the doses and length of treatment is necessary. Families should be intimately involved in weighing the benefits of the medication against the risk of academic or social delay. If used for sleep, the effect on next-day performance may be minimized by using short-acting agents.

Buspirone

The side effects of buspirone are seldom serious, but if intolerable, may require a reduction in dose or cessation of treatment. Dizziness, GI upset, and headaches are common reasons for discontinuing treatment. Gastrointestinal symptoms may be relieved by giving doses with meals. Headaches, if infrequent, may be managed with acetaminophen.

Antihistamines

If anticholinergic side effects predominate, consideration may be given to an alternative agent with fewer anticholinergic properties. Since these medications are appropriate only for very short-term uses, side effects are generally tolerable, if potentially unpleasant. Apart from reducing the dose or discontinuing treatment, there is no specific therapy for antihistamine side effects.

How to Withdraw Medication

Benzodiazepines

Several strategies for the withdrawal of BZP treatment have been advocated. Single-dose or intermittent single-dose prescription may require no special withdrawal program, but patients should be monitored closely for rebound insomnia even in these cases. With longer treatment, withdrawal symptoms include insomnia, anxiety, tremulousness, diaphoresis, irritability, muscle cramps, tinnitus, and nausea. Therefore, moderate- or long-term BZP use necessitates a gradual tapering of dosage. If treatment has been chronic, this tapering schedule may take weeks or months.[27] Since the risk of severe withdrawal is greatest with short-acting agents, it may be useful to switch to a long-acting agent such as diazepam or clonazepam at equivalent potency before tapering the drug.[23] One recent double-blind, placebo-controlled study of carbamazepine administered during a gradual tapering of long-term BZP yielded a higher success rate and milder withdrawal symptoms among adult patients who had a history of dependence.[132]

Buspirone and Antihistamines

No withdrawal syndromes have been described for these agents and, therefore, discontinuation does not usually require a tapering schedule. However, it may be prudent to discontinue buspirone gradually, since experience with this drug in children is still limited.

References

1. Adam, K., Oswald, I. (1986). The hypnotic effects of an antihistamine: Promethazine. *Br J Clin Pharmacol, 22(6)*, 715–717.

2. Aden, G.C., Thein, S.G. Jr. (1980). Alprazolam compared to diazepam and placebo in the treatment of anxiety. *J Clin Psychiatry, 41(7)*, 245–248.

3. Alessi, N., Bos, T. (1991). Buspirone augmentation of fluoxetine in a depressed child with obsessive-compulsive disorder. *Am J Psychiatry, 148(11)*, 1605–1606.

4. Aman, M.G., Werry, J.S. (1982). Methylphenidate and diazepam in severe reading retardation. *J Am Acad Child Psychiatry, 21*, 31–37.

5. Andersch, S., Rosenberg, N.K., Kullingsjo, H., et al. (1991). Efficacy and safety of alprazolam, imipramine and placebo in treating panic disorder: A Scandinavian multicenter study. *Acta Psychiatr Scand, 365(Suppl)*, 18–27.

6. Arana, G.W., Pearlman, C., Shader, R.I. (1985). Alprazolam-induced mania: Two clinical cases. *Am J Psychiatry, 142(3)*, 368–369.

7. Aronson, T.A., Shukla, S., Hirschowitz, J. (1989). Clonazepam treatment of five lithium-refractory patients with bipolar disorder. *Am J Psychiatry, 146(1)*, 77–80.

8. Azcarate, C. (1975). Minor tranquilizers in the treatment of aggression. *J Nerv Ment Dis, 160*, 100–107.

9. Bach-y-Rita, G., Lion, J.R., Climent, C.E., et al. (1971). Episodic dyscontrol: A study of 130 violent patients. *Am J Psychiatry, 127*, 1472–1478.

10. Ballenger, J.C., Carek, D.J., Steele, J.J., Cornish-McTighe, D. (1989). Three cases of panic disorder with agoraphobia in children. *Am J Psychiatry, 146(7)*, 922–924.

11. Balster, R.L. (1990). Abuse potential of buspirone and related drugs. *J Clin Psychopharmacol, 10*, 31S–37S.

12. Barbee, J.G., Black, F.W., Todorov, A.A. (1992). Differential effects of alprazolam and buspirone upon acquisition, retention, and retrieval processes in memory. *J Neuropsychiatry Clin Neurosci, 4(3)*, 308–314.

13. Bernstein, G.A., Garfinkel, B.D., Borchardt, C.M. (1990). Comparative studies of pharmacotherapy for school refusal. *J Am Acad Child Adolesc Psychiatry, 29*, 773–781.

14. Bernstein, G.A., Borchardt, C.M. (1991). Anxiety disorders of childhood and adolescence: A critical review. *J Am Acad Child Adolesc Psychiatry, 30(4)*, 519–532.

15. Biederman, J. (1987). Clonazepam in the treatment of prepubertal children with panic-like symptoms. *J Clin Psychiatry, 48(10, Suppl)*, 38–42.

16. Bond, W.S., Mandos, L.A., Kurtz, M.B. (1989). Midazolam for aggressivity and violence in three mentally retarded patients. *Am J Psychiatry, 146(7)*, 925–926.

17. Bonnet, M.H., Kramer, M., Roth, T. (1981). A dose response study of the hypnotic effectiveness of alprazolam and diazepam in normal subjects. *Psychopharmacology, 75(3)*, 258–261.

18. Bonnet, M.H., Dexter, J.R., Gillin, J.C., et al. (1988). The use of triazolam in phase-advanced sleep. *Neuropsychopharmacology, 1*, 225–234.

19. Bootzin, R.R., Perlis, M.L. (1992). Nonpharmacologic treatments of insomnia. *J Clin Psychiatry, 53(6 Suppl)*, 37–41.

20. Borbely, A.A., Youmbi-Balderer, G. (1988). Effect of diphenhydramine on subjective sleep parameters and on motor activity during bedtime. *Int J Clin Pharmacol Ther Toxicol, 26(8)*, 392–396.

21. Bradwejn, J., Shriqui, C., Koszycki, D., Meterissian, G. (1990). Double-blind comparison of the effects of clonazepam and lorazepam in acute mania. *J Clin Psychopharmacology, 10(6)*, 403–408.

22. Braun, P., Greenberg, D., Dasberg, H., Lerer, B. (1990). Core symptoms of posttraumatic stress disorder unimproved by alprazolam treatment. *J Clin Psychiatry, 51*, 236–238.

23. Busto, U., Sellers, E.M., Naranjo, C.A., et al. (1986). Withdrawal reaction after long-term therapeutic use of benzodiazepines. *N Engl J Med, 315(14)*, 854–859.

24. Carruthers, S.G., Shoeman, D.W., Hignite, C.E., Azarnoff, D.L. (1978). Correlation between plasma diphenhydramine level and sedative and antihistamine effects. *Clin Pharmacol Ther, 23(4)*, 375–382.

25. Chouinard, G. (1988). The use of benzodiazepines in the treatment of manic-depressive illness. *J Clin Psychiatry, 49(Suppl)*, 15–20.

26. Ciraulo, D.A., Sands, B.F., Shader, R.I. (1988). Critical review of liability for benzodiazepine abuse among alcoholics. *Am J Psychiatry, 145(12)*, 1501–1506.

27. Coffey, B. (1990). Anxiolytics for children and adolescents: Traditional and new drugs. *J Child Adolesc Psychopharmacol, 1(1)*, 57–83.

28. Coffey, B., Shader, R.I., Greenblatt, D.J. (1983). Pharmacokinetics of benzodiazepines and psychostimulants in children. *J Clin Psychopharmacol, 3(4)*, 217–225.

29. Cohn, J.B. (1981). Multicenter double-blind efficacy and safety study comparing alprazolam, diazepam and placebo in clinically anxious patients. *J Clin Psychiatry, 42(9)*, 347–351.

30. Cohn, J.B., Wilcox, C.S. (1986). Low-sedation potential of buspirone compared with alprazolam and lorazepam in the treatment of anxious patients: A double-blind study. *J Clin Psychiatry, 47*, 409–412.

31. Coleman, R.M., Roffwarg, H.P., Kennedy, S.J., et al. (1982). Sleep-wake disorders based on a polysomnographic diagnosis: A national cooperative study. *JAMA, 247*, 997–1003.

32. Cooper, A.J. (1987). Treatment of coexistant night-terrors and somnambulism in adults with imipramine and diazepam. *J Clin Psychiatry, 48(5)*, 209–210.

33. D'Amato, G. (1962). Chlordiazepoxide in management of school phobia. *Dis Nerv Sys, 23*, 292–295.

34. Dahl, R.E. (1992). The pharamacologic treatment of sleep disorders. *Pediatr Psychopharmacol, 15(1)*, 161–178.

35. De Roeck, J., Cluydts, R., Schotte, C., et al. (1989). Explorative single-blind study on the sedative and hypnotic effects of buspirone in anxiety patients. *Acta Psychiatr Scand, 79(2)*, 129–135.

36. DiMascio, A., Shader, R.I., Harmatz, J. (1969). Psychotropic drugs and induced hostility. *Psychosomatics, 10*, 27–28.

37. DiStefano, P., Case, K.R., Colello, G.D., Bosmann, H.B. (1979). Increased specific binding of [3H]diazepam in rat brain following chronic diazepam administration. *Cell Biol Int Rep, 3(2)*, 163–167.

38. Durand, V.M., Mindell, J.A. (1990). Behavioral treatment of multiple childhood sleep disorders. Effects on child and family. *Behav Modif, 14*, 37–49.

39. Eison, A.S. (1990). Azapirones: History of development. *J Clin Psychopharmacol, 10*, 2S–5S.

40. Feighner, J., Merideth, C., Hendrickson, G. (1982). A double blind comparison of buspirone and diazepam in outpatients with generalized anxiety disorder. *J Clin Psychiatry, 43*, 103–107.

41. Feldman, T.B. (1987). Alprazolam in the treatment of posttraumatic stress disorder. *J Clin Psychiatry, 48*, 216–217.

42. Fisher, C., Kahn, E., Edwards, A., Davis, D.M. (1973). A psychological study of nightmares and night terrors: The suppression of stage 4 night terrors with diazepam. *Arch Gen Psychiatry, 28*, 252–259.

43. France, K.G., Hudson, S.M. (1990). Behavior management of infant sleep disturbance. *J Appl Behav Anal, 23*, 91–98.

44. Gammons, R.E., Mayol, R.F., LaBudde, J.A. (1986). Metabolism and disposition of buspirone. *Am J Med, 80*, 41–51.

45. Gastfriend, D.R., Rosenbaum, J.F. (1989). Adjunctive buspirone in benzodiazepine treatment of four patients with panic disorder. *Am J Psychiatry, 146(7)*, 914–916.

46. Gillin, J.C. (1992). Relief from situational insomnia: Pharmacologic and other options. *Postgrad Med, 92(2)*, 157–170.

47. Gleser, C.G., Gottschalk, L.A., Fox, R., Lippert, W. (1965). Immediate changes in affect with chlordiazepoxide. *Arch Gen Psychiatry, 13*, 291–295.

48. Golbin, A.Z., Sheldon, S.H. (1992). Parasomnias. In S.H. Sheldon, J.P. Spire, H.B. Levy (Eds.) *Pediatric Sleep Medicine* (pp. 119–135). Philadelphia: W.B. Saunders.

49. Green, B.L., Korol, M., Grace, M.C., et al. (1991). Children and disaster: Age, gender, and parental effects on PTSD symptoms. *J Am Acad Child Adolesc Psychiatry, 30(6)*, 945–951.

50. Greenberg, G., Inman, W.H.W., Weatherall, J.A.C., et al. (1977). Maternal drug histories and congenital abnormalities. *Br Med J, 2*, 853–856.

51. Greenblatt, D.J. (1991). Benzodiazepine hypnotics: The interface of basic and clinical science. *J Clin Psychiatry, 52(9, Suppl)*, 3.

52. Greenblatt, D.J. (1991). Benzodiazepine hypnotics: Sorting the pharmacokinetic facts. *J Clin Psychiatry, 52(9, Suppl)*, 4–10.

53. Griest, J.H. (1990). Treatment of obsessive compulsive disorder: Psychotherapies, drugs, and other somatic treatment. *J Clin Psychiatry, 51(8, Suppl)*, 44–50.

54. Haefely, W. (1988). Endogenous ligands of the benzodiazepine receptor. *Pharmacopsychiatry, 21(1)*, 43–46.

55. Hewlett, W.A., Vinogradov, S., Agras, W.S. (1990). Clonazepam treatment of obsessions and compulsions. *J Clin Psychiatry, 51*, 158–161.

56. Hishikawa, Y. (1991). Appropriate use of benzodiazepines in insomnia: Clinical update. *J Clin Psychiatry, 52(7, Suppl)*, 10–13.

57. Imlah, N.W. (146). An evaluation of alprazolam in the treatment of reactive or neurotic (secondary) depression. *Br J Psychiatry, 146*, 515–519.

58. Jann, M.W. (1988). Buspirone: An update on a unique anxiolytic agent. *Pharmacotherapy, 8(2)*, 100–116.

59. Jenike, M.A., Baer, L. (1988). An open trial of buspirone in obsessive-compulsive disorder. *Am J Psychiatry, 145*, 1285–1286.

60. Kales, A., Manfredi, R.L., Vgontzas, A.N., et al. (1991). Rebound insomnia after only brief and intermittent use of rapidly eliminated benzodiazepines. *Clin Pharmacol Ther, 49(4)*, 468–476.

61. Kaplan, H.I., Sadock, B.J. (1991). *Synopsis of Psychiatry* (pp. 382, 619–626). Baltimore: Williams & Wilkins.

62. Kennedy, S.H., de Groot, J., Ralevski, E., Reed, K. (1991). A comparison of adinazolam and desipramine in the treatment of major depression. *Int Clin Psychopharmacol, 6(2)*, 65–76.

63. King, N.J., Gullone, E., Tonge, B.J., Ollendick, T.H. (1993). Self-reports of panic attacks and manifest anxiety in adolescents. *Behav Res Ther, 31(1)*, 111–116.

64. Koppel, C., Ibe, K., Tenczer, J. (1987). Clinical symptomatology of diphen-hydramine overdose: An evaluation of 136 cases in 1982 to 1985. *J Tox-icol—Clin Toxicol, 25(1-2)*, 53–70.

65. Kraft, I.A., Ardali, C., Duffy, J.H., et al. (1965). A clinical study of chlor-diazepoxide used in psychiatric disorders of children. *Int J Neuropsychiatry, 1*, 433–437.

66. Kranzler, H. (1988). Use of buspirone in an adolescent with overanxious disorder. *J Am Acad Child Adolesc Psychiatry, 27*, 789–790.

67. Kudo, Y., Kurihara, M. (1990). Clinical evaluation of diphenhydramine hydrochloride for the treatment of insomnia in psychiatric patients: A dou-ble-blind study. *J Clin Pharmacol, 30(11)*, 1041–1048.

68. Kutcher, S., MacKenzie, S. (1988). Successful clonazepam treatment of adolescents with panic disorder. *J Clin Psychopharmacol, 8*, 299–301.

69. Lader, M. (1983). *Introduction to Psychopharmacology* (pp. 96–101). Kala-mazoo, Mich.: Upjohn.

70. Lader, M. (1991). Can buspirone induce rebound, dependence or abuse? *Br J Psychiatry, 12(Suppl.)*, 45–51.

71. Last, C.G., Perrin, S., Hersen, M., Kazdin, A.E. (1992). DSM-III-R anxi-ety disorders in children: Sociodemographic and clinical characteristics. *J Am Acad Child Adolesc Psychiatry, 31(6)*, 1070–1076.

72. Lauerma, H. (1991). Nocturnal wandering caused by restless legs and short-acting benzodiazepines. *Acta Psychiatr Scand, 83(6)*, 492–493.

73. Lenox, R.H., Newhouse, P.A., Creelman, W.L., Whitaker, T.M. (1992). Ad-junctive treatment of manic agitation with lorazepam versus haloperidol: A double-blind study. *J Clin Psychiatry, 53(2)*, 47–52.

74. Litchfield, B.N. (1980). Complications of intravenous dizepam—adverse psychological reactions (an assessment of 16,000 cases). *Anesth Prog, 27*, 175.

75. Linscheid, T.R., Rasnake, L.K. (1990). Sleep disorders in children and ad-olescents. In B.D. Garfinkel, G.A. Carlson, E.B. Weller Eds., *Psychiatric Dis-orders in Children and Adolescents* (pp. 359–371). Philadelphia: W.B. Saunders.

76. Lippa, A.S., Critchett, D., Sano, M.C., et al. (1979). Benzodiazepine recep-tors: Cellular and behavioral characteristics. *Pharmacol Biochem Behav, 10*, 831–843.

77. Lucas, A.R., Pasley, F.C. (1969). Psychoactive drugs in the treatment of

emotionally disturbed children: Haloperidol and diazepam. *Comp Psychiatry, 10*, 376–386.

78. Maletzky, B.M. (1980). Anxiolytic efficacy of alprazolam compared to diazepam and placebo. *J Int Med Res, 8(2)*, 139–143.

79. Manfredi, R.L., Kales, A., Vgontzas, A.N., et al. (1991). Buspirone: Sedative or stimulant effect? *Am J Psychiatry, 148(9)*, 1213–1217.

80. Markovitz, P.J., Stagno, S.J., Calabrese, J.R. (1990). Buspirone augmentation of fluoxetine in obsessive-compulsive disorder. *Am J Psychiatry, 147*, 798–800.

81. Mauri, M.C., Percudani, M., Regazzetti, M.G., Altamura, A.C. (1990). Alternative prophylactic treatments to lithium in bipolar disorders. *Clin Neuropharmacol, 13(Suppl 1)*, S90–S96.

82. McLeer, S.V., Deblinger, E., Atkins, M.S., et al. (1988). Post-traumatic stress disorder in sexually abused children. *J Am Acad Child Adolesc Psychiatry, 27*, 650–654.

83. Mellinger, G.D., Balter, M.B., Uhlenhuth, E.H. (1985). Insomnia and its treatment. *Arch Gen Psychiatry, 42*, 225–232.

84. Meulman, J.R., Nelson, R.C., Clark, R.L., Jr. (1987). Evaluation of temazepam and diphenhydramine as hypnotics in a nursing-home population. *Drug Intell Clin Pharmacy, 21(9)*, 716–720.

85. Miller, L.G. (1991). Chronic benzodiazepine administration: From the patient to the gene. *J Clin Pharmacol, 31(6)*, 492–495.

86. Modell, J.G., Lenox, R.H., Weiner, S. (1985). Inpatient clinical trial of lorazepam for the management of manic agitation. *J Clin Psychopharmacol, 5(2)*, 109–113.

87. Mohler, H., Okada, T. (1977). Benzodiazepine receptor: Demonstration in the central nervous system. *Science, 198*, 849–851.

88. Monroe, R.R. (1975). Anticonvulsants in the treatment of aggression. *J Nerv Ment Dis, 160*, 119–126.

89. Moreau, D., Weissman, M.M. (1992). Panic disorder in children and adolescents: A review. *Am J Psychiatry, 149(10)*, 1306–1314.

90. Morselli, P., Principi, N., Tognoni, G., et al. (1973). Diazepam elimination in premature and full-term infants and children. *J Perinat Med, 1*, 6–14.

91. Nagy, L.M., Krystal, J.H., Woods, S.W., et al. (1989). Clinical and medication outcome after short-term alprazolam and behavioral group treatment in

panic disorder: 2. 5 year naturalistic follow-up study. *Arch Gen Psychiatry, 46*, 993–999.

92. Newton, R., Casten, G., Alms, D., et al. (1982). The side effect profile of buspirone in comparison to active controls and placebo. *J Clin Psychiatry, 43*, 100–102.

93. Pato, M.T., Pigott, T.A., Hill, J.L., et al. (1991). Controlled comparison of buspirone and clomipramine in obsessive-compulsive disorder. *Am J Psychiatry, 148(1)*, 127–129.

94. Payne, K., Mattheyse, F.J., Liebenberg, D., Dawes, T. (1989). The pharmacokinetics of midazolam in paediatric patients. *Eur J Clin Pharmacol, 37(3)*, 267–272.

95. Pedersen, W., Lavik, N.J. (1991). Adolescents and benzodiazepines: Prescribed use, self-medication and intoxication. *Acta Psychiatr Scand, 84(1)*, 94–98.

96. Petti, T.A., Fish, B., Shapiro, T., et al. (1982). Effects of chlordiazepoxide in disturbed children: A pilot study. *J Clin Psychopharmacol, 2(4)*, 270–273.

97. *Physician's Desk Reference (47th ed.)*. (1993). Oradell, N.J.: Medical Economics.

98. Pfefferbaum, B., Butler, P.M., Mullins, D., Copeland, D.R. (1987). Two cases of benzodiazepine toxicity in children. *J Clin Psychiatry, 48(11)*, 450–452.

99. Pfefferbaum, B., Overall, J.E., Boren, H.A., et al. (1987). Alprazolam in the treatment of anticipatory and acute situational anxiety in children with cancer. *J Amer Acad Child Adolesc Psychiat, 26(4)*, 532–535.

100. Pigott, T.A., L'Heureux, F., Hill, J.L., et al. (1992). A double-blind study of adjuvant buspirone hydrochloride in clomipramine-treated patients with obsessive-compulsive disorder. *J Clin Psychopharmacol, 12(1)*, 11–18.

101. Pishkin, V., Shurley, J.T., Wolfgang, A. (1967). Stress: Psychophysiological and cognitive indices in an acute double-blind study with hydroxyzine in psychiatric patients. *Arch Gen Psychiatry, 16*, 471–478.

102. Pohl, R., Balon, R., Yeragani, V.K., Gershon, S. (1989). Serotonergic anxiolytics in the treatment of panic disorder: A controlled study with buspirone. *Psychopathology, 22 (Suppl 1)*, 60–67.

103. Pollack, M.H., Tesar, G.E., Rosenbaum, J.F., et al. (1986). Clonazepam in the treatment of panic disorder and agoraphobia: A one-year follow-up. *J Clin Psychopharmacol, 6*, 302–304.

104. Popoviciu, L., Corfariu, O. (1983). Efficacy and safety of midazolam in the treatment of night terrors in children. *Br J Clin Pharmacol, 16 (Suppl 1)*, 97S–102S.

105. Quaison, N., Ward, D., Kitchen, T. (1991). Buspirone for aggression. *J Am Acad Child Adolesc Psychiatry, 30(6)*, 1026.

106. Quinn, D.M.P. (1986). Prevalence of psychoactive medication in childhood. *Can J Psychiatry, 31*, 575–580.

107. Ratey, J.J., Sovner, R., Mikkelsen, E., Chmielinski, H.E. (1989). Buspirone therapy for maladaptive behavior and anxiety in developmentally disabled persons. *J Clin Psychiatry, 50(10)*, 382–384.

108. Ratey, J., Sovner, R., Parks, A., Rogentine, K. (1991). Buspirone treatment of aggression and anxiety in mentally retarded patients: A multiple-baseline, placebo lead-in study. *J Clin Psychiatry, 52(4)*, 159–162.

109. Realmuto, G.M., August, G.J., Garfinkel, B.D. (1989). Clinical effect of buspirone in autistic children. *J Clin Psychopharmacol, 9(2)*, 122–125.

110. Reid, W.H., Haffke, E.A., Chu, C.C. (1984). Diazepam in intractable sleepwalking: A pilot study. *Hillside J Clin Psychiatry, 6(1)*, 49–55.

111. Rey, E., Delaunay, L., Pons, G., et al. (1991). Pharmacokinetics of midazolam in children: Comparative study of intranasal and intravenous administration. *Eur J Clin Pharmacol, 41(4)*, 355–357.

112. Richman, N. (1986). Recent progress in understanding and treating sleep disorders. *Adv Devel Behav Pediatr, 7*, 45–63.

113. Rickels, K., Amsterdam, J.D., Clary, C., et al. (1991). Buspirone in major depression: A controlled study. *J Clin Psychiatry, 52(1)*, 34–38.

114. Rickels, K., Morris, R.J., Newman, H., et al. (1983). Diphenhydramine in insomniac family practice patients: A double-blind study. *J Clin Pharmacol, 23(4–6)*, 234–242.

115. Rickels, K., Gingrich, R.L., Jr., Morris, R.J., et al. (1975). Triazolam in insomniac family practice patients. *Clin Pharmacol Ther, 18(3)*, 315–324.

116. Risse, S.C., Whitters, A., Burke, J., et al. (1990). Severe withdrawal symptoms after discontinuation of alprazolam in eight patients with combat-induced posttraumatic stress disorder. *J Clin Psychiatry, 51(5)*, 206–209.

117. Roehrs, T., Merlotti, L., Zorick, F., Roth, T. (1992). Rebound insomnia in normals and patients with insomnia after abrupt and tapered discontinuation. *Psychopharmacology, 108(1–2)*, 67–71.

118. Roehrs, T., Vogel, G., Sterling, W., et al. (1990). Dose effects of temazepam in transient insomnia. *Arzneimittelforschung, 40*, 859–862.

119. Roehrs, T., Merlotti, L., Zorick, F., Roth, T. (1992). Rebound insomnia and hypnotic self administration. *Psychopharmacology, 107(4)*, 480–484.

120. Roelofse, J.A., van der Bijl, P., Stegmann, D.H., et al. (1990). Preanesthetic medication with rectal midazolam in children undergoing dental extractions. *J Oral Maxillofac Surg, 48*, 791.

121. Roth, T., Kramer, M., Schwartz, J.L. (1974). Triazolam: A sleep laboratory study of a new benzodiazepine hypnotic. *Curr Ther Res Clin Exper, 16(2)*, 117–123.

122. Sachs, G.S. (1990). Use of clonazepam for bipolar affective disorder. *J Clin Psychiatry, 51(5, Suppl)*, 31–34.

123. Sachs, G.S., Rosenbaum, J.F., Jones, L. (1990). Adjunctive clonazepam for maintenance treatment of bipolar affective disorder. *J Clin Psychopharmacol, 10*, 42–47.

124. Sakol, M.S., Power, K.G. (1988). The effects of long-term benzodiazepine treatment and graded withdrawal on psychometric performance. *Psychopharmacology, 95(1)*, 135–138.

125. Salzman, C. (1991). The APA task force report on benzodiazepine dependence, toxicity, and abuse. *Am J Psychiatry, 148(2)*, 151–152.

126. Schatzberg, A.F. (1991). Overview of anxiety disorders: Prevalence, biology, course, and treatment. *J Clin Psychiatry, 52(7, Suppl)*, 5–9.

127. Schenck, C.H., Bundlie, S.R., Patterson, A.L., Mahowald, M.W. (1987). Rapid eye movement sleep behavior disorder. A treatable parasomnia affecting older adults. *JAMA, 257(13)*, 1786–1789.

128. Schenck, C., et al. (1986a). Chronic behavioral disorders of human REM sleep: A new category of parasomnia. *Sleep, 9*, 293.

129. Schenck, C.H., et al. (1986b). REM behavior disorder in a 10-year old girl and aperiodic TEM and NREM sleep movements in an 8-year old brother. *Sleep Res, 15*, 162.

130. Schubert, D.S. (1984). Hydroxyzine for acute treatment of agitation and insomnia in organic mental disorder. *Psychiatr J Univ Ottawa, 9(2)*, 59–60.

131. Schwartz, H.I., Blank, K. (1991). Regulation of benzodiazepine prescribing practices: Clinical implications. *Gen Hosp Psychiatry, 13(4)*, 219–224.

132. Schweizer, E., Rickels, K., Case, W.G., Greenblatt, D.J. (1991). Carbamazepine treatment in patients discontinuing long-term benzodiazepine ther-

apy. Effects on withdrawal severity and outcome. *Arch Gen Psychiatry, 48(5)*, 448–452.

133. Shalev, A.Y., Rogel-Fuchs, Y. (1992). Auditory startle reflex in post-traumatic stress disorder patients treated with clonazepam. *Isr J Psychiatry Related Sci, 29(1)*, 1–6.

134. Sheehan, D.V., Raj, A.B., Sheehan, K.H., Soto, S. (1990). Is buspirone effective for panic disorder? *J Clin Psychopharmacol, 10(1)*, 3–11.

135. Shorr, R.I., Bauwens, S.F. (1992). Diagnosis and treatment of outpatient insomnia by psychiatric and nonpsychiatric physicians. *Am J Med, 93(1)*, 78–82.

136. Simeon, G., Ferguson, H.B. (1987). Alprazolam effects in children with anxiety disorders. *Can J Psychiatry, 32*, 570–574.

137. Simons, F.E., Simons, K.J., Becker, A.B., Haydey, R.P. (1984). Pharmacokinetics and antipruritic effects of hydroxyzine in children with atopic dermatitis. *J Pediatrics, 104(1)*, 123–127.

138. Simons, K.J., Watson, W.T., Chen, X.Y., Simons, F.E. (1989). Pharmacokinetic and pharmacodynamic studies of the H1-receptor antagonist hydroxyzine in the elderly. *Clin Pharmacol Ther, 45(1)*, 9–14.

139. Simons, K.J., Watson, W.T., Martin, T.J., et al. (1990). Diphenhydramine: Pharmacokinetics and pharmacodynamics in elderly adults, young adults, and children. *J Clin Pharmacol, 30(7)*, 665–671.

140. Spier, S.A., Tesar, G.E., Rosenbaum, J.F., Woods, S.W. (1986). Treatment of panic disorder and agoraphobia with clonazepam. *J Clin Psychiatry, 47(5)*, 238–242.

141. Sunshine, A., Zighelboim, I., Laska, E. (1978). Hypnotic activity of diphenhydramine, methapyrilene, and placebo. *J Clin Pharmacol, 18(8–9)*, 425–431.

142. Tallman, J.F., Gallager, D.W. (1979). Modulation of benzodiazepine binding site sensitivity. *Pharmacol Biochem Behav, 10*, 809–813.

143. Terr, L.C. (1983). Chowchilla revisited: The effects of psychic trauma four years after a school-bus kidnapping. *Am J Psychiatry, 140*, 1543–1550.

144. Teutsch, G., Mahler, D.L., Brown, C.R., et al. (1975). Hypnotic efficacy of diphenhydramine, methapyrilene, and pentobarbital. *Clin Pharmacol Ther, 17(2)*, 195–201.

145. Tietz, E.I., Roth, T., Zorick, F.J., et al. (1981). The acute effect of quazepam on the sleep of chronic insomniacs. A dose-response study. *Arzneimittel-Forschung, 31(11)*, 1963–1966.

146. Tunnicliff, G. (1991). Molecular basis of buspirone's anxiolytic action. *Pharmacol Toxicol, 69(3)*, 149–156.

147. Uhthoff, H.K., Brunet, J.A., Aggerwal, A., Varin, R. (1981). A clinical study of quazepam in hospitalized patients with insomnia. *J Int Med Res, 9(4)*, 288–291.

148. Van Laar, M.W., Volkerts, E.R., van Willigenburg, A.P. (1992). Therapeutic effects and effects on actual driving performance of chronically administered buspirone and diazepam in anxious outpatients. *J Clin Psychopharmacol, 12(2)*, 86–95.

149. Van der Bijl, P., Roelofse, J.A. (1991). Disinhibitory reactions to benzodiazepines: A review. *J Oral Maxillofac Surg, 49(5)*, 519–523.

150. Vitiello, B., Ricciuti, A.J., Behar, D. (1987). P.r.n. medications in child state hospital inpatients. *J Clin Psychiatry, 48*, 351–354.

151. Vitiello, B., Hill, J.L., Elia, J., et al. (1991). P.r.n. medications in child psychiatric patients: A pilot placebo-controlled study. *J Clin Psychiatry, 52(12)*, 499–501.

152. Vogel, G. (1992). Clinical uses and advantages of low doses of benzodiazepine hypnotics. *J Clin Psychiatry, 53(6, Suppl)*, 19–22.

153. Wells, B.G., Chu, C.C., Johnson, R., et al. (1991). Buspirone in the treatment of posttraumatic stress disorder. *Pharmacotherapy, 11(4)*, 340–343.

154. Werry, J.S. (1982). An overview of pediatric psychopharmacology. *J Am Acad Child Psychiatry, 21*, 3–9.

155. Wolf, B., Guarino, J.J., Preston, K.L., Griffiths, R.R. (1989). Abuse liability of diphenhydramine in sedative abusers. *NIDA Res Mon, 95*, 486–487.

156. Wolf, B., Grohmann, R., Biber, D., et al. (1989). Benzodiazepine abuse and dependence in psychiatric inpatients. *Pharmacopsychiatry, 22*, 54–60.

157. Woods, S.W., Nagy, L.M., Koleszar, A.S., et al. (1992). Controlled trial of alprazolam supplementation during imipramine treatment of panic disorder. *J Clin Psychopharmacol, 12(1)*, 32–38.

158. Squires, R.F., Benson, D.I., Braestrup, C., et al. (1979). Some properties of brain specific benzodiazepine receptors: New evidence for multiple receptors. *Pharmacol Biochem Behav, 10*, 825–830.

159. Johnson, L.C., Chernik, D.A. (1982). Sedative-hypnotics and human performance. *Psychopharmacology, 76*, 101–113.

160. Glassman, J.N., Darko, D., Gillin, J.C. (1986). Medication-induced som-

nambulism in a patient with schizoaffective disorder. *J Clin Psychiatry, 47(10)*, 523–524.

161. Waters, B.G. (1990). Psychopharmacology of the psychiatric disorders of childhood and adolescence. *Med J Aust, 152(1)*, 32–39.

162. Schenck, C.H., Milner, D.M., Hurwitz, T.D., Bundlie, S.R. (1989). A polysomnographic and clinical report on sleep-related injury in 100 adult patients. *Am J Psychiatry, 146(9)*, 1166–1173.

163. Schenck, C.H., Mahowald, M.W., Kim, S.W., et al. (1992). Prominent eye movements during NREM sleep and REM sleep behavior disorder associated with obsessive-compulsive disorder. *Sleep, 15(3)*, 226–235.

Adrenergic Agents in Child and Adolescent Psychiatry

Clonidine

Clonidine, an alpha-2 adrenergic agonist with known antihypertensive efficacy, has no established FDA recommendations for use in child and adolescent psychiatry. Because it activates presynaptic alpha-2 receptors—which, through their negative feedback action, results in the postsynaptic inhibition of central noradrenergic neurons—clonidine may be a particularly useful agent in psychiatry. It is currently under active investigation better to discern its role in the treatment of children and adolescents. Thus far, it has been most studied with regard to Tourette's disorder, ADHD in children and adolescents, and the control of opiate withdrawal symptoms.

Clonidine appears to be most effective in reducing hyperarousal states with high levels of motoric activity and arousal, and less effective in ameliorating distractibility and impaired attention span.[1] The total number of children and adolescents who have participated in controlled studies is still too small to declare an outcome. Several ongoing studies comparing clonidine with placebo and other psychotropic medications are in progress.[1] In the meantime, many clinicians employ empirical trials of clonidine despite the lack of established criteria for patient selection or efficacy in children and adolescents.

Chemical Properties

See Table 11-1 and Figure 11-1.

Clonidine is a 9-carbon, two-ringed imidazoline derivative that, through its alpha-2 adrenergic receptor agonist activity, affects the locus ceruleus, the major noradrenergic center in the brain, resulting in a decrease in the amount of neurotransmitter released from the nerve terminal.[3] Oral clonidine is rapidly and almost completely absorbed from the GI tract.[1] Peak plasma concentrations are attained within one to three hours. Since it is so lipophilic, clonidine easily crosses the blood–brain barrier. It has no active metabolites, with 35% metabolized in the liver and 65% excreted unchanged in the urine.[2] Its elimination half-life is eight to 16 hours. Clonidine's behavioral effects last between three and six hours, while sedation effects are most prominent only 30 to 90 minutes after the last dose. This is in contrast to its antihypertensive and cardiac effects, which begin within a half to one hour of ingestion and last for six to eight hours.[1] Correlation of oral or skin patch clonidine dose with serum drug levels has not been established.[1,3]

Skin Patch
In addition to being available in an oral form, clonidine is also available as a skin patch known as the transdermal system. Absorption is a function of the surface area of the patch, while the plasma concentration of clonidine depends on the patient's renal function—specifically, the creatinine clearance.[1] In children, the behavioral effects are often noted within two to three days of applying the skin patch; this corresponds to its maximal antihypertensive effect, which also occurs two to three days after it is initiated.[1,3]

Indications

See Table 11-2.

Tourette's Disorder
Refer to Chapter 3 for a description of this disorder.

Neuroleptics have been the most frequently utilized medications for this condition (see Chapter 7). Fulton and colleagues[5] evaluated over 200 patients with Tourette's disorder and found that haloperidol was the medication most frequently used to treat these patients. Pimozide was used somewhat less frequently, and clonidine was the least commonly used of all the medications. These investigators also found that clonidine appeared to be less effective than the neuroleptics in the treatment of Tourette's disorder. It should be noted, however, that many studies have found clonidine to be helpful in this treatment,[6–9] with many patients treated with clonidine undergoing a 50% or greater decrease in their symptoms. Some practicing clinicians

357

Table 11-1

Pharmacokinetics of Adrenergic Agents in Children and Adolescents

Generic Name (Brand Name)	Selectivity	Peak Plasma Concentration (hours)	Plasma Half-Life (hours)	Metabolism and Excretion	Comments
Clonidine (Catapres)	Alpha-2	1–3	8–12	35% hepatic and 65% renal	Very lipophilic; easily penetrates blood–brain barrier
Propranolol (Inderal)	None	1–1½	4	Hepatic	Very lipophilic; potent central and peripheral effects

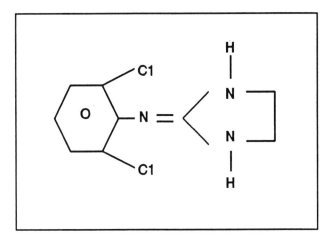

Figure 11-1
Clonidine

choose to start with clonidine when medication is required in the treatment of Tourette's disorder to avoid the serious, and sometimes irreversible, side effects associated with antipsychotic use, such as, tardive dyskinesia.

Case History
A 9-year-old boy with ADHD who had been started on methylphenidate by his pediatrician subsequently developed multifocal tics, and was re-

Table 11-2
Indications for Clonidine in Psychiatry

FDA-approved indications:
• None
Likely indications:
• Tourette's disorder
• ADHD in children and adolescents
• Opioid withdrawal
• Nicotine withdrawal
Possible indications:
• Anxiety and panic disorders
• Bipolar disorder in children and adolescents
• Psychosis
• Agitation (anxiety, hyperarousal)
• Neuroleptic-induced akathisia
• ADHD in adults
• Borderline personality disorder
• Social phobia
• PTSD

ferred to child psychiatry for evaluation. He was observed to have a combination of vocal and multiple motor tics. Coprolalia was also prominent. His parents and personnel at the school he attended were quite upset because, since being started on methylphenidate nine months earlier, he had exhibited a marked improvement in behavior. His tics had started three months prior to the psychiatric evaluation while on a dose of methylphenidate 15 mg t.i.d. The dose had been lowered to 10 mg t.i.d. without improvement in tic behavior. The medication was subsequently discontinued. Unfortunately, the patient's tics continued unabated, and his ADHD behavior recurred while he was off stimulant medication. A family history revealed a significant positive history of tics in two maternal uncles and one maternal grandfather. There was no history of seizure disorder. Neurologic examination of the patient was unremarkable except for periodic tics and vocalizations. An EEG was completely normal. In view of the patient's combined ADHD and probable Tourette's disorder, pharmacologic intervention was proposed. The treating psychiatrist was reluctant to prescribe haloperidol because it is not particularly effective in the treatment of ADHD and because of its potential side effects—extrapyramidal effects, tardive dyskinesia. Clonidine, which has been demonstrated to be effective in the treatment of ADHD, was initiated. Careful monitoring for orthostasis, sedation, and other side effects ensued. A test dose of clonidine 0.05 mg (one-half tablet) at bedtime was the initial starting dose. After tolerating this dose without side effects, his dose was increased to 0.05 mg b.i.d. It was increased by a 0.05-mg increment every five days to an ultimate dose of 0.1 mg t.i.d., at which he experienced a marked reduction of tic behaviors and a moderate improvement in ADHD behavior. No side effects were observed.

In addition to being an effective alternative when neuroleptic therapy has failed, clonidine has also been shown to be effective in decreasing the symptoms of tic disorder during haloperidol's withdrawal.[10] When comparing clonidine treatment with haloperidol treatment in 22 patients with Tourette's disorder, it was found that clonidine decreased tic symptoms in 68% of those studied.[11]

Clonidine has also been shown to be useful in augmenting the efficacy of neuroleptics in the treatment of Tourette's disorder, and it may allow for using lower doses of neuroleptics, which may decrease the risk of developing undesirable side effects.[10,19]

Troung and colleagues[21] studied 81 patients with multifocal tic disorders who were treated with haloperidol, clonazepam, or clonidine. They found that haloperidol was more effective than clonazepam, which was more effective than clonidine. Because of the severe adverse effects associated with antipsychotics, particularly tardive dyskinesia, these authors recommend that clonazepam be used as the initial treatment for these tics, followed by a combination of clonazepam and clonidine as a next step when necessary.[21] Although most efficacious, neuroleptics are best used as the last line of treatment when all else has failed, and only after it has been determined that the tic symptoms are significantly problematic and outweigh the risks inherent with neuroleptic use.

Clonidine appears to be particularly effective in certain subgroups of patients.[12,13,15] Mesulam and Peterson[14] reported that it may be particularly helpful in patients with mild tics and obsessive-compulsive symptoms, which are not infrequently associated with Tourette's disorder. Clonidine may also be a particularly good choice for the treatment of concomitant Tourette's disorder and disruptive behavior disorder, such as ADHD, for which it has also been demonstrated to be effective.[16–18,20,22] When clonidine is effective in controlling tic behavior, its discontinuation has been shown to result in the reemergence and/or worsening of the tics, which are ameliorated when the medication is reintroduced.[12,24]

In contrast with other clinicians, when child and adolescent psychiatrists are referred a patient with Tourette's disorder, it is not uncommon for there to be concomitant psychiatric problems, such as ADHD, obsessions and compulsions, sleep disturbances, depression, or conduct disorder.[22,23] Clonidine and methylphenidate have been used together to treat Tourette's disorder with coexistent ADHD[1,3] (see below).

It must be noted, however, that some studies of clonidine have failed to demonstrate significant clinical benefit from its use, including one placebo-controlled, double-blind study of 30 patients with Tourette's disorder.[25,26] Nonetheless, some patients who demonstrate no objective improvement in their tics have been reported to exhibit improved behavior, less hyperarousal, and decreased subjective distress.[1,3]

ADHD in Children and Adolescents

Currently, clonidine is considered an investigational medication in the treatment of ADHD in children and adolescents. Intense investigation, however, is currently in progress and is likely to delineate better the precise role of clonidine in this disorder.

Hunt and colleagues[3,18] have demonstrated that clonidine is significantly better than placebo in the treatment of disruptive behavior in children and adolescents. This was confirmed by parent, teacher, and clinician ratings of behavior.

When comparing the efficacy of clonidine with that of methylphenidate in the treatment of ADHD, Hunt[27] found that clonidine was as effective as methylphenidate based on parent, teacher, and clinician ratings of behavior. In contrast to the parents and clinicians, who expressed no preference for one medication over the other, the teachers appeared to slightly prefer the effects of methylphenidate over clonidine. Hunt and colleagues[18] further demonstrated that both clonidine and methylphenidate were more effective than placebo in decreasing hyperactivity and in increasing frustration tolerance and compliance. There were, however, some significant differences in the efficacy of the two medications regarding specific target symptoms.

The most clonidine-sensitive children appeared to be those with high rates of motoric overactivity, coexistent oppositional or conduct disorders, and early-age onset of their symptoms.[1,3] Clonidine decreases motor overactivity and hyperarousal states and improves the frustration tolerance in these children, often leading to their increased compliance with commands and expectations and significantly improved task performance, resulting in better learning and improved grades.[1,3] Clonidine does not appear to be effective for children with ADHD, whose primary problem is distractibility and impaired attention span.[20] Methylphenidate seems to be more effective than clonidine in ameliorating distractibility and attention difficulties. Clonidine is also not effective in the treatment of ADD without hyperactivity, where distractibility and poor attention span are the most prominent symptoms.[1,3]

As mentioned, clonidine has been shown to be particularly efficacious in children and adolescents with coexistent oppositional or conduct disorders. It has been shown to decrease physical and verbal aggression in nonpsychotic adolescents.[1,3] This likely is due, at least in part, to its sedating properties, which may also be why it has been found to be effective in other patient populations, such as manic patients with extreme hyperarousal. In contrast to methylphenidate, which is believed to affect primarily the dopaminergic system (which may play a key role in the ability to attend), clonidine is believed to affect primarily the noradrenergic system (which is thought to play an important role in arousal).[1,3] This may explain the fact that teachers more often prefer methylphenidate to clonidine, since sedation might hinder classroom performance in spite of decreased disruptive behavior. In fact, Hunt[18] found that clonidine's most common side effect was sedation, which usually appeared one hour after it was dispensed and lasted for as long as an hour. Fortunately, tolerance to this effect appears to occur within three weeks, so that discontinuation of the medication is seldom necessary (see "Side Effects").

Hunt[27] found that despite the relatively common occurrence of at least transient sedation when clonidine is used to treat ADHD, children have reported feeling more "normal" on clonidine than on methylphenidate. Hunt also found, in this same study, that the transdermal skin patch form of clonidine was as effective as oral clonidine. Seventy-five percent of the children and families involved in the study preferred the skin patch to oral administration because it avoided the embarrassment of having to take pills at school and was more convenient.[27]

The total number of children and adolescents enrolled in controlled studies is still too small to declare a definitive outcome. Certain symptom clusters that are common in ADHD children do appear to be more amenable to treatment with clonidine. While clonidine has been shown to be effective in treating ADHD characterized by hyperarousal states with increased motor activity, low frustration-tolerance states, and coexistent oppositional and conduct disorders, and in those who have responded poorly to CNS stimulants, it is not effective in the treatment of oppositional and conduct symptoms not associated with ADHD, nor is it useful in the treatment of distractibility in nonhyperactive ADD.[1,3] Clonidine and stimulants appear to be useful for different groups of patients with ADHD.[27]

Combination Therapy

Some individuals do seem to respond best when treated with a combination of methylphenidate and clonidine.[1,3] This regimen may be considered for children and adolescents whose symptoms do not respond sufficiently to either medication when used individually. When distractibility and hyperarousal states coexist, this combination may be particularly efficacious.[1,3] The approach is best achieved when methylphenidate dosages are gradually adjusted after the patient is on a stable dose of clonidine.[1,3,28] One notable advantage of this combination is that it often results in a reduction of 40% in the methylphenidate dose, while the side effects of the combination are usually minimal and may be better tolerated than when the medications are used by themselves.[1,3] Also, this combination has been shown to have a greater effect on parents' ratings of aggressive children than does either medication when used alone.[1,3] Methylphenidate–clonidine combination therapy may even prove to be the treatment of choice for patients with coexistent ADHD and conduct disorder. This may be due to the fact that methylphenidate improves attention span by reducing distractibility, while clonidine decreases hyperarousal, thereby improving frustration tolerance and task behavior.[1,3]

ADHD in Adults

Methylphenidate has been shown to be effective in the treatment of ADHD throughout life.[29] Clonidine has not been well studied in the treatment of ADHD in adults. Since the most prominent symptoms in adults tend to be poor attention focus and distractibility whereas the hyperactivity symptoms tend to dissipate with age, clonidine may not be effective for this population.[1,3] Dawson and colleagues,[30] however, have shown that clonidine is effective in the treatment of aggression in adults.

Opioid Withdrawal

Clonidine has been successful in helping patients to withdraw from narcotics[31,32] (see Chapter 14). It has been demonstrated to be more effective than morphine or placebo in decreasing the autonomic symptoms of opiate withdrawal, although not improving the subjective symptoms associated with withdrawal.[2] Clonidine can be used either alone or to facilitate the withdrawal from methadone, which is commonly employed in opiate detoxification protocols.[33–35] In adults, doses of 0.15 mg two times per day are used. Clonidine's use for this purpose has not been well studied in children and adolescents.

Nicotine Withdrawal

Although there had been some initial excitement regarding clonidine's facilitating the cessation of smoking in nicotine-dependent adults, Franks and colleagues[36] performed a randomized, controlled trial of clonidine for smoking cessation and demonstrated it to be of no benefit.

Bipolar Disorder in Adults

During the early 1980s, some reports began to suggest a potential role for clonidine in the treatment of bipolar disorder.[37–39] Patients were treated with clonidine 0.2 to 0.4 mg two times per day in combination with lithium and/or carbamazepine, and improved two to three days after an effective dose of clonidine was reached. Kontaxakis and colleagues[40] demonstrated that adults with bipolar disorder treated with antipsychotics and antidepressants experienced quick amelioration of symptoms without significant side effects when clonidine was added to the regimen. However, Giannini and his colleagues[41] conducted a double-blind crossover study of 24 patients with bipolar disorder in the midst of a manic episode and found lithium to be significantly more effective than clonidine. Clonidine's effectiveness in this disorder is far from clear, and several other alternative agents appear to be far more promising in the treatment of mania, such as valproic acid, carbamazepine, verapamil, and nifedipine.[31] No published data on clonidine exist for children and adolescents with bipolar disorder, but because of its very limited success in adult patients and the existence of more promising medications, it cannot be recommended for the treatment of children and adolescents.

Psychosis

Reports of clonidine's effectiveness in decreasing psychosis and anxiety in psychotic patients have appeared recently.[42,43] Van Kammen and colleagues[42] conducted a double-blind study and showed that four of 13 drug-free, relapsed paranoid schizophrenic adult patients improved significantly on clonidine. There has been further suggestion that clonidine may also ameliorate tardive dyskinetic movements in these schizophrenic patients. Van Kammen and colleagues[42] also found that an improvement in psychosis, anxiety, and negative symptoms correlated significantly with the response of growth hormone to a clonidine challenge test before treatment, suggesting that patients with "normal" CSF norepinephrine levels and normal or high alpha-2 activity might be more likely to respond to clonidine treatment. This lack of established efficacy makes it impossible to offer documented recommendations for its use in psychotic patients. There are no published data on clonidine's use for psychotic children and adolescents. Because of its potential antidyskinetic properties and its ability to decrease hyperarousal in children and adolescents, it would be valuable to conduct a controlled study using clonidine either alone or as an adjunct in the treatment of psychotic children and adolescents.

Anxiety and Panic Disorders

In general, clonidine has not been demonstrated to produce long-term benefit in adults with anxiety or panic disorders,[1,3] although it may temporarily decrease the intensity of an acute anxiety attack. Uhde and colleagues[43] showed that when oral clonidine was given chronically to 18 patients with panic disorder on a double-blind, flexible-dose schedule for 10 weeks, some patients reported improvement in anxiety symptoms, but this improvement was not reported by the group as a whole. Clonidine was also shown to produce a significant, acute reduction in the anxiety of 12 panic disorder patients as compared with 10 controls when 2 µg/kg IV clonidine and placebo were administered.[1,3]

Clonidine 0.15–0.7 mg/day was shown to quicken the tapering of alprazolam in panic disorder adult patients.[44] Although during the acute withdrawal period there was no relapse of panic symptoms, clonidine treatment did not prevent the subsequent recurrence of such symptoms. Moreover, Goodman and colleagues[45] reported the ineffectiveness of clonidine in the treatment of the benzodiapazine withdrawal syndrome in three patients. It seems doubtful that clonidine will prove to be a significantly beneficial treatment for the anxiety disorders. There are no data on children and adolescents.

Neuroleptic-Induced Akathisia

Clonidine doses of 0.15 to 2.0 mg/day have been reported to improve the subjective and objective signs and symptoms of akathisia.[31,46,47] This treatment has been limited because of clonidine's hypotensive side effects, which can be particularly troublesome when lower-potency neuroleptics (which can have significant hypotensive side effects of their own) are used at the same time. Further study is clearly warranted. Clonidine should be utilized only after all other treatment options have been explored, including neuroleptic dosage reduction, anticholinergic medications, beta-blockers, and benzodiazepines.[31] There are no data on children and adolescents. Because of its significant side-effect profile, we do not recommend that clonidine be used to treat akathisia.

Posttraumatic Stress Disorder

Friedman[48] showed that in adults with PTSD, clonidine reduced anxiety, hyperarousal, and intense and intrusive flashbacks of the precipitating trauma, but did not ameliorate avoidant-type behaviors. Kinzie and Leung[49] treated 68 Cambodian refugees diagnosed with chronic PTSD and depression with clonidine and imipramine, which helped to reduce depressive symptoms, anxiety, sleep disturbances, and nightmares. There are no data on children and adolescents.

Social Phobia

Clonidine has enjoyed some modest preliminary success in the treatment of social phobias.[48] Further study is needed before recommendations regarding the use of this medication for this disorder can be offered. There are no data on children and adolescents.

Borderline Personality Disorder

In view of the intense hyperarousal states that are frequently seen in patients with borderline personality disorder, clonidine may prove useful in its treatment.[1,3] There are no data on children and adolescents.

Contraindications

See Table 11-3.

Depression

Clonidine should be avoided for children and adolescents who have significant depressive symptoms and/or a family history of mood disorders.[1] Clonidine and other alpha-2 agonists, such as alpha-methyldopa, have been reported to have significant depressive side effects[50] (see "Side Effects").

Cardiovascular Disorders

Clonidine's only FDA-established indication is for hypertension, and it should, in general, be avoided for patients with cardiovascular disease be-

Table 11-3
Contraindications to Clonidine Use

Absolute:
• None
Relative:
• Depression (in patient or family history)
• Cardiovascular disorders
• Renal disease
• Skin disease/irritation (for skin patch only)

cause of its hypotensive side effects.[1,3] When its use is necessary, careful monitoring is required. This monitoring should consist of the taking of orthostatic blood pressure and pulse measurements prior to each dose when initiating clonidine, and at each dose increment until a stable dose is achieved. A baseline ECG, and subsequent ECGs if any clinical symptoms and/or significant blood pressure or pulse changes are noted, should be performed. Cardiology consultation is also indicated. The inpatient setting is the safest place for such a medication trial to be implemented. If this is not possible, frequent office monitoring is indicated. If the patient's family has access to a blood pressure cuff, family members can be taught to take these blood pressure and pulse measurements, and asked to notify their physician if there is any anomaly.

Renal Disease
Since clonidine is in part metabolized by the kidney (35%), it is relatively contraindicated for children and adolescents with kidney disease.[1]

History of Allergic Reaction to Clonidine
As with any medication, a history of an allergic reaction to clonidine should preclude its use.

Pregnancy
There is virtually no psychiatric indication for clonidine's use during pregnancy.

Skin Irritation/Disease—Skin Patch Only
Children and adolescents with significant problems with skin irritation and dermatologic conditions may not be candidates for the skin patch.[1] If the patient is a known responder to clonidine but refuses to take oral medication, as at school, and the teachers and parents are unable to enforce its ingestion, dermatologic consultation may be helpful. In general, however, the clonidine skin patch should be avoided in these patients.

Liver Disease

Since clonidine undergoes significant hepatic metabolism, it is relatively contraindicated for children and adolescents with liver disease.[1]

Side Effects

See Table 11-4.

Sedation

The most common side effect that children and adolescents experience while on clonidine is sedation, with complaints of lethargy and sluggishness.[1,3] This often is manifest as daytime sleepiness, and may be particularly problematic for children in school.[27] It is important to realize that many of the children receiving clonidine for ADHD, Tourette's disorder, and other disruptive behavioral disorders have extremely high baseline hyperarousal rates, so that sedation may be missed in this population because the parents and teachers may be so relieved that the child is not acting out. Similarly, children with high rates of baseline disruptive behavior may impress observers as being relatively sedated, when, in fact, their more "normal," less hyperactive behavior is such a marked change that it seems as though the child must be sedated.

Table 11-4
Side Effects of Clonidine

Common:
- Sedation
- Hypotension
- Cardiovascular
- Headache and dizziness
- Stomachache/nausea/vomiting

Uncommon:
- Depression
- Cardiac arrhythmias
- Rebound hypertension
- Retinal degeneration
- Skin irritation with skin patch
- Anticholinergic
- Vivid dreams/nightmares/disrupted sleep
- Appetite increase or decrease
- Sexual dysfunction
- Fluid retention
- Anxiety
- Increase blood glucose
- Raynaud's phenomenon

Sedation is most noticeable and problematic during the first month of treatment.[1,3] Fortunately, it usually remits progressively thereafter. In 15% of children on clonidine, however, the sedation persists, an effect that may be more pronounced in those who have lower baseline hyperarousal levels.[1,3] In 10% of children and adolescents on clonidine, dose adjustment is not successful in decreasing sedation, which often interferes with the patient's activities of daily living, and the medication, therefore, must be discontinued.

Hypotension
Children frequently experience a 10% decrease in systolic blood pressure, but this rarely results in clinical symptoms and is rarely significant.[1,3] Orthostasis occurs in less than 5% of children on clonidine.[1,3] Sedation appears to correlate with decreased blood pressure, but there do not appear to be any such correlations among decreased blood pressure, sedation, and improvement in behavior.

Cardiovascular Disease
Clonidine acutely reduces cardiac output by 10 to 20%, but during long-term treatment, the cardiac output returns to baseline.[1,3] Clonidine does not alter renal blood flow or GFR, but it does lower peripheral resistance and pulse. However, this is rarely clinically significant in physically healthy children and adolescents. As pointed out (see "Contraindications"), caution should be employed when utilizing this medication for patients with underlying cardiovascular disease.

Headache and Dizziness
Headache and postural dizziness are seen most commonly during the first month of treatment, and are most often short-term side effects that dissipate after the first month.[1,3] They seem to appear most commonly when the dose is rapidly increased.

Stomachache/Nausea/Vomiting
Gastrointestinal upset most commonly occurs at the very beginning of treatment and usually remits.[1,3]

Depression
The alpha-2 adrenergic agonists have been strongly associated with depressive side effects.[50] In fact, some clinicians now try to avoid these agents when treating hypertension in favor of other equally (or more) effective antihypertensive agents without alpha-2 activity. It is important to note that although clonidine causes depression in 5% of children and adolescents treated with this medication, most have significant depressive symptoms at the start of clonidine treatment, as well as a personal or family history of mood disorders.[1,3]

Cardiac Arrythmias

Dawson and colleagues[30] observed that clonidine can cause cardiac dysrhythmias in adults. They have not been reported in children and adolescents.

Rebound Hypertension

Caution is required when the patient is taking a beta-blocker, since a clonidine–beta-blocker combination can result in clinically significant rebound hypertension.[1,3] In addition, when clonidine has been administered chronically and/or at high dosages, abrupt withdrawal may result in a dangerous rebound hypertension. This hypertension is usually transient, but unless properly treated, it can jeopardize the child's safety. It is best never to withdraw clonidine abruptly, but to taper it prior to discontinuing it (see "Dosage and Administration"). When clonidine is abruptly withdrawn, other signs and symptoms, in addition to rebound hypertension, include anxiety, chest pain, increased and/or irregular pulse, headache, GI upset, sleeping problems, and tremor.[1]

Retinal Degeneration

A total of 353 adults treated with clonidine for 20 or more years showed no evidence of retinal degeneration.[1,3] There are no data on children, but this appears to be an unlikely risk.

Skin Irritation—Patch Only

It has been shown that the use of the transdermal clonidine skin patch can result in a localized contact dermatitis with itching and erythema in nearly 40% of children.[1,3] Even though the Band-Aid that can be placed over the patch may help keep the patch on, the Band-Aid appears to increase the frequency and symptoms of the contact dermatitis. This dermatitis often develops within the first three weeks of the patch's use, and may mandate its discontinuation. Hunt and colleagues[3] did find, however, that in contrast to adults who have been reported to be at increased risk for developing a generalized skin rash when they are switched from the patch to oral clonidine, this did not result in 50 children who were placed on oral clonidine after failing the patch.

Anticholinergic Effects

Approximately 50% of adult patients on clonidine report anticholinergic side effects such as dry mouth, especially during the first month of treatment.[31] Children, however, appear to be far less sensitive to these side effects.[1,3]

Vivid Dreams/Nightmares/Disrupted Sleep

Symptoms of sleep disturbance are not uncommonly seen in children and adolescents with underlying psychopathology, so differentiating the medication's side effect from the patient's disorder can be difficult. Approximately 10% of adults complain of sleep difficulties while taking clonidine.[1,3] This has not been well described in children and requires further study.

Appetite Increase or Decrease
Clonidine has been reported to increase or decrease both appetite and weight.[1,3] A weight gain of more than 5 pounds is, however, quite unusual. When it does take place, it tends to be observed in children with ADHD who had lost weight on methylphenidate and subsequently experienced a weight rebound on clonidine.[1,3]

Sexual Dysfunction
As with many psychotropic drugs, clonidine has been reported to result in decreased libido, impotence, or decreased sexual activity in adults receiving this medication.[50]

Fluid Retention
Fluid retention has been reported to occur, but it can be corrected with diuretic therapy.[1,3,31]

Anxiety
Anxiety and nervousness have been reported as occasional side effects of clonidine treatment.[50]

Increase in Blood Glucose
Increased blood glucose is rarely significant, and usually only for diabetic patients.[1,3]

Raynaud's Phenomenon
This syndrome, characterized by feelings of cold and pain in the fingers and toes, is a rarely observed side effect when clonidine is used.[50]

Important Conditions When Prescribing Clonidine

See Table 11-5.

Overdose
Overdose with clonidine can be a life-threatening medical emergency. Characteristic symptoms of clonidine overdose include decreased or absent reflexes, lethargy or somnolence, dilated pupils, hypotension and bradycardia, hypoventilation, and irritability.[50] Large overdoses may also present with seizures, apnea, reversible cardiac conduction defects, and arrhythmias. The treatment of clonidine overdose includes removing all clonidine systems,

Table 11-5
Important Considerations When Prescribing Clonidine

Use with caution in children and adolescents with:
- Hypertension/hypotension
- Cardiovascular disease
- Cerebrovascular disease
- Diabetes
- Depression
- Beta-blockade (i.e., on propranolol)

such as the skin patch. The use of IV fluids and/or pressors to treat hypotension, treatment with atropine for bradycardia, and careful monitoring of the patient's respiratory status are frequently required interventions after a clonidine overdose.[31,50]

Abuse
There is virtually no risk for the recreational abuse of clonidine.[4]

Drug Interactions
See Table 11-6.

Available Preparations and Cost

See Table 11-7.

Initiating and Maintaining Treatment

The practicing clinician who decides to start clonidine must ensure that a comprehensive baseline history is taken and the child or adolescent receives a physical examination. Blood pressure and pulse measurements should be documented. The clinician should also strongly consider obtaining a baseline CBC and differential, electrolytes, BUN and creatinine, thyroid function tests, LFTs, an ECG, and fasting blood glucose.[1,3]

While the child or adolescent is on clonidine, blood pressure and pulse measurements (preferably orthostatic measurements of both parameters) should be obtained each week until the dose is stabilized. After the dose is stabilized, blood pressure and pulse should be monitored every two months.[1,3] More frequent monitoring can be considered if sedation and/or other side effects are noted.

It is important to emphasize to the patient and family the very severe consequences that may result from the abrupt discontinuation of clonidine. Therefore, when prescribing clonidine, it is important to ensure that proper

Table 11-6
Clonidine Interactions

Increases drug effect of: • Heterocyclic antidepressants • Antipsychotics • Anticholinergic medications • CNS depressants (e.g., alcohol)
Decreases drug effect of: • Beta-blockers
Increases effect of clonidine: • Fenfluramine • Diuretics • Other antihypertensive medications • CNS depressants
Decreases effect of clonidine: • Heterocyclic antidepressants • Sympathomimetic drugs • Nonsteroidal anti-inflammatory analgesics
Increases: • Growth hormone levels (short-term) • Blood glucose
Decreases: • Urinary catecholamines
May Cause: • Abnormal LFTs • Wenckebach periods on ventricular trigeminy

Adapted from: Lowenthal, D.T., Matzek, K.M., MacGregor, T.R. (1988) Clinical pharmacokinetics of clonidine. *Clin Pharmacokinet, 14,* 287–310.

Table 11-7
Commercially Available Preparations of Clonidine

	Dosage Forms	Average Cost/Day
Generic	0.1 mg 0.2 mg 0.3 mg	$0.03 $0.04 $0.06
Catapres Transdermal (skin patch)	TTS-1 TTS-2 TTS-3	$1.18 $1.99 $2.75

Source: Red Book Annual Pharmacist Reference, 1989–1990. Oradell, NJ: Medical Economics.

follow-up takes place, and that the family does not let the prescriptions run out, use clonidine on a p.r.n. basis, or alter the medication regimen without physician consultation.

The patient and child should also be advised that long-term treatment may be required. Hunt and colleagues[3] reported on children treated with clonidine for as long as five years with continued beneficial effect and without significant dose alteration.

Clinical Practice

Dosage and Administration—Oral Clonidine

Tourette's Disorder (Table 11-8). To reduce daytime sleepiness and lethargy, clonidine is usually first initiated at bedtime.[1,3] The recommended starting dose is 0.05 mg at bedtime (half of the smallest available tablet). The dose should be increased very gradually by 0.05 mg every three to seven days to facilitate the child's adjustment to the medication. Even with this gradual increase in dosing, sedation is still usually the limiting factor in dose elevation.[1,3,51] Sedative effects have been found to peak one-half hour to one and a half hours after a dose of clonidine has been administered. Oral clonidine is best given in small divided doses, that is, three to four times per day with meals and at bedtime. Bruun[51] has noted that some patients experience a decrease in beneficial effects approximately five hours after the last dose, further arguing for the total daily dose to be administered in three to four divided doses. The treatment of Tourette's disorder usually requires 3 to 4 μgs/kg/day.[1,3] Dosages above this level may be required, but commonly produce unacceptable side effects, such as sedation and lethargy.

The patient and family should also be informed that during the initial treatment phase, the Tourette's symptoms, including motor and phonic tics, may

Table 11-8

Clinician's Guide to Using Clonidine for Tourette's Disorder and ADHD in Children and Adolescents

Tourette's Disorder	ADHD
• Start with 0.05 mg at bedtime, increase by 0.05 mg every three to seven days.	• Start with 0.05 mg at bedtime, increase by 0.5 mg every three to seven days.
• Optimal dose 3–4 μg/kg/day. three to four times a day (after meals and at bedtime).	• Optimal dose 3–6 μg/kg/day.
• After stable oral dose is achieved, may switch to skin patch (same dose).	• After stable oral dose, may switch to skin patch.
• Not FDA approved.	• Not FDA approved.

actually worsen.[1,3] Huk[52] has described how this transient exacerbation of tics in the treatment of Tourette's disorder with clonidine often dissipates once a stable dose has been achieved, usually two to four weeks after treatment has begun. A dose adjustment—a decrease, and possible reincrease after tolerance to clonidine's effects has resulted—is often necessary.

Cohen and colleagues[13] have developed a very useful paradigm, in which they describe five phases commonly experienced by patients on clonidine for Tourette's disorder. In the first phase, the patient often experiences decreased subjective distress, agitation, and anger, and, therefore, feels more tranquil and less aroused. The second phase begins approximately one month after clonidine has been started. During this phase, further behavior control is achieved, vocal and motor tics dissipate, and obsessive and compulsive behaviors also decrease. This usually corresponds to therapeutic dosages, 3 to 4 μg/kg/day. Phase 3 occurs approximately three months after treatment, when continued improvement is observed. Phase 4 is experienced by some (but not all) patients five or more months after clonidine was started. They may require further increases in their clonidine doses to prevent a relapse. Unfortunately, doses this high are often associated with intolerable side effects. Adjunctive therapy with clonazepam, or if this is unsuccessful, neuroleptics, might be considered, since their combined use sometimes allows lower dosages of clonidine to be used. These other medication have their own sedating side effects, however. Finally, phase 5 is characterized by further tolerance to clonidine, generally at dosages that cannot be increased further.

Tourette's disorder may require long-term treatment with clonidine.[1,3] It is very important that those children and adolescents who have been on chronic therapy be gradually tapered off clonidine to avoid rebound hypertension (see below).

Clonidine Treatment of ADHD (Table 11-8). The treatment of ADHD with clonidine usually requires doses of 3–4 μg/kg/day.[1,3] It is almost never necessary to exceed doses of 8 μg/kg/day. Intolerable side effects frequently make it impossible to attain such high doses. Children and adolescents with particularly high hyperarousal, agitation, and aggression baselines with poor frustration tolerance may be best able to tolerate high-dose clonidine. Dosage and administration should follow that described for Tourette's disorder, that is, starting with a bedtime dose of 0.05 mg and gradually increasing the dose every three to seven days by 0.05-mg increments. Divided doses given three to four times per day are preferred. Maximum doses may be higher than those required for Tourette's disorder, particularly for those children with high levels of hyperarousal. As with Tourette's disorder, sedation and other side effects are not uncommon, and frequently mandate clonidine's adjustment and dosage decrease, and sometimes even result in its discontinuation. For those who do respond, long-term treatment is often required. Clonidine may not exert its effect until two to three months after its initiation, and, therefore, no patient should be considered a treatment failure until this length of time has elapsed.

Management of Specific Side Effects of Oral Clonidine

Sedation
When sedation occurs during the first month of treatment, decreasing the rapidity with which the dose is increased may prove helpful.[1,3] The dose can be increased by 0.05-mg increments every 10 to 14 days instead of on a weekly basis. For smaller children, it might be advisable to increase the dose by 0.25 mg per week (one-fourth tablet). Sometimes, it may even be necessary to decrease the clonidine dose temporarily until the patient is capable of tolerating the lower dose. When this has been successfully achieved, a subsequent gradual increase of the dose may be initiated. Combination therapy often allows lower overall clonidine dosage, as when used in conjunction with methylphenidate to treat ADHD. Finally, sometimes the sedation and lethargy can be ameliorated by switching from oral clonidine to the skin patch, which produces a smaller dose pulse.[1,3]

Gastrointestinal Upset
Although GI upset is usually transient, it can be disconcerting; gradual dose increments and ingestion after meals may help ameliorate this side effect.[1,3]

Hypotension
Hypotension frequently is found in conjunction with sedation. If the systolic and/or diastolic blood pressure decreases by more than 10 mmHg, decreasing the dose is indicated.[1,3] If this is unsuccessful, switching from oral clonidine to the skin patch might reverse the blood pressure change. Performing an ECG and getting a cardiology consultation are advisable.

Depression
Depression has been found to occur most commonly in children who have had prior depressive episodes, current depressive symptoms, and/or a family history of mood disorders.[1,3] When clinical judgment deems clonidine treatment necessary, or in patients who develop a depressive episode de novo, decreasing the dose or switching to the skin patch are often effective in reducing the depressive symptoms.[1,3]

Dosage and Administration—Transdermal Therapeutic System

The clonidine skin patch is available only in proprietary form, the Catapress-TTS 1, 2, and 3, which correspond to oral clonidine doses of 0.1, 0.2, and 0.3 mg. While these are the only doses of the skin patch available, cutting the patch can produce intermediate doses so that oral doses can be achieved with the skin patch.[1,3]

It is, generally, not advisable to start clonidine treatment with the skin patch,[1] because oral clonidine can be used more easily to determine treatment response, making the switch to an equivalent dose of transdermal clonidine easier. Absorption via the skin patch is believed to be more variable than that after the oral administration of clonidine. It is important to emphasize that there is no fixed ratio of doses between routes of administration, and because of the significant variability between the two treatment approaches, modification and adjustment are frequently required when switching from one to the other.[1,3]

When selecting the site for administration of the clonidine patch in children and adolescents, it is important to choose an inaccessible area without hair on the lower back.[1] Children with ADHD and those who are just normally active might inadvertently (or intentionally) remove the patch, and either lose it or put it back on. In either case, the dosing regimen is affected, and accurate assessment of its efficacy versus toxicity is made considerably more difficult. The skin should be prepared by washing with soap and water and then drying. The 1.0- by 1.5-cm patch should be attached to the designated area like a Band-Aid. To make extra certain that the skin patch stays on the back, a protective 3-cm white adhesive strip may be applied over the patch. The problem with this is that the adhesive can exacerbate and increase the risk of developing skin irritation from the clonidine skin patch (see below).

One frequent concern of parents relates to what they should do when their child exposes the patch to water, as when swimming.[1] The clonidine skin patch is believed to be resilient to brief water exposure and does not have to be replaced after a shower or a bath.[1,3] But parents should be warned that the patch may require replacement during particularly humid summer days or when the child is exposed to water for extended periods, such as when swimming all day. This is not absolute, and the parents should be aware that they will have to monitor their child and assess the efficacy of the patch after long exposure to water.

The patch is believed to be effective for five days,[1] and should be replaced after this time. Many parents and children prefer this method of receiving medications, since it does not require pill taking and minimizes the risk of forgetting a dose of medication.

Nonspecific sedation may be noted soon after the skin patch is initiated. Clinical response is rarely observed before two weeks of treatment with clonidine,[1,3] and it usually takes a month before a significant clinical response occurs. It can take up to three months for the maximal therapeutic effect to occur, and a medication trial may necessitate two to three months of treatment before a child is considered to have failed the clonidine trial. Usually, after the primary response of decreasing hyperarousal, improvements in learning and attention span, compliance, social skills, irritability, and mood are seen.[1,3]

Management of Specific Side Effects of the Skin Patch

Skin Irritation

Hydrocortisone cream 1% can help ameliorate the skin irritation by decreasing erythema and itching.[1] In addition, not using the optional protective adhesive patch cover may reduce the skin irritation.[1,3] Consultation with a dermatologist may also be advisable. In some cases, however, it is necessary to return to oral clonidine. Fortunately, in contrast to adults, who not uncommonly are predisposed to adverse, generalized skin reactions when switched back to oral clonidine, this does not appear to happen in children and adolescents.[1,3]

How to Withdraw Clonidine

It is essential that clonidine be withdrawn gradually. In children, if clonidine has been given for less than one week, abrupt discontinuation of the 0.05 mg bedtime dose does not usually result in rebound hypertension or other problems.[1,3] When the medication has been dispensed for between two and three weeks, gradual tapering by 0.05 mg/day is required. After the child or adolescent has been on clonidine for one month or longer, an even more gradual tapering schedule is advised. In these patients, clonidine should be reduced by 0.05 mg every three to seven days. The more chronic the use, the more crucial it is that the clonidine taper be gradual.

Similarily to children on stimulants who have periodic drug holidays (see Chapter 3), some children on clonidine can be maintained at doses of one half to two thirds of the usual dose.[1,3] This should also be done gradually, as just described, to make sure that the child does not experience dangerous side effects, such as rebound hypertension. Thus it is probably not advisable to halve the dose over the Christmas recess, which is far shorter than children's summer vacations. In contrast to stimulants with their lack of sequelae from abrupt discontinuation and their short half-lives, clonidine, with its potentially dangerous side effects from abrupt withdrawal and a longer half-life than that of the stimulants, must always be gradually tapered, particularly when used over a long period.

One final caution is that if a child or adolescent is on both clonidine and a beta-blocker, the beta-blocker should be discontinued several days before initiating the clonidine taper in order to avoid rebound hypertension.[1,3]

Propranolol

Beta-Blockers

The beta-adrenergic blocking agents competitively antagonize epinephrine and norepinephrine actions at the beta-adrenergic receptors. These agents have many established indications for various cardiovascular disorders, but currently have no FDA-established indications for use in psychiatric disorders. Nonetheless, there continues to be great interest in, and hope for, the potential efficacy of these agents in the treatment of certain psychiatric disorders. Propranolol, a nonselective beta-1 and beta-2 antagonist, has thus far been the most investigated agent of its class, and will be the focus of discussion in this chapter.

There is some evidence suggesting that propranolol is efficacious for aggressive patients with brain damage.[53–55, 70] It has also been reported to be effective in the treatment of PTSD, anxiety and panic disorders, performance anxiety, and akathisia.[56–59] Thus far, it appears that propranolol's ability to decrease anxiety and agitation in certain psychiatric conditions is due more to its peripheral actions of slowing the increased heart rate characteristically associated with anxiety and hyperarousal states than to its central effects on noradrenergic beta-receptors. The total number of patients entered into controlled studies is still far too small to declare a definitive outcome. At present, some clinicians use propranolol to treat children and adolescents with impulsivity and aggression, especially when there is CNS damage such as mental retardation, or when they have failed first-line treatments of disruptive behavior disorders.[60] Because the efficacy and safety of propranolol have not been established in children and adolescents with psychiatric disorders, it is not possible to give documented recommendations regarding its use in this population. The few studies done involving this age group were not controlled and had very small sample sizes. In some cases, the beta-blocker was simply added to another psychoactive agent. Controlled studies comparing propranolol with placebo are necessary to determine its true role in the treatment of psychiatric disorders.

Comparison of Propranolol with Other Beta-Blockers

See Table 11-9.

Chemical Properties

See Figure 11-2.

Table 11-9
Pharmacokinetic Properties of Propranolol (Adults)

Drug (Brand Name)	Selectivity	Lipophilicity	Peak Effect (hours)	Plasma Half-Life (hours)	Elimination
Propranolol (Inderal)	None	High	1–1½	3–6	Hepatic
Atenolol (Tenormin)	B_1	Low	2–4	6–9	Renal
Nadolol (Corgard)	None	Low	3–4	14–24	Renal
Metoprolol (Lopressor)	B_1	High	1	3–4	Hepatic

Propranolol blocks both beta-1 and beta-2 receptors in the brain and peripherally. A derivative of propanol, it blocks the actions of norepinephrine and epinephrine at beta-adrenergic receptors. Since these catecholamines are associated with sympathetic arousal, propranolol exerts sympatholytic effects, such as reducing heart rate and blood pressure. It penetrates the

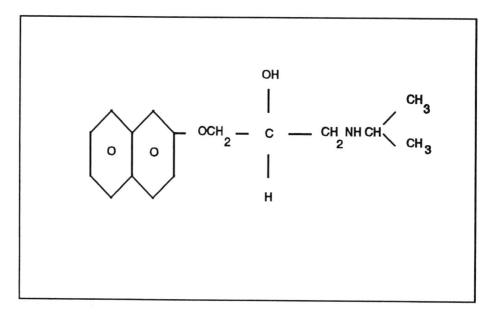

Figure 11-2
Propranolol

blood–brain barrier easily because of its high lipophilicity, and it is believed to have prominent central and peripheral effects. In the CNS, the noradrenergic receptors are mostly beta-1 receptors.[60] Beta-1 receptors in the periphery are known to stimulate the heart chronotropically and inotropically.[50] Beta-2 receptors are found most commonly in brain glial cells and peripherally in the lungs and blood vessels, where they produce bronchodilation and vasodilation. At the present time, the relative importance of the central versus peripheral effects of propranolol in the treatment of psychiatric disorders is not known. There is some evidence to suggest that the peripheral sympatholytic actions of propranolol may ameliorate anxiety and aggression more than its central activity.[60] Moreover, the beta-1 activity appears to be more involved in controlling anxiety and agitation than the beta-2 activity. Atenolol, a selective beta-1 antagonist that penetrates the blood–brain barrier in only very small amounts, has been reported anecdotally to reduce agitation and anxiety in adults, while the selective beta-2 receptor antagonists appear to have no obvious clinical use in the treatment of behavior disorders.

The pharmacokinetics of propranolol have not been described for children and adolescents. In adults, it is known that propranolol exerts its peak effect one to one and a half hours after oral administration.[50] Its serum half-life is three to six hours; therefore, it must be given more than once per day, in contrast to atenolol, which has a longer half-life and can often be given only once per day.[60] Propranolol, which is very highly protein bound, is predominantly metabolized by the liver and undergoes a significant first-pass effect.

Indications

See Table 11-10.

Aggression in Brain-Damaged Children and Adolescents

In the early 1980s, several investigators reported on propranolol's effectiveness in the treatment of violent behavior in adult patients with organic brain disease.[53–55] Williams and colleagues[61] gave propranolol in an open-label fashion to 30 patients, of whom 26 were children and adolescents. All subjects had exhibited uncontrolled rage and aggressive outbursts for at least six months and had failed to respond to other medications. Eighty percent of the children experienced moderate to marked improvement on a median dose of 160 mg of propranolol per day.[61] It should be noted that the highest daily dose of propranolol given was 1600 mg per day, and that the patient tolerated this without hypotensive or other side effects. In fact, in the entire sample studied, side effects were minimal, with only one child becoming depressed. It is important to point out, however, that 22 of the patients were receiving additional psychotropic medications, such as antipsychotics, anticonvulsants, and stimulants, while receiving propranolol.

Table 11-10
Indications for Propranolol in Children and Adolescents

FDA-established indications:
• None
Possible indications:
• Aggressive patients with CNS damage
• Lithium tremor
• Akathisia
• Performance anxiety
• Generalized anxiety disorder and panic disorder
• Hyperventilation attacks
• Alcohol withdrawal
• PTSD
Not indicated:
• Schizophrenia
• Tardive dyskinesia
• Extrapyramidal side effects of neuroleptics (except akathisia)

Subsequent open-label studies have reported propranolol to be effective in treating refractory aggression, particularly in brain-damaged pateints.[62,63]

Nevertheless, with the lack of placebo-controlled study, no definitive outcome can be declared at this time. Further study is necessary.

Posttraumatic Stress Disorder

Famularo and colleagues[58] treated 11 hyperaroused, treatment-refractory PTSD children with propranolol in an open study. Propranolol was initiated at 0.8 mg/kg/day and increased gradually to a maximum of 2.5 mg/kg/day. The dosage was maintained at this level for two weeks, and then gradually discontinued over the next three weeks. Side effects precluded raising the dose in only three children.[58] It is possible that lower doses of beta-blockers than those used in the treatment of anxiety disorders may be efficacious in the treatment of acute PTSD, and that p.r.n. doses prior to stressful situations may be particularly effective.[71] Propranolol and the beta-1 selective agents clearly merit further study in children and adolescents suffering from PTSD.

Performance Anxiety

Propranolol has been reported to be effective in the amelioration of performance anxiety in adults.[60,64] Performance anxiety, known in lay terms as stage fright, is a relatively common social phobia. In addition to impaired performance, characteristic physical symptoms often arise, such as dry mouth, hoarseness, increased heart rate, and difficulty in breathing. Propranolol has minimal central side effects and often improves performance,[64] in contrast to the benzodiazepines, such as diazepam, which can cause sedation and so tend to worsen performance. In adults, a single dose of propranolol 10–40 mg 30–60 minutes before the anxiety-producing event is often effective. It is wise to give a patient a test dose prior to a very important event to make sure that it helps and does not cause undue side effects in that particular patient. There are no data on children and adolescents, but this is a worthwhile area for study, since, like adults, they suffer from performance anxiety and may benefit from propranolol treatment.

Generalized Anxiety Disorder

When utilized in the treatment of adults with generalized anxiety disorders, propranolol has been found to be inferior to benzodiazepines and antidepressants.[55,56,64] Moreover, depressive disorders are common in such patients, and since one of propranolol's side effects is depression (see "Side Effects"), caution is advised when using this agent in this population of patients. Neppe,[71] however, reviewed 15 controlled studies of beta-blockers in the treatment of anxiety, 11 of which used propranolol, and determined that somatic anxiety (anxiety associated with cardiac and respiratory symptoms such as tachycardia and shortness of breath) responded well to these agents, while psychic anxiety (anxiety without somatic involvement) appears to be relatively unaffected by the beta-blockers. Gualtieri and colleagues[68] point out that while beta-blockers are not the first-line treatment for anxiety disorders, they can provide a useful second-line or adjunct treatment in certain types of anxiety disorder. There are no data on children, but this may be an important area worthy of further investigation.

Panic Disorder

Propranolol and the beta-blockers have been found to be largely ineffective in the treatment of panic disorder.[71] In contrast to antidepressant drugs, which are effective in treating adult panic disorder, the beta-blockers do not reduce lactate-induced panic attacks.[72] There are no data on children and adolescents, and because of the lack of efficacy in adults, their use in this population is not recommended.

Hyperventilation Attacks

Joorabchi[67] found that propranolol, 10–30 mg/day given in an open-label fashion, was effective in improving hyperventilation attacks in 13 of 14 adolescents.

Akathisia

Many clinicians believe that the beta-blockers such as propranolol are the drugs of choice for neuroleptic-induced akathisia in adults.[59,65,66] When akathisia is particularly refractory, or when extrapyramidal side effects coexist with the akathisia, propranolol can be given together with benzodiazepines or anticholinergic agents.[64] (See Chapter 7.) Propranolol is given at doses of 30–80 mg/day to treat akathisia and seems to work quickly once an effective dose is reached. It appears to have no effect on other parkinsonian symptoms. Alpert and colleagues[73] observed a significant improvement in both akathisia and aggression when nadolol was added to the treatment regimen of patients receiving antipsychotics, lending further support to the contention that a peripheral mechanism is responsible for the improvement in aggression and akathisia, that is, the decrease in hyperarousal. There are currently no data on children and adolescents. In children, where it is often difficult to differentiate akathisia from hyperactivity, beta-blockers are generally not recommended. Conservative measures, such as adjusting the antipsychotic medication, are preferred.

Lithium Tremor
Tremor is frequently seen in patients treated with lithium (see Chapter 8). The coarse tremor associated with lithium toxicity is particularly bothersome and easy to notice. Often, however, the fine tremor associated with therapeutic blood levels can be annoying and troublesome to patients. Before propranolol is initiated, it is important to make sure that the patient is on the lowest possible effective dose of lithium. Decreasing the dose may ameliorate the tremor to a sufficient degree so that it is no longer a problem, while still treating the psychiatric symptoms. In adults, tremor can be reduced by decreasing or eliminating caffeine consumption. Campbell and associates,[74] however, observed that although tremor was an untoward effect associated with lithium administration in children, it did not appear to be clinically significant and did not interfere with functioning. We do not recommend propranolol for the treatment of lithium-induced tremor in children and adolescents.

Alcohol Withdrawal
See Chapter 14.

Schizophrenia
High doses of propranolol of up to 4000 mg/day have been used to treat patients with schizophrenia without demonstrable benefit.[64] There are no data on children and adolescents. Because of its lack of efficacy in adults, its use in children and adolescents is not recommended.

Tardive Dyskinesia
Beta-blockers have been tried in the treatment of tardive dyskinesia in adults, but have not been found to be effective.[64] There are no data on chil-

dren and adolescents, but because of their lack of efficacy in adults, their use in children and adolescents is not recommended.

Contraindications

See Table 11-11.

Diabetes and Hypoglycemia
Propranolol is contraindicated for patients with diabetes. Particular caution is necessary in diabetics prone to hypoglycemia since beta-blockers may interfere with the normal response to hypoglycemia.[68]

Bronchospastic Disease
Propranolol is contraindicated for children and adolescents with bronchospastic diseases such as asthma.[68] Some clinicians believe that for patients with bronchospastic disease, selective beta-1 antagonists such as atenolol are preferable. It is important to remember, however, that even beta-1 selective agents have some risk of exacerbating the respiratory condition. Since there are few controlled studies assessing the efficacy of the beta-blockers, including the selective beta-1 agents, in psychiatric disorders, the risks of using any of these agents outweigh their potential benefits. Therefore, we strongly recommend avoiding the use of beta-blockers for children and adolescents with bronchospastic disease.

Cardiovascular Conditions
Propranolol is contraindicated for children and adolescents with heart disease.[60] It is, therefore, important to screen all patients for cardiovascular pathology by checking vital signs, giving them a physical examination, and taking a cardiogram before initiating treatment with propranolol.

Hyperthyroidism
Propranolol should generally be avoided in children and adolescents with hyperthyroidism.[60,68]

Table 11-11
Contraindications to Propranolol Use

● Bronchospastic disease (asthma)
● Diabetes/hypoglycemia
● Allergic reaction
● Medicated with MAOI
● Hyperthyroidism
● Depression
● Pregnancy

Depression

In general, propranolol should be avoided for children and adolescents with a depressive disorder, a history of depression, and/or a strong family history of affective disorders. A selective beta-1 antagonist such as atenolol may be indicated for these patients.[60] Atenolol may pose less of a risk for the development of depression than propranolol, possibly because of its poor penetration of the blood–brain barrier,[60] although its use also can be associated with depression.

Children and adolescents with anxiety disorders pose a dilemma. Patients with such disorders have a higher occurrence of comorbid depressive disorders than the general population. It may behoove the clinician in this instance to recommend the use of atenolol instead of propranolol.

Pregnancy

There is virtually no psychiatric indication for propranol or any beta-blocker's use during pregnancy.

Patients on MAOIs

Propranolol and the other beta-blockers are absolutely contraindicated for children and adolescents receiving MAOIs.[68]

History of Allergic Reaction

As with any medication, a history of allergic reaction to the beta-blockers precludes their use.

Side Effects

See Table 11-12.

Decreased Heart Rate

Propranolol can decrease the pulse to less than 50 beats per minute.[60,68,71] It is, therefore, essential to get baseline vital signs and monitor cardiovascular function while the patient is on propranolol. It is best to increase the dose gradually in children and adolescents. Bradycardia is much less likely to occur when atenolol is used instead of propranolol.[60]

Raynaud's Phenomenon

Propranolol administration, by decreasing the peripheral circulation, can lead to the development of Raynaud's phenomenon, which is characterized by tingling, numbness, and pain in the fingers.[60]

Table 11-12
Side Effects of Propranolol

Common: • Decreased heart rate   • Raynaud's phenomenon   • Lethargy   • Impotence
Uncommon: • Bronchoconstriction   • Congestive heart failure   • Depression   • Hallucinations
Rare: • Hypoglycemia   • Hypotension/dizziness   • Nausea/diarrhea   • Vivid dreams and nightmares

Tiredness and Weakness

Patients treated with propranolol rather commonly experience the side effects of tiredness and weakness.[60]

Sexual Impotence

Impotence is considered a common side effect of propranolol.[60]

Congestive Heart Failure

This is a relatively uncommon side effect of propranolol, and the risk is extremely low for those without preexisting cardiovascular disease.[60]

Bronchoconstriction

Bronchoconstriction is a relatively uncommon but very serious and potentially life-threatening side effect of propranolol. It is believed to be less common with atenolol,[60] but as we have pointed out, we recommend immediate discontinuation of all beta-blockers when this side effect is encountered since the risks outweigh the possible benefits.

Depression

Depression is a potentially serious side effect of propranolol treatment and appears to be less of a problem when atenolol is used instead of propranolol.[60] We recommend discontinuing propranolol in depressed patients and switching to atenolol.

We do not subscribe to the view of some clinicians that depression induced by propranolol can be treated with an antidepressant, thus obviating the need for discontinuing propranolol. Since the antidepressants have not yet been proved to be effective in the treatment of child and adolescent depression (see Chapter 4), we believe that their addition to the treatment regimen is not warranted and only serves to place the child or adolescent on added medication, exposing the patient to the risk of polypharmacologic side effects. Depression as a result of beta-blocker administration requires discontinuation of the beta-blocker and *not* treatment with TCAs.

Hallucinations
Hallucinations are an uncommon side effect of propranolol that has rarely been reported.[60] It is believed to be practically nonexistent in patients treated with atenolol.

Hypoglycemia
Hypoglycemia is a rare side effect and, as mentioned, is mainly of concern in diabetic patients.[60]

Hypotension/Dizziness/Nausea/Diarrhea
These problems are occasional side effects of propranolol.[60]

Vivid Dreams and Nightmares
Sleep disruption is an occasional adverse side effect of propranolol.[60] When insomnia and nightmares appear, propranolol is most frequently the beta-blocker being administered, since these problems appear to be almost nonexistent with the other beta-blockers.[60]

Overdose and Toxicity
Beta-adrenergic blockade can be a medical emergency, resulting in bradycardia, hypotension, cardiac arrest, and respiratory distress.[60] Gastrointestinal symptoms such as nausea and diarrhea may also be experienced. Peripheral cyanosis, psychosis, and seizures may occur after overdose.

Propranolol is not dialyzable, and when a patient overdoses, immediate evacuation of gastric contents is necessary. When bradycardia occurs, atropine 0.25–1.0 mg should be administered. If there is no response to vagal blockade, cautious administration of isoproterenol is recommended.[50,64] In the event of cardiac failure, digitalization and diuretics are necessary. In the event of hypotension, vasopressors such as epinephrine are indicated. When bronchospasm is encountered, the administration of isoproterenol and aminophylline is necessary.[50,64]

Abuse

There appears to be relatively no risk for the recreational abuse of propranolol.

Drug Interactions

See Table 11-13.

Available Preparations and Cost

See Table 11-14.

Initiating and Maintaining Treatment

The practicing clinician who decides to start propranolol must ensure that the child or adolescent has a comprehensive baseline history and a physical

Table 11-13
Drug Interactions

Propranolol may increase effects of: • Anesthetics • Antipsychotics • Calcium blockers • Clonidine • Epinephrine • Lidocaine • MAOIs • Phenytoin • Thyroxine
Propranolol may decrease effects of: • Insulin • Oral hypoglycemia
Drugs that increase effect of propranolol: • Cimetidine • Molindone
Drugs that decrease the effect of propranolol: • Carbamazepine • Estrogens (birth control pills) • Nicotine • Nonsteroidal anti-inflammatory analgesics
When used together, shared inhibition of propranolol and: • Aminophylline • Narcotic analgesics • Sympathomimetics • Theophylline

Table 11-14
Available Preparations and Cost

Drug	Preparations	Average Cost/Day
Propranolol	Generic (scored tablets): 10, 20, 40, 60, 80, 90 mg Inderal: 1 mg/ml injectable	$0.11
Atenolol	Tenormin (scored tablets): 50, 100 mg	$0.74

Source: *Red Book Annual Pharmacist Reference, 1989–1990.* Oradell, NJ: Medical Economics.

examination. Documentation of cardiovascular function must be obtained. Baseline vital signs also must be obtained, and careful monitoring of cardiovascular functioning must be implemented while the child or adolescent is receiving propranolol. Starting with low-dose propranolol and increasing the dose gradually so as to ensure that blood pressure and pulse drop as little as possible is advisable. If the blood pressure decreases to below 90/60 mmHg and/or if the pulse falls to less than 60, the next dose of propranolol should not be given.[60] Consideration of decreasing subsequent dosages of propranolol is also indicated. An ECG should be performed. If there is any abnormality or if the vital signs do not return to normal, consultation with a cardiologist is advisable.

As was mentioned earlier, if the child or adolescent with a psychiatric disorder has asthma or a potential for asthma, propranolol is contraindicated since its safety has not been established in this population. If the child develops an asthmatic condition while on propranolol, the medication must be discontinued immediately and the asthma treated appropriately. The propranolol should not be reinstituted once the asthma attack subsides. We also believe that all beta-blockers, regardless of selectivity, should be avoided in such patients.

The hypoglycemic side effects of propranolol usually do not require any intervention in patients who are not diabetic.[60] Propranolol should be avoided, however, if the patient has a history of diabetes. When there is a family history of diabetes, propranolol is not absolutely contraindicated, but fasting blood sugars and a glucose tolerance test are recommended to evaluate fully how much risk is involved.[60] When there is a doubt or concern, we recommend avoiding propranolol. It would be our recommendation, for example, that a child with a significant family history of diabetes and normal fasting blood sugars and glucose tolerance tests be started on atenolol rather than propranolol. In the event of any abnormality of the fasting blood sugar and/

or glucose tolerance test, we advise using another medication and avoiding beta-blocking agents. If the clinician feels that a beta-blocker is essential to treatment, consultation with the child or adolescent's medical doctor is strongly recommended.

It is also important to inform both male and female adolescents about the risk for sexual dysfunction with propranolol, since this is a relatively common side effect. It is important to talk with the adolescent prior to starting the medication and to monitor this during treatment. Moreover, the female adolescent should be asked about sexual activity and her chances of becoming or plans to become pregnant.

It is important to monitor closely for propranolol-induced depressive side effects. It is particularly important when taking the history to determine whether there is a personal or family history of depression, and if so, it is best to avoid using propranolol for these children and adolescents. Atenolol may be a better choice in such patients. When depressive side effects are encountered during propranolol therapy, switching to atenolol may be warranted since this agent is less commonly associated with depression, probably because of its poor penetration of the blood–brain barrier. We do not recommend the initiation of TCA therapy in combination with propranolol for these children and adolescents, since these agents can have significant side effects, including cardiac complications, and have not been demonstrated to be superior to placebo in the treatment of child and adolescent depression.

The sleep disturbances that are occasionally seen with propranolol use can often be easily ameliorated by changing the time of the last daily dose of the medication to earlier in the day.[60]

Clinical Practice

Dosage and Administration
No firm guidelines have been established for the dosing and administration of propranolol and other beta-blockers in child and adolescent psychiatry, nor has any age limit been specified for their use. But since these agents have been utilized in the treatment of many medical disorders, there are some guidelines that may be appropriate for psychiatric patients as well.[69] The normal dose range for adolescents treated with propranolol is 20–300 mg/day.[60] The dose is generally started at 10 mg two times per day and increased by 10–20 mg every three to four days. Prepubertal children are usually started on a dose of propranolol of 10 mg/day, with the dose being increased by 10 mg increments every three to four days.[60] The normal dose range for these children is 10–120 mg/day. No one has determined a maximal dose for children and adolescents. The FDA guidelines for the dose limit

for propranolol in the treatment of medical conditions affecting adults and children is 16 mg/kg/day for children and 640 mg four times per day for adults.[69] Even less information exists on the use of atenolol. Here, the FDA guidelines for the treatment of medical disorders have set a dose limit of 200 mg four times per day in adults. There is no specification for children.

Withdrawal of propranolol in children and adolescents should be done gradually, especially if the patient has been receiving the medication chronically. Rebound sympathomimetic side effects such as hypertension, tachycardia, and arrythmias have been reported in adult patients with cardiac disorders when propranolol is abruptly discontinued after chronic use.[60] Although these risks appear to be less in healthy children and adolescents as compared with adult cardiac patients, caution is recommended, particularly if the child or adolescent is being treated as an outpatient and so close monitoring is more difficult. Generally, the patient should be withdrawn by 10–20 mg decrements every three or four days, making sure that vital signs remain stable.

References

1. Hunt, R.D., Capper, L., O'Connell, P. (1990). Clonidine in child and adolescent psychiatry. *J Child Adolesc Psychopharmacol, 1*, 87–101.

2. Kaplan, H.I., Sadock, B.J. (Eds.) (1991). *Synopsis of Psychiatry Behavioral Sciences* (6th ed.) (pp. 636–637). Baltimore: Williams & Wilkins.

3. Hunt, R.D., Cohen, D.J., Anderson, G., et al. (1988). Noradrenergic mechanisms in ADHD. In L.M. Bloomingdale (Ed.), *Attention Deficit Disorder: New Research in Attention, Treatment, and Psychopharmacology*. New York: Pergamon.

4. Lowenthal, D.T., Matzek, K.M., MacGregor, T.R. (1988). Clinical pharmacokinetics of clonidine. *Clin Pharmacokinet, 14*, 287–310.

5. Fulton, W.A., Shady, G.A., Champion, L.M. (1988). An evaluation of Tourette syndrome and medication use in Canada. *Neurosci Biobehav Rev, 12*, 251–254.

6. Leckman, J.F., Walkup, J.T., Cohen, D.J. (1988). Clonidine treatment of Tourette's syndrome. In D.J. Cohen, R.D. Bruun, J.F. Leckman (Eds.) *Tourette's Syndrome and Tic Disorders: Clinical Understanding and Treatment*. New York: Wiley.

7. Leckman, J.F., Detlor, J., Harcherik, D.F., et al. (1985). Short- and long-term treatment of Tourette's syndrome with clonidine: A clinical perspective. *Neurology, 35*, 343–351.

8. Leckman, J.F., Cohen, D.J., Detlor, J., et al. (1982). Clonidine in the treatment of Tourette's syndrome: A review of data. In A.J. Friedhoff, T.N. Chase (Eds.) *Gilles de la Tourette Syndrome* (pp. 391–401). New York: Raven Press.

9. Leckman, J.F., Cohen, D.J. (1983). Recent advances in Gilles de la Tourette's syndrome: Implications for clinical practice and future research. *Psychiatr Dev, 1*, 301–306.

10. Max, J.E., Rasmussen, S.A. (1986). Clonidine in the treatment of Tourette's syndrome exacerbation due to haloperidol withdrawal. *J Nerv Ment Dis, 174*, 243–246.

11. Borison, R.L., Ang, L., Hamilton, W.J., et al. (1983). Treatment approaches in Gilles de la Tourette's syndrome. *Brain Res Bull, 11*, 205–208.

12. Singer, H.S., Gammon, K., Quaskey, S. (1986). Haloperidol, fluphenazine, and clonidine in Tourette's syndrome: Controversies in treatment. *Pediatr Neurol Sci, 12*, 71–74.

13. Cohen, D.J., Detlor, J., Young, J.G., et al. (1980). Clonidine ameliorates Gilles de la Tourette's syndrome. *Arch Gen Psychiatry, 37*, 1350–1354.

14. Mesulam, M.M., Peterson, R.C. (1987). Treatment of Gilles de la Tourette's syndrome: Eight-year practice based experience in a predominantly adult population. *Neurology, 37*, 1828–1833.

15. Bond, W.S. (1986). Psychiatric indications for clonidine: The neuropharmacologic and clinical basis. *J Clin Psychopharmacol, 6*, 81.

16. Hunt, R.D. (1988). Treatment of ADHD with clonidine: Guidelines for physicians. *Psychiatr Times*, September.

17. Caine, E.D., McBride, M.C., Chiverton, P., et al. (1988). Tourette's syndrome in Monroe County school children. *Neurology, 38*, 472–475.

18. Hunt, R.D., Minderaa, R.B., Cohen, D.J. (1985). Clonidine benefits children with attention deficit disorder and hyperactivity: Report of a double-blind placebo-controlled crossover study. *J Am Acad Child Psychiatry, 24*, 617–629.

19. Bruun, R.D. (1984). Gilles de la Tourette's syndrome: An overview of clinical experience. *J Am Acad Child Psychiatry, 23*, 126–133.

20. Hunt, R.D., Minderaa, R.B., Cohen, D.J. (1986). The therapeutic effect of clonidine in attention deficit disorder with hyperactivity: A comparison with placebo. *Psychopharmacol Bull, 22*, 229–236.

21. Troung, D.D., Bressman, S., Shale, H., et al. (1988). Clonazepam, haloperidol, and clonidine in tic disorders. *South Med J, 81*, 1103–1105.

22. Jankovic, J., Rohardy, H. (1987). Motor, behavioral, and pharmacologic findings in Tourette's syndrome. *Can J Neurol Sci, 14(Suppl 3)*, 541–546.

23. Golden, G.S. (1986) Tourette syndrome: Recent advances. *Pediatr Neurol, 2*, 189–192.

24. Ernberg, G. (1988). Pharmacologic therapy of tics in childhood. *Pediatr Ann, 17*, 395–404.

25. Abuzzahab, F.S. (1981). Clonidine HCI in Gilles de la Tourette syndrome. First International Gilles de la Tourette Syndrome Symposium; 17(Abstract).

26. Goetz, C.G., Tanner, C.M., Wilson, R.S., et al. (1987). Clonidine and Gilles de la Tourette syndrome: Double-blind study using objective rating methods. *Ann Neurol, 21*, 307–310.

27. Hunt, R.D., (1987) Treatment effects of oral and transdermal clonidine in relation to methylphenidate: An open pilot study in ADDH. *Psychopharmacol Bull, 23*, 111–114.

28. Hunt, R.D., Clopper, L., Ebert, M.H. (1989, October). Clonidine and methylphenidate: Combined use in treatment of selected ADHD children. Presentation, Annual Meeting, American Academy of Child and Adolescent Psychiatry, New York.

29. Wender, P. (1987). *The Hyperactive Child, Adolescent, and Adult: Attention Deficit Disorder Through the Lifespan.* New York: Oxford University Press.

30. Dawson, P.M., Vander-Zanden, J.A., Werkman, S.L., et al. (1989). Cardiac dysrhythmia with the use of clonidine in explosive disorder. *DICP, 23*, 465–466.

31. Arana, G.W., Hyman, S.E. (Eds.) *Handbook of Psychiatric Drug Therapy (2nd ed.)* (pp. 177–180). Boston: Little Brown.

32. Gold, M.S., Redmond, D.E., Kleber, H.D. (1978). Clonidine blocks acute opiate withdrawal symptoms. *Lancet, 2*, 599.

33. Charney, D.C., Heninger, G.R., Kleber, H.D. (1986). The combined use of clonidine and naltrexone as a rapid, safe, and effective treatment of abrupt withdrawal from methadone. *Am J Psychiatry, 143*, 831.

34. Hoder, E.L., Leckman, J.F., Paulsen, J. (1984). Clonidine treatment of neonatal narcotic abstinence syndrome. *Psychiatry Res, 13*, 243.

35. Jasinski, D.R., Johnson, R.E., Kocher, T.R. (1985). Clonidine in morphine withdrawal. *Arch Gen Psychiatry, 42*, 1063.

36. Franks, P., Harp, J., Bell, B. (1989). Randomized, controlled trial of clonidine for smoking cessation in a primary care setting. *JAMA, 262*, 3011.

37. Zubenko, G.S., Cohen, B.M., Lipinski, J.F., et al. (1984). Clonidine in the treatment of mania and mixed bipolar disorder. *Am J Psychiatry, 141*, 1617.

38. Hardy, M.D., Lecrubien, Y., Widlocher, D. (1983). Efficacy of clonidine in 24 patients with acute mania. *Am J Psychiatry, 143*, 1450.

39. Jovent, R., Lecrobier, Y., Puech, A.J., et al. (1980). Antimanic effect of clonidine. *Am J Psychiatry, 137*, 1275.

40. Kontaxakis, V., Markianos, M., Markidis, M., et al. (1989). Clonidine in the treatment of mixed bipolar disorder. *Acta Psychiatr Scand, 47*, 108–110.

41. Giannini, A.J., Pascarzi, G.A., Loiselle, R.H., et al. (1986). Comparison of clonidine and lithium in the treatment of mania. *Am J Psychiatry, 143*, 1608.

42. Van Kammen, D.P., Peters, J.L., Van Kammen, W.B., et al. (1989). Clonidine treatment of schizophrenia: Can we predict treatment response? *Psychiatry Res, 27*, 297–311.

43. Uhde, T.W., Stein, M.B., Vittone, B.J., et al. (1989). Behavioral and physiologic effects of short-term and long-term administration of clonidine in panic disorder. *Arch Gen Psychiatry, 46*, 170–177.

44. Fyer, A.J., Liebowitz, M.R., Gorman, J.M., et al. (1988). Effects of clonidine on alprazolam discontinuation in panic patients: A pilot study. *J Clin Psychopharmacol, 8*, 270–274.

45. Goodman, W.K., Charney, D.S., Price, L.H., et al. (1983). Ineffectiveness of clonidine in the treatment of the benzodiazepine withdrawal syndrome: Report of three cases. *Am J Psychiatry, 143*, 1450.

46. Zubenko, G.S., Cohen, B.M., Lipinski, J.F., et al. (1984). Use of clonidine in treating neuroleptic-induced akathisia. *Psychiatry Res, 13*, 253.

47. Adler, L.A., Angrist, B., Peselow, E., et al. (1987). Clonidine in neuroleptic-induced akathisia. *Am J Psychiatry, 144*, 235.

48. Friedman, M.J. (1988). Toward rational pharmacotherapy for post traumatic stress disorder: An interim report. *Am J Psychiatry, 145*, 281–285.

49. Kinzie, J.D., Leung, P. (1989). Clonidine in Cambodian patients with posttraumatic stress disorder. *J Nerv Ment Dis, 177*, 546–550.

50. *Physicians' Desk Reference* (45th ed.) (1991). Oradell, N.J.: Medical Economics.

51. Bruun, R. (1983). TSA medical update. Treatment with clonidine. *Tourette Syndrome Association Newsletter*, Spring.

52. Huk, S.G. (1989). Transient exacerbation of tics in treatment of Tourette's syndrome with clonidine. *J Am Acad Child Adolesc Psychiatry, 28*, 583–586.

53. Yudofsky, S., Williams, D., Gorman, J. (1981). Propranolol in the treatment of rage and violent behavior in patients with chronic brain syndrome. *Am J Psychiatry, 138*, 218.

54. Greendyke, R.M., Schuster, D.B., Wooton, J.A. (1984). Propranolol in the treatment of assaultive patients with organic brain disease. *J Clin Psychopharmacol, 4*, 282.

55. Ratey, J.J., Morrill, R., Oxenkrug, G. (1983). Use of propranolol for provoked and unprovoked episodes of rage. *Am J Psychiatry, 140*, 1356.

56. Kathol, R., Noyes, R., Slymen, D.J., et al. (1981). Propranolol in chronic anxiety disorders: A controlled study. *Arch Gen Psychiatry, 37*, 1301.

57. Granville-Grossman, K.L. (1974). Propranolol, anxiety, and the central nervous system. *Br J Clin Pharmacol, 1*, 361.

58. Famularo, R.A., Kinscherff, R., Fenton, T. (1988). Propranolol treatment for childhood post traumatic stress disorder, acute type. *Am J Dis Child, 142*, 1244–1247.

59. Lipinski, J.F., Zubenko, G.S., Cohen, B.M., Barreira, P.J. (1984). Propranolol in the treatment of neuroleptic-induced akathisia. *Am J Psychiatry, 141*, 412.

60. Coffey, B.J. (1990). Anxiolytics for children and adolescents: Traditional and new drugs. *J Child Adolesc Psychopharmacol, 1(1)*, 57–83.

61. Williams, D., Mehl, R., Yudofsky, S., et al. (1982). The effect of propranolol on uncontrollable rage outbursts in children and adolescents with organic brain dysfunction. *J Am Acad Child Adolesc Psychiatry, 21*, 129–135.

62. Kuperman, S., Stewart, M.A. (1987). Use of propranolol to decrease aggressive outbursts in younger patients. *Psychosomatics, 28*, 315–319.

63. Grizenko, N., Vida, S. (1988). Propranolol treatment of episodic dyscontrol and aggressive behavior in children (Letter). *Can J Psychiatry, 33*, 776, 778.

64. Arana, G.W., Hyman, S.E. (1991). *Handbook of Psychiatric Drug Therapy* (2nd ed.) (pp. 173–174). Boston: Little Brown.

65. Ratey, J.J., Sorgi, P., Polakoff, S. (1985). Nadolol as a treatment for akathisia. *Am J Psychiatry, 142*, 640.

66. Adler, L., Angrist, B., Peselow, E., et al. (1986). A controlled assessment of propranolol in the treatment of neuroleptic-induced akathisia. *Br J Psychiatry, 149*, 42–45.

67. Joorabchi, B. (1977). Expressions of the hyperventilation syndrome in childhood. *Clin Pediatr, 16*, 1110–1115.

68. Gualtieri, C.T., Golden, R.N., Fahs, J.J. (1983). New developments in pediatric psychopharmacology. *Dev Behav Pediatr, 4*, 202–209.

69. Forsythe, W., Gilles, D., Silles, M. (1977). Propranolol (Inderal) in the treatment of childhood migraine. *Dev Med Child Neurol, 26*, 237–241.

70. Arnold, L.E., Aman, M.G. (1991). Beta blockers in mental retardation and developmental disorders. *J Child Adolesc Psychopharmacol, 1(5)*.

71. Neppe, V.M. (1989). *Innovative Psychopharmacotherapy*. New York: Raven Press.

72. Gorman, J.M., Levy, G.F., Liebowitz, M.R., et al. (1983). Effect of acute beta-adrenergic blockade on lactate-induced panic. *Arch Gen Psychiatry, 40*, 1079–1082.

73. Alpert, M., Allan, E.R., Citrone, L., et al. (1990). A double-blind, placebo-controlled study of adjunctive nadolol in the management of violent psychiatric patients. *Psychopharmacol Bull, 26*, 367–371.

74. Campbell, M., Small, A.M., Green, W.H., et al. Behavioral efficacy of haloperidol and lithium carbonate: A comparison in hospitalized aggressive children with conduct disorder. *Arch Gen Psychiatry, 41*, 650–656.

Atypical and Adjunctive Agents

If a psychopharmacologic agent is a drug that alters the course of emotional illness, then the choice of subjects for a psychopharmacology textbook depends on what one considers a drug. Several substances that have been tried in childhood psychiatric disorders are not psychoactive drugs in the traditional sense, but include foods, exogenous hormones, and pharmacologic agents that have little or no effect in the normal population. However, some have been widely publicized or are in current use, making it necessary for the practitioner to be familiar with the evidence supporting or refuting their use. Several atypical approaches to child and adolescent psychiatric disorders are discussed here, both pharmacologic and nonpharmacologic. Only treatments that have received some degree of experimental scrutiny will be covered, including opiate antagonists, nutritional therapy, high-dose vitamin therapy, and thyroid hormone analogues. Due in part to inadequate testing and in part to lackluster results, few of these treatments have a significant place in the physician's armamentarium.

Opiate Antagonists

Of the treatments discussed in this chapter, opiate antagonists have gained the greatest clinical and experimental favor. Naloxone (Narcan) and other parenteral opiate antagonists have long been used as tools to study the role of endogenous and exogenous opiates in animal physiology and behavior.

Naloxone was marketed for human use to treat iatrogenic and recreational opiate toxicity (see Chapter 14). However, several behavioral effects suggested other uses for the drug. Animal studies showed that opiate antagonists reverse the hyperphagia and obesity associated with elevations in endogenous opiate levels,[66] decrease social aggression,[58] and attenuate drug- or stress-induced stereotypy.[23,88] These observations, along with the recent availability of an oral opiate antagonist (naltrexone), have led to human trials for obesity, eating disorders, autistic disorder, and self-injurious behavior.

Chemical Properties

Opium may be the oldest psychotropic medication still in use. It was considered indispensable by ancient Greek physicians and its earliest recorded use may have been in Mesopotamia around 5000 B.C.[2,96] The modern use of opium derivatives is limited to analgesic agents (morphine, meperidine, codeine) and drugs of abuse (heroin). The study of opiate antagonists began with the use of nalorphine as an antidote to intoxication with such drugs.[96]

Absorption and Metabolism

Two forms of opiate antagonist are used in psychiatry, parenteral naloxone (Narcan) and oral naltrexone (Trexan). Naloxone may be administered IV or IM, and the onset of action is within minutes from either route. Oral naltrexone is variably absorbed, with more than 90% of the drug being converted to active (6-beta-naltrexol) and inactive metabolites, and it reaches peak concentrations in one hour. The approximate mean elimination half-lives for naloxone and naltrexone are one and four hours, respectively, although 6-beta-naltrexol has a longer half-life of 12.9 hours. The half-life of naloxone is extended in neonates, but has not been well studied in children.[77]

Mechanism of Action

Opiate antagonists clearly block the effects of exogenous opiate drugs such as morphine and heroin (see Chapter 14). In the absence of exogenous opiates, clinical effects are mediated by blocking endogenous opioids. Morphine-like substances (endorphins and enkephalins) are present naturally in the CNS and are released during times of physical pain or stress, accounting for the phenomena of posttraumatic analgesia and euphoria following intense exercise. Dysregulation of endogenous opioids is hypothesized in each of the disorders for which opiate antagonists have been tested and forms the theoretical basis for the mechanism of action. However, the precise role of endogenous opioids in self-injurious behavior, autistic disorder, and other conditions is hypothetical.

Indications

Opiate antagonists are not FDA approved for any psychiatric disorder that does not involve intoxication with opiate drugs. However, used independently, naloxone and naltrexone are remarkably safe medications with few side effects. Therefore, they are acceptable, albeit unproved, for use in child and adolescent psychiatric disorders.

Self-Injurious Behavior

Self-injurious behavior (SIB) is a common symptom of psychiatric illness, especially in children with severe developmental disability. One logical pathogenetic theory is that affected children either are less sensitive to pain or are behaviorally reinforced by the release of endogenous opioids. If accurate, this theory would predict that blocking endogenous opioids would either increase pain during SIB (providing an aversive stimulus) or block reinforcement for SIB (leading to extinction).

Several placebo-controlled studies have reported the reduction of SIB with naloxone or naltrexone treatment, but these were conducted on very small samples and were of short duration.[95] Sandman and associates[83,85] reported an acute, dramatic decrease in self-injury 10–80 minutes after injections of 0.1–0.4 mg naloxone in three adults with long histories of SIB. In a later, controlled trial of naltrexone in four mentally retarded adults, they found a significant dose-dependent reduction of SIB at doses between 0.36 and 2.53 mg/kg/day. In one subject (a 23-year-old male), SIB returned to baseline at a dose of 1.43 mg/kg/day. In all subjects, stereotypy was slightly increased on 0.7–1.3 mg/kg/day and hyperactivity measures were unaffected.[84] Barrett and associates[7] found a paradoxical increase of SIB with naloxone, but a significant decrease with naltrexone (1.2 mg/kg/day) under double-blind conditions in a 12-year-old female with mental retardation and autism. Herman and colleagues[40] have extensively studied the effects of opiate antagonists in animals. And in three adolescent humans (aged 10, 17, and 17 years), they found a threefold decrease in mean SIB frequency at doses of 0.5–1.5 mg/kg, but no improvement at a higher dose of 2.0 mg/kg. Another placebo-controlled study on an 18-year-old male also demonstrated dose dependency, with an optimal dose of 50 mg daily.[10] However, there are also negative reports.[9,24] Kars and associates[50] used a fixed dose of 50 mg of naltrexone daily (0.6–1.5 mg/kg) in a double-blind trial of six males aged 15 to 31 years. One subject (a 31-year-old man with Down's syndrome) had a threefold decrease in the frequency of SIB over the three weeks of active treatment. Another subject had a statistically significant reduction in SIB, but had relatively low baseline rates. The remaining four subjects did not show significant improvement. Similarly, Szymanski and colleagues[94] found that 50 or 100 mg of naltrexone under double-blind conditions had no effect on the SIB, self-stimulatory behavior, or agitated behavior of two young adults with mental retardation.

In summary, there is preliminary evidence for the short-term efficacy of opiate antagonists in treating SIB, but the data are inconclusive because of the use of fixed dosing schedules in some studies and the small sample sizes. In controlled studies, the cumulative sample was 24 subjects, 15 of whom improved significantly. Szymanski and associates[94] point out that there are undoubtedly many etiologic factors that produce SIB and that opiate antagonists may be effective in a subset of patients. Therefore, larger trials using variable, weight-adjusted doses of naltrexone would help to define those patients who may respond. Only one controlled case report indicated the successful treatment of SIB for as long as six months.[98] The demonstration of long-term clinical benefit is essential, since SIB typically persists for years and the possibility of tolerance to opiate antagonism has been unexplored. Finally, if one returns to the theory that SIB may be reinforced by endogenous opioid release, then further clinical trials of opiate antagonists must allow for an initial persistence or worsening of SIB (the extinction burst), which has been reported in two cases.[54]

Autistic Disorder

Autistic children often exhibit SIB, but also have other characteristics that have been loosely compared to opiate intoxication. Opiates can induce social withdrawal, stereotypy, and sensory hyper- or hyposensitivity, leading to the hypothesis that endogenous opioids may play an etiologic role in autism.[26,47] More compelling are the effects of opiate drugs on the early social development of animals. Morphine reduces maternal–offspring separation distress and attachment in young mammals and chicks[42,70] and decreases social exploratory behavior without affecting nonsocial exploratory behavior in young rodents.[56] These observations have given rise to a pathogenetic theory of autism analogous to an endogenous opioid "addiction."[82]

The first systematic study of naltrexone in autistic children was conducted by Campbell and associates.[17,18,20] Ten children aged 3 to 7 years were treated with 0.5, 1.0, or 2.0 mg/kg/day in an open trial with structured outcome measures. The results indicated significant improvements in some autistic symptoms (withdrawal, underproductive speech, and stereotypy) and some nonautistic symptoms (restlessness and tantrums). Abnormal object relations, aggression, and SIB improved slightly, and the only adverse effect was mild sedation.[18,20] This group recently repeated this study on 18 autistic children (aged 3–8 years) under double-blind conditions. The treatment group improved significantly on a global assessment scale, but not on the specific symptom scales employed in the earlier studies. The most consistent improvements were in social withdrawal and communicative speech.[17] Leboyer and colleagues[57] recently published a double-blind trial of naltrexone in four autistic children, three of whom were declared responders based on improved social relatedness, verbalization, and withdrawal. However, one child had the fragile X genotype and the data were incomplete for two children. One additional open trial reported similar effects in four children that persisted for up to one year.[69]

In summary, animal studies support a possible role of endogenous opioids in the pathogenesis of autistic disorder. Preliminary clinical trials of opiate antagonists indicate that these agents may improve several "core" autistic symptoms, such as social withdrawal and communicative speech. Although controlled studies are needed, no other agents reliably improve these features of autism, and naltrexone appears to be very safe in doses of 0.5 to 2.0 mg/kg/day. Therefore, early clinical use may be warranted. Interestingly, the opioid "addiction" hypothesis would predict that treatment would have the greatest effect on social development when started at a young age. This was not the observation of Campbell and colleagues,[17] who noted the greatest symptomatic improvement in older autistic children. Further controlled comparison of the effects of naltrexone across age groups is desirable.

Obesity and Eating Disorders

Opiate antagonists inhibit hyperphagia in some strains of genetically obese rodents and rodents with high endogenous opioid levels.[55] This effect was also noted in three patients with the Prader-Willi syndrome,[55] although later studies did not support that finding.[99] However, other reports of decreased appetite or weight on naltrexone suggested its trial in obesity and bulimia.[93] Although human studies of obesity suggest that naltrexone may affect food preference,[28,90] it does not appear to reduce weight significantly under double-blind conditions.[63] In one double-blind, multiple-dose study of 60 obese subjects, no weight loss was evident across the entire sample, but female subjects lost an average of 1.7 kg.[5] Similarly, naltrexone is probably not superior to placebo at reducing binge eating and vomiting in bulimic patients,[64] although several authors have suggested that a subset of bulimics with abnormal endorphin levels may respond.[3,44–46] Although research into the role of endogenous opioids in obesity and eating disorders continues, current data do not support the clinical use of naltrexone to treat these disorders.

Contraindications

At doses of 300 mg/day, test subjects developed elevated hepatic enzymes on naltrexone. Therefore, the manufacturer recommends monitoring transaminases and considers preexisting hepatic disease to be a contraindication to naltrexone treatment. The only additional contraindications relate to the concurrent use of, withdrawal from, or dependence on opiate drugs, since naltrexone may cause precipitous opiate withdrawal in such cases. As with all medications, a known hypersensitivity to naltrexone is a contraindication to treatment.[77]

Side Effects

In the studies cited above, mild sedation was the only reported adverse effect in children. The manufacturer of naltrexone and naloxone (DuPont) also reports mild hepatic toxicity at high doses, but not at doses that effectively block opioid receptors. Insomnia, anxiety, and GI upset are listed as infrequent side effects, but have not been reported in clinical studies. Abuse of and dependence on these agents are not described. There are no reported cases of overdose.[77]

Available Preparations and Cost

Naloxone is available only as an injection, so has no outpatient application. Naltrexone (Trexan) is available only as 50-mg tablets, with an average wholesale price of $209.40 per 50 tablets. Since the most effective dose for both SIB and autistic disorder appears to be 1.5 mg/kg/day, a 50-kg child would require approximately 75 mg per day at a (wholesale) cost of $6.29. An 80-kg adult would require approximately 125 mg at a cost of $10.48 per day.[78]

Initiating and Maintaining Treatment

The clinical use of naltrexone for SIB and autistic disorder is not approved, but is acceptable in treatment-resistant cases based on the results of preliminary trials and the apparent safety of this agent in children.[41] The use of opiate antagonists in substance-abuse disorders is discussed in Chapter 14. However, even in patients who are not known to use exogenous opiate drugs, a small test dose of naltrexone should be administered before treatment, followed by close observation for signs of opiate withdrawal. Baseline and periodic LFTs are recommended, and the drug should be discontinued in the unlikely event of hepatic toxicity.

The manufacturer does not provide dosing guidelines for children, since naltrexone is not approved for use for patients under 18 years of age. Available

studies suggest that some autistic children and children with SIB will respond to a low dose of 0.5 mg/kg/day. Since even lower doses have not been
tested, clinical use should start at 0.25 mg/kg/day in a single dose, with
gradual increases every one or two weeks. The 50-mg scored tablet may be
quartered or crushed to allow for fine increments. The average effective dose
in studies of children is 1.5 mg/kg/day. Some autistic children have further
symptom reduction at 2.0 mg/kg/day, but several studies have reported that
SIB returns to baseline at this dose. Therefore, 2.0 mg/kg should be considered the maximum dose until further studies are available.

Nutritional Therapy

The motivation for developing nonpharmaceutical treatments for child and
adolescent emotional illness is high. Such therapies are attractive because
they do not incur the social distaste that accompanies the use of mood-altering drugs in children. Nutritional therapy in particular is advocated as a
more natural alternative to medication, and if effective would help, on some
level, to disavow the existence of serious pathology in affected children. It is
much more attractive to see one's child as suffering from a food allergy than
as having a mental illness.

Indications

Attention-Deficit Hyperactivity Disorder
Perhaps the most widely publicized nutritional therapy is the dietary treatment of ADHD. Feingold[30,31] hypothesized that hyperactivity could result
from allergic reactions to food additives and natural salicylates. There is little evidence for a causal relationship, as naturalistic studies have failed to
detect a difference in the diets of hyperactive and nonhyperactive children.[49]
However, the therapeutic effect of restricting food additives is still debated.
Most studies of the Feingold diet in the treatment of hyperactivity report no
effect, although some indicate that parents report subjective improvement,
which is not supported by objective measures.[51,61,81] One recent study restricted additives in the diets of 24 hyperactive boys even more stringently
than was recommended by Feingold. A majority of parents reported improvement during the treatment phase, but the study suffers from a lack of
adequate objective measures and the inability to blind parents to
treatment conditions.[48]

It seems clear that if there is a therapeutic effect of additive-free diets, it is
modest in magnitude and restricted to a subgroup of hyperactive children.
Furthermore, the effort required to eliminate all such substances from children's diets is prohibitive for most families. Less regimented approaches

have included the reduction of refined sugar, caffeine, and other naturally occurring stimulants (e.g., phenylethylamine in chocolate) in children's diets. The evidence is stronger that refined sucrose can produce or exacerbate motor hyperactivity and aggression. A naturalistic study of diet in hyperactive children found high correlations between sugar intake and both motor activity and aggression.[79] Under double-blind conditions, both sucrose and fructose produced a significant increase in motor activity and inappropriate behavior when compared with an aspartame placebo.[22] Low dietary sugar is much easier to maintain than restrictive nonadditive diets, and may be a useful adjunct to standard behavioral and pharmacologic therapy in some cases. Neither nonadditive nor low-sugar diets are known to have any adverse side effects.

Failure to consume an adequate breakfast produces a well-studied impairment in children's attention and school performance.[22] However, this effect is by no means exclusive to children with ADHD. Rather, adequate morning calorie intake should be considered an essential part of mental hygiene, and is especially vital for children with ADHD.

Substance Abuse

A unique variant of nutritional therapy has been developed as an adjunct to alcohol and drug treatment. Supplemental amino acids (phenylalanine, glutamine, tryptophan, and pyridoxal) are postulated by one research group to enhance neurotransmitter repletion and are reported to reduce depressive symptoms, tremors, and requests for benzodiazepines in subjects undergoing rehabilitation.[12–14] Although these effects have been tested in double-blind, placebo-controlled designs, no effect on relapse rate after rehabilitation has been demonstrated. Since relapse is the most important outcome measure in substance-abuse treatment, this treatment must be considered experimental. No studies on adolescents or children are available. See Chapter 14 for further information on the treatment of substance abuse in children and adolescents.

High-Dose Vitamin Therapy

Vitamins have been used at pharmacologic doses to treat all manner of disease, sometimes with severe adverse consequences. There is no doubt that vitamins are psychoactive. Pyroxidine (B_6) toxicity, for example, is associated with severe neurologic impairment. Deficiencies of B_6 and niacin produce neuropsychiatric symptoms, including nerve degeneration, seizures, delirium, and psychosis.[62] On the other hand, studies that examined nutritional status in childhood psychiatric disorders did not find direct relationships with vitamin deficiencies.[87]

405

The prescription of vitamins at pharmacologic doses (megavitamin or ortho-molecular therapy) is a strategy that has received a great deal of attention in the popular press since the early 1970s. Linus Pauling has served as one highly visible proponent for the use of high-dose vitamin C in viral infections,[76] hepatitis,[73] psychiatric disorders,[72,74,75] cancer,[71] and AIDS.[37] In psychiatry the main areas of interest have been the treatment of ADHD, schizophrenia, and autism. There is no evidence that high-dose vitamin therapy is effective in these psychiatric disorders, but the attention paid to it in the lay press, the ready availability of vitamins for self-medication, and their potential toxicity make it important for the practitioner to be well informed.

Indications

Attention-Deficit Hyperactivity Disorder

High doses of vitamin A and other vitamins have been proposed for the treatment of ADHD. Few controlled studies are available that both standardize pretreatment diagnosis and use objective outcome measures. However, two well-designed and controlled trials with a cumulative sample of 72 hyperactive children showed no improvement based on objective outcome measures.[4,39] On the contrary, there was a statistically significant 25% *increase* in disruptive classroom behavior in children treated with a combination of vitamin B_6, vitamin C, niacin, and calcium pantothenate.[39] Severe toxicity to vitamin A has been reported in children treated for ADHD.[86] In their recent review of 53 trials of megavitamin therapy, Kleijnen and Knipschild[53] concluded that there was no evidence for a therapeutic effect of B_6 in ADHD, or at least not sufficient evidence to warrant the risk of toxicity.

Schizophrenia

A theoretical vitamin regimen was proposed for the treatment of schizophrenia in one of the first applications of orthopsychiatric methods.[6,74] The use of high-dose niacin and B_6 was vigorously tested between 1955[67] and 1977,[27] and case reports of the success of B_6 and B_{12} in both adult and child schizophrenics have appeared.[15,25,100] Again, in a broad review of all controlled trials, Kleijnen and Knipschild[53] found no evidence for the efficacy of vitamin therapy in schizophrenia. No study since 1970 has shown a significantly positive result, and no study with a follow-up longer than three months has ever shown such a result. There is stronger support for including folate at physiologic doses when red cell folate is demonstrated to be low or marginal.[34] However, this must be considered an appropriate correction of a vitamin deficiency, rather than an independent treatment.

Fragile X Syndrome

Unlike the other megavitamin therapies, there is some heuristic support for the treatment of the fragile X syndrome with folic acid. The fragile X defect is revealed in vitro in chromosomes cultured in a folate-free medium, and the percentage of cultured cells expressing the fragile X site may be reduced by folate enrichment.[33] Sporadic reports of improved mentation or behavior were followed by a number of controlled studies that showed no significant group effect.[16,33,36,59] When Fisch and colleagues[32] used non–fragile X control subjects, there was no difference in behavior on folic acid. The positive results, therefore, may be attributed to nonblind, noncontrolled study designs.

Autism

Rimland and associates[80] conducted the first controlled study of B_6 in autism, after successful case reports had appeared. They reported statistically significant improvement in the behavioral measures of 15 children on 3 g/day of pyridoxine. However, this study has been criticized on the grounds that few of the children studied met the research criteria for autism and that the sample was preselected for sensitivity to vitamins.[65] The only other controlled trial available in the English-language literature found no effect.[60]

Mental Retardation

Reports of increased IQ scores after vitamin supplementation generated an enthusiastic response from the media 10 to 15 years ago. One double-blind trial on a group of 16 mentally retarded children (IQ range 17–70) treated with four months of broad vitamin supplementation reported a mean IQ gain of 10 points.[38] The researchers also noted improved visual acuity and increased growth rates in two children. However, several methodologic problems with this study cannot be overlooked. First, since vitamins were used at physiologic rather than pharmacologic doses and the children's nutritional status was not assessed prior to treatment, it seems likely that some improvements were due to the correction of nutritional rather than intellectual deficiencies. This is suggested by the increased growth rate. More important, IQ tests are not designed to be dynamic measures of intellectual ability. Retesting within one year, in fact, may elevate scores owing to a practice effect, even if a different test is used.

A later open trial of broad vitamin supplementation in young adults with mental retardation and Down's syndrome produced no effect.[21] High-dose vitamin therapy was tested in a double-blind, placebo-controlled trial of 56 mentally retarded children with Down's syndrome and showed no demonstrable effect on several measures of intelligence.[89] Kleijnen and

Knipschild[53] found no support for a direct effect of orthomolecular therapy on intelligence in a review of all published trials.

Thyroid Hormone Treatment

Thyroid hormone and analogues have been tried at physiologic or supraphysiologic doses for unipolar depression, bipolar affective disorder, and autism with mixed results. Experimental validation of this treatment is complicated by the immediate, stimulatory effects of iatrogenic hyperthyroid states. For this reason, the evaluation of successful reports must pay particular attention to the length of follow-up and the appropriateness of the outcome measures.

Indications

Unipolar Depression
One of the first well-controlled studies of thyroid-releasing hormone (TRH) examined its effect in nonendogenous depression[52] and found it to be countertherapeutic. An open Japanese trial of T4 in 20 subjects with major depression indicated extreme variability in response, from marked improvement to mild worsening.[68] Based on these and similar studies, thyroid analogues are probably not an effective treatment for depression when prescribed alone.[92]

In contrast, triiodothyronine (T3) effectively augmented TCA response in a double-blind study of 12 cases of adult major depression.[35] Improvement was independent of changes in the plasma level of the TCA (mean = 252.5 mg/ml), and each subject had been treated with imipramine or amitriptyline for at least three weeks prior to the addition of T3. In a one-month follow-up period, most subjects had a statistically significant improvement on a global depression scale, although only four of the 12 had a change of three points or more, which the authors considered clinically significant.[35] Most controlled studies of T3 as an adjunct to TCAs are similarly positive.[92] In their review of thyroid hormone treatment in tricyclic nonresponders, Extein and Gold[29] estimate that 50% of patients will improve on 25 µg of T3 per day. This is a physiologic dose of thyroid hormone, so it is not associated with serious side effects and does not significantly suppress thyroid gland function. A recent comparison indicated that T3 may be marginally superior to T4 for tricyclic augmentation.[43]

No well-controlled studies are available on children, although the adult studies are promising. The low incidence of side effects and the high frequency of tricyclic-resistant depression in children and adolescents make the evaluation of thyroid analogues in childhood depression a high priority for future research. This strategy cannot be currently recommended for euthyroid children and adolescents, since the effects of prolonged T3 use in this age group are unknown. However, prolonged therapy may not be necessary, as several authors note that thyroid may be discontinued after several weeks without a loss of effect.[92]

Bipolar Affective Disorder

After several successful case series,[91,92] one controlled trial of supraphysiologic thyroxine in rapid-cycling bipolar disorder has appeared. Bauer and Whybrow[8] examined 11 subjects in an open trial and found an improvement in 10 of them. A subsequent double-blind, placebo-controlled crossover study of four of the responders confirmed the benefit, although half of the original 10 responders relapsed eventually. Although promising, only four patients were studied in a controlled design. Furthermore, the use of supraphysiologic doses of thyroxine probably increases the chance of undesirable side effects. Much more research is needed before this becomes an accepted practice and before it is attempted in youngsters.

Autism

Studies of thyroid status in autistic individuals have not yielded any durable abnormalities.[1] However, controlled trials of thyroid analogues have been conducted. Campbell and associates[19] administered T3 to 30 nondepressed autistic children and found no benefit as compared with placebo.

Down's Syndrome

An increased incidence of subclinical TSH elevation and a correlation with global level of function has been reported in patients with Down's syndrome.[11] However, Tirosh and associates[97] tested thyroid supplementation in a group of 44 Down's syndrome patients with borderline thyroid status under double-blind, placebo-controlled conditions and found no clinical benefit.

Conclusions

Countless nontraditional therapeutic agents have been tried for child and adolescent psychiatric disorders. Of those that have been subjected to experimental scrutiny, only two remain promising: opiate antagonists for the treatment of autistic disorder and self-injurious behavior, and thyroid analogues as adjuncts to antidepressants. Opiate antagonists are acceptable for limited clinical use because of their success in limited studies and the very low incidence of adverse effects. However, the positive results of thyroid analogues must be viewed with care. Nearly all successful trials have been carried out in severe refractory cases, and trials of thyroid analogues as a primary treatment for depression have been largely unsuccessful. Furthermore, the long-term effects of prescribing thyroid to euthyroid children and adolescents are unknown, and could adversely affect growth and intellectual development, particularly in prepubertal children. Therefore, the clinical use of thyroid analogues for children cannot be recommended.

Paradoxically, nutritional and vitamin therapies have been passionately supported in the popular press, despite disappointing research findings. Nutritional studies have demonstrated the beneficial effect of limiting refined sugars and providing adequate morning calories on the behavior and attention of schoolchildren, but these measures should be considered matters of standard hygiene for all children. They do not afford a treatment for any specific psychiatric disorder. The most effective nonpharmacologic ways of treating child and adolescent emotional illness are not simple cures, but involve comprehensive behavioral programming, lavish social support services, and effective psychotherapy.

References

1. Abbassi, V., Linscheid, T., Coleman, M. (1978). Triiodothyronine (T3) concentration and therapy in autistic children. *J Autism Child Schizophr, 8(4)*, 383–387.

2. Alexander, F.G., Selesnick, S.T. (1966). *The History of Psychiatry* (p. 285). New York: Harper & Row.

3. Alger, S.A., Schwalberg, M.D., Bigaouette, J.M., et al. (1991). Effect of a tricyclic antidepressant and opiate antagonist on binge-eating behavior in normoweight bulimic and obese, binge-eating subjects. *Am J Clin Nutr, 53(4)*, 865–871.

4. Arnold, L.E., Christopher, J., Huestis, R.D., Smeltzer, D.J. (1978). Megavitamins for minimal brain dysfunction. A placebo-controlled study. *JAMA, 240(24)*, 2642–2643.

5. Atkinson, R.L., Berke, L.K., Drake, C.R., et al. (1985). Effects of long-term therapy with naltrexone on body weight in obesity. *Clin Pharmacol Ther, 38(4)*, 419–422.

6. Ban, T.A., Lehmann, H.E., Deutsch, M. (1977). Negative findings with megavitamins in schizophrenic patients: Preliminary report. *Commun Psychopharmacol, 1(2)*, 119–122.

7. Barrett, R.P., Feinstein, C., Hole, W.T. (1989). Effects of naloxone and naltrexone on self-injury: A double-blind, placebo-controlled analysis. *Am J Ment Retard, 93(6)*, 644–651.

8. Bauer, M.S., Whybrow, P.C. (1990). Rapid cycling bipolar affective disorder. II. Treatment of refractory rapid cycling with high-dose levothyroxine: A preliminary study. *Arch Gen Psychiatry, 47(5)*, 435–440.

9. Beckwith, B.E., Couk, D.I., Schumacher, K. (1986). Failure of naloxone to reduce self-injurious behavior in two developmentally disabled females. *Appl Res Ment Retard, 7(2)*, 183–188.

10. Bernstein, G.A., Hughes, J.R., Mitchell, J.E., Thompson, T. (1987). Effects of narcotic antagonists on self-injurious behavior: A single case study. *J Am Acad Child Adolesc Psychiatry, 26(6)*, 886–889.

11. Bhaumik, S., Collacott, R.A., Garrick, P., Mitchell, C. (1991). Effect of thyroid stimulating hormone on adaptive behaviour in Down's syndrome. *J Ment Defic Res, 35(6)*, 512–520.

12. Biery, J.R., Williford, J.H., Jr., McMullen, E.A. (1991). Alcohol craving in rehabilitation: Assessment of nutrition therapy. *J Am Diet Assoc, 91(4)*, 463–466.

13. Blum, K., Trachtenberg, M.C., Elliott, C.E., et al. (1988). Enkephalinase inhibition and precursor amino acid loading improves inpatient treatment of alcohol and polydrug abusers: Double-blind placebo-controlled study of the nutritional adjunct SAAVE. *Alcohol, 5(6)*, 481–493.

14. Blum, K., Trachtenberg, M.C., Ramsay, J.C. (1988). Improvement of inpatient treatment of the alcoholic as a function of neurotransmitter restoration: A pilot study. *Int J Addict, 23(9)*, 991–998.

15. Brooks, S.C., D'Angelo, L., Chalmeta, A., et al. (1983). An unusual schizophrenic illness responsive to pyridoxine HCI (B6) subsequent to phenothiazine and butyrophenone toxicities. *Biol Psychiatry, 18(11)*, 1321–1328.

16. Brown, W.T., Cohen, I.L., Fisch, G.S., et al. (1986). High dose folic acid treatment of fragile (X) males. *Am J Med Genet, 23(1–2)*, 263–271.

17. Campbell, M., Anderson, L.T., Small, A.M., et al. (1990). Naltrexone in autistic children: A double-blind and placebo-controlled study. *Psychopharmacol Bull, 26(1)*, 130–135.

18. Campbell, M., Overall, J.E., Small, A.M., et al., (1989). Naltrexone in autistic children: An acute open dose range tolerance trial. *J Am Acad Child Adolesc Psychiatry, 28(2)*, 200–206.

19. Campbell, M., Small, A.M., Hollander, C.S., et al. (1978). A controlled crossover study of triiodothyronine in autistic children. *J Autism Child Schizophr 8(4)*, 371–381.

20. Campbell, M., Adams, P., Small, A.M., et al. (1988). Naltrexone in infantile autism. *Psychopharmacol Bull, 24(1)*, 135–139.

21. Coburn, S.P., Schaltenbrand, W.E., Mahuren, J.D., et al. (1983). Effect of megavitamin treatment on mental performance and plasma vitamin B6 con-

411

centrations in mentally retarded young adults. *Am J Clin Nutr, 38(3)*, 352–355.

22. Conners, C.K., Blouin, A.G. (1982–1983). Nutritional effects on behavior of children. *J Psychiatr Res, 17(2)*, 193–201.

23. Cronin, G.M., Wiepkema, P.R., van Ree, J.M. (1985). Endogenous opioids are involved in abnormal sterotyped behaviors of tethered sows. *Neuropeptides, 6(6)*, 527–530.

24. Davidson, P.W., Kleene, B.M., Carroll, M., Rockowitz, R.J. (1983). Effects of naloxone on self-injurious behavior: A case study. *Appl Res Ment Retard, 4(1)*, 1–4.

25. Denson, R. (1976). Vitamin B$_{12}$ in late-onset psychosis of childhood. *Can Med Assoc J, 114(2)*, 113.

26. Deutsch, S.I. (1986). Rationale for the administration of opiate antagonists in treating infantile autism. *Am J Ment Defic, 90(6)*, 631–635.

27. Deutsch, M., Ananth, J.V., Ban, T.A. (1977). Nicotinic acid in the treatment of chronic hospitalized schizophrenic patients: A placebo controlled clinical study. *Psychopharmacol Bull, 13*, 21–23.

28. Drewnowski, A., Krahn, D.D., Demitrack, M.A., et al. (1992). Taste responses and preferences for sweet high-fat foods: Evidence for opioid involvement. *Physiol Behav, 51(2)*, 371–379.

29. Extein, I.L., Gold, M.S. (1988). Thyroid hormone potentiation of tricyclics. *Psychosomatics, 29(2)*, 166–174.

30. Feingold, B.F. (1975). *Why Your Child Is Hyperactive*. New York: Random House.

31. Feingold, B.F. (1973). *Introduction to Clinical Allergy*. Springfield, Ill: Charles C Thomas.

32. Fisch, G.S., Cohen, I.L., Gross, A.C., et al. (1988). Folic acid treatment of fragile X males: A further study. *Am J Med Genet, 30(1–2)*, 393–399.

33. Gillberg, C., Wahlstrom, J., Johansson, R., et al. (1986). Folic acid as an adjunct in the treatment of children with the autism fragile-X syndrome (AFRAX). *Dev Med Child Neurol, 28(5)*, 624–627.

34. Godfrey, P.S., Toone, B.K., Carney, M.W., et al. (1990). Enhancement of recovery from psychiatric illness by methylfolate. *Lancet, 336(8712)*, 392–395.

35. Goodwin, F.K., Prange, A.J., Jr., Post, R.M., et al. (1982). Potentiation of antidepressant effects by L-triiodothyronine in tricyclic nonresponders. *Am J Psychiatry, 139(1)*, 34–38.

36. Hagerman, R.J., Jackson, A.W., Levitas, A., et al. (1986). Oral folic acid versus placebo in the treatment of males with the fragile X syndrome. *Am J Med Genet, 23(1–2)*, 241–262.

37. Harakeh, S., Jariwalla, R.J., Pauling, L. (1990). Suppression of human immunodeficiency virus replication by ascorbate in chronically and acutely infected cells. *Proc Nat Acad Sci USA, 87(18)*, 7245–7249.

38. Harrell, R.F., Capp, R.H., Davis, D.R., et al. (1981). Can nutritional supplements help mentally retarded children? An exploratory study. *Proc Nat Acad Sci USA, 78(1)*, 574–578.

39. Haslam, R.H., Dalby, J.T., Rademaker, A.W. (1984). Effects of megavitamin therapy on children with attention deficit disorders. *Pediatrics, 74(1)*, 103–111.

40. Herman, B.H., Hammock, M.K., Arthur-Smith, A., et al. (1987). Naltrexone decreases self-injurious behavior. *Ann Neurol, 22(4)*, 550–552.

41. Herman, B.H., Hammock, M.K., Arthur-Smith, A., et al. (1989). Effects of acute administration of naltrexone on cardiovascular function, body temperature, body weight and serum concentrations of liver enzymes in autistic children. *Dev Pharmacol Ther, 12(3)*, 118–127.

42. Herman, B.H., Panksepp, J. (1978). Effects of morphine and naloxone on separation distress and approach attachment: Evidence for opiate mediation of social affect. *Pharmacol Biochem Behav, 9(2)*, 213–220.

43. Joffe, R.T., Singer, W. (1990). A comparison of triiodothyronine and thyroxine in the potentiation of tricyclic antidepressants. *Psychiatry Res, 32(3)*, 241–251.

44. Jonas, J.M., Gold, M.S. (1987). Naltrexone treatment of bulimia: Clinical and theoretical findings linking eating disorders and substance abuse. *Adv Alcohol Substance Abuse, 7(1)*, 29–37.

45. Jonas, J.M., Gold, M.S. (1986–1987). Treatment of antidepressant-resistant bulimia with naltrexone. *Int J Psychiatry Med, 16(4)*, 305–309.

46. Jonas, J.M., Gold, M.S. (1988). The use of opiate antagonists in treating bulimia: A study of low-dose versus high-dose naltrexone. *Psychiatry Res, 24(2)*, 195–199.

47. Kalat, J.W. (1978). Speculations on similarities between autism and opiate addiction. *J Autism Child Schizophren, 8(4)*, 477–479.

48. Kaplan, B.J., McNicol, J., Conte, R.A., Moghadam, H.K. (1989). Dietary replacement in preschool-aged hyperactive boys. *Pediatrics, 83(1)*, 7–17.

49. Kaplan, B.J., McNicol, J., Conte, R.A., Moghadam, H.K. (1989). Overall nutrient intake of preschool hyperactive and normal boys. *J Abnorm Child Psychol, 17(2)*, 127–132.

50. Kars, H., Broekema, W., Glaudemans-van Gelderen, I., et al. (1990). Naltrexone attenuates self-injurious behavior in mentally retarded subjects. *Biol Psychiatry, 27(7)*, 741–746.

51. Kavale, K.A., Forness, S.R. (1983). Hyperactivity and diet treatment: A meta-analysis of the Feingold hypothesis. *J Learning Disabilities, 16*, 324–330.

52. Kiely, W.F., Adrian, A.D., Lee, J.H., Nicoloff, J.T. (1976). Therapeutic failure of oral thyrotropin-releasing hormone in depression. *Psychosom Med, 38(4)*, 233–241.

53. Kleijnen, J., Knipschild, P. (1991). Niacin and vitamin B6 in mental functioning: A review of controlled trials in humans. *Biol Psychiatry, 29(9)*, 931–941.

54. Knabe, R., Schulz, P., Richard, J. (1990). Initial aggravation of self-injurious behavior in autistic patients receiving naltrexone treatment. *J Autism Dev Disord, 20(4)*, 591–593.

55. Kyriakides, M., Silverstone, T., Jeffcoate, W., Laurance, B. (1980). Effect of naloxone on hyperphagia in Prader-Willi syndrome. *Lancet, 1(8173)*, 876–877.

56. Landauer, M.R., Balster, R.L. (1982). Opiate effects on social investigatory behavior in male mice. *Pharmacol Biochem Behav, 17(6)*, 1181–1186.

57. Leboyer, M., Bouvard, M.P., Launay, J.M., et al. (1992). Brief report: A double-blind study of naltrexone in infantile autism. *J Autism Dev Disord, 22(2)*, 309–319.

58. Lynch, W.C., Libby, L., Johnson, H.F. (1983). Naloxone inhibits intermale aggression in isolated mice. *Psychopharmacology, 79(4)*, 370–371.

59. Madison, L.S., Wells, T.E., Fristo, T.E., Benesch, C.G. (1986). A controlled study of folic acid treatment in three fragile X syndrome males. *J Dev Behav Pediat, 7(4)*, 253–256.

60. Martineau, J., Barthelemy, C., Garreau, B., Lelord, G. (1985). Vitamin B_6, magnesium, and combined B_6-Mg: Therapeutic effects in childhood autism. *Biol Psychiatry, 20*, 467–478.

61. Mattes, J.A. (1983). The Feingold diet: A current reappraisal. *J Learning Disabilities, 16*, 319–323.

62. Menolascino, F.J., Donaldson, J.Y., Gallagher, T.F., et al. (1988). Ortho-molecular therapy: Its history and applicability to psychiatric disorders. *Child Psychiatry Hum Dev, 18(3)*, 133–150.

63. Mitchell, J.E., Morley, J.E., Levine, A.S., et al. (1987). High-dose naltrex-one therapy and dietary counseling for obesity. *Bio Psychiatry, 22(1)*, 35–42.

64. Mitchell, J.E., Christenson, G., Jennings, J., et al. (1989). A placebo-con-trolled, double-blind crossover study of naltrexone hydrochloride in outpa-tients with normal weight bulimia. *J Clin Psychopharmacol, 9(2)*, 94–97.

65. Moss, N., Boverman, H. (1978). Megavitamin therapy for autistic chil-dren. *Am J Psychiatry, 135(11)*, 1425–1426.

66. O'Brien, C.P., Stunkard, A.J., Ternes, J.W. (1982). Absence of naloxone sensitivity in obese humans. *Psychosom Med, 44(2)*, 215–223.

67. O'Reilly, P.O. (1955). Nicotinic acid therapy and the chronic schizo-phrenic. *Dis Nerv Sys, 16*, 67–72.

68. Okuno, Y., Nakayasu, N. (1988). Thyroid function and therapeutic effi-cacy of thyroxine in depression. *Jpn J Psychiatry Neurol, 42(4)*, 763–770.

69. Panksepp, J., Lensing, P. (1991). Brief report: A synopsis of an open-trial of naltrexone treatment of autism with four children. *J Autism Dev Disord, 21(2)*, 243–249.

70. Panksepp, J., Herman, B.H., Vilberg, T., et al. (1980). Endogenous opi-oids and social behavior: *Neurosci Biobehav Rev, 4(4)*, 473–487.

71. Pauling, L., Moertel, C.A. (1986). Proposition: Megadoses of vitamin C are valuable in the treatment of cancer. *Nutr Rev, 44(1)*, 28–32.

72. Pauling, L. (1979). Dietary influences on the synthesis of neurotransmit-ters in the brain. *Nutr Rev, 37(9)*, 302–304.

73. Pauling, L. (1981). Vitamin C prophylaxis for posttransfusion hepatitis. *Am J Clin Nutr, 34(9)*, 1978–1980.

74. Pauling, L., Wyatt, R.J., Klein, D.F., Lipton, M.A. (1974). On the ortho-molecular environment of the mind: Orthomolecular theory. *Am J Psychia-try, 131(11)*, 1251–1267.

75. Pauling, L. (1979). Treating mental disorders. *Science, 206(4417)*, 404.

76. Pauling, L. (1973). Ascorbic acid and the common cold. *Scott Med J, 18(1)*, 1–2.

77. *Physicians' Desk Reference* (47th ed.) (1993). Montvale, N.J.: Medical Eco-nomics.

78. *Prescription Pricing Guide.* (1992). Indianapolis: Medi-Span.

79. Prinz, R.J., Roberts, W.A., Hartman, E. (1980). Dietary correlates of hyperactive behavior in children. *J Consult Clin Psychol, 48,* 760–769.

80. Rimland, B., Callaway, E., Dreyfus, P. (1978). The effect of high doses of vitamin B_6 on autistic children: A double-blind crossover study. *Am J Psychiatry, 135,* 472–475.

81. Rowe, K.S. (1988). Synthetic food colourings and "hyperactivity": A double-blind crossover study. *Aust Paediatr J, 24(2),* 143–147.

82. Sahley, T.L., Panksepp, J. (1987). Brain opioids and autism: An updated analysis of possible linkages. *J Autism Dev Disord, 17(2),* 201–216.

83. Sandman, C.A., Datta, P.C., Barron, J., et al. (1983). Naloxone attenuates self-abusive behavior in developmentally disabled clients. *Appl Res Ment Retard, 4(1),* 5–11.

84. Sandman, C.A., Barron, J.L., Colman, H. (1990). An orally administered opiate blocker, naltrexone, attenuates self-injurious behavior. *Am J Ment Retard, 95(1),* 93–102.

85. Sandman, C.A., Barron, J.L., Crinella, F.M., Donnelly, J.F. (1987). Influence of naloxone on brain and behavior of a self-injurious woman. *Biol Psychiatry, 22(7),* 899–906.

86. Shaywitz, B.A., Siegel, N.J., Pearson, H.A. (1977). Megavitamins for minimal brain dysfunction. A potentially dangerous therapy. *JAMA, 238(16),* 1749–1750.

87. Siva Sankar, D.V. (1979). Plasma levels of folates, riboflavin, vitamin B6, and ascorbate in severely disturbed children. *J Autism Dev Disord, 9(1),* 73–82.

88. Skorupska, M., Langwinski, R. (1989). Some central effects of opioid antagonists. Part 1. *Pol J Pharmacol Pharm, 41(5),* 401–411.

89. Smith, G.F., Spiker, D., Peterson, C.P., et al. (1984). Use of megadoses of vitamins with minerals in Down syndrome. *J Pediatr 105(2),* 228–234.

90. Spiegel, T.A., Stunkard, A.J., Shrager, E.E., et al. (1987). Effect of naltrexone on food intake, hunger, and satiety in obese men. *Physiol Behav, 40(2),* 135–141.

91. Stancer, H.C., Persad, E. (1982). Treatment of intractable rapid-cycling manic-depressive disorder with levothyroxine. Clinical observations. *Arch Gen Psychiatry, 39(3),* 311–312.

92. Stein, D., Avni, J. (1988). Thyroid hormones in the treatment of affective disorders. *Acta Psychiatr Scand, 77(6),* 623–636.

93. Sternbach, H.A., Annitto, W., Pottash, A.L., Gold, M.S. (1982). Anorexic effects of naltrexone in man. *Lancet, 1(8268)*, 388–389.

94. Szymanski, L., Kedesdy, J., Sulkes, S., et al. (1987). Naltrexone in treatment of self injurious behavior: A clinical study. *Res Dev Disabilities, 8(2)*, 179–190.

95. Taylor, D.V., Hetrick, W.P., Neri, C.L., et al. (1991). Effect of naltrexone upon self-injurious behavior, learning and activity: A case study. *Pharmacol Biochem Behav, 40(1)*, 79–82.

96. Thompson, T., Schuster, C.R. (1968). *Behavioral Pharmacology* (pp. 48–51). Englewood Cliffs, N.J.: Prentice-Hall.

97. Tirosh, E., Taub, Y., Scher, A., et al. (1989). Short-term efficacy of thyroid hormone supplementation for patients with Down syndrome and low-borderline thyroid function. *Am J Ment Retard, 93(6)*, 652–656.

98. Walters, A.S., Barrett, R.P., Feinstein, C., et al. (1990). A case report of naltrexone treatment of self-injury and social withdrawal in autism. *J Autism Dev Disord, 20(2)*, 169–176.

99. Zipf, W.B., Berntson, G.G. (1987). Characteristics of abnormal food-intake patterns in children with Prader-Willi syndrome and study of effects of naloxone. *Am J Clin Nutr, 46(2)*, 277–281.

100. Zucker, D.K., Livingston, R.L., Nakra, R., Clayton, P.J. (1981). B12 deficiency and psychiatric disorders: Case report and literature review. *Biol Psychiatry, 16(2)*, 197–205.

Chapter 13

Consultation–Liaison Psychiatry–Pharmacologic Approaches

Child and adolescent psychiatrists are playing an increasingly important role on consultation–liaison services. Psychiatrists are often consulted on and participate in the treatment and management of children and adolescents who might not otherwise have access to psychiatric care. Important developments in child and adolescent consultation–liaison psychiatry in the medical and surgical setting have led to an expanded role for the psychiatric practitioner in the management and care of this population. Currently, there is a paucity of literature on child and adolescent consultation psychiatry. This is especially true with regard to psychopharmacologic interventions in the consultation–liaison setting. The American Psychiatric Press's *Review of Psychiatry*[1] contains an excellent, well-written and well-researched section on consultation–liaison psychiatry discussing the current state of scientific and clinical knowledge for adult consultation-liaison psychiatry. We refer the reader to this excellent source, and advocate the need for a similar manual for child and adolescent consultation–liaison psychiatry.

We will address the following areas that we believe to be especially relevant to the child and adolescent psychiatrist in the medical and surgical setting: (1) psychiatric consultation to neurology, (2) psychiatric consultation to pediatrics, (3) psychiatric consultation to oncology, (4) psychiatric consultation to organ transplant services, and (5) psychiatric consultation to obstetrics and gynecology.

Psychiatric Consultation to Neurology

Neurologic conditions are associated with a high prevalence of psychiatric dysfunction. Epilepsy, one of the most common chronic illnesses of childhood, has a very high prevalence of associated psychiatric dysfunction.[2,3] Other neurologic disorders necessitating psychiatric consultation include patients who, after brain trauma, develop aggressive, disruptive, and/or depressed behavior.[1] Some patients have exacerbations or recurrences of psychiatric symptoms.[1] It is often difficult to discern whether the condition is attributable to an emotional reaction, is caused by neurologic disability, is directly due to the neurologic pathology, or results from a combination of all three.[4] There are other patients in whom neurologic and physical examination fails to find an organic basis for the symptoms, and the psychiatrist is called in to determine whether there is a psychogenic cause, that is, a somatization disorder, conversion disorder, or the like.[1] On the other hand, in some cases, emotional disturbances exacerbate the preexisting neurologic condition. Consultation is often required to evaluate altered states of consciousness, alertness, perception, language, and memory, such as delirium and Down's syndrome (or other cases of mental retardation).

Epilepsy

In the Isle of Wight study, the rate of psychiatric disorder was higher among epileptic children than in healthy controls or in children with other chronic illnesses.[5] It also appears that epileptic patients have a distinctive personality profile. Bear and Fedio[6] found that patients with temporal lobe epilepsy (TLE) had distinctive features of behavior, emotion, and thought (Table 13-1).

Organic Personality Disorder

Garyfallos and colleagues[7] noted that organic personality disorder occurred in 20% of TLE patients as opposed to 0% in patients with non-TLE. Predictors of the development of organic personality disorder were an early age of onset of epilepsy and protracted course of the illness.

419

Table 13-1
Personality Profile of Temporal Lobe Epilepsy Patients

Behaviors	*Thought*	*Mood*
• Obsessionalism	• Philosophical	• Mood swings
• Circumstantiality	• Religious	• Anger
• Hypergraphia	• Humorlessness	• Sadness
• Dependence		

Source: Bear, D.M., Fedio, P. (1977). Quantitative analysis of interictal behavior in temporal lobe epilepsy. *Arch Neurol, 34,* 454–467.

Mood Disorders and Suicide

The association of epilepsy, particularly TLE, with mood disorders has been well documented. Flor-Henry[8] found that bipolar disorder symptoms are associated with right TLE. Mendez and colleagues[9] found that 30% of epileptics had attempted suicide, with the suicide rate for epileptics believed to be about four times that of the general population.[10] Brent[11] found an overrepresentation of epileptics in a consecutive series of suicide attempters seen at the Children's Hospital of Pittsburgh, 1978–1983.[11] Out of 131 consecutive suicide attempts, nine of the patients were epileptic, which is 15 times more frequent than would be expected, given the prevalence of epilepsy in school-age children. Epileptic attempters made more medically serious attempts, had more premeditation prior to the attempt, and had a higher suicide intent before and after the attempt than did nonepileptic attempters. This confirmed two earlier studies that reported an increased suicide rate for children with epilepsy as compared with nonepileptic children.[12,13] Brent[11] also found that eight of the nine epileptic suicide attempters had been treated with phenobarbital, and hypothesized a possible relationship between phenobarbital usage and suicidal behavior. This view, that a portion of the psychiatric morbidity in childhood epilepsy may be due to the effects of antiepileptic medications, has only recently begun to receive close attention.[14–17]

Phenobarbital-Induced Psychiatric Dysfunction

Brent and colleagues[18] assessed the prevalence and severity of psychopathology in 15 epileptic children treated with phenobarbital and 24 patients treated with carbamazepine. The groups were carefully matched across a wide range of demographic, seizure-related, and family-environmental variables. Those patients treated with phenobarbital as compared with carbamazepine showed a significantly higher prevalence of major depressive disorder (40% versus 4%) and suicidal ideation (47% versus 4%). The differential prevalence of depression between the two groups was only noted in patients with a family history of mood disorder among first-degree relatives. The authors recommended closely monitoring patients treated with phenobarbital for depression and suicidal ideation. Alternative treatment (i.e., carbamazepine) was advocated for patients with newly diagnosed epilepsy and a personal or family history of mood disorder.

Treatment of children and adolescents with phenobarbital has been associated with an increased risk of psychological disturbances in addition to depression and suicidal ideation, including hyperactivity, irritability, sleep difficulties, poor self-esteem, mood fluctuations, neurotic symptoms, and conduct problems[19–25] (see "Psychiatric Effects of Anticonvulsants"). This causal relationship between phenobarbital and psychiatric difficulties is in part supported by the improvements in mood and concentration seen following the substitution of carbamazepine for phenobarbital in an open clinical trial.[24]

Case History

A 14-year-old boy, following an orthotopic liver transplant, was referred to child and adolescent psychiatry to evaluate him for possible depression. The patient had no past psychiatric history, but three days prior to the psychiatric consultation, had appeared more sluggish and lethargic, and, according to the nursing staff, had "less get up and go." His sleep and appetite were also recorded as being abnormal. His mother confirmed that he appeared more "worn out." She also told the psychiatrist that on the previous day her son had not recognized her and had seemed "really out of it." The patient admitted to having less energy because of his surgery, but denied suicidal ideation. No psychotic symptoms were endorsed. There was no history of drug or alcohol use or abuse. He had been observed to be anxious and was receiving lorazepam 2 mg every six hours for anxiety. For his insomnia, he was receiving triazolam 0.125 mg q.h.s. In addition, he was on high-dose steroids (prednisone and cyclosporine) to prevent rejection of his liver. For pain, he was receiving morphine. Cyclosporine levels were reported as being within the therapeutic range. On mental status examination, he was observed to alternate between being alert and responsive to questions and periods of five to 15 minutes during which he was unable to respond appropriately to questions, had difficulty attending to the conversation, and on two occasions spoke to a friend from school who was not present in the room. On another occasion, he asked his grandmother, who had died three years earlier, for something to drink. He did not appear to be depressed or unduly anxious. On formal testing of his cognition and sensorium, he was unable to perform serial 7s or 3s, and was only able to count back to 17 from 20 before making errors. On immediate recall, he repeated one of three objects on his first effort and two of three on his second effort. After five minutes, he was unable to recall any of the three objects. He was unable to name the hospital where he was staying or the year, although he did know his name and the city where the hospital was located. He was unable to connect several numbered dots drawn out for him.

The boy was diagnosed as having a delirium secondary to recent surgery and/or a current medication regimen that was likely impairing cognition (i.e., steroids, benzodiazepines, pain medications, and cyclosporine). Computed tomography of the head was entirely normal, as was CSF analysis. An EEG slowing with a grade II dysrhythmia was observed, which helped to confirm the diagnosis of delirium. The triazolam was discontinued and the lorazepam was tapered and discontinued since benzodiazepines can impair cognition in vulnerable patients. In addition, prednisone dosing was carefully monitored, as was the dispensing of pain medications. The nurses were alerted to perform frequent "reality checks" to determine the patient's state of awareness. They would quiz him on time, place, name, and other current topics several times during the day and evening. Upon discontinuation of the lorazepam, the patient appeared noticeably more anxious, particularly before procedures. However, just being in the hospital frightened him and he admitted to being afraid that he was going to die. Since his mental status had improved to baseline with the aforementioned interventions, and because of lorazepam's potential for exacerbating the patient's cognitive function, lorazepam therapy was not reinitiated to treat his anxiety. Relaxation training methods, including daily 20-minute back massages, listening to relaxation training tapes, and instruction in breathing techniques to reduce anxiety, were commenced. Unfortunately, these behavioral interventions were only minimally effective. A trial of buspirone was then initiated. The patient was started on buspirone 10 mg b.i.d. This dose was subsequently increased to 10 mg t.i.d., which resulted in a moderate amelioration of the patient's anxiety symptoms.

Panic Attacks

Epileptic patients may have panic attacks that often prove difficult to delineate from the primary seizure disorder.[26] Silver and colleagues[33] have found that some patients with panic disorder respond to standard antipanic treatment, while others require both anticonvulsant and antipanic medication, such as clonazepam, alprazolam, or antidepressants. There are no data on children and adolescents.

Psychosis

McKenna and colleagues[27] have found that about 7% of adult patients with epilepsy may have persistent psychosis and that brief episodic psychoses in epileptics are not uncommon. Psychosis is most often associated with TLE. Antipsychotic medication may be warranted to treat such patients. There are no data on children and adolescents.

Aggression

The association of epilepsy with aggressive and violent behavior has been an area of great controversy. Stevens and Hyman[28] reviewed the literature on the association of TLE with violent behavior and concluded that the most significant factor leading to violence is damage of the limbic area of the brain, rather than the epilepsy.

Seizures That Are Uncontrolled

The psychiatrist is frequently called in to evaluate patients whose seizures have not been controlled by standard anticonvulsant medications. Referring physicians will often ask for psychiatric help when they believe that the seizure is psychogenic. Non–mental health care professionals often refer to these episodes as "pseudoseizures." It is important, however, that the consulting psychiatrist remember that this often is not an all-or-none phenomenon. That is, psychogenic seizures can complicate a true seizure disorder. In addition, stress can exacerbate or induce genuine seizures in vulnerable patients. Sleep deprivation has been associated with increased seizures. Thus a patient who is depressed and consequently is having difficulty falling or staying asleep may have increased seizure attacks despite treatment with appropriate doses of anticonvulsants.

Differentiation of these various types of seizures can often be based on clinical criteria, along with 24-hour video and EEG monitoring. The psychiatrist can play an important role here because the treatment team and/or the patient and family may have become frustrated at the lack of success in treating the seizures. At this point, some are tempted to take refuge in psychiatry and consider the patient's problem to be entirely psychogenic. Nonetheless, psychiatric diagnoses remain diagnoses of exclusion only when an organic factor has been definitively ruled out as the cause of the disturbance. This is not to say that psychiatric phenomena do not interact with organic phenomena, and vice versa. The psychiatrist, however, may have to use both medical and psychiatric knowledge in evaluating and assessing the patient to ensure an adequate and complete workup. If a psychiatric condition is diagnosed (e.g., panic disorder), appropriate psychopharmacologic intervention may be warranted (see Chapters 4 and 10).

Psychiatric Effects of Anticonvulsants

Anticonvulsants are discussed in detail in Chapter 9. One of the key roles of the consultation–liaison psychiatrist in all medical–surgical settings is to be aware of the potential behavioral, psychiatric, and cognitive effects of medications used to treat medical conditions. This is especially true of the anticonvulsants. For example, polydrug therapy is associated with more adverse neuropsychiatric and behavioral side effects than is monodrug therapy. Hoare[29] found that polydrug anticonvulsant therapy of epileptic children resulted in increased behavioral problems. Benzodiazepines, which are used to treat certain epileptic conditions, can produce behavioral disinhibition leading to increased irritability and aggression in these children. All anticonvulsants can potentially affect behavior and cognition, but phenytoin and phenobarbital appear to have more profound effects than carbamazepine or valproic acid.[30] Fortunately, many of these side effects are reversible when the medication is tapered and discontinued. Cognitive impairment has been observed in children receiving chronic treatment with phenytoin and/or phenobarbital.[31]

As we have mentioned, antipsychotics and antidepressants have been reported to lower the seizure threshold. Before rushing in to treat specific psychiatric syndromes such as depression, bipolar disorder, and psychosis, careful evaluation of the patient's medication is warranted. An epileptic child who has a first-degree relative with a major mood disorder and who is on phenobarbital and exhibiting depressive symptoms and suicidal ideation may benefit more by having the phenobarbital discontinued and switching to another antiepileptic such as carbamazepine or valproic acid than by adding another antidepressant. As a last resort, if the depressive symptoms and suicidal ideation remain prominent, antidepressant agents may be warranted. The reader is referred to Chapters 4 and 9 for dosing strategies for these agents. Bupropion, a new nonheterocyclic antidepressant, should probably be avoided in epileptic and brain-damaged patients because of an increased incidence of seizures (see Chapter 4).

Psychotic and aggressive patients who present a clear danger to themselves and/or others may require antipsychotic intervention. If a child is on an effective anticonvulsant regimen, antipsychotics can be cautiously introduced.[32] Antipsychotic medications must be used judiciously in patients with epilepsy, particularly in those not being treated with an anticonvulsant. Molindone and fluphenazine have been shown to have the lowest potential for decreasing the seizure threshold, so these agents may be particularly warranted in psychotic epileptic children and adolescents.[34]

The psychiatrist, primary physician, and patient and family may encounter a dilemma when an epileptic child who has long been refractory to treatment of his or her seizures finally achieves seizure control, but develops significant psychiatric complications such as depression. The parents and the child, for example, may be unwilling or reluctant to discontinue phenobarbital if it is the only medication that adequately controls the seizure disorder. Chronic epileptic crises are very stressful and unpleasant for both the patient and family. If an epileptic child becomes depressed on phenobarbital and this is the only medication that controls his or her seizures, discontinuation may not be feasible. The child and family should be alerted to the possible increased risk of major mood disturbance and suicidal ideation. An attempt should be made to lower the anticonvulsant to the lowest possible dose that controls the seizure disorder. When frank suicidal ideation and/or behavior is encountered, this is an emergency situation and inpatient hospitalization is required. In the safety of the inpatient setting, gradual weaning of the patient from the phenobarbital and the cautious initiation of trials with other anticonvulsants can be undertaken. In addition, psychotropic agents can be cautiously introduced into the medication regimen if depression and suicidal ideation prove refractory to medication adjustment. In addition, sedative and anticholinergic side effects of antipsychotic and antidepressant medications, which occur at lower than ordinary doses in neurologically impaired patients, can be more closely monitored in the hospital setting.

Brain Tumors

Mood and neuropsychiatric complications are seen far less commonly in children with brain tumors than in adults.[35] There are, however, significant issues that the child and family must face with neurosurgery. All may benefit from a thorough psychiatric assessment.[1,35] In addition, some patients with CNS tumors will develop convulsions and be placed on anticonvulsants. As we have discussed, these agents can cause behavioral and psychiatric disturbances that may require intervention.

Traumatic Brain Injury

Head injury can result in a number of psychiatric and behavioral sequelae. Such children, for example, may appear depressed, anxious, agitated, manic, psychotic, or hyperactive, or exhibit conduct problems. Moreover, they are more prone to other neurologic sequelae, such as seizures, which can further exacerbate the psychiatric symptomatology. There are no data on the psychopharmacologic treatment of children experiencing psychiatric disturbances. Clinical guidelines should be employed when pharmacologic intervention is instituted.

Metabolic Diseases of the Nervous System

Child and adolescent psychiatrists are playing an increasingly important role in the treatment of children and adolescents with these often rare disorders. In this section, we will discuss only those syndromes that most frequently result in psychiatric consultation. The same strategies and interventions can be used for most of the other conditions, and indeed for the majority of all chronic medical illnesses.

Phenylketonuria

Phenylketonuria (PKU) is an inborn error of metabolism with the inability to convert phenylalanine into tyrosine because of the absence or inactivity of phenylalanine hydroxylase. The majority of PKU patients are severely mentally retarded. Hyperactivity and erratic and unpredictable behavior are frequently observed.[35] The patients can be very difficult to manage and may have frequent temper tantrums. They may exhibit bizarre movements of their extremities, and at times their behavior may resemble that of autistic or schizophrenic patients. These children have many perceptual difficulties, often have difficulty with communication, and appear to be uncoordinated. The psychiatrist may be asked to evaluate this problematic behavior. It is essential to realize that convulsions are present in approximately one third of all cases.[36] This may affect the decision as to the appropriateness of psychopharmacologic intervention.

Hyperactivity or full-fledged ADHD may require pharmacologic intervention. Behavioral interventions should be instituted first. If these are unsuccessful, however, pharmacologic intervention with stimulants, antidepressants, and so on is warranted (see Chapter 3). It is important to remember that mentally retarded children may be more susceptible to the side effects of psychostimulant medications than are nonretarded patients (see Chapter 3). Initiation of treatment at a low dose and then gradually increasing the dosage are warranted. Therapeutic doses of methylphenidate have not been associated with an increased risk of seizure. Antidepressants have been reported to lower the seizure threshold, so caution is required when administering these agents. Severe behavioral problems and/or psychotic ideation involving danger to the child or others may require pharmacologic intervention with a benzodiazepine or neuroleptic. It is always important to investigate the medications the patient is currently receiving and to assess their risk of contributing to the problem behaviors.

Wilson's Disease

Wilson's disease is an autosomal recessive disorder that results in liver dysfunction, jaundice, and Kayser-Fleischer rings in the cornea. Psychiatric symptoms are often prominent, may precede medical or neurologic signs, and include irritability, depression, psychosis, and hepatic encephalopathy with profound mental changes.[186] Mood swings are common and can be explosive. Patients may become combative and symptoms sometimes may resemble schizophrenia. Memory loss may occur and may be particularly upsetting to the patient. Pharmacologic intervention may be necessary.

Lesch-Nyhan Syndrome

This syndrome is a disorder of purine metabolism and is characterized by hyperuricemia associated with spasticity and severe choreoathetosis. These patients often self-mutilate, such as by involuntarily biting their fingers, arms, and lips, or pulling out clumps of their hair.[187] Physical restraint is often required. These children are often quite distressed by their compulsion to mutilate themselves. Pharmacologic intervention, including neuroleptics, is frequently necessary. Trials with agents such as fluoxetine, propranolol, lithium, and carbamazepine have been found anecdotally to be helpful in the treatment of self-injurious behavior (see Chapters 8, 9, 11, and 12).

Tourette's Syndrome

The pharmacologic treatment of this disorder is covered in great detail in other chapters (e.g., Chapters 3 and 7).

Down's Syndrome/Chromosome Abnormalities

Mental retardation is prominent in Down's syndrome patients, but behavior problems are uncommon. Those patients with more severe and profound deficits in IQ may exhibit behavioral disturbances, which are managed as discussed previously.[1]

Prader-Willi Syndrome

The pharmacologic treatment of this disorder is covered in Chapter 4.

Spina Bifida

Spina bifida refers to meningocele, myelomeningocele, and other cystic lesions. This is often a lifelong disorder, with considerable psychiatric morbidity and psychosocial adjustment problems experienced by the patient and family.[188] There are no data on the psychopharmacologic treatment of those patients who experience psychiatric symptoms.

Psychopharmacologic Treatment of Psychiatric Sequelae of Neurologic Disease

It is very important that the prescribing psychiatrist be cognizant of the fact that neurologically impaired patients are more exquisitely sensitive to the side effects of psychotropic medications than are neurologically intact patients. Thus it is important to begin with a low dose and increase doses in small increments over longer periods.[1] Neurologically impaired patients are likely to be more sensitive to the sedative and anticholinergic side effects of medications such as antipsychotics, so it is crucial when prescribing these agents to follow the "start low, go slow" strategy.

Depression

In contrast to adults, TCAs have not been shown to be superior to placebo in the treatment of child and adolescent depression, but clinicians continue to prescribe these agents because the number of patients enrolled in controlled studies is too low to declare a definitive outcome. The MAOIs are rarely used in children and adolescents. Electroconvulsive therapy, a highly effective and safe treatment modality of depression in adulthood, merits consideration. Although it appears to be safe and efficacious in neurologically impaired depressed adults, it is rarely used for children and adolescents.

Mania

Mania associated with head trauma/injury and other CNS lesions has, in adults, been successfully treated with lithium, carbamazepine, valproic acid, and ECT.[38–41] It is important to remember that these medications and ECT can exacerbate confusion and induce mental-status changes in patients with CNS impairment.[42] Moreover, these patients appear to be more susceptible to the side effects of these medications, such as nausea, ataxia, tremor, and lethargy.[1,42] Mania, irritability, and aggression have been reported in patients treated with carbamazepine.[43] While there are no data on children and adolescents with brain injury who develop mania, our experience confirms that it does occur. Silver and colleagues[33] recommend that in adults the use of lithium should be reserved for patients with mania and those with recurrent depressive illness that preceded brain damage. Moreover, they recommend that carbamazepine or valproic acid be utilized in the treatment of patients with mania and seizure disorder.

Although there are no data on children and adolescents, we recommend similar strategies for them. Important caveats in this population include administering the medication in small divided doses (see Chapter 7), starting at low dosages and increasing gradually, while monitoring closely for side effects. Frequent drug blood levels should be drawn to check for toxicity. In children and adolescents, we advocate the use of carbamazepine in the treatment of mania and epilepsy, since this allows for monodrug therapy, which can help minimize medication side effects, while the same drug targets both disorders. This may also help with compliance, since patients taking multiple medications may have a more difficult time being compliant. We do not, however, advocate the use of lithium in depressive illness that precedes brain injury unless there has been evidence of mood swings, hypomania, or actual mania (current or by history). Lithium alone has not been shown to be effective in depressive illness, and because of brain-damaged patients' increased susceptibility to lithium-induced side effects, we do not believe that the risk/benefit ratio favors its use.

Psychosis

The reader is referred to Chapter 7, which discusses in detail the psychopharmacologic management of psychotic children and adolescents with neurologic disorders. Here we will discuss some key concepts that particularly apply to the child and adolescent consultation–liaison psychiatrist.

Psychotic children and adolescents with neurologic disorders should be treated with antipsychotic medications when their behavior is dangerous to themselves or others, or when their behavior is interfering significantly with their social and occupational functioning and with the treatment of their medical disorder. It is crucial that the prescribing psychiatrist be cognizant of the potential side effects, as neurologically impaired patients may be more susceptible to the side effects of these medications (see Chapter 7), and that the consulting psychiatrist warn the patient, the family, and the medical staff, including the neurologist, nursing staff, and other ancillary staff, of this possibility. An acute dystonic reaction is easily treatable with diphenhydramine or benztropine mesylate, but can be enormously disconcerting and frightening to patients, their families, and staff members who are unaware of this side effect of neuroleptic medication. Moreover, in brain-damaged patients, a dystonic reaction may be mistaken for a convulsion or seizure-like activity. Thus it can have important treatment ramifications. Prevention and ensuring that antiparkinsonian agents are available should side effects occur are recommended.

Another concern that arises with neuroleptics is the possibility that they may hinder neuronal recovery.[44] Thus, whenever possible, these drugs should be avoided in the acute phases of recovery after brain injury.[33] Silver and colleagues[33] recommend low-dose haloperidol, 0.5 mg b.i.d. or fluphenazine, 0.5 mg b.i.d. A low-dose neuroleptic strategy is recommended for all patients.[45] We believe that these agents can be used in children and adolescents provided careful monitoring is available. In our clinical experience, children and adolescents treated with haloperidol not uncommonly exhibit unsettling extrapyramidal side effects and/or dystonic reactions. Low-potency medications such as chlorpromazine and thioridazine, which have fewer extrapyramidal side effects, have increased anticholinergic and sedating effects. Middle-potency neuroleptics such as perphenazine may be more suitable for these patients, as they have fewer anticholinergic and sedating properties than do the lower-potency neuroleptics and fewer parkinsonian

429

side effects than do high-potency neuroleptics such as haloperidol. See Chapter 7 for dosing and administration.

It is important to emphasize that anticonvulsants are not always effective in treating psychosis in patients with epilepsy.[1] In fact, psychosis may ensue as the seizures are being controlled. Molindone and fluphenazine have been shown to have the lowest potential for decreasing the seizure threshold.[45] Ojemann and colleagues[46] point out, however, that this side effect may not be clinically important if the patient is already maintained on adequate anticonvulsant doses and plasma levels.

Anxiety

We recommend that, whenever possible, behavioral, psychosocial, cognitive, and psychotherapeutic interventions be instituted in favor of psychopharmacologic interventions in this population. Sleep in brain-damaged patients is often disrupted, so it is generally best to avoid tranquilizers for these patients. For acute panic attacks, however, benzodiazepines may be required. If so, their use should be short-term and on an as-needed basis, and at the lowest possible dosages necessary to control panic symptoms. Behavioral interventions should be instituted concomitantly, and as soon as possible, the benzodiazepine should be tapered and withdrawn. It is also important that patients be advised to avoid over-the-counter sleep or cold preparations because of their significant anticholinergic side effects.[1]

One anxiolytic that may be of use in relieving anxiety is buspirone. There are no data on children and adolescents, but this agent has a favorable side-effect profile and is not addictive. This agent is being used more commonly for a number of psychiatric conditions in children and adolescents, including autistic disorder, OCD, and various organic brain syndromes (see Chapter 10 for possible indications and dosing). Further study is clearly warranted.

Aggression

The major classes of medications utilized to treat aggression in children and adolescents with neurologic disorders—including antipsychotics, anxiolytics, antidepressants, lithium, anticonvulsants, beta-blockers, and clonidine—have been described in detail in the appropriate chapters and will not be discussed here.

Psychiatric Consultation to Pediatrics

The role of the consultation–liaison psychiatrist in the general pediatric setting continues to grow. We will focus on those clinical conditions and situations in which this professional is likely to play the greatest part.

Endocrine Disorders

A wide variety of endocrine disorders have been directly linked to psychiatric symptomatology. The following discussion will cover the most common of these endocrinopathies.

Diabetes

Pharmacologic intervention is a last resort in these patients. Mental status changes (delirium, anxiety, irritability, etc.) often resolve once the underlying medical disturbance is corrected. The key to treatment is maintaining compliance and good medical and personal self-care after the medical disturbance is corrected. If psychiatric symptoms such as psychosis or depression persist, treatment can be considered. Psychotic patients who present an active and clear danger to the self can be treated with low-dose neuroleptics (see Chapter 7). If depression persists after resolution of the medical condition and cognitive, behavioral, and psychosocial interventions have been unsuccessful, treatment with TCAs and nonheterocyclic antidepressants may be considered (see Chapter 3).

Thyroid Disease

Hypothyroidism   In adults, hypothyroidism is the most common endocrine disorder associated with psychiatric symptoms. This condition has received a great deal of attention, since it not uncommonly presents with apathy or depressive symptoms without accompanying physical symptoms. Subclinical hypothyroidism affects about 5% of the population.[47] Although the prevalence is believed to be lower in children and adolescents, screening, including thyroid function tests and especially TSH, is often performed on young people with unexplained psychiatric symptoms. In general, when hypothyroidism is encountered, pediatric and/or endocrine consultation is merited. We recommend first treating the underlying condition (with thyroid replacement therapy), and then monitoring to determine whether the psychiatric symptoms will abate. Occasionally, psychiatric symptoms may persist after thyroid replacement therapy. Antidepressants may be considered in depression refractory to psychosocial interventions, with short-term benzodiazepine use indicated for acute anxiety and/or panic states. The reader is referred to the appropriate chapters for guidelines.

Lithium-induced hypothyroidism is covered in Chapter 8.

Hyperthyroidism   As in hypothyroidism, medical management of the thyroid illness does not always result in complete resolution of the psychiatric symptoms. If psychosocial and behavioral interventions prove unsuccessful,

431

psychopharmacologic management may be indicated. We believe that TCAs are contraindicated for children and adolescents with hyperthyroidism and depression because of the risk of cardiac arrhythmias.[48] If symptoms persist four to six weeks after resolution of the thyroid abnormality and after psychosocial interventions have been instituted, pharmacologic alternatives such as nonheterocyclic antidepressants can be considered. Early in the course of treatment and for time-limited periods, benzodiazepines or beta-blockers may be warranted in patients with significant anxiety.

Gastrointestinal Disorders

Gastrointestinal patients not uncommonly require psychiatric consultation. We will discuss the role of the consulting psychiatrist and emphasize necessary pharmacologic adjustments required in patients with GI disturbances.

Abdominal Pain
The precipitation and exacerbation of abdominal pain are often partially related to psychiatric disturbance.[49-51] It is important to emphasize, however, that a significant proportion of these patients may be suffering undiagnosed medical illnesses.[33,52,53]

Irritable Bowel Syndrome
A positive relationship between emotional and physical symptoms exists in the irritable bowel syndrome (IBS).[54] These patients have been reported to have a high frequency of depression. A plethora of medical and psychiatric treatments have been utilized, including behavioral relaxation training techniques, biofeedback, and anticholinergics. Anxiolytics and antidepressants also have been used in the treatment of IBS.[55,56] Greenbaum[57] found desipramine to be effective in the treatment of diarrhea-prominent IBS when compared with placebo and atropine.

Inflammatory Bowel Disease
Inflammatory bowel diseases (IBD) such as ulcerative colitis and Crohn's disease have been associated with psychiatric symptoms. Helzer and colleagues[58] observed a high frequency of depression in patients with IBD as compared with controls. Andrews and associates[59] found that the coexistence of psychiatric illness with IBD adversely affected physical recovery. While much remains to be learned in this population, it does appear that these children and adolescents are also more vulnerable to psychiatric disturbances, and that such dysfunctions can have a negative impact on the underlying medical condition. There are no data on the psychopharmacologic management of such children and adolescents. We recommend a similar approach to that advocated in the other sections of this chapter. The TCAs

should be avoided because of their anticholinergic effects, which may exacerbate the underlying medical condition. Similarly, other psychotropic agents such as lithium and carbamazepine, which often have GI side effects, can be problematic in the treatment of this population. Low-dose therapy accompanied by medical treatment of the GI symptoms can help when these agents are necessary.

Liver Disease

Liver diseases are not uncommonly associated with a wide variety of psychiatric conditions that can result in, among others, fatigue, apathy, mental status changes, and depression. Such patients require special pharmacologic attention with regard to such factors as drug choice and dosing and administration. Most psychotropic drugs are metabolized by the liver. Thus, in patients with liver failure, medications may rise to toxic levels owing to the inability of the liver to metabolize the drug. Antidepressants and antipsychotics that rely on hepatic clearance when administered to patients with liver failure will result in an increase in drug bioavailability.[60] It is, therefore, essential that lower doses of these drugs be utilized—especially for children, who, because of their increased liver-to-whole-body ratio, usually metabolize medications far more quickly than do adults. Thus the clinician must be cognizant of the effect of liver disease on drug metabolism and recognize that significantly higher drug blood levels may accumulate because of the lack of function of this organ in these patients.

Lithium, which is metabolized by the kidney, may be particularly indicated for patients with psychiatric symptoms, particularly if mood lability is prevalent. Barbiturates and most benzodiazepines will have longer half-lives in patients with liver disease. We recommend avoiding such agents in favor of benzodiazepines that are metabolized by glucuronide conjugation, such as oxazepam, temazepam, or lorazepam, because liver-dependent mechanisms for longer-acting drugs such as diazepam are impaired.[78]

Specific Pharmacologic Strategies in GI Patients

Gastrointestinal conditions other than liver disease frequently require psychopharmacologic adjustment and manipulation. For example, the H_2-blockers, such as cimetidine, ranitidine, and famotidine, have been reported to cause depression and delirium.[61,62] Sucralfate, a gastric mucosal coating agent that is not systematically absorbed, is an alternative treatment to the H_2-blockers when psychiatric side effects are problematic.[78] When antacids are used, it is important to remember that gel-type antacids that contain aluminum and magnesium may slow the absorption of neuroleptics.[61,62,78]

Cimetidine can prolong the half-lives of benzodiazepines metabolized by oxidation, such as diazepam, but does not affect the half-life of benzodiazepines metabolized by conjugation, such as lorazepam, temazepam, and oxaze-pam.[78] As in patients with liver disease, we recommend that those who are on cimetidine and require benzodiazepine treatment receive such agents as lorazepam, temazepam, or oxazepam as opposed to medications metabolized by oxidation, such as diazepam. Another alternative is to try the nonbenzodi-azepine anxiolytic buspirone, which has a favorable side-effect profile and is not known to interact with cimetidine. If a benzodiazepine metabolized by oxidation must be the drug of choice, ranitidine can be used, as it does not alter diazepam metabolism.[63]

In adults, TCAs have weak H_2 blocking effects,[64] and thus we cannot en-dorse their use in peptic ulcer disease (PUD). Moreover, this condition is far less common in children and adolescents than in adults. If clinicians do pre-scribe cimetidine and a TCA, it must be remembered that cimetidine raises serum TCA levels.[78]

Finally, it is important to remember that agents such as metoclopramide (Reglan) and prochloperazine (Compazine), which are used in the treatment of nausea and vomiting and delayed gastric emptying syndromes, are dopa-mine antagonists and may cause typical neuroleptic side effects (i.e., seda-tion, akathisia, extrapyramidal syndromes, and tardive dyskinesia).[65,66] Metoclopramide has also been linked to depression.[78]

Connective Tissue Disease

Systemic Lupus Erythematosus
Systemic lupus erythematosus (SLE) is the best known of the connective tis-sue diseases that cause psychiatric disturbances. Diagnostic and therapeutic issues are frequently compounded and clouded by the use of steroids to treat this condition. Patients with SLE are particularly vulnerable to delirium be-cause of multisystem involvement.[78] Delirium induced by steroids is not un-commonly seen in SLE patients, since high doses of steroids are often used to treat disease exacerbations. It is most likely to occur when the steroid dose is abruptly altered and at steroid doses equal to 40 mg of prednisone.[68] The treatment of choice for steroid-induced delirium is first to lower the ste-roid dose to the lowest possible effective dose, and then, when necessary, to use a low-dose neuroleptic such as haloperidol, 1–2 mg/day.[69] The neurolep-tic should be administered only during the acute psychosis and discontinued as soon as possible.[78]

Steroids and adrenocorticotropic hormones are known to have prominent psychiatric side effects, including mood variability, depression, mania, psy-chosis, delirium, and agitation. The treatment strategy is similar to that out-lined above. The first step is to decrease the steroid medication to the lowest possible dose, and then to utilize psychotropic medications only if the symptoms do not resolve with this adjustment. It is important to emphasize that the use of steroids does not contraindicate antidepressant, antipsychotic, lithium, or most other psychotropic drug use (see Chapter 14). There have been reports that lithium may have both a prophylactic and a stabilizing effect on steroid-induced manic states.[78] We recommend avoiding benzodiazepines and over-the-counter anticholinergic medications such as diphenhydramine, since these agents can exacerbate steroid-induced delirium. (See Chapter 14 for a more detailed description of the management and treatment of the psychiatric sequelae of steroid use.)

Renal Disease

Patients with renal failure who require dialysis and/or are awaiting kidney transplant not uncommonly exhibit neuropsychiatric symptoms (depression, anxiety, psychosis, delirium, cognitive impairment) that merit psychiatric consultation.[70,78] There are very limited data on children and adolescents with renal failure, but as with many other medical conditions, they appear to be more susceptible to psychiatric complications, including depression, anxiety, psychosis, and delirium.

Pharmacologic Considerations in Renal Failure
Lithium is the main psychotropic whose drug levels are primarily dependent on renal clearance mechanisms (see Chapter 8). When lithium carbonate is indicated for treatment, it is usually given in a single dose of 300–600 mg immediately after dialysis because lithium levels should not fall until the next dialysis.[78] It should be noted that lithium levels drawn immediately after dialysis do not accurately reflect true serum lithium levels and will increase as reequilibration with tissue stores occurs within two hours of dialysis.[78] Vincent and colleagues[71] also observed that in renal transplant patients, cyclosporine can increase lithium levels by decreasing its clearance.

To avoid some of these difficulties, alternative antimanic agents such as carbamazepine or valproic acid may be considered. Indeed, since most psychotropic drugs are hepatically metabolized, they can be administered without adjustment to the patient's renal disease. In addition, uremic patients are more sensitive to the anticholinergic side effects of psychotropic medications,[78] which can further exacerbate impairment of delirious patients' cognitive functioning. There is a theoretical concern that the active polar metabolites of some benzodiazepines, such as diazepam and chlordiazepoxide, would normally be excreted by the kidneys and might result in renal failure, causing delirium and increased sedation.[72] In reality, however, even with very severe renal disease, dose adjustments are unnecessary for most benzodiazepines. Primary exceptions include chlordiazepoxide and midazo-

435

lam, which should be decreased by 50%.[72,78] Full doses of TCAs, fluoxetine, bupropion, MAOIs, and buspirone can be used for patients with renal failure.[72]

Cardiac Disorders

Child and adolescent psychiatrists are not infrequently consulted concerning patients with heart disease. This relates in part to the devastating impact of such a disease on the patient and family, since heart disease is so much rarer in children and adolescents than it is in adults. Moreover, psychological factors affecting the course of heart disease may exacerbate the cardiac problems. For example, these patients and their families, because of their depression and hopelessness, may be less compliant with medical treatment and may suffer increased morbidity and mortality as a result. Moreover, anxious patients may present with cardiac symptoms despite no objective evidence of heart disease.

Hypertension

Hypertension is far less common in children and adolescents than in adults, but it can occur, particularly in association with certain medical conditions. Psychiatric side effects are of particular concern with some of the antihypertensive medications that are used. In fact, CNS symptoms are the most common side effects of antihypertensives and are seen to varying extents with all antihypertensives.[73,74] Recent attention has been generated regarding the beta-blocker propranolol's neuropsychiatric side effects, including depression, cognitive impairment, and nightmares. It has been shown that hydrophilic beta-blockers such as atenolol, which do not penetrate the blood–brain barrier (in contrast to propranolol), cause fewer CNS side effects than lipophilic beta-blockers, such as propranolol, metoprolol, and pindolol.[75] We advocate the use of atenolol rather than propranolol in the treatment of hypertensive patients with depression. In addition, as a preventative measure, we would recommend its use for any child or adolescent with either a personal history of depression or a family history of mood disorder. Since atenolol is generally felt to be as effective as propranolol in the treatment of hypertension, it may be advisable to use this agent first, regardless of psychiatric history, since it does not penetrate the blood–brain barrier and has less chance of causing neuropsychiatric complications.

It must be emphasized that not only the use of beta-blockers, but also their withdrawal, can result in psychiatric symptoms.[78] Withdrawal symptoms such as severe anxiety, restlessness, palpitations, and nightmares, and medical symptoms such as angina, hypertension, headache, and vomiting, are commonly seen when beta-blockers are discontinued over a week or less.[76] The abrupt withdrawal of other antihypertensives may cause similar symptoms (see Chapter 11). The major caveat is that all of these medications should be withdrawn gradually over at least two weeks.[78]

With all of the attention regarding the neuropsychiatric side effects of antihypertensive medications, an investigation to determine whether certain antihypertensives had more favorable psychiatric side-effect profiles was begun. Croog and colleagues[77] compared the effects of captopril, methyldopa, and propranolol on the quality of life of hypertensive patients in a multicenter, randomized, double-blind clinical trial. They found that the patients receiving captopril reported fewer side effects and better well-being than those receiving propranolol or methyldopa. It should be noted, however, that there were some inherent flaws in the study. The doses of the three drugs were not equivalent, since hydrochlorothiazide was added more often to the medication regimens of patients receiving captopril than to those in the other groups.[78] Further study in this area is warranted before definitive recommendations can be given.

Psychiatric Side Effects of Cardiac Medications
Cardiac drugs not uncommonly cause psychiatric side effects (see Table 13-2).

Pharmacologic Considerations in Cardiac Patients
It was originally believed that many psychiatric drugs and ECT were absolutely contraindicated for adults with heart disease, but recent study has shown this not to be the case. Levenson[74] demonstrated that TCAs can be used safely for most patients with stable heart disease. Orthostatic hypotension is the most common adverse side effect of TCAs in adults that necessitates medication cessation, but it is seldom seen in children.[78] No TCA has proved to be safer than any other with regard to risk in patients with preexisting conduction disease (see Chapter 4).

The MAOIs have little effect on cardiac conduction. Their major limitations in adult cardiac patients are orthostatic hypotension and interactions with

Table 13-2
Psychiatric Side Effects of Cardiac Drugs

Tocainamide, Mexiletin, Lidocaine	Flecainide	Amiodarone	Captopril, Enalapril, Lisinopril	Digitalis
Anxiety Psychosis Dizziness Agitation	Anxiety or dizziness	Depression, confusion	Elevation or depression of mood	Illusions Depression Delirium

other medications (see Chapter 6). Serotonin reuptake inhibitors such as fluoxetine and sertraline do not appear to cause cardiac side effects, but there are no studies in this respect on patients with cardiac disease. Bupropion is another nonheterocyclic antidepressant that, because of its side-effect profile (lack of cardiac complications), may be appropriate for treating cardiac patients who are depressed. However, there are also no data on this population. Finally, ECT has been used safely in patients with cardiovascular disease,[80] but there are no data on children and adolescents. Children may be more susceptible to some of the cardiac side effects of TCAs (i.e., arrhythmias—see Chapter 4). Consultation with a cardiologist is recommended for any child or adolescent with cardiac dysfunction. If tricyclic therapy is contraindicated, alternative agents such as bupropion or fluoxetine may be considered.

Electroconvulsive therapy is not currently used for children and adolescents, except as a last resort. This may be an area deserving further attention, particularly if alternative antidepressants such as the SSUIs and bupropion fail to show a significant effect in treating child and adolescent depression.

Antipsychotic medications can generally be used when necessary for children and adolescents with cardiac disease. However, these agents, particularly those of low potency, have more potential cardiovascular side effects, including orthostasis and tachycardia (see Chapter 7), and caution is required when dispensing them. In addition, clozapine, a new antipsychotic, may produce tachycardia and orthostatic hypotension and has been associated, though rarely, with serious cardiac complications.[79,80] There are no data on children and adolescents. Nonetheless, clinicians are beginning to use this medication in these young patients who have failed other neuroleptic therapy and/or have developed intolerable extrapyramidal side effects on standard agents.

Lithium has been rarely associated with cardiac conduction abnormalities (see Chapter 8), and can be used for patients with mania who also have cardiac disease. Careful monitoring for side effects and close attention to blood levels are recommended.

For drug interactions between psychiatric and cardiac drugs, see Table 13-3.

Pulmonary Diseases

Psychiatric consultation with regard to these patients predominantly involves asthma and its complications and the psychiatric side effects of pulmonary medications.

Table 13-3

Drug Interactions Between Psychiatric and Cardiac Drugs

Beta-blockers:
  ● Benzodiazepines—possible benzodiazepine toxicity
  ● Phenothiazines—increase effects of both

Verapamil:
  ● Lithium—decrease effect lithium
  ● Carbamazepine—carbamazepine toxicity

Amiodarone: ● Benzodiazepines—cardiac toxicity
Digoxin: ● Fluoxetine—increase effects of both
Sublingual nitrates: ● TCAs—decrease effect of nitrate

See references 76–78.

Asthma

Asthma has had a long association with stress. Adequately treating the underlying physical condition and medication regimens are first priorities. Assessment of the patient's medications is essential (discussed below).

Psychotropic Drugs and Asthma

Stress can bring on or exacerbate an asthmatic attack. In some cases, children who have had life-threatening asthma attacks necessitating intubation and who require frequent hospitalizations may experience chronic anxiety and/or panic attacks. Fear when away from home or far from a hospital setting can be stressful for patients who have almost died of their asthma. The clinician may be faced with a dilemma when trying to treat anxiety in these patients. As benzodiazepine use can depress ventilation and can be life-threatening, for asthmatic patients, particularly those in the midst of an acute exacerbation, these agents should be avoided. Benzodiazepines also have addictive potential. If their use is deemed essential by the treatment team, careful monitoring of the patient's respiratory status with blood gases, preferably in an intensive-care setting, is recommended.

One alternative anxiolytic is buspirone, which may be safer than benzodiazepines in the treatment of anxiety in children and adolescents with asthma. Normal adult subjects treated with buspirone 10 mg and diazepam 10 mg showed no effect on resting ventilation or ventilatory response to mechanical loading, but buspirone did not appear to have diazepam's depressant effect on ventilation driven by exogenous carbon dioxide.[79] There are no data on children and adolescents, and controlled trials in this population are needed. We recommend a trial of buspirone in chronically anxious asthmatic children and adolescents, particularly where the anxiety is interfering with treatment, starting with a low test dose of 10 mg/day and increasing the dose gradually by 10 mg increments every five to seven days.

The TCAs and MAOIs have adverse interactions with sympathomimetic drugs (see Chapters 4 and 6). The MAOIs should not be used when sympathomimetic drugs such as ephedrine are being administered because hypertensive crises can result.[78] Selective beta-2 agonists such as terbutaline, albuterol, and metaproterenol can be used safely with TCAs and MAOIs.

Nonselective beta-blockers such as propranolol, which are sometimes used in psychiatry to treat anxiety and aggression (see Chapter 11), are absolutely contraindicated for patients with asthma. Although selective beta-blockers such as atenolol are felt to be safer, most authorities caution against their use for asthmatics with anxiety and aggression until further evaluation has taken place.

Important Theophylline Drug Interactions
See Table 13-4.

Psychiatric Side Effects of Respiratory Drugs
See Tables 13-5 through 13-12.

Anticholinergic Agents. Anticholinergic agents are found in a wide variety of prescription and nonprescription medications. These agents are not uncommonly associated with neuropsychiatric side effects.

Expectorants, Mucolytic Agents. See Table 13-11.

Calcium Channel Blockers. In addition to being effective in treating cardiovascular disease, preliminary investigation has shown them to be effective in treating asthma.[107–109] Psychiatric side effects associated with these medications are believed to be minimal.

Table 13-4
Bronchodilator Drug Interactions

Theophylline:
• Increases renal clearance lithium.[89–92]
• May cause anxiety, jitteriness, nervousness when combined with CNS stimulants.[88]

Table 13-5
Side Effects of Theophylline

- Anxiety[86–91]
- Mental status changes and seizures[86]
- Depression[92]
- ADHD—not proven
- Learning disabilities—not proven[81,82,84,85]

Table 13-6
Neuropsychiatric Side Effects of Albuterol

- Anxiety[86]
- Psychosis[93–96]
- Mania[96,97]
- Antidepressant—not proven[98–101]

Table 13-7
Aerosol-Inhaler–Induced Psychiatric Side Effects

- Psychological addiction
- Anxiety
- Agitation
- Disorientation
- Greater risk of toxicity to children[86]

Table 13-8
Psychiatric Side Effects of Decongestants

Ephedrine[103]
- Anxiety
- Dysphoria
- Irritability
- Restlessness
- Insomnia
- Psychosis
- Mania

Phenylpropanolamine[86]
- Psychosis
- Agitation and restlessness
- Irritability
- Aggressiveness
- Organic brain syndromes
- Children especially vulnerable

Naphazoline[86,104]
- Sedation
- Coma

Table 13-9

Cautions When Using Decongestants

Use decongestants with caution
- When prescribing CNS psychostimulants due to possible potentiation of side effects.
- Be alert for psychosis and mania.
- Avoid phenylpropanolamine for children and adolescents.
- Phenylpropanolamine absolutely contraindicated if patient is receiving MAOI.
- Naphazoline contraindicated in children less than 6 years old.[104]

Table 13-10

Psychiatric Side Effects of Anticholinergic Agents

Central anticholinergic syndrome
- Peripheral muscarinic blockade
- Acute psychosis
- Ataxia
- Myotonic twitching
- Increased muscle tone and muscular weakening
- Toxic delirium
- Impaired GI motility (paralytic ileus)

See references 102, 105.

Table 13-11

Side Effects of Expectorant Mucolytic Agents

- Goiter/hypothyroidism
- Nervousness
- Insomnia

See reference 86.

Table 13-12

Psychiatric Side Effects of Central Cough Suppressants

Codeine
- Agitation
- Combative behavior
- Sedation

Dextromethorphan
- Excitation
- Confusion
- Opiatelike respiratory depression
- Hypomania

See references 86, 106.

Neuropsychiatric Side Effects of Calcium Channel Blockers. See Table 13-13.

Cromolyn Sodium. Psychiatric side effects associated with cromolyn sodium are rare.[83] There have been, however, two questionable reports in which psychosis was associated with the use of cromolyn sodium.[110,111] Both cases were complicated by the fact that the patients were simultaneously receiving sympathomimetic medications in addition to the cromolyn sodium. Thus a cause-and-effect relationship between cromolyn sodium and psychosis cannot be established at this time. Although this compound appears to be relatively safe, the clinician is urged to be cautious and to monitor for this possible side effect.

AIDS

As of 1990, over 2000 AIDS cases had been reported in children less than 13 years of age.[112] In children, the most common manifestation of AIDS is failure to thrive, with loss of developmental milestones.[113] The human immunodeficiency virus (HIV) can directly infect CNS cells, and can cause encephalopathy, motor dysfunction, meningitis, seizures, and cerebral tumors.[114–118] Children can also experience profound neuropsychological impairment characterized by a gross deterioration in cognitive functioning.[119] Neurovegetative symptoms of depression, including apathy and psychomotor retardation, can also be presenting symptoms of children infected with the AIDS virus.

Preexisting or coexistent psychiatric disorders are common in adolescents with AIDS.[113] AIDS dementia complex with primary HIV infection of the brain is believed to be a leading cause of cognitive, motor, and behavioral deterioration,[120,121] which may be preceded by psychiatric and behavioral symptoms.[113] Organic brain syndromes caused by HIV infection of the brain can mimic such psychiatric disorders as major depression, psychosis, mania, and

Table 13-13
Neuropsychiatric Side Effects of Calcium Channel Blockers

- Mood changes (nifedipine only)
- Lightheadedness
- Giddiness
- Jitteriness
- Tremulousness
- Sleep disturbance
- Ataxia
- Incoordination

See references 107–109.

OCD.[122–130] Young males with AIDS (20–39 years of age) have been shown
to be at a significantly increased risk of suicide.[131,132] Since suicide is already known to be the second leading cause of death in adolescents, HIV-infected adolescents would be expected to be at a significantly increased risk.

Psychiatric Intervention

The mainstay of the treatment of HIV-infected children and adolescents is,
of course, ensuring that they receive proper medical consultation and care.
Hospitalization is often necessary when such patients become suicidal. Pharmacotherapy is generally an intervention of last resort.

Pharmacotherapy in Children and Adolescents with AIDS

Depression   The TCAs have anticholinergic side effects that can be problematic in AIDS patients, who often suffer from organic mental syndromes.
Even TCAs with fewer anticholinergic side effects, such as desipramine or
nortriptyline as opposed to amitripyline or doxepin, pose a risk. In addition,
anticholinergic effects can result in atropine psychosis (see "Anticholinergic
Syndrome").

Serotonin reuptake inhibitors, such as fluoxetine and sertraline, and other
available antidepressants that have no anticholinergic side effects may be
more appropriate for these patients.

Other agents that can be considered are bupropion (see Chapter 4) and trazodone. When administering bupropion, it is important to remember that it
has a higher risk of seizure than many other antidepressants, and that
HIV-infected patients may be at increased risk of seizure. Trazodone can be
quite sedating, and it may have orthostatic side effects, which may be of concern in motorically/neurologically and cognitively impaired HIV-infected patients. It should be emphasized that there has been no systematic study of
the use of any of the aforementioned agents for children and adolescents
with AIDS.

Psychosis   As with antidepressants, antipsychotics have anticholinergic side
effects. Nonetheless, cases of severe psychosis with danger to the patient or
others may require pharmacologic intervention. A high-potency neuroleptic
such as haloperidol is preferred to low-potency agents such as thioridazine
and chlorpromazine, which have more anticholinergic side effects, since the
former is less likely to exacerbate an organic mental syndrome. We recommend starting with low-dose haloperidol, 0.5 mg b.i.d. and 1 mg at bedtime.
Careful monitoring for extrapyramidal side effects, dystonia, and tardive dyskinesia is necessary. Standard antiparkinsonian agents may be problematic
in AIDS patients because of their anticholinergic actions. Thus careful titra-

tion of the neuroleptic dose is recommended to minimize the risk of untoward side effects so that polydrug therapy can be avoided.

Agitation/Aggression Low-dose haloperidol may also be indicated for patients with severe agitation (not necessarily due to psychosis). In non–AIDS-infected patients, a benzodiazepine such as lorazepam may be indicated for the short-term treatment of acute anxiety and agitation. Benzodiazepines however, may, exacerbate the patient's mental status and worsen or induce an existing delirium and cognitive impairment. Low-dose haloperidol, which is less likely to impair cognition and/or exacerbate delirium, may be warranted.

AIDS patients who are having acute anxiety and/or panic attacks may require short-term benzodiazepine intervention, particularly if the anxiety is compromising the patient's medical/respiratory status. Agents such as alprazolam should be avoided because they often are difficult to taper once a patient has been receiving such medication. Low-dose lorazepam may be warranted in these situations, with doses of 1–2 mg as needed for acute attacks. Careful monitoring of the patient's mental status is essential. Around-the-clock doses of lorazepam (i.e., every four hours) are to be avoided to ensure that the patient receives no more medication than is absolutely necessary. Finally, for patients with more generalized anxiety and who have proved refractory to behavioral and relaxation training, the non-benzodiazepine anxiolytic buspirone may be considered. This agent is less sedating than benzodiazepines and is less likely to cause or exacerbate impaired cognition. It can be started at a dose of 10 mg b.i.d.–t.i.d. It should be noted, however, that it frequently takes two to four weeks to exert a full effect (see Chapter 10).

Mania In the event that an HIV-infected patient becomes manic, it is advisable to review the patient's current treatment to ascertain whether he or she has been receiving any medications, such as corticosteroids, that might cause mania. This includes antidepressants used to treat depression. Sometimes decreasing or discontinuing the offending agent may attenuate the manic symptoms. If this is not possible or such medication alterations prove unsuccessful, treatment with lithium may be warranted. Caution is required when using lithium in AIDS patients as they may be sensitive to its neurologic side effects (see Chapter 8 and "Psychiatric Consultation to Neurology"). Carbamazepine or valproic acid may be warranted if lithium is not completely successful, is not effective, or is contraindicated. Agents such as valproic acid or carbamazepine may be especially helpful for patients with CNS injury (see Chapter 9). Nonetheless, careful monitoring for mental-status side effects of these medications is necessary.

Psychiatric Consultation to Oncology

The association of psychiatric disorders with cancer has been well documented. Approximately one half of adult patients with cancer develop a psychiatric disorder, most commonly depression.[131] In addition, many of the chemotherapy regimens can cause psychiatric complications of patient mood, affect, cognition, and thought content.

The use of pharmacologic interventions, including neuroleptics and antidepressants, for children and adolescents with cancer is based on principles similar to those discussed in the sections on neurology and general pediatrics. Thus we will not discuss the pharmacologic management of specific syndromes. Instead, we will briefly discuss features that are unique to the pediatric oncologic patient with a coexistent psychiatric condition.

Pharmacologic Interventions in Children and Adolescents with Cancer

Neuroleptics

Medically ill patients may be more susceptible to neuroleptic side effects, especially the serious one of the neuroleptic malignant syndrome (NMS).[133] Therefore, in cancer patients who are psychotic, it is advisable to keep neuroleptic doses low by adding benzodiazepines for the management of delirium and agitation.[133] It is important to remember, however, that benzodiazepines can adversely affect a patient's mental status, so careful monitoring is essential when administering these agents with neuroleptics. As NMS is a life-threatening condition that can afflict children and adolescents, it is preferable to use as low a dose of neuroleptic as possible. Careful titration of the benzodiazepine and neuroleptic dose is advisable. Lorazepam is the benzodiazepine of choice because it is metabolized by conjugation, has no active metabolites, has a short duration of action, can be given parenterally, and is less affected by illness than are other benzodiazepines. Agents such as alprazolam, which frequently require prolonged weaning, are to be avoided.

For neuroleptics such as metoclopramide, which are frequently used as antiemetics during chemotherapy, close monitoring for adverse side effects is needed.[133] Cancer patients who receive high doses of the drug and repeated exposure to it are susceptible to developing disabling and possibly lifelong side effects. Akathisia and tardive dyskinesia have been reported.[134] Lorazepam has been used successfully in antiemetic regimens for sedation and to attenuate akathisia.

Benzodiazepines

Benzodiazepines for the treatment of anxiety and panic disorder were discussed in the previous section.

Antidepressants

As with other medical illnesses, TCAs should be used with caution in depressed children and adolescents with cancer. Moreover, their anticholinergic side effects make them particularly unattractive agents for pediatric cancer patients with depression. Alternative agents such as SSUIs (i.e., fluoxetine, sertraline) or bupropion may deserve consideration.

Pain Management

Pharmacologic management of pediatric pain in children and adolescents is in its infancy, but investigation is under way and much is being learned. Shannon and Berde[136] present a comprehensive review of key principles regarding the pharmacology of pediatric pain.

Nonopioid Peripherally Acting Analgesics
See Table 13-14.

This category consists of salicylates such as aspirin, nonsteroidal anti-inflammatory agents (NSAIDs), and acetaminophen. These agents do not produce tolerance or physical dependence. There have, however, been case reports of rebound sequelae after prolonged use for chronic headaches.[136]

Table 13-14
Nonopioid Peripherally Acting Analgesics

Acetaminophen
- Most common analgesic for children and adolescents in the United States.
- First medication used in mild–moderate pain.
- Combination with codeine (Tylenol 3) treats severe pain.
- High therapeutic ratio.[137]
- Give in doses 10–20 mg/kg every four hours.[136]
- Does not cause gastritis and bleeding.
- Neuropathy and liver damage unlikely at therapeutic doses.

Salicylates
- Associated with Reye's syndrome.
- Can cause gastritis and platelet dysfunction.
- Should not be used in pediatric population.

NSAIDs
- Minimal study in children.
- Give with food to decrease GI upset.
- Relieve pain by inhibiting prostaglandin synthesis.[136]
- Concern about bleeding problem in children.[136]

447

Opioids

Opioids are the primary agents utilized in the treatment of chronic cancer pain.[138] They are also frequently used to ameliorate postoperative pain, post-traumatic pain, sickle-cell crises, and so on.

Opioids bind to opioid receptors in the CNS, and their action is considered to be "morphine-like." Opiates such as morphine and codeine, which are derived from opium, are phenanthrene alkaloids.[139] Synthetic opioids such as fentanyl, methadone, and meperidine are structurally different from morphine, even though their actions are similar. The term narcotic is most often used to refer to opioid analgesics.[133,138]

Opioids produce analgesia by binding to CNS receptors, thus mimicking the effects of endogenous opioids.[136] Their action on the mμ-receptor is generally correlated with analgesia.

Pain has two discrete components—the physical sensation of pain and the emotional distress of experiencing pain. Opioids alleviate both forms of pain. They also attenuate autonomic hyperreactivity such as tachycardia, sweating, and hypertension.[136]

Administration   Opioids can be administered orally, IV, subcutaneously, IM, transdermally, transmucosally, or directly into the epidural and subarachnoid space.[140] The oral route is preferred whenever possible, as it is less frightening to children, who resent being stuck with needles. When an IV is in place, administration by this route is possible, particularly if the child is having difficulty tolerating oral administration. Intramuscular injections can be extremely frightening and painful to children, who may deny that they have pain in order to avoid such shots.[136]

Physiologic Effects of Opioids   Opioids can produce sedation, respiratory depression, GI intolerance, cough suppression, and vasodilation.[136] The adverse effects of opioids have received a great deal of attention, but can often be managed by appropriate supervision and dosage adjustment.[136] Careful titration of opioids is necessary, monitoring closely for efficacy versus toxicity. As there is tremendous variability in response to these agents, individual dosage titration is essential in treating patients with opioids.

PCA Pump

The computer-driven, patient-controlled analgesia (PCA) pump provides a dramatic and very effective way for patients to titrate opioids by regulating their own analgesic administration.[141–146] Patients receive small IV doses of opioid when they push a button. After each dose, there is an interval during which they cannot receive additional doses. There is also a maximum amount that can be administered in a four-hour period. This technique has been found to be very effective for adolescents and for children as young as 5 years old who are experiencing pain. The patients get a sense of control in managing their pain.

Opioids differ from benzodiazepines in that they do produce dose-related sedation, but there is a range of dosage and plasma levels that result in analgesia without impairing cognition.[136] Opioids, however, affect mood and can cause depression and/or euphoria—that is, organic mood disorders. It should be noted that the administration of sedative hypnotics with opioids can significantly increase the sedative and respiratory depressant effects of the opioids.[147]

Respiratory depression is a dose-related side effect of opioid administration and is believed to be related to the patient's clinical condition, the type of disease, the severity of pain, and the patient's age.[136] Opioid use can result in hypoxemia and hypercapnia. Fortunately, most patients have a wide margin between doses that cause analgesia and those that cause respiratory depression. Respiratory depression more commonly occurs as a side effect of opioid administration in patients with respiratory insufficiency or neurologic dysfunction, and in infants less than 3 months of age.[148,149] Opioid use is not contraindicated for such patients, provided adequate medical monitoring is available and reduced dosages are used. It should be noted that respiratory depression is seen very rarely in patients being treated with opioids for pain from cancer.[150]

Pure Opiate Agonists (Morphine, Methadone, Fentanyl)
See Table 13-15.

Table 13-15
Opiate Agonists and Antagonists

Pure opiate agonists   • Include morphine, methadone, fentanyl.   • No ceiling effect.[136]   • Increased dose results in increased pain relief.[136]
Mixed agonist–antagonists   • Include pentazocine, butorphanol, propoxyphene.   • Have ceiling effect.[135,151]   • Can antagonize and reverse actions of pure agonists.[151,152]   • Associated with high rate of dysphoria.[136]   • May precipitate opiate withdrawal.[136]
Opiate antagonists   • Include naloxone, naltrexone.   • Reverse opiate-induced analgesia, sedation, and respiratory depression.[153,154]   • Chronic administration can result in anxiety, depression, nausea, vomiting, and pulmonary edema.[136]

Tolerance and Physical Dependence

For a full description of tolerance and physical dependence, see Chapter 14.

Specific Opioids

See Table 13-16.

Opiate Antagonists

See Chapters 12 and 14.

Table 13-16

Specific Opiods

Morphine
- Effective in ameliorating pediatric pain.
- In opioid-naïve patients, starting doses are 0.1 mg/kg IV every two hours, or 0.1 mg/kg IM or SQ every three to four hours.[136]
- Acute oral-to-parenteral ratio 6:1.[136]
- Chronic oral-to-parenteral ratio 3:1.[136]
- Time-release oral preparations of morphine allow b.i.d. or t.i.d. dosing.[136]
- Need to monitor neuropsychiatric function.

Codeine
- Most commonly administered oral opioid for moderate pain.[136]
- Starting dose 0.5 mg/kg PO every four hours.[136]

Methadone
- Longer duration of action than morphine or heroin.[155–157]
- Metabolized very slowly.
- Unlike heroin, can be given orally.[136]
- Somnolence relatively common and necessitates dosage reduction.
- In children, oral administration of methadone every six to eight hours or IV every four to six hours following a loading dose yields consistent clinical effect in children.[136]
- Initial oral doses: 0.1 mg/kg every four hours and then every six to eight hours.[136]

Fentanyl
- Much shorter duration of action after bolus administration than morphine.[158]
- Useful when analgesia is required for brief but painful procedures.[136]
- Doses for painful procedures: 102 μg/kg or increasing dose by 0.5 μg/kg every 1–2 minutes p.r.n.[136]

Meperidine (Demerol)
- Shorter duration of action than morphine.
- Active metabolite normeperidine associated with convulsions and dysphoria.[159,160]

Hydromorphine (Dilaudid)
- Eight times more potent than morphine.[136]
- Oral-to-parenteral ratio 3–4:1.[136]
- Oral preparation better tolerated than oral morphine preparation.[136]

Naloxone Administration
See Table 13-17.

Tricyclic Antidepressants
See Chapter 4.

Stimulants
Methylphenidate and dextroamphetamine have been shown to decrease narcotic requirements and narcotic-induced CNS depression.[136,161]

Cocaine had been proposed as an effective agent in the treatment of chronic pain, but its use results in less pain relief and more dysphoric reactions than does amphetamine use.[136] Cocaine is not recommended for the treatment of pain. Marijuana has been used in some adult patients with chronic pain, but there are no data on children and adolescents. Trials of stimulants such as dextroamphetamine or methylphenidate to attempt to reduce narcotic requirements and CNS depression may be useful.

Sedative-Hypnotics
Whenever possible, these agents should be avoided. Children and adolescents with pain are better treated with opioid agents. The goal is to provide pain relief, not to make the child too sedated to report his or her pain.[136]

Antipsychotics
Phenothiazines and butyrophenones have been used in the treatment of nausea and vomiting associated with cancer chemotherapy.[161] The doses of neuroleptics necessary to ameliorate nausea and vomiting postoperatively are significantly lower than those used for chemotherapy-induced nausea and vomiting. These agents have significant side effects that can be quite debilitating, such as NMS, dystonias, and tardive dyskinesia (see Chapter 7). They have little analgesic effect, but can decrease a patient's ability to re-

Table 13-17
Naloxone Administration

- Used in emergency treatment of opioid overdose.
- Doses of 0.01–0.02 mg/kg cause complete reversal of opiate agonist effects.[136]
- When possible, give lower dose of 0.002 mg/kg to attenuate respiratory depression without completely reversing sedative and analgesic effects.[136]
- Duration action 30–45 minutes.
- Monitor closely for relapse respiratory depression.[136]

port pain.[163] Neuroleptics have been combined with opioids for sedation for certain procedures. We agree with Shannon and Berde[136] that neuroleptics should not be used for chemical restraint, particularly for children and adolescents.

Phenothiazines have also been used alone or in combination with antidepressants to treat intractable pain in adults.[162] These agents have such severe and chronic side effects (NMS, tardive dyskinesia) that we do not recommend their use for children and adolescents. Moreover, when a neuroleptic is used with an antidepressant, the two increase each other's blood concentration, further raising the risk of toxicity (see Chapters 4 and 7).

Benzodiazepines

Benzodiazepines produce little pain relief,[136] although they are useful preoperatively and for some procedures. When administered with opioids, they increase sedative and respiratory depressant side effects.[136] Their use for chronic pain is limited, and they should be employed only as time-limited temporary adjuncts. They should not be routinely used to facilitate sleep.

Barbiturates

Barbiturates do not produce pain relief, and in some cases can be antianalgesic.[136] Physical dependence and tolerance are important concerns. These agents should not be used in the management of children and adolescents with chronic pain.[136]

Antihistamines

Antihistamines have relatively little analgesic effect and primarily cause sedation. They can treat opioid side effects such as pruritus.[164] Anticholinergic side effects can be problematic. They do, however, have a high margin of safety as sedative agents.[136] Cyproheptadine, which has antihistamine properties in addition to its serotonergic effects, has been used to treat migraine headaches.[165,166]

Membrane-Stabilizing Drugs

Anticonvulsants. Anticonvulsants such as phenytoin, carbamazepine, and clonazepam are frequently prescribed for patients with migraine and neuropathy.[167–169] These medications are given without utilizing loading doses, and dosage increments are dependent on plasma drug levels and are limited by side effects.[136] The most common side effects (see Chapter 9) are dysphoria, ataxia, sedation, disorientation, and GI upset. It is very important to monitor hematologic and hepatic function.

These agents have been shown to help some adult patients with pain, particularly of the shooting and stabbing variety, but it is difficult to predict which patients will respond to them.[136] There are no data on children and adolescents, and we cannot recommend their routine use for these conditions.

Local Anesthetics.   The data on the use of these agents to treat chronic pain in children and adolescents are very limited. The administration of local anesthetics such as lidocaine or 2-chloroprocaine IV has been proposed as a potential treatment of neuropathic pain.[136] Diagnostic trials with these agents are often conducted, and if the patient responds, he or she is given an oral analogue, mexiletin or tocanide.[136] These agents can produce toxic reactions, so caution is necessary when they are administered. Again, as there are no data on children and adolescents, this procedure cannot be endorsed for this population at this time.

Corticosteroids.   The corticosteroids relieve the pain associated with swelling and inflammation, such as pain from headaches caused by brain tumors, pain from bony metastases, and joint pain due to rheumatologic disorders.[136] These agents have also been used in cancer patients with refractory nausea. It is important to monitor for psychiatric side effects (see Chapter 14).

Psychiatric Consultation to Organ Transplant Services

Trzepacz and associates[171] found that liver transplant candidates who were delirious were significantly more emotionally stressed than were nondelirious candidates. Adjustment disorders with depressed and/or anxious features are rather common in transplantation candidates and patients.[172–174]

It is important to remember that the very presence of medical disease is a risk factor for major depression.[172] Studies of transplant candidates have revealed that up to 16% experience depression.[175,176] In adults, medications are frequently necessary to treat the depression.[170] However, lower doses of antidepressant often are required for transplant patients because of their impaired hepatic and/or renal metabolism.[177,178] Close monitoring of plasma drug levels is recommended. In adult depressed transplant patients, TCAs are the medications of choice. Nortriptyline is preferred since it has fewer side effects than many of the other TCAs, and has a therapeutic window of effective serum levels that facilitates monitoring.[179]

The SSUIs such as fluoxetine or sertraline may also be considered for these patients, since they lack anticholinergic side effects and so may be less likely to exacerbate cognitive function. Caution must be exercised when utilizing these agents as they are metabolized by the liver. Thus lower dosing regimens are recommended for children and adolescents with liver failure.

Mood Instability/Bipolar Disorder

The treatment of mood instability and bipolar disorder has been discussed. In liver transplant patients, treatment with lithium may be especially indicated since this medication is metabolized by the kidney and not by the liver (see Chapter 8). If there is evidence of kidney failure, lithium should probably not be used unless the patient has demonstrated a prior positive response to the medication. The lowest possible dose should be utilized, and the careful monitoring of kidney function is necessary. It is also imperative that careful attention be paid to mental status and that neurologic status be maintained, since these patients may be at increased risk for lithium's CNS side effects (see Chapter 8). Careful monitoring of lithium plasma levels is necessary.

It also behooves the clinician to be cognizant of important lithium drug interactions, as with ibuprofen and chlorothiazid, which can increase the lithium to toxic levels (see Chapter 8). Alternative agents to treat mood instability and bipolar disorder, such as carbamazepine and valproic acid, may be indicated when lithium therapy is unsuccessful or contraindicated. Caution is necessary, however, in patients with liver failure, since these agents are metabolized by the liver. They may be warranted in bipolar patients with kidney failure. We wish to emphasize that the first intervention in such children and adolescents is to assess their current medical regimen and attempt to discern whether medications such as prednisone, cyclosporine, or narcotics are causing the mood disorder. The lowest possible effective doses of these agents should be used.

Delirium

Studies of delirium in transplant candidates have demonstrated incidences as high as 50%.[170] When such delirious patients become agitated or psychotic, and while an etiology is being delineated, the patients can be treated symptomatically with a neuroleptic. Haloperidol is used most commonly because of its lower risk of exacerbating delirium due to its minimal anticholinergic side effects. Low dosing regimens are important; 0.5 mg–3.0 mg in small divided doses is recommended. Haloperidol can be used orally, IM, or IV in equivalent doses.[180] Extrapyramidal side effects are far less common at such low doses. Haloperidol should probably be given IV only when the patient is in a monitored bed, as in an ICU setting. This medication has been used safely in patients with many different types of organ failure.[180]

Substance Abuse

Drug and alcohol abusers may need liver or cardiac transplants. Intravenous drug abuse may, for example, result in hepatitis and require liver transplantation. Acetaminophen overdose can cause liver toxicity and necessitate transplantation. It is also important to evaluate patients for the presence of withdrawal states, which can present as autonomic dysfunction and can be confused with other medical problems, such as delirium, apathy, agitation, anxiety, depression, and even psychosis.[170] The patient should be given time for detoxification before transplantation is performed.[170] Benzodiazepine intervention may be warranted (see Chapter 14).

Anxiety

Anxiety as a symptom can be found in up to 39% of organ transplant patients.[173] As mentioned earlier, when benzodiazepines are necessary, those that have short half-lives and do not require oxidative hepatic metabolism, such as lorazepam and oxazepam, are preferred. Lorazepam has the added advantage of being absorbed when given IM. Long-acting benzodiazepines such as alprazolam and diazepam should be avoided. It is important to use the lowest effective dose. These medications should be used for discrete time-limited periods. Around-the-clock dosing should be avoided, the medication given on an as-needed basis instead. It is important to emphasize that all benzodiazepines can cause confusion and sedation in medically compromised patients.[181] Agents such as triazolam and temazepam, which are frequently dispensed as sleeping pills and have short half-lives, are not recommended for children and adolescents (see "Treatment of Chronic Sleep Disruption in Children and Adolescents"). Buspirone, a new anxiolytic, has not been extensively studied in transplant patients. It is not addictive and is less sedating than the benzodiazepines, so a trial may be warranted in chronic, refractory anxiety (see prior section).

Psychiatric Consultation to Obstetrics and Gynecology

In this section, we discuss the premenstrual syndrome and pregnancy and perinatal issues. Teenage females may be at particular risk with the added stressors of adolescence. For a thorough review of the assessment, evaluation, and management involved in the psychiatric consultation to obstetrics and gynecology, the reader is referred to the American Psychiatric Press's *Review of Psychiatry*.[182]

Premenstrual Syndrome

Studies of patients with the premenstrual syndrome (PMS) have shown depression rates of 45–60%.[183] Since premenstrual symptoms are linked to hormonal cycles, estrogen, progesterone, endorphins, neurotransmitters, prostaglandins, and pyridoxine have been used to treat PMS, with no controlled studies demonstrating the etiologic or curative activity of any of these agents.[182]

Treatment
There is, as yet, no known successful PMS treatment. Controlled studies have not shown any medication to be effective.

Pregnancy and Perinatal Issues

Pregnancy is by definition a normative life crisis for the woman, her mate, and the family,[184] and it can represent an even greater crisis for an adolescent female, whose pregnancy may be unexpected, unwanted, and the cause of family consternation and anger.

Psychiatric Complications
In the United States, 50–80% of new mothers suffer "postpartum blues." The condition consists of crying, anxiety, forgetfulness, and impaired concentration; becomes evident a few days postpartum; and lasts about 10 days.[185] It lessens in severity each postpartum day. Reassurance and support are the mainstays of treatment. Pharmacologic intervention is not warranted.

Postpartum Psychosis
Postpartum psychosis is seen with one to two of every 1000 deliveries. The risk is increased if the patient has a history of mood disorder or if the patient's mother had a postpartum illness. The symptoms usually occur by the third postpartum day. This condition is a psychiatric emergency. Patients are at increased risk for killing themselves and their babies.

The aggressive treatment of major mood disorders is recommended.[182] Neuroleptics can help the agitated and psychotic patient, and TCAs have been found effective in adult women with major depression.

There is, of course, controversy over the danger of using psychotropic medications for the nursing mother. One possible way to circumvent this is to recommend bottle feeding, which may even be a relief to some women.

Managing pregnant patients is one of the great challenges facing psychiatry. Common consultations of the psychiatrist involve the onset of a major psychiatric condition in pregnancy and/or the feasibility of maintaining a patient on medication during pregnancy. In addition, some adolescents may not communicate to the health-care provider that they are pregnant, and they often do not present for prenatal care until late in their pregnancy. Currently, the knowledge about teratogenic effects and other adverse side effects of psychotropic medications is inadequate,[182] and it is not likely further data will be acquired. It is not possible ethically to perform controlled studies on humans, and it is not known how well studies on pregnant animals will generalize to humans.[182] For the use of specific psychotropic agents in pregnancy, refer to the appropriate medication chapters.

The consultation–liaison psychiatrist must also be aware that untreated major psychiatric illness is associated with a significantly increased risk of obstetric complications.[182] Depressed patients, because of neurovegetative symptoms such as apathy and decreased energy level, take poorer care of themselves, become less compliant, and become dangerous to themselves or others.[182] Psychotic patients may have compliance problems and not show up for clinic appointments. It is necessary for the psychiatrist to weigh the risks versus the benefits of prescribing psychotropic medications in this situation. When the decision is made to prescribe medication, the lowest possible effective dose should be used.

References

1. Hales, R.E., Thompson, T.L. (1991). Consultation-liaison psychiatry. In A. Tasman, S.M. Goldfinger, C.A. Kaufmann (Eds.), *Review of Psychiatry (volume 9)* (pp. 433–566). Washington, D.C.: American Psychiatric Press.

2. Hauser, W., Kurland, L. (1975). The epidemiology of epilepsy in Rochester, Minnesota: 1935 through 1967. *Epilepsia, 16*, 1–66.

3. Cavazutti, G.B. (1980). Epidemiology of different types of epilepsy in school age children of Modena, Italy. *Epilepsia, 21*, 51–62.

4. MacKinnon, R.A., Yudofsky, S.C. (1986) *The Psychiatric Evaluation in Clinical Practice*. Philadelphia: J.B. Lippincott.

5. Rutter, M., Graham, P., Yule, W. (1970). *A Neuropsychiatric Study in Childhood: Clinics in Developmental Medicine, no. 35–36*. London: Spastics International Medical Publications/Heinemann Medical Books.

6. Bear, D.M., Fedio, P. (1977). Quantitative analysis of interictal behavior in temporal lobe epilepsy. *Arch Neurol, 34*, 454–467.

7. Garyfallos, G., Manos, N., Adamopoulou, A. (1988). Psychopathology and personality characteristics of epileptic patients: Epilepsy, psychopathology and personality. *Acta Psychiatr Scand, 78*, 87–95.

8. Flor-Henry, P. Determinants of psychosis in epilepsy: Laterality and forced normalization. *Biol Psychiatry, 18*, 1045–1057.

9. Mendez, M.F., Cummings, J.L., Benson, D.F. (1986). Depression in epilepsy: Significance and phenomenology. *Arch Neurol, 43*, 766–779.

10. Matthews, W., Barabas, G. (1981). Suicide and epilepsy: A review of the literature. *Psychosomatics, 22*, 515–524.

11. Brent, D.A. (1986). Overrepresentation of epileptics in a consecutive series of suicide attempters seen at Children's Hospital, 1978–1983. *J Am Acad Child Psychiatry, 25(2)*, 242–246.

12. Keviatkowska, E., Bichonski, R. (1967). The Ehbecke syndrome in the course of epilepsy in children. *Psychatr Pol, 1*, 159–164.

13. Silanpaa, M. (1973). Medico-social prognosis of children with epilepsy. *Acta Paediatr Scand, 62:(suppl 237)*, 6–93.

14. Corbett, J., Timble, M. (1983). Epilepsy and anticonvulsant medication. In M. Rutter (Ed.), *Developmental Neuropsychiatry* (pp. 112–129). New York: Guilford Press.

15. Stores, G. (1975). Behavioral effect of anti-epileptic drugs. *Dev Med Child Neurol, 17*, 647–658.

16. Timble, M., Reynolds, E. (1976). Anticonvulsant drugs and mental symptoms: A review, editorial. *Psychol Med, 6*, 169–198.

17. American Academy of Pediatrics, Committee on Drugs. (1985). Behavioral and cognitive effects of anticonvulsant therapy. *Pediatrics, 76*, 644–647.

18. Brent, D.A., Crumrine, P.K., Varma, R.R., et al. (1987). Phenobarbital treatment and major depressive disorder in children with epilepsy. *Pediatrics, 80*, 909–917.

19. Ounsted, C. (1955). The hyperkinetic syndrome in epileptic children. *Lancet, 2*, 303.

20. Wolf, S., Forsythe, A. (1978). Behavioral disturbance, phenobarbital and febrile seizures. *Pediatrics, 61*, 728–731.

21. Thorn, I. (1975). A controlled study of prophylactic long-term treatment of febrile convulsions with phenobarbital. *Acta Neurol Scand, 60(suppl)*, 67–73.

22. Camfield, C., Cahplen, S., Doyle, A.B., et al. (1979). Side effects of phenobarbital in toddlers: Behavioral and cognitive aspects. *J Pediatr, 95*, 361–365.

23. Ferrari, M., Barabas, G., Matthews, W. (1983). Psychologic and behavioral disturbance among epileptic children treated with barbiturate anticonvulsants. *Am J Psychiatry, 140*, 112–113.

24. Schain, R., Ward, J., Guthrie, D. (1977). Carbamazepine as an anticonvulsant in children. *Neurology, 27*, 476–480.

25. Corbett, J.A., Trimble, M.R., Nichol, T.C. (1985). Behavioral and cognitive impairments in children with epilepsy: The long-term effects of anticonvulsant therapy. *J Am Acad Child Psychiatry, 24*, 17–23.

26. Weilberg, J.B., Bear, D.M., Sachs, G. (1989). Three patients with concommitant panic attacks and seizure disorder: Possible clues to the neurology of anti-anxiety. *Am J Psychiatry, 144*, 1053–1056.

27. McKenna, P.J., Kane, J.M., Parrish, K. (1985). Psychotic syndromes in epilepsy. *Am J Psychiatry, 142*, 895–904.

28. Stevens, J.R., Hyman, B.P. (1981). Temporal lobe epilepsy, psychopathology, and violence: The state of the evidence. *Neurology, 31*, 1127–1132.

29. Hoare, P. (1984). The development of psychiatric disorder among school children with epilepsy. *Dev Med Child Neurol, 26*, 3–13.

30. Gallassi, R., Morreale, A., Lorusso, S., et al. Carbamazepine and phenytoin: Comparison of cognitive effects in epileptic patients during monotherapy and withdrawal. *Arch Neurol, 45*, 892–894.

31. Corbett, J.A., Trimble, M.R., Nichol, T.C. (1985). Behavioral and cognitive impairments in children with epilepsy: The long-term effects of anticonvulsant therapy. *J Am Acad Child Psychiatry, 24*, 17–23.

32. Ojemann, L.M., Baugh-Bookman, C., Dudby, D.L. (1987). Effect of psychotropic medications on seizure control in patients with epilepsy. *Neurology, 37*, 1525–1527.

33. Silver, J.M., Hales, R.E., Yudofsky, S.C. (1990). Psychiatric consultation to neurology. In A. Tasman, S.M., Goldfinger, C.A., Kaufmann (Eds.), *Review of Psychiatry (volume 9)* (pp. 433–465). Washington, D.C.: American Psychiatric Press.

34. Oliver, A.P., Luchins, D.J., Wyatt, R.J. (1982). Neuroleptic-induced seizures: An in vitro technique for assessing relative risk. *Arch Gen Psychiatry, 39*, 206–209.

35. Menkes, J.H. (1990). Tumors of the nervous system. In J.H. Menkes (Ed.), *Textbook of Child Neurology (4th ed.)* (pp. 526–582). Philadelphia: Lea & Febiger.

36. Jaffe, J. (1987). The subjective experience of brain surgery: The mind at risk. In R.S. Blacher (Ed.), *The Psychological Experiences of Surgery* (pp. 435–450). New York: Wiley.

37. Kaplan, H.I., Sadock, B.J. (1991). Mental retardation. In H.I. Kaplan, B.J. Sadock (Eds.), *Synopsis of Psychiatry* (6th ed.) (pp. 691–692). Baltimore: Williams & Wilkins.

38. Stewart, J.T., Nemsath, R.H. (1988). Bipolar illness following traumatic brain injury: Treatment with lithium and carbamazepine. *J Clin Psychiatry, 49*, 74–75.

39. Pope, H.G. Jr., McElroy, S.L., Satlin, A., et al. (1988). Head injury, bipolar disorder, and response to valproate. *Compr Psychiatry, 29*, 34–38.

40. Kahn, D., Stevenson, E., Douglas, C.J. (1988). Effect of sodium valproate in three patients with organic brain syndromes. *Am J Psychiatry, 145*, 1010–1011.

41. Clark, A.F., Davison, K. (1987). Mania following head injury: A report of two cases and a review of the literature. *Br J Psychiatry, 150*, 841–844.

42. Schiff, H.B., Sabin, T.D., Geller, A., et al. (1982). Lithium in aggressive behavior. *Am J Psychiatry, 139*, 1346–1348.

43. Pleak, R.R., Birmaher, B., Gavrilescu, A. (1988). Mania and neuropsychiatric excitation following carbamazepine. *J Am Acad Child Adolesc Psychiatry, 27*, 500–503.

44. Feeney, D.M., Gonzalez, A., Law, W.A. (1982). Amphetamine, haloperidol, and experience interact to affect rate of recovery after motor cortex injury. *Science, 217*, 855–857.

45. Silver, J.M., Yudofsky, S.C. (1988). Psychopharmacology and electroconvulsive therapy. In J.A. Talbott, R.E. Hales, S.C. Yudofsky (Eds.), *American Psychiatric Textbook of Psychiatry* (pp. 767–853). Washington, D.C.: American Psychiatric Press.

46. Ojemann, L.M., Baugh-Bookman, C., Dudley, D.L. (1987). Effect of psychotropic medications on seizure control in patients with epilepsy. *Neurology, 37*, 1525–1527.

47. Tunbridge, W.M.G., Evered, D.C., Hall, R., et al. (1977). The spectrum of thyroid disease in a community survey. *Clin Endocrinol, 7*, 481–493.

48. Blackwell, B., Schmidt, G.L. (1984). Drug interactions in psychopharmacology. *Psychiatr Clin N Am, 7*, 625–636.

49. Craig, T.K.J., Brown, G.W. (1984). Goal frustration and life events in the aetiology of painful gastrointestinal disorder. *J Psychosom Res, 28*, 411–421.

50. Rose, J.D.R., Thoughton, A.H., Giardina, E.G.V., et al. (1986). Depression and functional bowel disorders in gastrointestinal outpatients. *Gut, 27,* 1025–1028.

51. Talley, N.J., Fung, L.H., Gilligen, I.J., et al. (1986). Association of anxiety, neuroticism, and depression with dyspexsia of unknown cause: A case control study. *Gastroenterology, 90,* 886–892.

52. Vatn, M.H., Mogstad, T.E., Gjone, E. (1985). A prospective study of patients with uncharacteristic abdominal disorders. *Scand J Gastroenterol, 20,* 407–414.

53. Stoudemire, A., Sandhu, J. (1987). Psychogenic/idiopathic pain syndromes. *Gen Hosp Psychiatry, 9,* 79–86.

54. Creed, F., Guthrie, E. (1987). Psychological factors in the irritable bowel syndrome. *Gut, 28,* 1307–1318.

55. Kasich, A.M. (1968). A double-blind study of heteronium bromide and amobarbital in the management of gastrointestinal conditions associated with anxiety. *Curr Ther Res, 10,* 508–513.

56. Rhodes, J.B., Abrams, H.J., Manning, R.T. (1978). Controlled clinical trial of sedative-anticholinergic drugs in patients with irritable bowel syndrome. *J Clin Pharm, 18,* 340–345.

57. Greenbaum, D.S., Mayle, J.E., Vanegreen, L.E., et al. (1987). Effects of desipramine on irritable bowel syndrome compared with atropine and placebo. *Dig Dis Sci, 32,* 257–266.

58. Helzer, J.E., Chammas, S., Norland, C.C., et al. (1984). A study of the association between Crohn's disease and psychiatric illness. *Gastroenterology, 86,* 324–440.

59. Andrews, H., Barczak, P., Allan, R.N. (1986). Psychiatric illness in patients with inflammatory bowel disease. *Gut, 28,* 1600–1604.

60. Sellers, E.M., Bendoyan, R. (1987). Pharmacokinetics of psychotropic drugs in selected patient populations. In H.Y. Meltzer (Ed.), *Psychopharmacology: The Third Generation of Progress* (pp. 1397–1406). New York: Raven Press.

61. Silverstone, P.H. (1984). Ranitidine and confusion. *Lancet, 1,* 1071.

62. Hennan, N.E., Carpenter, D.U., Janda, S.M. (1988). Famotidine-associated mental confusion in elderly patients. *Drug Intell Clin Pharm, 22,* 976–978.

63. Abernathy, D.R., Greenblatt, D.J., Eshelman, F.N., et al. (1984). Ranitidine does not impair oxidative or conjugative metabolism: Noninteraction

with antipyrine, diazepam, and lorazepam. *Clin Pharmacol Ther, 35,* 188–192.

64. Shrivastava, R.K., Shah, B.K., Siegal, H. (1985). Doxepin and cimetidine treatment in duodenal ulcer: A double-blind comparative study. *Clin Ther, 7,* 181–189.

65. Henaver, S.A., Hollister, L.E. (1984). Cimetidine intervention with imipramine and nortriptyline. *Clin Pharmacol Ther, 35,* 183–186.

66. Lazzara, R.R., Stoudemire, A., Manning, D., et al. (1986). Metoclopramide-induced tardive dyskinesia. *Gen Hosp Psychiatry, 8,* 107–109.

67. Stoudemire, A., Fogel, B.F. (1987). *Principles of Medical Psychiatry.* Orlando, Fla.: Grune & Stratton.

68. Hall, R.C.W., Popkin, M.K., Stickney, S.K., et al. (1979). Presentation of the steroid psychoses. *J Nerv Ment Dis, 167,* 229–239.

69. Hall, R.C.W., Stickney, S.K., Gardner, E.R. (1981). Psychiatric symptoms in patients with systemic lupus erythematosus. *Psychosomatics, 22,* 15–24.

70. Hart, R.P., Kreutzen, J.S. (1988). Renal system. In R.E. Tarter, D.H. Van Thiel, K.L. Edwards (Eds.), *Medical Neuropsychology* (pp. 99–120). New York: Plenum.

71. Vincent, H.H., Wentiag, G.J., Schalekamp, M.A.D.H., et al. (1987). Impaired functional excretion of lithium: A very early marking of cyclosporine nephrotoxicity. *Transplant Proc, 19,* 4147–4148.

72. Bennett, W.M., Aronoff, G.R., Golper, T.A., et al. (1987). *Drug Prescribing in Renal Failure.* Philadelphia: American College of Physicians.

73. Gengo, F.M., Gabos, C. (1988). Central nervous system considerations in the use of β-blockers, angiotensin-converting enzyme inhibitors, and thiazide diuretics in managing essential hypertension. *Am Heart J, 116,* 305–310.

74. Levenson, J.L. (1987). Cardiovascular disease. In A. Stoudemire, B.F. Fogel (Eds.), *Principles of Medical Psychiatry* (pp. 477–493). Orlando, Fla.: Grune & Stratton.

75. Medical letter (1986). Choice of a beta blocker. *Med Lett, 28,* 20–22.

76. Houston, M.C., Hodge, R. (1988). Beta-adrenergic blocker withdrawal syndromes in hypertension and other cardiovascular diseases. *Am Heart J, 116,* 515–522.

77. Croog, S., Levine, S., Testa, M.A., et al. (1986). The effects of antihypertensive therapy on the quality of life. *N Engl J Med, 314,* 1657–1664.

78. Stoudemire, G.A., Levenson, J.L. (1991). Psychiatric consultation to internal medicine. In A. Tasman, S.M. Goldfinger, C.A. Kaufmann (Eds.), *Review of Psychiatry (volume 9)* (pp. 460–490). Washington, DC: American Psychiatric Press.

79. Donosky, T. (1988). Mead-Johnson Pharmaceuticals, December 7. Personal communication.

80. Furukawa, C.T., Shapiro, G.G., DuHamel, T., et al. (1984). Learning and behavioral problems associated with theophyline therapy (letter). *Lancet, 1*, 621.

81. McLoughlin, J., Nall, M., Isaacs, B., et al. (1983). The relationship of allergies and allergy treatment to school performance and student behavior. *Ann Allergy, 51*, 506–510.

82. Rachelefsky, G.S., Wo, J., Adelson, J., et al. (1986). Behavior abnormalities and poor school performance due to oral theophylline use. *Pediatrics, 78*, 1133–1138.

83. Springer, C., Goldenberg, B., Dou, I.B., et al. (1985). Clinical, physiologic, and psychologic comparison of treatment by cromolyn or theophylline in childhood asthma. *J Allergy Clin Immunol, 76*, 64–69.

84. Creer, T.L., Gustafson, K.E. (1989). Psychological problems associated with drug therapy in childhood asthma. *J Pediatr, 115*, 850–855.

85. Creer, T.L., Kotses, H., Gustafson, K.E., et al. (1988). A critique of studies investigating the association of theophylline to psychological or behavioral performance. *Pediatr Asthma Allergy Immunol, 2*, 169–184.

86. Hall, R.C., Beresford, T.P., Stickney, S.K., et al. (1985). Psychiatric reactions produced by respiratory drugs. *Psychosomatics, 26(7)*, 605–616.

87. Marley, E., Nistico, G. (1972). Effects of catecholamines and adenosine derivations given into the brain of foculs. *Br J Pharmacol, 46*, 619–636.

88. Haulica, I., Ababei, D., Branisteanu, D., et al. (1973). Preliminary data on the possible hypnogenic role of adenosine. *J Neurochem, 21*, 1019–1020.

89. Maitre, M., Crexielski, L., Lehmann, A., et al. (1974). Protective effect of adenosine and nicotinamide against audiogenic seizure. *Biochem Pharmacol, 23*, 2807–2816.

90. Weiner, M., Olson, J.W. (1977). Single-dose tolerance to the behavioral effects of dibutyryl cyclic AMP in mice. *Psychopharmacology, 54*, 61–65.

91. Snyder, S.H., Bruns, R.F., Daly, J.W., et al. (1981). Multiple neurotransmitter receptors in the brain: Amines, adenosine and cholecystokinin. *Fed Proc, 40*, 142–146.

92. Murphy, M.B., Dillon, A., Fitzgerald, M.X. (1980). Theophylline and depression. *Br Med J, 281*, 1322.

93. Gluckman, L. (1974). Ventolin psychoses. *NZ Med J, 80*, 411.

94. Feline, A., Jouvent, R. (1977). Manifestations of psychosensoriellos observees choz des psychotiques soumises a des medications beta-mimetiques. *L'Encephale, 3*, 149–158.

95. Ray, I., Evans, J.C. (1978). Paranoid psychosis with ventoline (salbutamol tablets)(letter). *Can Psychiatr Assoc J, 23*, 427.

96. Jacquot, M., Bottari, R. (1981). Manic state provoked by salbutamol via oral route. *L'Encephale, 7*, 45–49.

97. Abensour, P., Jouvent, R., Lecrubier, Y. (1982). Noradrenergic drugs and affective disorders. *Am J Psychiatry, 139*, 142–143.

98. Widlocher, D., Lecrubier, Y., Jouvent, R., et al. (1977). Antidepressant effect of salbutanol. *Lancet, 2*, 767–768.

99. Jouvent, R., Lecrubier, Y., Puech, A.T., et al. (1977). De l'etude experimentale d'un stimulant beta-adrenergique a la mese en evidence de son activite anti-depressive chez l'homme. *L'Encephale, 18*, 330–336.

100. Simon, P., Lecrubier, Y., Jouvent, R., et al. (1978). Experimental and clinical evidence of the antidepressant effect of a beta-adrenergic stimulant. *Psychol Med, 8*, 335–338.

101. Lecrubier, Y., Puech, A.J., Jouvent, P., et al. (1980). A beta-adrenergic stimulant (salbutinol) versus clomipramine in depression: A controlled study. *Br J Psychiatry, 136*, 354–358.

102. Johnson, A.L., Hollister, L.E., Berger, P.A., et al. (1981). The anticholinergic intoxication syndrome: Diagnosis and treatment. *J Clin Psychiatry, 42*, 313–317.

103. Weiner, N. (Ed.) (1980). *Pharmacological Basis of Therapeutics* (p. 163). New York: Macmillan.

104. *Physicians' Desk Reference* (45th ed.). (1991). Oradell, NJ: Medical Economics (p. 771).

105. Holst, P.E., et al. (1978). A long-term trial of ipratropium in asthmatic patients. *Aust NZ J Med, 6*, 367–368.

106. Chakravarty, N.K., Matallana, A., Jensen, R., et al. (1956). Central effect of antitussive drugs on cough and respiration. *J Pharmacol Exp Ther, 117*, 127–135.

107. Patel, K.E. (1981). Calcium antagonists in exercise-induced asthma. *Br Med J, 282*, 932–933.

108. Barnes, P.J., Wilson, N.M., Brown, M.J. (1981). A calcium antagonist, nefedepine, modifies exercise-induced asmtha. *Thorax, 36*, 726–730.

109. Cerrina, J., Denjean, A., Alexandre, G., et al. (1981). Inhibition of exercise-induced asthma by a calcium antagonist, nifedipine. *Am Rev Respir Dis, 123*, 156–160.

110. Williams, S.E. (1974). Psychosis associated with sympathomimetic and cromoglycate therapy (Letter). *Med J Aust, 2*, 180.

111. Gale, A.E. (1974). Psychoses associated with sympathomimetic and cromoglycate therapy (Letter). *Med J Aust, 2*, 420.

112. Centers for Disease Control. (1990, Feb.). HIV/AIDS Surveillance Reports.

113. Belfer, M.L., Munir, K. (1991). Acquired immunodeficiency syndrome. In J.M. Wiener (Ed.), *Textbook of Child and Adolescent Psychiatry* (1st ed.) (pp. 495–506). Washington, D.C.: American Psychiatric Press.

114. Barnes, D.M. (1986). Brain function decline in children with AIDS. *Science, 232*, 1196.

115. Ho, D.D., Rota, T.R., Schoolely, R.T., et al. (1985). Isolation of HTLV-III from cerebrospinal fluid and neural tissues of patients with neurological syndromes related to AIDS. *N Engl J Med, 313*, 1493–1497.

116. Shaw, G.M., Harper, M.E., Hahn, B.E., et al. (1985). HTLV-III infection in brains of children and adults with AIDS encephalopathy. *Science, 227*, 177–181.

117. Ammana, A.J. (1987). Pediatric acquired immunodeficiency syndrome. Information on AIDS for the practicing physician. *AMA Nat Council Drugs, 2*, 17–23.

118. Rogers, M.F., Ou, C.Y., Rayfield, M., et al. (1989). Use of polymerase chain reaction for early detection of the proviral sequences of human immunodeficiency virus in infants born to seropositive mothers. *N Engl J Med, 320*, 1649–1654.

119. Belman, A.L., Diamond, G., Dickson, D., et al. (1988). Pediatric acquired immunodeficiency syndrome: Neurologic syndromes. *Am J Dis Child, 149*, 29–35.

120. Grant, I., Atkinson, J.H., Hesselink, J.R., et al. (1987). Evidence for early CNS involvement in AIDS and other HIV infections: Studies with neu-

ropsychologic testing and magnetic resonance imaging. *Ann Intern Med, 107*, 828–836.

121. Navia, B.A., Jordan, B., Price, R.W. (1986). The AIDS dementia complex: I. Clinical features of the AIDS dementia complex. *Ann Neurol, 19*, 525–535.

122. Beckett, A., Summergrad, P., Manscreck, T., et al. (1987). Symptomatic HIV infection of the CNS in a patient without clinical evidence of immunodeficiency. *Am J Psychiatry, 144*, 1342–1344.

123. Ostrow, D., Grant, I., Atkinson, H. (1988). Assessment and management of the AIDS patient with neuropsychiatric disturbances. *J Clin Psychiatry, 49(suppl)*, 14–22.

124. Faulstich, M.E. (1987). Psychiatric aspects of AIDS. *Am J Psychiatry, 144*, 551–556.

125. Thomas, C.T., Szabaldi, E. (1987). Paranoid psychoses as the first presentation of a fulminating lethal case of AIDS. *Br J Psychiatry, 151*, 693–695.

126. Gabel, R.H., Barnard, N., Norko, M., et al. (1986). AIDS presenting as mania. *Compr Psychiatry, 27*, 251–256.

127. Fenton, T.W. (1987). AIDS-related psychiatric disorder. *Br J Psychiatry, 151*, 579–588.

128. Nurnberg, H.G., Prodic, J., Fiori, M., et al. (1984). Psychopathology complicating AIDS. *Am J Psychiatry, 141*, 95–96.

129. Perry, S., Jacobsen, P. (1986). Neuropsychiatric manifications of AIDS-spectrum disorders. *Hosp Community Psychiatry, 37*, 135–142.

130. Rundell, J.R., Wise, M.G., Ursano, R.S. (1986). Three cases of AIDS-related psychiatric disorders. *Am J Psychiatry, 143*, 777–778.

131. American Psychiatric Association (1987). *Diagnostic and Statistical Manual of Mental Disorders* (3rd edition, rev.). Washington, D.C.: American Psychiatric Association.

132. Holland, J.C., Rowland, J.H. (Eds.). (1989). *Handbook of Psychooncology: Psychological Care of the Patient with Cancer.* New York: Oxford University Press.

133. Lederberg, M.S., Massie, M.J., Hollard, J.C. (1991). Psychiatric consultation to oncology. In A. Tasman, S.M. Goldfinger, C.A. Kaufmann (Eds.), *Review of Psychiatry (volume 9)* (pp. 491–514). Washington, D.C.: American Psychiatric Press.

134. Breitbart, W. (1986). Tardive dyskinesia associated with high dose IV metoclopramide. *N Engl J Med, 315*, 518–519.

135. Bonica, J.J. (1978). Cancer pain: A major national health problem. *Cancer Nurs J, 4*, 313–316.

136. Shannon, M., Berde, C.B. (1989). Pharmacologic management of pain in children and adolescents. *Pediatr Clin North Am, 36(4)*, 855–870.

137. Rumack, B.H. (1978). Aspirin versus acetaminophen: A comparative view. *Pediatrics, 62*, 943–946.

138. Foley, K.M. (1979). Pain syndromes in patients with cancer. *Adv Pain Res Ther, 2*, 59–75.

139. Martin, W.R. (1984). Pharmacology of opioids. *Pharm Review, 35*, 285–373.

140. Payne, R. (1987). *Principles of Analgesic Use in the Treatment of Acute Pain and Chronic Cancer Pain.* Washington D.C.: American Pain Society.

141. Bennett, R.C., Batenhorst, R.L., Bivens, B.A., et al. (1981). Patient-controlled analgesia: A new concept of postoperative pain relief. *Ann Surg, 195*, 700–705.

142. Dodd, E., Wang, J.M., Rauck, R.L. (1988). Patient-controlled analgesia for post-surgical pediatric patients ages 6-16 years. *Anesthesiology, 69*, A372.

143. Graves, D.A., Foster, T.S., Batenhorst, R.L., et al. (1983). Patient-controlled analgesia. *Ann Intern Med, 99*, 360–366.

144. Harnes, M., Rosen, M., Vickers, M.D. (1985). *Patient Controlled Analgesia.* London: Blackwell Scientific Publications.

145. Keeri-Szanlo, M., Heamon, S. (1972). Postoperative demand analgesia. *Surg Gynecol Obstet, 134*, 647–651.

146. Means, L.J., Allen, H.M., Lookabill, S.J., et al. (1989). Recovery room initiation of patient controlled analgesia in pediatric patients. *Anesthesiology, 69*, A772.

147. Klotz, U. (1983). Interactions of analgesics with other drugs. *Am J Med, 75*, 133–138.

148. Hertzka, R.E., Fisher, D.M., Gauntlett, I.S., et al. (1987). Are infants sensitive to respiratory depression from fentanyl? *Anesthesiology, 67*, A512.

149. Koren, G., Butt, W., Chinyanga, H., et al. (1985). Postoperative morphine infusion in newborn infants: Assessment of disposition characteristics and safety. *J Pediatr, 107*, 963–967.

150. Jaffe, J.H. (1985). Drug addiction and drug abuse. In L.S. Goodman, A. Gilman (Eds.), *Goodman and Gillman's The Pharmacological Basics of Therapeutics* (pp. 522–574). New York: Macmillan.

151. Reed, D.A., Schnoll, S.H. (1986). Abuse of pentazocine-naloxone combination. *JAMA, 256*, 2562–2564.

152. Wood, A.J.J., Moir, D.C., Campbell, C., et al. (1974). Medicines evaluation and monitoring group: CNS effect of pentazocine. *Br Med J, 1*, 305–307.

153. Fossel, M., Rosen, P. (1984). Naloxone treatment for codeine-induced gastrointestinal symptoms. *J Emerg Med, 2*, 107–110.

154. Handal, K.A., Schauben, J.L., Salamone, F.R. (1983). Naloxone. *Ann Emerg Med, 12*, 438–445.

155. Berde, C.B., Holzman, R.S., Sethana, N.F., et al. (1988). A comparison of methadone and morphine for postoperative analgesia in children and adolescents. *Anesthesiology, 69*, A768.

156. Berde, C.B., Sethna, N.F., Holzman, A.S., et al. (1987). Pharmacokinetics of methadone in children and adolescents in the perioperative period. *Anesthesiology, 67*, A519.

157. Newman, R.G., Gourlay, G.K., Wilson, P.R., Glynn, C.J. (1982). Pharmachodynamics and pharmacokinetics of methadone during the perioperative period. *Anesthesiology, 57*, 458–467.

158. Rosow, C.E., Moss, J., Phisbin, D.M., et al. (1982). Histamine release during morphine and fentanyl anesthesia. *Anesthesiology, 56*, 93–96.

159. Goettling, M.G., Thirma, M.J. (1985). Neurotoxicity of meperidine. *Ann Emerg Med, 14*, 1007–1009.

160. Morisy, L., Platt, D. (1986). Hazards of high-dose meperidine. *JAMA, 255*, 467–468.

161. Arana, G.W., Hyman, S.E. (Eds.) (1991). *Handbook of Psychiatric Drug Therapy (2nd Ed.)* (p. 168). Boston: Little Brown.

162. Monks, R., Mersky, H. (1984). Psychotropic drugs. In P.D. Wall, R. Melzack, J.J. Bonica (Eds.), *Textbook of Pain* (p. 537). Edinburgh Scotland: Churchill Livingstone.

163. McGee, J.L., Alexander, M.R. (1979). Phenothiazine analgesia: Fact or fantasy? *Am J Hosp Pharm, 36*, 633–640.

164. Rumore, M.M., Schlichting, D.A. (1985). Analgesic effects of antihistamines. *Life Sci, 36*, 403–416.

165. Barlow, C.F. (1977). Migraine in childhood. *Res Clin Stud Headache, 5,* 34–36.

166. Bille, B., Luduigsson, J., Sanner, G. (1977). Prophylaxis of migraine in children. *Headache, 17,* 61–63.

167. Swerdlow, M. (1984). Anticonvulsant drugs and chronic pain. *Clin Neuropharmacol, 7,* 51–82.

168. Swerdlow, M., Candell, J.G. (1981). Anticonvulsant drugs used in the treatment of lancinating pain: A comparison. *Anesthesiology, 56,* 1129–1132.

169. Wilbur, M. (1986). Pharmacology of diphenylhydantoin and carbamazepin reaction and voltage sensitive sodium channels. *Trends Neurosci, 9,* 147–151.

170. House, R.M., Trzepacz, P.T., Thompson, T.L. (1991). Psychiatric consultation to organ transplant services. In A. Tasman, S.M. Goldfinger, C.A. Kaufmann (Eds.), *Review of Psychiatry (volume 9)* (pp. 515–536). Washington, D.C.: American Psychiatric Press.

171. Trzepacz, P.T., Brenner, R., Van Theil, D.H. (1989). A psychiatric study of 247 liver transplantation candidates. *Psychosomatics, 30,* 147–153.

172. Freeman, A.M., Watts, D., Karp, R. (1984). Evaluation of cardiac transplant candidates: Preliminary observations. *Psychosomatics, 25,* 197–207.

173. Mai, F.M., McKenzie, F.N., Kostuk, W.J. (1986). Psychiatric aspects of heart transplantation: Preoperative evaluation and postoperative sequelae. *Br Med J, 292,* 311–313.

174. Watts, D., Freeman, A.M., McGriffin, D.G., et al. (1984). Psychiatric aspects of cardiac transplantation. *J Heart Transplant, 3,* 243–247.

175. Hong, B.A., Smith, M.D., Robson, A.M., et al. (1987). Depressive symptomatology and treatment in patients with end-stage renal disease. *Psychol Med, 17,* 185–190.

176. Kuhn, W.F., Myers, B., Brennan, A.F., et al. (1988). Psychopathology in heart transplant candidates. *J Heart Transplant 7,* 223–226.

177. Levy, N.B. (1985). Use of psychotropics in patients with kidney failure. *Psychosomatics, 26,* 699–709.

178. Rosser, R. (1990). Depression during renal dialysis and following transplantation. *Proc R Soc Med, 69,* 20–21.

179. Roose, S.P., Glassman, A.H., Giardinia, E.G., et al. (1991). Tricyclic antidepressants in depressed patients with cardiac conduction disease. *Arch Gen Psychiatry, 44,* 273–275.

180. Ayd, F. (1984). IV Haloperidol-lorazepam therapy for delirium. *Int Drug Ther Newsletter, 19*, 1–3.

181. Berlin, R.M. (1986). Hypnotics in renal failure. *Psychosomatics, 27*, 537–538.

182. Stotland, M.L., Smith, T.E. (1991). Psychiatric consultation to obstetrics and gynecology: Systems and syndromes. In A. Tasman, S.M. Goldfinger, C.A. Kaufmann (Eds.), *Review of Psychiatry (volume 9)* (pp. 537–563). Washington, D.C.: American Psychiatric Press.

183. Roy-Byrne, P.P., Hoban, M.C., Rubinow, D.R. (1987). The relationship of menstrually related mood disorders to psychiatric disorders. *Clin Obstet Gynecol, 30*, 386–395.

184. Nadelson, C.C. (1978). "Normal" and "special" aspects of pregnancy: A psychological approach in the woman patient. In C.C. Nadelson, M.T. Notman (Eds.), *Medical and Psychological Interfaces (volume 1): Sexual and Reproductive Aspects of Women's Health Care* (pp. 73–86). New York: Plenum.

185. Jacobson, S.J., Jones, K., Johnson, D., et al. (1992). Prospective multicenter study of pregnancy outcome after lithium exposure during first trimester. *Lancet, 1*, 530–533.

186. Menkes, J.H. (1990). *Textbook of Child Neurology (4th ed.)* (pp. 114–121). Philadelphia: Lea & Febiger.

187. Lesch, M., Nyham, W.L. (1964). A familiar disorder of oric acid metabolism and central nervous system function. *Am J Med, 36*, 561.

188. Menkes, J.H., Till, K., Gabriel, R.S. (1990). Malformations of the central nervous system. In J.H. Menkes (Ed.), *Textbook of Child Neurology (4th ed.)* (pp. 218–231). Philadelphia: Lea & Febiger.

Pharmacologic Treatment of Substance Abuse Disorders

Accidents, suicide, and homicide account for 80% of adolescent deaths,[1] with substance abuse the major precipitant for most of this premature mortality and morbidity.[2] Drugs and alcohol are involved in 50% of these deaths.[1,3] Adolescents and young adults between the ages of 15 and 24 are now the only group in the United States whose life span is decreasing, and driving while drunk is the most common cause of death in this population.[2] The problem has reached epidemic proportions. Indeed, its extent most likely has been underestimated, since many psychiatrists and other physicians receive little training in the recognition and treatment of adolescent substance abuse.

A detailed description of the diagnosis and nonpharmacologic treatment of adolescent substance abuse is beyond the scope of this book, but we will briefly delineate the key relevant issues as they relate to potential psychopharmacologic treatment in this population. For a more comprehensive overview, the reader is referred to Bailey's chapter on substance use and abuse in Wiener's *Textbook of Child and Adolescent Psychiatry*.[5]

In this chapter, we will discuss (1) the basic conceptualization of the disorder; (2) an understanding of basic pharmacologic concepts relevant to substance abuse; (3) diagnostic issues and problems unique to adolescents; (4) intoxication, tolerance, and dependence, as they relate to the adolescent population; (5) drugs as reinforcers; (6) treatment strategies for withdrawal, reinforcement reduction or aversion development, and pharmacologic attenuation of craving; (7) pharmacotherapy of concomitant psychiatric disorders in adolescent substance abusers; (8) other concerns, such as teenage steroid use/abuse and the effects of prenatal exposure to alcohol, opiates, and other substances; and (9) alternative treatment options.

Conceptualization of the Disorder

The clinical psychopharmacologic treatment of substance-abuse disorders is an underdeveloped area.[6] And this is especially true in the adolescent population where, in contrast to adults, virtually no studies (controlled or uncontrolled) have been conducted. Moreover, treating adolescent substance abusers with the same psychopharmacologic interventions used for adults may not necessarily result in the same desired effects. Developmental issues must be taken into account. Antidepressants, for example, which have been proven to be effective in the treatment of depressed adult patients, have not been shown to be superior to placebo in the treatment of depressed children and adolescents (see Chapter 4). It also appears that, when compared with adults, adolescents have an increased vulnerability to substance abuse and/or dependence.[2] Risk factors for adolescent substance abuse or dependence include (1) a positive family history of substance abuse, (2) friends who use drugs, (3) physical and sexual abuse, and (4) having a comorbid psychiatric condition such as conduct disorder, ADHD, or depression.[2,10–14]

Moreover, adolescents more commonly engage in polydrug use, further complicating diagnosis and therapy. Concomitant psychiatric disorders in adolescent substance abusers, such as depression, suicidality, anxiety, conduct disorders, and organic mental syndromes, are not uncommon.[7–9] It is often difficult to treat these patients effectively. Currently, psychosocial interventions are the mainstay of treatment in the adolescent population.

An added challenge facing clinicians treating adolescent substance abusers is the introduction in recent years of more potent and dangerous forms of existing drugs of abuse and of new "designer drugs"—chemically altered and redesigned psychoactive substances.[6,15]

Crack cocaine has received the most publicity; it comes in small chunks referred to as rocks, which are smoked, resulting in a more rapid and intense high.[182] When crack is smoked, it easily penetrates the blood–brain barrier. Compulsive use often follows, making this a very expensive vice.[15] Ice, a very potent form of the stimulant methamphetamine, is also smoked. It delivers a highly potent dose directly to the brain, but unlike crack, its effects last for hours instead of minutes.[15] Lysergic acid diethylamide (LSD) use among adolescents has increased in recent years after a period of decline.[15]

Marijuana is often considered by parents, many of whom have tried it, to be more benign and less dangerous than other, "more serious" drugs. However, hybrid forms of marijuana have been introduced that contain many times the active ingredient, tetrahydrocannabinol (THC), found in even the most potent forms of cannabis.[15] Moreover, persistent, heavy marijuana use by cannabis-dependent adolescents results in significant and long-lasting short-term memory deficits.[16] This likely is due to the fact that the marijuana smoked today is nearly 600% more potent than the marijuana used in early studies in the 1970s.[16-22] Hallucinogenic mushrooms received much press, but were used only relatively rarely in the 1970s. Phencyclidine (PCP) is another hallucinogenic agent with a very dangerous side-effect profile. Heroin, designer opioids, methylenedioxymethamphetamine (MDMA—street name "ecstasy"), prescription stimulants, and sedative hypnotic drugs—drugs that had been primarily used by adults—are increasingly being used by adolescents.

Ecstasy use has increased in recent years among adolescents, particularly in large urban centers such as New York and Los Angeles. "Raves," or all-night dance parties, have become popular in this subculture, and ecstasy is consumed in an attempt to stay up all night. Interestingly, there has been speculation that MDMA may be toxic to serotonergic neurons, although no one knows the actual clinical ramifications.

Look-alike drugs made from nonprescription, over-the-counter substances such as caffeine and ephedrine are being consumed by adolescents in order to get "high."[15,23] These compounds, which have novel pharmacologic properties, have prompted investigators to study them in great detail, looking particularly at the biological mechanisms of drug action, drug reinforcement, the psychobiology of addiction, and the clinical syndromes commonly associated with their use and abuse.[6] In addition, clinicians are being forced to become familiar with the trends and the different names used by adolescents to describe the drugs they are using. The use of terms like weed in referring to marijuana, for example, is outdated, and thus the clinician treating adolescents should become familiar with the current teenage drug jargon. This will facilitate more accurate assessment and diagnosis of adolescent substance abusers and lead to more appropriate therapeutic interventions.

According to the National Institute of Mental Health (NIMH) Epidemiologic Catchment Area program, alcoholism is currently the most common psychiatric disorder among men.[24] This takes on added significance for adolescents, since they are starting to use and abuse alcohol and other drugs at younger ages than did adolescents and young adults in the 1960s and 1970s.[15] The average age of initiation in California children is believed to range from 10.7 to 18.8 years.[15]

Epidemiology

The National Institute on Drug Abuse undertook a study of alcohol and drug use among high school seniors, college students, and other young adults from 1975 to 1990 in order to document the trends and extent of drug and alcohol use and abuse in this population.

Alcohol

Nearly all American high school seniors, college students, and young adults report having tried alcohol (90%),[182] and more than half are defined as being current users, that is, as having ingested alcohol within the past month. Daily alcohol use for this age group is 3.7%, but occasional heavy drinking is substantially more prevalent, with almost a third of all high school seniors reporting that on at least one occasion during the prior two-week interval, they had had five or more consecutive drinks.[182] Frequent use of alcohol tends to be disproportionately seen in males. Drinking large quantities of alcohol in one setting is also much more common in males than in females. On the other hand, there are practically no differences between males and females in the lifetime, annual, or monthly prevalence of alcohol use. Thus it is the frequency and the quantity of drinking that best differentiate these two groups.

Frequent alcohol use does appear to be more prevalent among non–college-bound students than in those going on to attend college.[182] Noncontinuation rates for alcohol are very low, and of the 90% of all seniors who have tried it, almost all continue to use alcohol during their senior year (and often beyond).

Nicotine

Almost two thirds of high school seniors report having tried cigarettes, and almost one third are current users. Cigarettes are used daily by this group more than any other drug group. Alarmingly, over 10% admit to smoking one-half pack or more per day.[182] In contrast to other drugs, of which respondents were considered daily users if they had used the drug on 20 or more occasions in the 30 days prior to the survey, respondents were considered daily cigarette users if they smoked one or more cigarettes per day. Moreover, for cigarettes, noncontinuation is defined as the percentage of those who report having smoked regularly at one time, but who also report not smoking at all during the past month. Very few of the regular smokers surveyed (less than 20%) met this criterion.

In recent years, young teenage females have become the only age group demonstrating an increased incidence of cigarette smoking. This has important clinical ramifications in that lung cancer has recently surpassed breast cancer as the cancer most commonly causing death in females. It should be noted, however, that equal proportions of males and females report some smoking in the past month (just under 30%), and that more males report smoking at the rate of one-half pack or more per day (11.6% versus 10.8% for females). The largest difference in substance use between the college-bound and non–college-bound high school students involves cigarette smoking—7.5% of the college-bound seniors smoke one-half pack or more daily as compared with 19% of non–college-bound seniors.[182] There is also a large regional difference for regular cigarette smoking. Fourteen percent of seniors in the northeastern and north central states report smoking one-half pack or more a day versus only 9% in the South and 8% in the West.

Marijuana

Marijuana is the most commonly used illicit drug, with 41% of those surveyed reporting some use in their lifetime, 27% reporting some use within the past year, and 14% reporting some use in the past month.[183] Although almost one half of all high school seniors report having used illicit drugs at some point in their lives, a significant proportion (19% of all those sampled and 39% of illicit drug users) have used only marijuana. Nonetheless, almost one third of all high school seniors do report using an illicit drug other than marijuana at some time.

Approximately one in 45 (2%) high school seniors report the daily use of marijuana, as compared with daily alcohol use by 3.7%. Marijuana has one of the lowest noncontinuation rates in the senior year of high school, since a large number of users continue to use it and to be exposed to its use at some level over an extended period.[182] The proportion of young people ever using marijuana is only slightly higher among males than among females, but daily use of marijuana is three times higher in males than in females. Marijuana use is also more frequent in non–college-bound than in college-bound seniors. Daily use is almost four times higher in those not planning to go to college.

Cocaine

Nine percent of all high school seniors report having tried cocaine.[185] Cocaine also has a relatively low noncontinuation rate of 44%, but this may be due to its relatively late age of onset of use. Male–female prevalence rates are approximately 1.5–2.0:1.0. Cocaine use is also more common among non–college-bound than among college-bound high school seniors.

Crack Cocaine

Some 3.5% of high school seniors report having tried crack at some time in their lives.[182] The noncontinuation rate is 46%. It should be noted that of those who have ever used crack, only one fifth are current users and only 0.1% of the entire sample are daily users. Thus, while crack is known to be very addictive, there is evidence to support its not usually being addictive on the first use. Crack use in males is about twice as common as in females. Annual prevalence rates are highest in the West. College-bound seniors have lower prevalence rates than do non–college-bound seniors.

Inhalants and Nitrites

In recent years, it has been necessary to adjust inhalant lifetime prevalence rates upward, since not all users of one subtype of inhalants, amyl nitrite, report themselves as inhalant users. Common inhalants such as glue and aerosols, which are more likely to be discontinued prior to the senior year of high school, were included in the most recent survey of drug use among young Americans, and therefore nitrite use becomes proportionately more common in later years.[182] The specific classes of inhalants and amyl and butyl nitrites, referred to on the street as poppers or snappers, are sold legally and have been tried by approximately 2% of high school seniors.[182] Only 0.3% report daily use of inhalants. Nitrites, which have a relatively late age of onset of use, have low noncontinuation rates of 33%. Inhalants, however, have a high rate of noncontinuation by the senior year of 60%, and are often used at younger ages. One and a half to two times as many males as females use inhalants. Use is more common by non–college-bound than by college-bound seniors. The north central states rank relatively high in the use of inhalants.

Hallucinogens

The lifetime prevalence of PCP is 2.8%, which is considerably lower than the 8.7% lifetime prevalence of LSD.[182] Some 0.3% of high school seniors report the daily use of hallucinogens. Hallucinogens have a relatively high noncontinuation rate, and approximately twice as many males as females use them. The current prevalence of use is higher in non–college-bound than in college-bound high school seniors. The West ranks highest in the use of hallucinogens, especially LSD.

Opiates

Opiates other than heroin have been used by approximately 8% of high school seniors.[182] Only 1.3% admit to have ever used heroin, the most infrequently used drug. It should be remembered, however, that the marked stigma associated with heroin makes it likely that its use is underreported.[182] The highest noncontinuation rates reported were those for heroin, 62%, and quaaludes, 70%. Males report a somewhat higher annual incidence of use of opiates other than heroin, and a one and a half to two times higher annual incidence of the use of heroin. It should be noted that males account for a larger proportion of the frequent and heavy users of opiates, including heroin. Opiate use is more common among non–college-bound than among college-bound high school seniors. The West shows the highest rate of the use of opiates, except for heroin, for which it shows the lowest level of use. Heroin use is highest in the Northeast.

Sedatives

The general class of sedatives may be broken down into the specific drug methaqualone and the barbiturates. Methaqualone use has a 2.3% lifetime prevalence among high school seniors, while barbiturates have a 6.8% lifetime prevalence.[182] Quaaludes are no longer available by prescription in the United States. Thus methaqualone must be obtained through the black market, which raises obvious questions about the purity of the substance and, in fact, its very identity, or whether it was smuggled in from Canada or Mexico, where quaaludes are legally dispensed with a physician's prescription. The noncontinuation rate for tranquilizers is 51%. Compared with females, males report a slightly higher annual rate of use of barbiturates. Annual prevalence rates of tranquilizer and methaqualone use by females match or exceed those for males. Their use also is higher among non–college-bound than among college-bound high school seniors. The South shows the highest rate of use of barbiturates, tranquilizers, and sedatives. Methaqualone use is highest in the Northeast. Tranquilizer use ranks lower in terms of current use than it does for lifetime use.

Alcohol and Drug Abuse and Dependence

The costs of alcohol and drug abuse and dependence to the abusers, their families, and society are large. Among adults, alcohol abuse results in increased rates of liver disease, CNS damage, GI disease, cardiac disease, nutritional deficiencies, poisonings, cancers, metabolic anomalies, and motor vehicle injuries.[25] Despite these risks and dangers and the increasing incidence of early-onset alcoholism, parents are still often relieved when they discover that their child is "only" using alcohol and tobacco, as opposed to the "more dangerous" illegal drugs.[15]

Subtly, and perhaps unconsciously, parents may even encourage the use of these substances as being "normal teenage things" or facts of life in the development of adolescents as they become adults. What these parents do not know is that physicians treating substance-abusing adolescents are discovering more teenagers with enlarged livers, marijuana-induced memory deficits, and increased liver enzymes.[3,16,26] It must be emphasized, however, that there is much less evidence regarding the occurrence in adolescents of many of these complications, such as CNS damage. As will be elaborated below, alcohol abuse and dependence appear to be different phenomena in children and adolescents than in adults. Further investigation is clearly necessary.

This ignorance about the detrimental effects of drugs previously believed to be relatively safe is not limited to parents of adolescents. Physicians need to be aware that all mood-altering substances have the capability of being highly addictive. Experimentation with cigarettes and alcohol can lead to more serious dependence.[2] Alcohol and tobacco have been referred to as "gateway drugs" because their use markedly increases the likelihood of subsequent use of other substances.[2,27-29] For this reason, we have included nicotine dependence and potential pharmacologic interventions to treat withdrawal and nicotine craving in this section (see below).

Economically, alcohol abuse alone is estimated to cost society in excess of $89 billion per year, while other drug abuse is estimated to cost an additional $50 billion yearly.[30] It is expected that these figures will continue to increase, since more children and adolescents are abusing alcohol and drugs at an earlier age and in increasing numbers than ever before.[15]

Basic and clinical research has resulted in an enhanced understanding of mechanisms of action of alcohol and, to a lesser extent of other drugs. Genetic mechanisms involved in the development of alcohol and drug addiction are being elucidated. A family history of substance abuse or dependence is the best predictor of substance abuse or addiction in children and adolescents, particularly in males.[2,31-34]

In adults, research has yielded pharmacologic treatment approaches for drug and alcohol withdrawal syndromes, for drug and alcohol craving, and for achieving abstinence.[6] Investigators are continuing to be challenged by the aforementioned changing trends in drug and alcohol abuse. Nonetheless, these new pharmacotherapies proposed for the treatment of substance abuse disorders require further investigation so that their true role and value in this area may be properly determined. It is also clear that these new pharmacologic interventions are best used as adjuncts to psychosocial interventions.[6] Although advances in research may potentially result in a new psychopharmacologic armamentarium, it is doubtful that the successful treatment of substance-abusing and dependent children and adolescents can neglect the social, cultural, and psychological factors involved, while concentrating solely on the biological and pharmacologic aspects of these disorders. As in other areas of child and adolescent psychiatry, a biopsychosocial approach is necessary.

Pharmacologic Concepts Relevant to Substance Abuse

The concepts of intoxication, dependence, and tolerance, and the intrinsic reinforcing properties of drugs and alcohol, are central to the psychopharmacologic approach and treatment of substance abuse disorders.[6] Although these entities are observed in children and adolescents, some important differences in their expression and occurrence exist, and will be elaborated on in the following.

Intoxication

Intoxication is defined as the disturbance of normal CNS function caused by the particular pharmacologic characteristics of a drug.[6] This state is characterized by alterations in consciousness, cognition, mood, and motor and sensory functions. Different drugs produce unique and varied patterns of disruption of brain function based on the specific properties of the particular drug. For example, adolescents who abuse or are dependent on alcohol may experience blackouts, mood swings, depression, impaired judgment, incoordination, attentional difficulties, sedation, and impairment in the performance of various tasks.[6,26,35] Drug effects may vary from individual to individual, and depend on the dose ingested, how the drug was administered, when (what time of day) the drug was taken, gender, body habitus, liver and kidney function, rate of gastric emptying, and prior exposure to the drug.[6]

Tolerance

Tolerance is defined as the change that occurs in an individual as a result of repeated exposure to a drug or closely related compound so that less effect is produced by taking the same amount of drug and an increased amount is required to produce the same effect.[36] There are two types of tolerance, metabolic and functional. Changes in drug absorption, distribution, biotransformation, elimination, and excretion that lead to a decrease in the degree and duration of exposure of a particular organ (e.g., the CNS) to a drug is referred to as metabolic tolerance.[6] Functional tolerance, on the other hand, is

479

a term used to characterize changes in the target organ that make it less sensitive to the drug. Tabakoff and colleagues[37] have proposed further dividing functional tolerance into environment-dependent and environment-independent tolerance, to account for the role of conditioned learning in the development of functional tolerance.

Dependence

The definition of dependence as given in DSM-III-R[38] has changed markedly from that in previous editions. According to DSM-III, a patient was considered to be alcohol or drug dependent if he or she was tolerant to the substance and experienced withdrawal upon its discontinuation, with alleviation attained only by its (or a similar compound's) reinstitution.[39] The DSM-III-R has expanded the definition so that dependence now is defined as "a syndrome of clinically significant behaviors, cognitions, and other symptoms that indicate loss of control of substance use and continued substance use despite adverse consequences." Thus DSM-III-R emphasizes the compulsive aspects of the substance's use and the resultant impairment in personal, social, and occupational functioning, while diminishing the importance of specific physiologic sequelae. In other words, it places less emphasis on physical dependence and increases the emphasis on psychological dependence.

Adolescent substance abusers appear to display some unique characteristics. For example, for various reasons, they have to be more surreptitious when they use drugs and alcohol, including the fact that they have to hide this use from their parents and that they must spend much of their time in school where, theoretically, it is more difficult to abuse drugs. This does not, of course, stop adolescents from using and abusing drugs and alcohol, but instead forces such use to be more episodic and out of the view of adults. Adults, in contrast, often find it easier to use and abuse drugs and alcohol for prolonged and uninterrupted periods, thus increasing their likelihood of becoming chemically dependent.

Moreover, adolescents appear not to experience the life-threatening side effects of withdrawal from alcohol (and from other drugs, as well) that adults do (Vingelis and Smart[40] and unpublished data, University of Pittsburgh, Western Psychiatric Institute and Clinic). In fact, our inpatient adolescent dual-diagnosis unit (alcohol and/or drug abuse comorbid with a DSM-III-R psychiatric disorder) has not found it necessary to use pharmacologic prophylaxis in adolescents for withdrawal symptoms. No evidence of alcohol withdrawal, such as delirium tremens (DTs) or alcohol withdrawal seizures, has been observed. While they are in hospital, the adolescents are closely monitored 24 hours a day with frequent vital sign checks and neurologic examinations to assess physical status, but thus far in our experience, medication has not been needed. There have been rare instances of blood pressure changes, but these have not been severe enough to warrant pharmacologic intervention, and vital signs have subsequently normalized.

Despite the fact, however, that adolescents are less likely than adults to become dependent on alcohol or other drugs, chemical dependence in this population is by no means impossible. The number of high school dropouts is increasing in the United States, and the remaining students often skip classes to use drugs and alcohol. Further study is clearly warranted before definitive recommendations can be made concerning the correct diagnosis and therapy of chemical dependence in adolescents.

Whether or not the term dependence or abuse actually is used, the practicing clinician who treats adolescents must be constantly alert to the possibility of their presence. Substance-abusing teenagers experience significant impairments in psychological, occupational, health, legal, financial, and spiritual functioning.[26,38] Denial is particularly common among adolescents, who often believe that they are indestructible. They frequently come from dysfunctional families and may be experiencing significant emotional problems, and their use of drugs or alcohol may be an attempt to self-medicate to alleviate the stress or depression they are undergoing. Moreover, children and their parents may not look at alcohol or tobacco use as substance abuse. The U.S. tobacco and alcohol industries have spent billions of dollars advocating that these substances are enjoyable and that, after working hard, people deserve them as an effective way to relax. Thus the physician is often put in the difficult position of having to make the diagnosis of a substance abuse disorder by history, while the adolescent (and possibly the parents) are not being entirely truthful in his or her report.

Drugs as Reinforcers

As early as 1956, evidence from animal studies suggested that drugs may be self-administered for their reinforcing effects.[41] Subsequent application of behavioral and pharmacologic techniques has confirmed that the inherent reinforcing properties of certain drugs contributes to drug-seeking behavior in human beings.[6] The most highly reinforcing drugs of abuse—alcohol, cocaine, morphine, nicotine, heroin, and marijuana—have been found to produce high rates of self-administration.[42-47] Interestingly, it is believed that these effects may occur independently of pharmacologic dependence and withdrawal.[6] Caution is required in generalizing these data to naturalistic clinical settings, since most of the data were generated by laboratory assessment of human operant behavior, and most of the patients studied were drug abusers. Obviously, substance abusers may have certain characteristics that make them especially susceptible and sensitive to the reinforcing properties of alcohol and drugs.[6]

Diagnostic Issues and Problems

A number of instruments and rating scales are available for diagnosing substance abuse disorders. The construct validity of these taxonomic systems has frequently, however, been without empirical validation.[6] Three contemporary diagnostic criteria for alcohol dependence, the Research Diagnostic Criteria (RDC), the Feigner Criteria, and the DSM-III criteria, have not been found to be concordant for classifying alcohol-dependent individuals.[48] The DSM-III criteria for alcohol abuse have also been found to correlate poorly with self-reported drinking patterns and quantities and consequences of alcohol use.[49] It is possible that the DSM-III-R criteria may be found to be more concordant with the other two instruments in classifying alcoholic individuals, since the DSM-III-R has significantly broadened the definition of dependence and has dichotomized substance abuse disorders into two discrete categories: substance abuse and substance dependence (see "Dependence").

In DSM-III, a significant effort was made to distinguish between substance "abuse" and "dependence." A diagnosis of abuse was given when the patient showed a pathologic pattern of use and impairment in psychological, social, and occupational functioning. Dependence, on the other hand, was diagnosed when tolerance and withdrawal were present in addition to the features seen in abuse. The implication was that dependence was the more severe disorder, but this may not, in fact, be the case.[6] It is, for example, possible for an individual to be dependent on nicotine, and yet not suffer any adverse psychosocial consequences. We have already mentioned the unique problematic inconsistencies of these criteria in the adolescent population (see "Dependence").

What is most important to remember is that for either of these diagnoses, the presence of a maladaptive, deleterious, and compulsive pattern of use that is viewed as undesirable across most cultural boundaries is central.[6] Physiologic signs and symptoms are now downplayed as criteria for dependence. The DSM-III-R lists nine criteria, three of which must be met for the diagnosis of dependence to be made.[38] There are, however, problems with this construct. Tarter and associates[49] found that this framework yields over 80 potential subtypes of alcohol dependence. Another drawback to this method of diagnosing dependence is that the clinician treating such a patient may not be aware of the possibility of an impending withdrawal syndrome, since physiologic symptoms are no longer sine que non for the diagnosis.[6] Adolescents, as mentioned, appear to experience withdrawal less frequently than do adults, and when withdrawal is experienced, the symptoms tend to be less prominent and life-threatening. Nonetheless, this is an underdeveloped area, and it is too early to conclude definitively that adolescents do not experience life-threatening withdrawal phenomena such as seizures and DTs.

Substance abuse by adolescents is a disorder that affects these young people in all areas of their functioning. However, the symptoms observed in adolescent substance abusers are often vague, and may not always be associated with drug use in the mind of the practitioner.[26] It is essential, therefore, that the clinician treating adolescents be on the alert for substance abuse, as its presentation may be variable and relatively nonspecific. Rogers and colleagues[35] found that fatigue, sore throat, cough, chest pain, conjunctivitis, headaches, and school or behavioral problems are the most common symptoms of adolescent drug use.

Denial, a mechanism by which a person keeps out of conscious awareness any aspects of reality that, if acknowledged, would produce anxiety,[183] is often a key defense mechanism employed by both the adolescent and his or her parents. Adolescent substance abusers often feel that they are invincible.[26] They are often uncooperative and resistant with physicians, whom they see as adversaries who wish to take away their primary way of feeling good, or less bad. Thus it is crucial to talk with family members, and to order a urine drug screen for any adolescent suspected by the clinician of abusing drugs or alcohol.

It should be noted, however, that the members of an adolescent substance abuser's family are not always able to provide reliable data. Adolescent substance abusers often come from dysfunctional families. Moreover, because of the genetic component of drug and alcohol abuse, many of these adolescents' parents may have their own substance abuse problems. This often results in the parents' not noticing their child's abuse patterns.[38]

Another major difficulty in assessing adolescents for substance abuse is distinguishing substance abuse from other emotional problems. Studies have shown that adolescents with substance abuse disorders often have comorbid psychiatric disorders.[50-57] Those who have emotional problems may turn to drugs and alcohol to self-medicate in order to relieve the emotional pain they are suffering.[38] Thus the coexistence of psychiatric disorders with substance abuse disorders complicates diagnostic and therapeutic issues in adolescents.

Dual-diagnosis patients have been found to be heterogeneous as to their comorbid psychiatric disorders and the substances that they abuse.[7] This not only is of diagnostic interest, but also influences prognostic and therapeutic considerations. There is a growing body of evidence to suggest that symptom severity and the specific type of psychiatric comorbid disorder may have predictive value in the response to treatment of patients with substance abuse disorders.[57–60]

Recent investigation has also shown that children and adolescents who experience an early depressive or anxiety disorder are at increased risk for subsequent substance abuse disorders.[13,14,31] Stowell[7] conducted a pilot study of 226 adolescents entering inpatient treatment because of a primary substance abuse disorder, and found that 82% met the DSM-III-R criteria for an Axis I psychiatric disorder, and that 74% had two or more psychiatric disorders in addition to a substance abuse disorder (unpublished data, 1990). Comorbid mood disorders were most common (61%), followed by conduct disorders (54%), anxiety disorders (43%), and, finally, organic mental disorders (61%). These data support the growing contention among experts in psychiatry and addiction research that a simultaneous evaluation for both substance abuse disorders and comorbid psychiatric disorders is necessary.

One important finding in Stowell's pilot study[7] was that nicotine abuse preceded alcohol and marijuana use, suggesting that nicotine may be the prime "entry" substance that results in a stepwise progression to alcohol, marijuana, and so on (also, unpublished data). Stowell also reports that his clinical impression from his pilot study was that among those adolescents who relapsed after being drug-free, a significant number returned first to their nicotine dependence.

Defining patterns of substance abuse in adolescence is not always easy. In other words, delineating use from abuse is not a simple task. There is some evidence that adolescents who completely abstain from alcohol may have more social adjustment problems than have adolescents who are light drinkers.[62–66] Hughes and colleagues[62] attempted to define patterns of drinking in adolescence in a comprehensive way so as to assess measures of social context, as well as the frequency and quantity of alcohol use. The subjects' scores on frequency, quantity, and five social-context variables were cluster analyzed, and revealed that there were four socially appropriate drinking patterns and three problem drinking patterns. Socially appropriate patterns (i.e., normative developmentally) for both sexes were light drinking, light party drinking, family drinking, and drinking while on dates. Problem drinking patterns were school drinking and solitary/with a stranger drinking for males and solitary/school drinking for females.[62] These groups also showed significant differences in their reasons for drinking and drinking consequences, even after differences due to frequency and quantity were statistically controlled. Thus it may not be appropriate to label all adolescents who use alcohol or marijuana as substance abusers. Indeed, the desire for acceptance by peers is very pronounced in this age group. The occasional use of alcohol, tobacco, or even marijuana, an illicit substance, may be socially "appropriate" among teenagers. Adolescents who totally abstain from alcohol or drug experimentation may, for a variety of reasons, be less socialized than their peers, and may suffer social adjustment difficulties. This is not meant to condone alcohol or illicit drug use by adolescents, but rather to give a realistic picture of teenage norms and rites of passage into adulthood. Obviously, adolescents who experiment with drugs and alcohol are at risk of becoming substance abusers and/or chemically dependent, particularly if they have other inherent vulnerabilities.

As has been discussed, adolescents who have a positive family history for substance abuse disorders are themselves at increased risk for substance abuse. Unfortunately, there are but limited data on the existence of substance abuse disorders and/or psychiatric disorders among the family members of adolescents. Mirin and associates[52] have demonstrated the importance of such information. They found that approximately 30% of 160 adult substance abusers met the DSM-III-R criteria for at least one Axis I psychiatric diagnosis during their lifetime. Gfeerer[61] has also shown that there is a strong correlation between drug use by teenagers and drug use by older family members. Family studies of substance-abusing adolescents are clearly warranted to increase our understanding of the genetics of comorbidity and the correlation between substance abuse and the comorbid psychiatric disorder.[53]

Suicide is now the second leading cause of death in adolescents 15 to 19 years of age.[185] Moreover, the rate of adolescent suicide has tripled in the past three decades.[184,185] This increased rate may be attributable in part to the parallel increases in the rates of alcohol abuse and depression in youths born after World War II.[185,186] The rate of suicide by firearms—the most common method of suicide for both sexes in adolescence—appears to be increasing faster than the suicide rate by other methods, and shooting oneself is an especially common suicide method when the adolescent has also been drinking alcohol.[184–187] Indeed, adolescent suicide victims are frequently intoxicated with alcohol at the time of death.[185,188] Many adolescent suicides and attempts are highly impulsive acts,[127] with the motives often compounded by substance use/abuse, which can decrease inhibitions while increasing impulsivity. Two thirds of adolescent suicide attempters engage in suicidal behavior for reasons other than wanting to die.[128] When alcohol and other drugs are involved, the risk to the adolescent's life increases. The most common method of suicide attempt in adolescents is intentional overdose.[129,130] Obviously, an adolescent who is abusing alcohol and/or drugs increases the likelihood of harming himself or herself when intentionally overdosing. Moreover, the adolescent may become more careless in general when intoxicated, and even though not wanting to die, may be less "careful" when making an attempt. About one third of the victims of substance abuse by others had difficulties with substance abuse themselves, often in combination with an affective disorder.[127,133]

It is important, therefore, that the clinician look for symptomatology that most places adolescents at risk for suicidal behavior. Substance abuse, depression, and conduct disorder have been found to be most closely related to suicidal behavior.[131,132] When these conditions coexist, the risk may be even higher. It is crucial to obtain a thorough family history, since relatives of adolescent suicide attempters and completers have a high prevalence of alcohol and drug abuse.[132] In addition, if family members are abusing alcohol and/or drugs, they may be less able to discern substance use and abuse in their children. Thus it is crucial when evaluating suicidal behavior in an adolescent to search for evidence of substance abuse/dependence in both the primary patient and family members.

One controversial issue is how to categorize adolescents with dual diagnoses of substance abuse disorders and other psychiatric disorder(s). An accurate history regarding the development of the substance abuse and psychiatric diagnosis is essential. Most commonly, primary psychiatric disturbances such as conduct disorders, depression, and anxiety precede substance abuse in adolescents.[7] Less commonly, substance abuse precedes the onset of psychiatric symptoms. There is also a third category that must be considered—the "pure" form of dual diagnosis where both disorders appear independently of each other.[7]

These categorizations have theoretical, prognostic, and therapeutic implications, in addition to their diagnostic importance. Treatment of the primary psychiatric disorder in adolescents whose psychiatric disorder precedes their substance abuse might be expected to result in ameliorating not only the primary psychiatric disorder, but the substance abuse problems as well. Conversely, treating the primary substance abuse disorder in adolescents whose substance abuse disorder precedes their psychiatric disturbance would be expected to alleviate the substance abuse disorder, and also to reduce the psychiatric symptoms. A different approach, however, would be required for those adolescents with dual primary disorders. Theoretically, this group would need treatment that focuses on both of the disorders. A family history of substance abuse disorders, psychiatric disorders, and dual diagnoses can be helpful diagnostically and therapeutically. Nonetheless, there are very limited data in this area. It has not yet been demonstrated that dividing adolescents into these three categories is valid or useful therapeutically. It can be argued that since both psychiatric disorders and substance abuse disorders have significant morbidity and mortality associated with them, it behooves clinicians to attend to both disorders simultaneously in all three groups (see following section).

Treatment Strategies

Strategies applied to substance abuse and dependence have primarily concentrated on (1) suppressing and/or attenuating withdrawal symptoms, (2) altering the drug's stimulus properties to decrease drug-seeking behaviors, and (3) reducing drug craving.[6]

Attenuation of Withdrawal Symptoms

Drug-seeking behavior was previously felt to be motivated primarily by the desire and need to avoid the symptoms encountered when withdrawing from the particular substance. This view has been challenged by recent evidence that has shown that not all abusable drugs produce withdrawal upon discontinuation, while some drugs produce a withdrawal state that is clinically insignificant.[6] The focus of the pharmacologic control of withdrawal states is now, therefore, specifically directed at decreasing the morbidity and mortality associated with acute abstinence, and making patients more comfortable as they withdraw so that they are better able to participate in and derive benefit from the psychosocial interventions being administered. In adults, the most severe form of alcohol withdrawal, DTs, was associated with a 15% death rate prior to pharmacologic advances in the form of benzodiazepines, which have decreased this death rate significantly.[67] Adolescents appear to be somewhat less susceptible to these severe forms of alcohol (and other drug) withdrawal, but there is a paucity of available literature on the subject.

Alteration of the Stimulus Properties of the Drug

Another strategy employed in the pharmacologic approach to chemical dependency involves altering the stimulus properties of the drug so that it no longer causes drug-seeking behavior.[6] This takes the form of utilizing either substances that reduce the reinforcement from alcohol or drug use ("antagonist" drugs) or substances that make such use aversive ("deterrent" drugs). Naltrexone therapy and high-dose methadone maintenance for opiate abuse are examples of reinforcement-reduction techniques. Disulfiram (Antabuse) is the best-known and most widely used example of an aversive approach used to treat alcohol dependence. There are no data on children and adolescents (see below).

Reducing Drug Craving

Recent investigation has begun to focus on the use of medications to decrease the craving for an abused substance. Rankin and colleagues[68] discuss the theoretical concept of craving as representing the internal drive state inducing drug-seeking or alcohol-seeking behavior. Craving, although increased during withdrawal, persists beyond the physical withdrawal period into the postwithdrawal period. Various clinicians have reported the existence of a subacute, prolonged abstinence syndrome, extending weeks after the physiologic signs of withdrawal have ceased, but empirical studies are lacking.[69] It has been postulated that neuroadaptive changes continue to occur even beyond the classic withdrawal period. Williams and Rundell[70] observed that the sleep disturbances of newly abstinent alcoholics may not normalize for from nine to 21 months. Khan and colleagues[71] also showed that nonsuppression on the dexamethasone suppression test may persist for more than three weeks after classical physical alcohol withdrawal. Interestingly, this craving appears to peak during the postwithdrawal period. There are no data on children and adolescents.

In an attempt to reduce this craving, two approaches have been utilized: (1) drug substitution, and (2) correction of the underlying physiologic disturbances produced by the drug.

Drug Substitution

Drug substitution has been the more frequently used method of attempting to modify or eradicate craving and drug-seeking behavior.[6] A classic example of this approach is methadone maintenance for heroin addicts. Substitutes for tobacco in the form of nicotine-containing gum and, more recently, the nicotine patch (Prostat, Nicoderm, and Habitrol) are other examples.[72] Kissin[73] suggested using chronic benzodiazepine treatment for alcohol-dependent patients. The problem with this approach is that it involves readdicting the patient to another drug, followed by the subsequent tapering of the substituted drug. This technique may result in short-term benefits, such as retaining the patient in treatment or decreasing any involvement in criminal activities, but eventually the patient is still required to undergo withdrawal of the drug and some degree of drug craving.[6] Buprenorphine also recently received a great deal of attention as an agent that alters cocaine craving among opiate addicts. Mello and colleagues[134] found that buprenorphine suppressed cocaine self-administration by rhesus monkeys for 30 consecutive days. The effects of the buprenorphine were dose dependent. Importantly, the suppression of cocaine self-administration by buprenorphine did not reflect a generalized suppression of behavior. These data suggest that buprenorphine may be a useful pharmacologic therapy for cocaine abuse.[134] In addition, because buprenorphine is a safe and effective pharmacotherapy for heroin dependence, such treatment may also attenuate the concomitant abuse of cocaine and heroin. There are no data on this in children and adolescents. Further investigation is clearly warranted.

Correction of the Underlying Physical Disturbance

Following an investigation into correcting the underlying physiologic disturbances produced by the chronic presence of a drug in the body, cocaine craving was reported to be attenuated with bromocriptine, a dopamine agonist, and with desipramine, a TCA.[74,75] These approaches are believed to work by reversing the cocaine-induced pathophysiology in the central dopaminergic and noradrenergic systems. Borg[76] also reported bromocriptine to be effective in the treatment of alcohol craving. The data on these and other agents in reducing drug craving are still very limited, however, and further research, particularly double-blind, placebo-controlled studies, is needed. There are no data on children and adolescents, and the role of such agents in the treatment of drug craving in this population is likely to be limited until more is known about their use in treating adults. Thus, we cannot recommend a specific dosing regimen for children and adolescents, since such treatment would necessarily rely on extrapolation from data generated on adults. We advocate that when clinicians prescribe these agents, they adhere to the caveats applicable to child and adolescent pharmacotherapy (i.e., starting with a low dose, increasing the medication gradually, and using a divided-dosage schedule whenever possible). In addition, because of children's and adolescents' enhanced metabolism of psychotropic medications as compared with adults, higher maximal doses may be required.

Pharmacologic Treatment of the Withdrawal Syndrome

Opiate Withdrawal

Adult inpatients undergoing opiate withdrawal are most commonly treated by the substitution method. Methadone, a long-acting opiate with a half-life of 15–22 hours, is substituted for heroin, morphine, and other opioids. The rationale for methadone use is based on its prolonged half-life as compared with other opiates, its cross-tolerance with other opiates, and the fact that it is easily and well absorbed from the GI tract.[77-79] When withdrawal symptoms are noted, patients are given an initial oral dose of 15 to 20 mg of methadone. Doses are then titrated upward to target withdrawal symptoms to a maximum daily dose of 80 mg. When stabilization on an adequate amount of methadone is achieved so that the patient is symptom-free for a 24-hour period, a gradual reduction in the methadone dose may ensue. In general, dose reductions of 20% per day are well tolerated.[77-79] Methadone substitution protocols typically take anywhere from 10 days to one month for successful detoxification.

There are no data on children and adolescents. Many practitioners are hesitant to prescribe methadone in this population, since it, too, is addictive. Moreover, adult guidelines may not be applicable when administering methadone to adolescent heroin abusers who are undergoing withdrawal. Just because adults have been found to respond well to a particular pharmacologic intervention does not mean that children and adolescents will necessarily respond to the same intervention. Depressed children and adolescents, for example, respond no better to TCAs than to placebo, while up to 80% of depressed adults will experience significant symptom reduction on these same agents (see Chapter 4). Furthermore, in contrast to other drugs, such as barbiturates, opiate withdrawal, albeit uncomfortable, does not result in death if pharmacologically untreated. However, trying methadone in adolescents who are experiencing significant withdrawal symptoms that are interfering with their competent participation in psychosocial treatment programs may be warranted. Further study is clearly indicated.

It recently was discovered that clonidine, an alpha-2 adrenergic receptor agonist, effectively reduces the signs and symptoms of opiate withdrawal in adults.[80] Oral clonidine daily doses of 1 to 2 mg are used to treat withdrawal symptoms in opiate abusers. Clonidine administration may be required for up to 10 days, especially if a long-acting opiate is the drug abused or when clonidine is used to treat methadone withdrawal.[81] To effect a more rapid opiate detoxification regimen, a combination of clonidine and the long-term opiate antagonist naltrexone has been found of value.[82] This combination works because it is more effective in precipitating and then attenuating a withdrawal syndrome so that detoxification can be started sooner. Detoxification from methadone can be accomplished within four to five days by using these two agents simultaneously to precipitate and suppress opiate withdrawal. Clonidine and naltrexone have the further advantage over methadone of their not being addictive. There are no data on children and adolescents. Although the use of opiates appears to be increasing in adolescents, withdrawal syndromes in this population are uncommon. Clonidine also has significant side effects that often make its use unpleasant for children and adolescents. Naltrexone, too, is not without its side effects (see Chapter 12). Further investigation and assessment are clearly required.

Alcohol Withdrawal

Isbell and associates[83] conducted a study in which six adult volunteers were put on a nutritious diet for 48 days while drinking large quantities of alcohol. When alcohol ingestion was abruptly halted, these volunteers developed a broad spectrum of alcohol withdrawal symptoms, including seizures, hallucinations with an intact sensorium, and DTs. Since a nutritional deficiency could be ruled out by the nutritionally correct dietary intake, the authors concluded that alcohol alone was responsible for this syndrome. Since that time, a wide variety of pharmacologic interventions to suppress alcohol withdrawal syndromes have been utilized. The two most successful treatments have involved (1) substituting drugs that are cross-tolerant with alcohol, but that have a different pharmacokinetic profile, and (2) using pharmacologic agents that reduce sympathetic nervous system activity. The safety of benzodiazepines in the treatment of the alcohol withdrawal syndrome in adults has been well established, and clinical trials have demonstrated their superiority in such treatment over antipsychotics, anticonvulsants, paraldehyde, hydroxyzine, and meprobamate.[67,84-87] Nonetheless, as has been mentioned, the probability of seeing these withdrawal phenomena in adolescents appears to be quite low, so that the use of these agents is usually unnecessary.

Chlordiazepoxide (Librium), the first introduced benzodiazepine, has been the standard for treating the alcohol withdrawal syndrome. Establishing an appropriate dosing regimen is often difficult, however. Chlordiazepoxide's slow rate of absorption following oral administration frequently produces a delay of several hours for peak plasma concentrations to be achieved. Consequently, overmedication with this agent is not uncommon. Baskin and Easdale[88] reported that patients often remain lethargic, ataxic, or confused for several days after resolution of the withdrawal state.

A more rational approach proposed by Sellers and associates,[89] which involves diazepam (Valium) loading, simplifies the treatment of alcohol withdrawal. Diazepam is very lipid soluble, and consequently peak plasma concentrations are achieved within about one hour. The major advantage of this agent, therefore, is that it allows the physician who is administering the diazepam to quickly observe its effect on the alcohol withdrawal syndrome. The favorable pharmacokinetic profile of diazepam also allows oral loading of the drug on the first day of treatment.[6] Since diazepam's half-life is approximately 33 hours and that of its active metabolite desmethyldiazepam is approximately 50 hours, after only one day's loading, therapeutic plasma concentrations will be present for more than the 72 hours' duration of a typical adult alcohol withdrawal syndrome. In this method, oral diazepam doses of 20 mg are administered every two hours until the patient is asymptomatic. After the first day, the patient may continue on diazepam, with additional medication given only on an as-needed basis. It must be emphasized that even this pharmacologic approach has its limitations and is best conducted in the setting of good supportive psychosocial care. In addition, a recent report suggested that 80% of adult patients with alcohol withdrawal syndromes were capable of being managed by nonpharmacologic means. This percentage appears to be even higher in adolescents.

A limitation to the diazepam method is that patients with severe liver dysfunction do not metabolize the drug, which results in its excess accumulation. Lorazepam (Ativan) may be a safer medication for these patients, since it depends on both renal and hepatic biotransformation for its excretion, so that, in the presence of liver disease, it is still cleared adequately. The oral form of lorazepam has a delay in absorption similar to that of chlordiazepoxide, but there is a rapidly absorbed sublingual preparation, and IM and parenteral forms are available.[90,91]

More recently, clonidine was shown to have efficacy in treating alcohol withdrawal.[92] Clonidine stimulates presynaptic alpha-adrenoreceptors, which decreases noradrenergic transmission and decreases sympathetic nervous system activity. Baumgartner and Rowen[93] found clonidine to be superior to chlordiazepoxide in decreasing the cardiovascular symptoms of alcohol withdrawal, and as effective in improving cognitive capacity, decreasing anxiety, and decreasing subjective complaints of withdrawal. It does, however, lack anticonvulsant properties, but in contrast to the benzodiazepines, it has no abuse potential. Thus many clinicians believe that clonidine deserves future study and should be considered as a potential alternative to benzodiazepines in the treatment of alcohol withdrawal. It should be noted, however, that, unlike the benzodiazepines, clonidine does not ameliorate or affect insomnia or agitation, which are often important features of the withdrawal syndrome. Moreover, the benzodiazepines are safer, and thus have a higher therapeutic index, than clonidine. Benzodiazepines remain the treatment of choice in treating alcohol withdrawal.

Adolescents, as mentioned, appear to be less prone to drug withdrawal syndromes, and currently, do not receive pharmacologic prophylactic treatment for withdrawal. There are no data on treating adolescents who do experience pronounced physical withdrawal symptoms. Inpatient adolescent alcohol abusers, therefore, should be closely monitored, and if physiologic withdrawal occurs and the patient appears to be decompensating medically (significant orthostasis, hypertension, tremor, anxiety, etc.), benzodiazepines should be administered. Continued careful monitoring of the patient's vital signs and neurologic and physical status is required. Further investigation and assessment in the adolescent population are clearly warranted.

Cocaine Withdrawal

Until recently, cocaine was not felt to be addictive, and hence the recognition of a physical cocaine withdrawal syndrome ("crash") is relatively new. But even with the new recognition that cocaine is addictive, some still doubt the existence of a cocaine withdrawal syndrome. This controversy is in large part fueled by recent observations that cocaine "withdrawal" symptoms last

only 24 hours.[135] The symptoms observed in cocaine withdrawal are the opposite of those seen in cocaine intoxication. They include intense drug craving, anergy, hypersomnia, hyperphagia, decreased libido, irritability,
psychomotor retardation, lack of motivation, and a decrease in attention and
concentration.[74] The subjective discomfort of cocaine withdrawal is also felt
to act as a negative reinforcer, thereby increasing drug-seeking behavior.

The catecholaminergic system, particularly the dopaminergic and noradrenergic, is felt to be involved both in cocaine's actions and in the development
of the withdrawal syndrome. Cocaine releases dopamine from nerve termi-
nals, and is a potent inhibitor of dopamine and other catecholamines.[94,95]
Chronic cocaine ingestion results in the depletion of catecholamines. Taylor
and Ho[96] noted that chronic cocaine administration resulted in a decrease in
brain dopamine levels. Subsequent study in rats revealed that chronic cocaine use caused a compensatory increase in the number of dopamine receptors in rat brain.[97] Tennant[98] also observed a decrease in the primary
urinary metabolite of central and peripheral norepinephrine (MHPG) in
chronic cocaine abusers. Increases in the number of beta-adrenoreceptors
have also been reported.[99] Consequently, the cocaine withdrawal syndrome
has been suggested as resulting from a decrease of dopaminergic and/or noradrenergic neurotransmission produced by the chronic effects of cocaine.

Thus far, two successful clinical psychopharmacologic approaches to adult cocaine withdrawal have been reported.[74,75] Low-dose bromocriptine, a dopamine receptor agonist (D1), has been effective in treating cocaine
withdrawal.[74] The rationale for using bromocriptine is based on its serving
as a physiologic replacement for cocaine in which a dopamine agonist com-
pensates for the presynaptic dopamine depletion and down-regulates postsynaptic dopamine receptors until natural physiologic dopamine synthesis is
able to catch up with its losses. As mentioned, buprenorphine has been observed to suppress cocaine self-administration by rhesus monkeys for 30
straight days, and these observations have led to further investigation and
consideration of its use in the pharmacotherapy of cocaine craving and
abuse. There are no data on children and adolescents. Further study on
adults is also necessary, and should include placebo-controlled, double-blind
trials before this approach is applied to children and adolescents. Again,
thus far, the available data and anecdotal reports suggest that children and
adolescents have withdrawal syndromes less frequently, and when they do
experience cocaine withdrawal, it is often less severe than the withdrawal
of adults.

Tricyclic antidepressants such as desipramine and imipramine have been
shown to down-regulate supersensitive beta-adrenoreceptors and dopamine
receptors.[100,101] Desipramine and imipramine have, in fact, been used suc-

cessfully in the treatment of cocaine withdrawal.[75] In addition, TCAs appear to be effective independently of the presence of a depressive disorder in the cocaine abuser. The goal of this approach is not to treat depression, but to produce pharmacologic normalization of the catecholaminergic system. There are no data on children and adolescents. If an adolescent were to experience significant physiologic withdrawal symptoms upon discontinuing cocaine, this approach might be worth trying. The observation that the TCAs such as desipramine and imipramine appear to be effective in treating adult cocaine withdrawal independently of the depressive disorder in the substance abuser may be applicable to the child and adolescent population. Thus far, antidepressants have not been shown to be superior to placebo in the treatment of child and adolescent depression, so that, if this were the mechanism by which TCAs ameliorate cocaine withdrawal, one would not postulate much success in the child and adolescent population. But since effecting pharmacologic normalization of the catecholaminergic system is the goal of TCA therapy in cocaine withdrawal, it stands to reason that children and adolescents with a disrupted catecholaminergic system may benefit from this approach. Moreover, TCAs such as desipramine and imipramine have been shown to be superior to placebo in childhood ADHD (see Chapter 4). One mechanism suggested for this efficacy is normalizing a presumed alteration of the catecholaminergic system in childhood ADHD. Further investigation is necessary.

Reinforcement Reduction or Aversion Development

Lithium Carbonate

Chronic lithium pretreatment has been observed to attenuate the euphoria and activation associated with amphetamine, cocaine, and IV methylphenidate.[102–105] Subsequent trials, however, have revealed less consistency in its effectiveness.[106] Gawin and Kleber[107] compared lithium and desipramine in an open trial of the treatment of cocaine abuse, and found that lithium was not clinically effective. Thus lithium's use for routine stimulant abuse cannot be recommended.

Lithium has also been proposed as a potential treatment for alcohol abuse (see also Chapter 8), but early reports, suggested that it might be of benefit only in depressed alcoholics.[108,109] Studies on normal volunteers, however, suggested that lithium decreases the subjective intoxication "high" from alcohol, and also alcohol-induced psychomotor performance deficits.[110,111] Judd and Huey[112] conducted a double-blind, placebo-controlled study of detoxified alcoholics receiving chronic lithium treatment and demonstrated that such patients had significantly less intoxication, less desire to continue drinking, and fewer cognitive and psychomotor performance deficits when challenged with doses of alcohol. A subsequent double-blind, placebo-controlled trial of lithium therapy for alcohol dependence found that subjects with therapeutic lithium levels had a better treatment outcome than did the placebo group.[113] These results were all the more impressive since it was shown that they were independent of the presence of affective symptoms. Dorus and colleagues,[135] however, came to a different conclusion when they assessed the efficacy of lithium carbonate in the treatment of 457 male alcoholics in a double-blind, placebo-controlled Department of Veteran Affairs Cooperative Study. They evaluated its effects on alcohol-dependent patients either without depression or with a history of major depression, a current episode, or dysthymic disorder, and found that lithium treatment did not affect the course of alcoholism in either depressed or nondepressed alcoholics. There are no data on children and adolescents. In view of this recent large comprehensive study, which conclusively showed lithium carbonate's ineffectiveness in treating alcoholic adults, its role in treating adolescent alcohol abusers appears limited.

Methadone and Naltrexone

Because methadone is cross-tolerant with heroin, methadone maintenance was developed as a method for treating opiate dependence in an attempt to stop heroin addicts from abusing illegal opiates.[114] Methadone theoretically works by blocking the effects of street drug opiates and by attenuating drug-seeking activity and resultant criminal activity. It is believed to block the effects of other opiates both by saturating the opiate receptors and by inducing tolerance. Methadone maintenance was, therefore, originally intended to decrease both opiate and nonopiate drug use and the addict's criminal behavior to obtain drugs.[115] Subsequent investigation, however, revealed that methadone's ability to attenuate the reinforcing effects of heroin is primarily a dose-dependent phenomenon.[78,116] Inadequate plasma levels of methadone and/or lower doses may allow opiate-seeking behavior to continue unabated.

It has been suggested that for those patients on methadone who continue to engage in illicit drug use and criminal behavior, both higher oral doses (greater than 80 mg/day) and careful monitoring of methadone plasma levels may be necessary.[78,116] There are no data on children and adolescents. Since opiate drugs seem to be making a resurgence among adolescent substance abusers, this area may merit further exploration. Currently, it is difficult to give guidelines for methadone's use for adolescents, since it is by no means certain that they will respond similarly to adults. To reiterate, however, if heroin or other opiate abuse is continuing despite psychosocial interventions, and the adolescent is engaging in criminal behavior to support the habit, a trial of methadone may be warranted. Further study is necessary.

Naltrexone is a pure opiate antagonist, which is effective when given orally, and is structurally similar to oxymorphine. When patients are pretreated with naltrexone and then given morphine, heroin, or other opiates, the naltrexone has been observed to significantly block and reduce the pharmacologic effects of these opiates, such as the subjective high that results, the drug craving, and the production of physical dependence. Naltrexone pretreatment thus blocks much of the intrinsically reinforcing properties of opiates.[6] It has also been shown to decrease alcohol consumption in rats taught to drink alcohol, appearing significantly to decrease alcohol craving in these animal models. Volpicelli et al.[190] conducted a 12-week double-blind, placebo-controlled trial of naltrexone 50 mg/day as an adjunct to the treatment of 70 male alcohol-dependent patients following detoxification. Naltrexone-treated patients reported significantly less alcohol craving and fewer days during which any alcohol was consumed. Only 23% of the naltrexone-treated patients met the criteria for relapse, while 54% of the placebo-treated subjects relapsed. The primary effect of naltrexone was seen in subjects who drank any alcohol while attending outpatient treatment. Of the placebo-treated patients, 95% relapsed after they sampled alcohol, while only 50% of the naloxone-treated patients exposed to alcohol met relapse criteria. It is important to note that naltrexone was not associated with mood symptoms or other psychiatric symptoms. Side effects were minimal. The authors concluded that naltrexone may be a safe and effective adjunct in the treatment of alcohol dependence, especially in preventing relapse.[190]

O'Malley et al.[191] treated 97 alcohol-dependent patients for 12 weeks in a double-blind, placebo-controlled study evaluating the efficacy of naltrexone and two manual guided psychotherapies in the treatment of alcohol dependence. Patients were randomized to receive either naltrexone or placebo and either coping skills/relapse prevention therapy or a supportive therapy designed to support the patient's effort at abstinence without teaching specific coping skills. Naltrexone was found to be superior to placebo on measures of drinking and alcohol-related problems, including abstention rates, number of drinking days, relapse, and severity of alcohol-related problems. Naltrexone interacted with the type of psychotherapy received.[191] The cumulation rate of abstinence was highest for subjects treated with naltrexone and supportive therapy. Of the patients who sampled alcohol again, those who received naltexone and coping skills therapy were the least likely to relapse.

The clinical utility of naltrexone has been called into question because poor patient compliance is often seen in naltrexone-treated opiate abusers. Ginzburg[116] reported that in one multicenter trial of naltrexone therapy for opiate abuse and addiction, the duration of client compliance in the program was as short as six weeks. Nonetheless, Resnik and associates[117] observed that programs that combine pharmacotherapy with psychosocial support services fared better with respect to naltrexone compliance, with improved treatment outcome and better clinical retention in the program. There are no data on children and adolescents. Compliance in this population is often a problem. Still, a comprehensive program that utilizes a multimodal approach combining pharmacotherapy with psychosocial interventions, together with cooperative parents, may make this a feasible option for some adolescents. Further study is clearly necessary, however, before this treatment can be recommended.

Disulfiram

Disulfiram remains the only pharmacologic therapy that is specifically indicated for the treatment of alcohol dependence.[118] It acts by altering the intermediate metabolism of alcohol through its inhibitory effect on the enzyme acetaldehyde dehydrogenase. When alcohol is ingested, blood acetaldehyde concentrations increase, resulting in what is referred to as an acetaldehyde reaction. This disulfiram–alcohol interaction is extremely unpleasant; it consists of vasodilation, sweating, intense throbbing in the head and neck often causing a severe headache, respiratory problems, nausea and vomiting, vertigo, chest pain, and hypotension, which may be severe enough to cause postural syncope. Thus it is an aversion reaction, which lasts from half an hour to several hours.

The reaction serves to decrease the reinforcing aspects of alcohol use. Unfortunately, this often proves to be of more use theoretically than practically. That is, most alcohol-dependent persons never consume alcohol while taking disulfiram, since the very knowledge that they will have a reaction is sufficient to deter them from drinking. In other words, disulfiram acts, in a sense, as an "active placebo."[6]

It must be noted that the efficacy of disulfiram is far from clear, despite its having been available as a treatment for alcoholism since 1948 in Europe[182] and since 1949 in the United States. In fact, its use is quite controversial. Fuller and Williford[119] and Fuller et al.[120] used actuarial methods to describe the outcome of three randomly assigned alcoholic groups of patients who were being counseled in addition to receiving medical care. One group was given a daily therapeutic dose of disulfiram of 250 mg; the second group was told that they would be receiving disulfiram, but were given a markedly subtherapeutic dose of 1 mg; and the third group was told that they would not be treated with the drug. Both disulfiram groups had superior outcomes when compared with the no-drug group. However, there was no significant difference in clinical outcome between the group treated with a therapeutic dose of disulfiram and that treated with the subtherapeutic dose. This suggests that therapeutic doses may be no better than placebo, since the group receiving the subtherapeutic dose was told that they would be receiving disulfiram. A large-scale multicenter study conducted at the Veterans Administration hospitals also looked at the effects of counseling in addition to disulfiram therapy, and found that there were no differences among any of the three groups in terms of abstinence.[119,120] Counseling alone was observed to be as effective as disulfiram or the low-dose active placebo. It should be noted, however, that among the patients who relapsed, those receiving therapeutic doses of disulfiram had fewer drinking days than did those in the counseling-only and subtherapeutic disulfiram dose groups.

Disulfiram is associated with many significant side effects, including hepatotoxicity, carbon disulfide poisoning with polyneuropathy, psychotic reactions, acute organic brain syndrome, and a worsening of preexisting schizophrenia.[121-126] Most of these side effects appear to be dose related. Early dosing schedules frequently exceeded the 250–500 mg dose range now recommended. Christensen and colleagues[139] and Branchey and associates,[140] in investigating side effects seen at this lower dose range, did not implicate disulfiram in the production of physical or psychiatric complications. The study conducted by Christensen and colleagues was marred by its duration of only six weeks, but Branchey and associates' investigation was noteworthy in that it carefully screened out all patients who had a history of organic mental disorder, schizophrenia, mood disorder, or psychotropic drug abuse. Thus a longer duration of treatment, the use of higher doses, and the utilization of patients who have preexisting psychiatric disorders may account for the earlier reports of excess side effects. Until further study helps to clarify these important issues, physicians who wish to prescribe this compound should prescribe lower doses for a limited time, and should avoid its use or use it with extreme caution for patients with hepatic, cardiac, or neuropsychiatric disorders.[6] There are no data on children and adolescents.

Because of the many unclarified issues regarding disulfiram's use, and because of its potential to cause or exacerbate potentially life-threatening side effects, this agent cannot be recommended for use in children and adolescents. The reaction to disulfiram plus alcohol also makes this a less attractive treatment option for adolescent patients, who may succumb to peer pressure in spite of the aversive sequelae of drinking alcohol while on disulfiram, and thereby suffer a potentially severe adverse reaction. We do not believe that disulfiram will prove to be useful for child and adolescent alcohol abusers.

Serotonin Reuptake Inhibitors

Serotonin selective reuptake-inhibiting (SSUI) antidepressant medications, including zimelidine, citalopram, fluoxetine, paroxetine (SKFB), and fluvoxamine, appear to be effective in attenuating alcohol consumption, independently of their effects on depression.[141,142] Zimelidine's manufacturer has withdrawn it from clinical trials because of its side effects. The other agents, however, appear to have relatively favorable side-effect profiles and are continuing to be studied. Moreover, the introduction of the new SSUI sertraline (Zoloft), which is now FDA approved, has generated a great deal of excitement owing to the fact that its half-life is shorter than that of fluoxetine and its side-effect profile is more favorable.

The exact mechanism of action of these drugs is unknown, but it has been suggested that they inhibit the neurobiological substrate for positive reinforcement that maintains alcohol-consuming behavior.[143] There are no data on children and adolescents. These agents appear promising because of their relative safety (lethal overdose by fluoxetine and sertraline are rare to nonexistent) and favorable side-effect profile as compared with the standard TCAs. Moreover, serotonin deficiency has been implicated in impulsivity, a characteristic that applies to many adolescent substance abusers. Serotonin reuptake inhibitors such as fluoxetine and sertraline increase CNS serotonin levels. Thus far, however, controlled studies have not shown fluoxetine to be beneficial in abating alcohol consumption. Study of the other serotonergic agents has not been reported. Further investigation is necessary.

Pharmacologic Attenuation of Craving

Cocaine Craving

As mentioned previously, two approaches—bromocriptine and TCAs such as desipramine and imipramine—have been reported to be effective in decreasing cocaine craving during the postwithdrawal period.[74,144] Dackis and Gold[74] observed a dramatic reduction in cocaine craving with oral bromocriptine doses of 0.625 mg three times a day. They believe that bromocriptine is effective because it functionally reverses the dopamine depletion resulting from chronic cocaine use. The subjective craving is hypothesized to be a response to this dopaminergic deficit, and when bromocriptine, a dopamine agonist, reverses this deficit, drug-craving behavior is reduced. There are no data on children and adolescents. Because cocaine use is increasing among adolescents, this treatment approach merits further exploration. One limitation of its use may be in those patients who become psychotic after using cocaine. Psychosis is often induced by a hyperdopaminergic state, and the pharmacologic treatment of choice is generally a dopamine receptor blocker such as haloperidol (see Chapter 7). Administering a dopamine agonist that might exacerbate the hyperdopaminergic state might be contraindicated.

Tennant and Rawson[144] first reported that therapeutic doses of desipramine were helpful in effecting successful cocaine withdrawal. Subsequently,

Gawin and Kleber[107] reported that desipramine was effective in decreasing cocaine craving in the postwithdrawal period in a group of psychotherapy-only treatment failures. They later suggested that beta-adrenergic supersensitivity was the biological substrate for craving, and that tricyclics induce down-regulation, thus decreasing craving.[75]

Recent investigation, however, has cast doubt on desipramine's usefulness in this population. Arndt et al.[192] conducted a double-blind, placebo-controlled, randomized 12-week trial of desipramine treatment of cocaine dependence among methadone-maintained subjects. Fifty-nine patients completed the 12-week medication trial, 36 receiving desipramine and 23 receiving placebo. There were significantly more dropouts in the desipramine-treated group than in the placebo-treated group.[192] Baseline to 12-week comparisons of Addiction Severity Index interview data indicated that both groups demonstrated improvements. At 12 weeks, the desipramine group showed significantly better psychiatric status than the placebo group, but did not differ from the placebo group on any of the 21 other outcome measures, including cocaine use. During the 12-week medication phase and at the one-month follow-up evaluation, urine toxicology screenings were not significantly different between the groups. The placebo group, however, had significantly less cocaine use at both the three- and six-month follow-up points. The authors concluded that desipramine had few benefits with regard to the control of cocaine use in this population.

In a double-blind, placebo-controlled 12-week randomized clinical trial, Kosten et al.[193] compared amantadine (300 mg/day; $n = 33$), desipramine (150 mg/day; $n = 30$), and placebo ($n = 31$) in the treatment of cocaine-abusing methadone-maintained patients. Over 75% of the patients completed the full 12-week trial. Although reported cocaine use was significantly lower in the medicated groups as compared with the placebo group at the fourth week, no significant difference was found at the eighth week, and no difference was found in cocaine-free urine samples.[193] The authors emphasized the need for further study and the selection of more homogeneous subgroups, such as depressed cocaine abusers. There are no data on children and adolescents. Because of the absence of clear evidence supporting desipramine's use in cocaine-abusing/craving adults, we cannot endorse its use in cocaine-abusing/craving children and adolescents.

Opiate Craving

Drug substitution has been the primary successful method utilized in attenuating opiate craving. Unfortunately, methadone, the drug of choice for treating opiate craving, itself results in tolerance and dependence. Methadone maintenance does not decrease the desire to use opiates, nor does it ameliorate the psychological symptoms of addiction; instead, it utilizes a more pro-social drug therapy to attenuate the use of illicit opiates.[145] The hope is that psychosocial interventions can begin to take effect while the patient is on methadone maintenance, resulting in the addict's subsequent implementation of these new skills he or she has learned so that he or she may then be successfully tapered off methadone and become drug-free. This is often more successful in theory than in practice. Milby and colleagues[146] reported that 20% to 30% of patients on chronic methadone maintenance acquire a morbid fear of detoxification, which makes subsequent methadone detoxification more difficult and less successful. There are no data on children and adolescents.

Because methadone maintenance still results in drug tolerance and dependence, and does not decrease the desire to use cocaine or relieve the psychological symptoms associated with addiction, we recommend its consideration only as a last resort. That is, if all other interventions have failed, (e.g., psychosocial) and the adolescent is continuing to use illicit opiates and engage in criminal behavior, a methadone trial may be worthwhile. We also wonder whether treatments used in opiate withdrawal, such as clonidine and/or naltrexone, might merit trials for opiate craving. We know of no such studies on children and adolescents, and recognize that these treatments have not always been successful in ameliorating opiate withdrawal in adults, so that limitations to this approach may exist. We also know of no studies on children and adolescents using TCAs such as desipramine or imipramine or the SSUIs such as fluoxetine and sertraline to treat opiate craving. In addition to reducing alcohol and cocaine craving, these agents, which have the advantage of being nonaddictive, may also help to reduce opiate craving, and reduce the psychological symptoms imposed by opiate addiction as well.

Alcohol Craving

The use of chronic benzodiazepine therapy to reduce alcohol craving has been proposed.[73] The argument in favor of this type of treatment asserts that many patients are not able to deal with a prolonged withdrawal syndrome, and that benzodiazepines would decrease alcohol craving and thereby help retain patients in therapy. Subsequent clinical experience has shown that this is often not a good treatment approach. Alcohol-dependent patients are at increased risk for abusing benzodiazepines. In fact, benzodiazepines are now relatively contraindicated in alcohol- or other drug-dependent patients outside the acute alcohol withdrawal period. Benzodiazepines potentiate the effects of alcohol, and cross-addiction to benzodiazepines is not uncommon.[6] There are no data on children and adolescents, but this would not appear to be a useful therapy in this population. Moreover, children and adolescents have been noted not uncommonly to experience behavioral rebound and disinhibition when receiving benzodiazepines. Alcohol-abusing children and adolescents often have impulsive and relatively disinhibited personalities, and would, therefore, be poor candidates for this type of treatment.

Buspirone, a nonbenzodiazepine medication used in the treatment of anxiety, has been suggested as a potential treatment for alcohol craving because of its reported lack of abuse potential and its lack of potentiation of the effects of alcohol.[147] Since buspirone is an anxiolytic, it may relieve some of the psychological symptoms imposed by addiction. There are little data on the effects of buspirone on alcohol craving in adults, and no data on children and adolescents. Because of its anxiolytic properties and reported lack of abuse potential, buspirone merits further study. Its serotonergic activity may make it a useful adjunct to TCAs or SSUIs in both attenuating alcohol consumption and reducing alcohol craving. Further study is clearly necessary.

It must be emphasized that the risk of benzodiazepine abuse when using these agents for adolescents must always be considered. Ciraulo and colleagues[136] showed that parental alcoholism is a risk factor in benzodiazepine use. Nine of 12 men with a family history of alcoholism but only two of 12 control subjects had euphoric responses to alprazolam. The authors concluded that children of alcoholics may be at high risk of abusing benzodiazepines such as alprazolam. A review of the literature also suggests that the prevalence of benzodiazepine use among alcoholics is greater than in the general population, and that the liability for abuse may also be greater for alcoholics.[137] Because anxiety disorders and benzodiazepine use are common among alcoholics, their potential for abuse must be considered. Thus caution is necessary when using benzodiazepines in the treatment of alcoholic patients, since they appear to be more reinforcing among alcoholics and their offspring, and so chronic benzodiazepine therapy for these patients should be avoided. Kissin[138] has argued that the ideal anxiolytic to use in the treatment of alcoholic patients should effectively maintain patients in treatment, have a low potential for abuse, and not potentiate the effects of alcohol. Buspirone, an agent that is believed not to be addictive and should not potentiate the effects of alcohol, has received increasing attention as an ideal anxiolytic in the treatment of anxiety in alcoholic patients. There are no data on children and adolescents.[189] Further study is necessary.

Dopamine agonists such as bromocriptine and apomorphine may have some use in reducing alcohol craving.[76,148] Both agents have been reported to control withdrawal symptoms and to decrease alcohol craving for two to 26 weeks after detoxification. It should be noted, however, that Wadstein and colleagues[149] failed to find any clinical benefit of apomorphine for postintoxication symptoms. More controlled studies are necessary, better to define the roles of apomorphine and bromocriptine in the treatment of alcohol craving. There are no data on children and adolescents. This area merits further investigation.

Nicotine Craving

Nicotine is known to be one of the most addictive substances, with female adolescents having an even greater prevalence of nicotine dependence than males. Thus far, few approaches have been effective in helping patients discontinue smoking once they have become addicted. Alcoholics who finally become abstinent frequently are unable also to become tobacco abstinent. Alcoholics Anonymous (AA) meetings are infamous for the amount of cigarette smoking observed during sessions dealing with alcohol abstinence. One of the most difficult aspects of becoming nicotine abstinent is the intense craving experienced by smokers when they stop smoking. Nicotine withdrawal is also characterized by nervousness, irritability, restlessness, mood lability, anxiety, drowsiness, sleep disturbances, impaired concentration, increased appetite, headache, myalgia, constipation, fatigue, and weight gain. Withdrawal from nicotine is so unpleasant, in fact, that it makes many patients loath to quit smoking "cold turkey." Moreover, other psychosocial interventions have not been found very effective in the long-term accomplishment of nicotine abstinence. Psychotherapy, hypnosis, behavioral modification therapy, and the like have all been tried, but with little consistent success. One hears reports of nicotine-dependent patients who are dying of lung cancer and are on respirators, and yet risk their lives to smoke a cigarette.

Pharmacologic approaches, until recently, have not proved effective in decreasing nicotine craving. Nicotine-replacement therapy using polacrilex chewing gum often resulted in patients' becoming dependent on the gum. Many patients relapsed or continued to smoke cigarettes while they were chewing nicotine gum (Nicorette).

A cause for recent excitement among smokers and practitioners was the introduction of the nicotine transdermal system (Nicoderm, Prostep, and Habitrol). The system involves patches that provide the systemic delivery of nicotine for 24 hours following their application to intact skin. The patches come in varying strengths—7, 14, 21, and 22 mg. Nicotine is the active ingredient in this compound, while other components of the system are inactive. The rate of delivery of nicotine to the patient from each system is proportional to the surface area. Over 70% of the total amount of nicotine remains in the system 24 hours after application. Nicotine transdermal systems are labeled by the dose actually absorbed by the patient, which represents 68% of the amount released within 24 hours. The other 32% (e.g., 9 mg/day for the 21-mg/day system) volatizes from the edge of the system. Following the second daily application, steady-state plasma nicotine concentrations are achieved, and are about 30% higher than with single-dose applications. Plasma nicotine concentrations are proportional to dose.

Nicotine kinetics are similar for all sites of application on the upper body and outer arm. Following removal of the nicotine transdermal system, plasma nicotine concentrations decline, with a mean half-life of three to four hours. The systems are believed to have relatively low abuse potential because of their much slower absorption, much smaller fluctuations in blood levels, lower blood levels of nicotine, and less frequent use (once daily) as compared with cigarettes. To minimize the risk of dependence, it is recommended that patients be withdrawn gradually from the system after at least six weeks of use. As the patch is worn all day and then discarded, this can be a rather expensive intervention (over $150 per month).

Clinical studies thus far have been limited, and have mainly been performed by the drug companies marketing the system, such as Marion Merrell Dow, Inc. This company conducted two placebo-controlled, double-blind trials on 756 otherwise healthy patients who smoked at least one pack of cigarettes a day, and showed the nicotine transdermal system to be more effective than placebo in producing smoking cessation. The trials consisted of six weeks of active treatment, six weeks of weaning off the system, and 12 weeks of follow-up on no medication. Quitting was defined as total abstinence from smoking as determined by patient diary and expired carbon monoxide. All doses of the transdermal system were found to be superior to placebo, and doses of 21 mg/day resulted in significantly higher quit rates than did 14 mg/day and placebo treatments. Quit rates were still significantly different after an additional six-week weaning period and at follow-up three months later. It should be noted that all patients received weekly supportive care.

In a study conducted by Marion Merrell Dow on smokers with coronary artery disease (CAD), which compared 77 patients treated with the nicotine transdermal system with 78 placebo-treated patients, those patients receiving the system treatment had a significantly higher quit rate than did those receiving placebo. The transdermal system did not affect angina frequency or the occurrence of arrhythmias.

Patients in both studies who used the nicotine transdermal system were reported to have a significant reduction in their craving for cigarettes as compared with placebo-treated patients.

The goal of nicotine transdermal system therapy is complete abstinence. Patients need to be counseled not to continue to smoke cigarettes while they are on the patch. Reports have appeared in the lay press about patients who continued to smoke under treatment, resulting in a nicotine overdose with ensuing vasoconstriction that led to hypotension, prostration, and other problems. That is, side effects similar to those seen in nicotine poisoning may occur when patients smoke cigarettes while they are on the patch. Such patients should have the patch discontinued immediately. Careful prescreening is essential to determine how reliable the patient will be in complying with the no-smoking regimen, and, more important, how likely it is that the patient will inform his or her physician if he or she should begin to smoke while still on the patch.

Currently, a six-week trial of the nicotine transdermal system is felt to be most effective. The dosing strategy recommended is 21 mg for six weeks, followed by incremental tapering of the dose to 14 mg for two weeks, then to 7 mg for two weeks, and then discontinuing the dose. It has been suggested that this dosing regimen increases the likelihood of achieving abstinence and minimizing nicotine craving. Further study is clearly warranted before this drug can be recommended for all cigarette smokers. Even if future investigation reveals it to be successful, it is doubtful that such an approach can work alone without the patient's participation in supportive-care settings and formal smoking-cessation programs.

There are no data on children and adolescents. Because of the need for future studies in adults, and because of the potentially severe side effects from noncompliance (i.e., smoking while on the patch), we do not recommend using the nicotine transdermal system for adolescent nicotine abusers. Adolescents are susceptible to peer pressure, and an adolescent who has smoked in the past and is offered a cigarette by a peer may find it difficult to abstain from smoking in spite of the risk, and in spite of his or her not actually craving tobacco since he or she is wearing a patch that reportedly minimizes craving.

Smokeless Tobacco

Snuff and chewing tobacco are used by adolescents. This is an area that has not received much attention, but one that we feel merits further investigation. These substances are known to be addictive. And since they expose the adolescent to tobacco, the future risks cannot be discounted, such as mouth or throat cancer. In addition to focusing on the treatment of cigarette smoking, we believe that programs should be developed to focus on treating smokeless-tobacco use, since it potentially can cause severe complications.

Dual-Diagnosis Treatment Issues

This is a burgeoning area in both adult and adolescent psychiatry. Currently, there are no studies of depressed, affectively disordered, or psychotic (i.e., schizophrenic) adolescents who are also substance abusers, and few adequately designed studies on adults.[150-153] Making matters more difficult is the fact that non–substance-abusing adolescents with depression, bipolar disorder, and schizophrenia do not necessarily respond to pharmacologic treatment as adults do. Tricyclic antidepressant superiority over placebo in depressed adolescents has not been demonstrated (see Chapter 4). This has prompted the search for alternative agents to treat these disorders, such as the SSUIs, including fluoxetine, sertraline, and fluvoxamine. These agents may prove to be of particular value in child and adolescent depression because recent study has shown significant correlations between alterations in the serotonergic system (i.e., decreases in CNS serotonin levels) and impulsivity, aggression, depression, and suicidal behavior.[154,155]

Serotonin reuptake inhibitors such as fluoxetine, which differ both chemically and pharmacologically from standard TCAs, increase CNS serotonin levels (see Chapter 4). This has led to increased anticipation that these agents may be more effective in adolescent depression, which is frequently characterized by impulsivity. Nonetheless, there are no controlled studies to support this. Moreover, controlled studies are lacking in most areas of child and adolescent psychopharmacology, including the treatment of bipolar disorder and schizophrenia (see Chapters 4 and 8). Although the antipsychotics and lithium are believed to be effective in the treatment of adolescents with these disorders, double-blind, placebo-controlled studies performed to support this belief are limited.[156] Further complicating the issue is that it is not possible to distinguish between a drug-induced behavior that will be self-limiting and a drug-induced first episode of bipolar disorder or schizophrenia.[157] This obviously has particular relevance to substance-abusing patients.

There are significant differences involved when choosing a treatment approach for the dually diagnosed adolescent as opposed to one for the dually diagnosed adult patient. These factors include the incomplete personality development of the adolescent; signs, symptoms, and behaviors that are relatively specific to adolescents, such as the profound effect of peer pressure; dependence on parents/family; age-specific use of defense mechanisms such as denial, rationalization, splitting, isolation, projection, and sublimation; and specific risk factors, including perceived peer approval of drug and alcohol use, perceived adult drug and alcohol use, and poor academic achievement.[7] These developmental, psychological, and social differences emphasize the need for a treatment approach specifically geared to adolescent substance abusers. This goes beyond translating and modifying adult treatment strategies. Treatment strategies unique to adolescents that are designed to address these psychiatric, learning, and developmental issues are essential.

A very important issue in dually diagnosed adolescent patients is the use of psychotropic medication. Nonphysician clinicians and other special interest groups are often opposed to the use of psychoactive drugs for children and adolescents regardless of their substance abuse history, and are even more adamant with regard to substance-abusing teenagers. Alcoholics Anonymous and Narcotics Anonymous (NA), for example, warn their members about the dangers of becoming dependent on physician-prescribed or illicit psychoactive drugs as a substitute for their original addiction. Specifically, AA warns its members about the danger of becoming addicted to sedatives and hypnotics.[158] Adolescent substance abusers frequently have substance-abusing family members who may be members of AA or NA. Thus, when discussing psychopharmacologic interventions with the adolescent and family members, opposition may be encountered. Moreover, it is often difficult to convince patients and their families that certain psychotropic agents do not cause addiction. They tend to believe that all drugs are dangerous and potentially addictive, and they often are not aware of the differences between addictive benzodiazepines and nonaddictive antidepressants, for example. Since they have learned that even society-approved substances such as alcohol are potentially life-threatening for them, it is difficult for them to accept the fact that other drugs do not carry a similar risk.

In general, all adolescent substance abusers with or without positive urine and blood studies require a detoxification period in which medications are withheld, where possible, during the first two weeks of evaluation of a dually diagnosed patient.[7,157] There can be a significant overlap of psychiatric and substance abuse symptoms during this period. Substance abuse, intoxication, and withdrawal can mimic/cause/exacerbate many psychiatric conditions, including depression, mood swings/mania, psychosis, hyperactivity, and irritability. The two-week detoxification period increases the likelihood of being able to distinguish between psychiatric and substance abuse disorders and to define whether or not both conditions coexist. Whenever possible, waiting an additional one to three months for further observation and evaluation of the efficacy of psychosocial, nonpharmacologic interventions is recommended.[7] The lack of controlled pharmacologic studies on adolescents and the lack of definitive evidence supporting medication efficacy in many psychiatric disorders further support this approach.

There are also specific medical/psychiatric issues that need to be taken into account when prescribing psychotropic agents to dually diagnosed adolescents. Marijuana and all TCAs may elevate the heart rate,[159,160] and their additive effect could result in serious tachycardia or arrhythmia. Hillard and Vieweg[161] reported the occurrence of marked sinus tachycardia resulting from the synergistic effects of marijuana and nortriptyline. Thus it is essential that when using psychotropic medications in adolescents, abstinence from all other drugs must continue through the initiation and maintenance phase of pharmacologic treatment.[7] There are no controlled studies on dually diagnosed adolescents documenting the efficacy of psychotropic agents in this population. Further investigation and assessment are necessary.

Important considerations when treating substance-abusing adolescents include hepatic induction in those using alcohol and drugs on a chronic basis. This necessitates careful monitoring of plasma blood levels of psychotropic medications. Hepatic induction can result in a significant decrease in the plasma half-lives of drugs, so that it may be necessary to use lower doses of psychotropic medications in adolescent substance abusers. As it may be weeks before the cytochrome P-450 system returns to normal, it is imperative that blood levels of psychotropic medications be monitored at least once a week to dose adolescent substance abusers most effectively and safely. Once hepatic induction and liver microsomal enzymes do return to normal, if proper monitoring is not continued, the risk of drug overdose increases, especially in the early stages of treatment.

Alcohol, for example, is known to inhibit the binding of drugs to cytochrome P-450. Therefore, if an adolescent is drinking and taking psychotropic medications at the same time, particularly in the case of medications without a high therapeutic index, peak or toxic levels of the medications may be reached because biotransformation is not occurring due to the adolescent's alcohol use. Alcohol produces diuresis through its inhibitory effect on vasopressin. This takes on considerable importance for adolescents being treated with lithium, since, if they are drinking alcohol, they are likely to urinate large volumes while retaining lithium salts, resulting in increased lithium levels. It should be emphasized that clinicians treating adolescent substance abusers must evaluate all medications being taken, since nonpsychotropic medications such as warfarin and oral hypoglycemics, when ingested with alcohol, can be life-threatening as a result of drug interactions and the alteration of hepatic induction.

Currently, there are only a limited number of possible indications for medication intervention in dually diagnosed adolescents. As mentioned, detoxification/withdrawal in adolescents very rarely requires medical intervention, and adolescents appear, on the whole, to be less susceptible to drug and alcohol withdrawal. With the lack of controlled studies and knowledge in this area, the regular use of pharmacologic interventions cannot be endorsed at this time. We advocate withholding medication whenever possible, and using it only in medically compromising situations.

Indications for Pharmacologic Intervention

Major Depression

Major depression may be an indication for psychopharmacologic treatment in the dually diagnosed patient. Yet TCAs have not been shown to be superior to placebo in the treatment of depressed adolescents. Moreover, as we have mentioned, if an adolescent continues to use certain recreational drugs, such as marijuana, while he or she is receiving TCAs, potentially dangerous side effects may ensue. Thus it is difficult to justify TCA therapy in adolescents with depression as the risk/benefit ratio is not clearly in favor of the benefits. We advocate trying psychosocial interventions, such as cognitive and behavioral therapy.

Suicidal patients present the physician with a dilemma, particularly if non-pharmacologic interventions are proving unsuccessful. Suicidal ideation is obviously a psychiatric emergency that requires prompt treatment. Inpatient treatment is, of necessity, a time-limited intervention, and, practically speaking, many suicidal patients (e.g., those without an organized plan or those who report only passive death wishes) frequently are not hospitalized and are treated as outpatients. It is necessary to continue looking for pharmacologic alternatives, including ECT, for this population.

The SSUI antidepressants may be an attractive alternative. Some very preliminary data suggest that fluoxetine may be useful in some treatment-refractory depressed adolescents and young adults (see Chapter 4). The side-effect profiles of these agents also may be more favorable than that of standard TCAs. Fluoxetine and sertraline do not, for example have anticholinergic and cardiovascular side effects. Therefore, although it is preferred that all adolescents receiving psychotropic medications be abstinent, it is to be expected that some of them (possibly a significant number) will continue, at least sporadically, to use recreational substances such as marijuana. Urine and blood drug screens can monitor for this, but the possibility of an adolescent's circumventing such monitoring and/or indulging in sporadic use at parties and so on cannot be discounted. While we still recommend impressing on adolescents and their parents the importance of abstinence, and facilitating it by psychosocial interventions, we find it difficult to recommend discontinuing a pharmacologic intervention that is successful just because an adolescent uses marijuana at one party. Each patient requires individualized treatment and assessment. In addition, if a patient were to use marijuana while using fluoxetine or sertraline, the additive effects on the heart rate that are seen with marijuana and tricyclic use would not occur.

Two other important considerations regarding the potential utility of the SSUI antidepressants deserve mention. These agents may be particularly in-

509

dicated for the impulsive behavior that is frequently seen in depressed, substance-abusing alcoholics. Moreover, they have been shown to have some efficacy in the attenuation of alcohol consumption independently of their antidepressant effects.[141–143] Thus these agents may reduce alcohol (and possibly other drug) consumption in dually diagnosed patients, which, in addition, to their potential antidepressant effects, may make them the ideal agents for treatment of adolescent patients with dual diagnoses. It is possible that this may be a safer and more effective pharmacologic intervention directed toward both comorbid conditions simultaneously. Further study and investigation are clearly warranted.

Another issue that deserves mention is that MAOIs have also been mentioned as being potentially effective agents in the treatment of adolescent depression, but there have been no controlled studies with these agents in this population. We currently believe that they are, therefore, contraindicated for adolescent substance abusers, who are by nature impulsive. The potential medically life-threatening interactions that MAOIs have with a variety of substances, including wine and meperidine, result in a very poor risk/benefit ratio. Although new selective MAOIs are being developed that appear to be relatively safer and sparing of the "hypertensive-cheese" effect (see Chapters 4 and 6), until further investigation documents their safety, MAOIs should be avoided in depressed adolescent substance abusers.

Bipolar Disorder: Manic, Depressed, or Mixed Types

Lithium treatment for substance-abusing bipolar-disorder patients may be recommended. Although controlled studies are limited, the available literature to date suggests that adolescents with bipolar disorder respond about as well to lithium as do bipolar adults (see Chapter 8). Lithium has also been reported to reduce the subjective "intoxication" high and to attenuate the craving associated with a variety of substances of abuse, including alcohol, cocaine, amphetamines, and IV methylphenidate.[102–109] Lithium, therefore, may be an ideal agent to treat adolescent substance abusers with coexistent bipolar disorder. But since not all studies confirm its efficacy in treating substance abuse in adults, and there are no studies on adolescents, further study is necessary before firm pharmacologic treatment recommendations can be given.

As previously discussed, recent investigation has found lithium to be ineffective in treating alcoholics with or without an affective disorder, although it has been proved effective for bipolar disorder (see Chapter 8). Therefore, in adolescents who have undergone detoxification and receive a discrete diagnosis of bipolar disorder, lithium would be indicated to treat the bipolar disorder, but would not be expected to be helpful in the treatment of the substance abuse disorder. It is also important that the clinician remember the potential danger involved in administering lithium if the adolescent continues to ingest alcohol. In summary, lithium's role in treating substance-abusing adolescents appears limited.

Acute Psychosis

Acute psychosis, regardless of whether it stems from substance abuse or is a primary psychiatric disorder, may require urgent pharmacologic intervention. It is not always possible to wait for the patient to be detoxified when he or she is actively psychotic and represents a danger to the self or others. An antipsychotic medication such as haloperidol may be warranted in such situations (see Chapter 7). Treatment for these patients should be initiated using the lowest effective dose of antipsychotic, and other doses as needed in addition to the regular doses. When the psychosis resolves, tapering of the antipsychotic should be instituted.

If the psychosis does not resolve and it is determined that the patient has an underlying psychiatric disorder that accounts for the psychotic symptoms, it is important accurately to delineate the specific psychiatric condition—depression, bipolar disorder, schizophrenia, and so on. Antipsychotics are generally employed in all of these conditions, with or without an adjunctive agent such as an antidepressant or lithium (see Chapter 7). Further study is much needed in this very important area where chemical intervention is often required.

Severe Agitation and Aggression

Adolescents displaying dangerous aggression and combative behavior often require pharmacologic interventions for the safety of others and themselves. Agents employed to treat these behaviors include benzodiazepines such as lorazepam. However, their use may be problematic in adolescent substance abusers, who can become dependent on them. Moreover, benzodiazepines can produce paradoxical behavior rebound and disinhibition in adolescents. Unfortunately, neuroleptics are contraindicated until it is determined what substances the adolescent has been abusing. Antipsychotics used with certain drugs, such as PCP, can result in severe cardiovascular complications. Thus alternative agents should be tried first.

In some cases, the patient is so violent and combative that neuroleptics are necessary. Fortunately, this usually occurs in emergency rooms and/or inpatient settings where the patient can be closely monitored, and should he or she suffer an adverse medical or psychiatric complication (dystonic reaction, extrapyramidal side effects, etc.), prompt treatment can be instituted. The treating clinicians, however, must be alert to these side effects, as they can be difficult to detect in an aggressive, combative, and intoxicated substance-abusing adolescent. Further study in this area is much needed.

Attention-Deficit Hyperactivity Disorder

This disorder is known to be associated with an increased risk for the development of alcohol abuse and alcohol dependence (see Chapter 3). Thus adolescents with dual diagnoses of ADHD and a substance abuse disorder require treatment. Behavioral approaches should be tried first in children and adolescents with ADHD, but these are frequently insufficient, necessitating pharmacologic intervention. The drugs of choice for the treatment of ADHD are the psychostimulants methylphenidate, dextroamphetamine, and pemoline. But stimulants are also drugs of abuse, and concern has been raised about prescribing them to substance-abusing patients.

Although children and adolescents with ADHD do exhibit a twofold to fourfold increased risk for substance abuse, current data show no evidence that the use of correctly prescribed stimulant medications results in an increased risk for the abuse of and dependence on recreational or prescription drugs, or in dependence on and addiction to the stimulants themselves (see Chapter 3). These data, however, were not obtained on ADHD patients who are abusing drugs and/or alcohol. Thus when stimulants are prescribed correctly by a physician for a child with ADHD who is not abusing alcohol or drugs, it appears that such use does not represent an increased risk for substance abuse. No studies have assessed this risk in ADHD patients who have a co-existent substance abuse disorder.

Dextroamphetamine has the highest risk for abuse, with methylphenidate having a lower risk and pemoline the lowest risk for abuse of all the stimulants. These agents produce euphoria, which initially may be quite pleasing to adolescents with ADHD and/or conduct disorders, who commonly suffer from feelings of low self-esteem (see Chapter 3). This may be even more problematic in substance-abusing adolescents with these conditions.

We caution against using psychostimulants in adolescents with a coexistent substance abuse disorder, as their risk for abuse would seem to be higher than that for the general non–substance-abusing adolescent population, even when prescribed by an experienced physician. Moreover, these adolescents frequently have family members who are substance abusers as well. The risk of other family members abusing the adolescent patient's stimulant must be appraised. In addition, if the adolescent observes family members abusing his or her medication, he or she may be more inclined to do so as well. Peers may also tell an adolescent about the highs that can result from using stimulants. Thus suggestion and peer pressure may increase the risk for abuse in adolescents with a history of substance abuse.

We recommend treating ADHD unresponsive to behavioral management alone with TCA, such as desipramine and imipramine, which have proved to be more effective than placebo in the treatment of ADHD (see Chapter 4). Preliminary studies have shown that other, alternative antidepressants such as bupropion and fluoxetine may also be effective in the treatment of ADHD. We advocate starting with a tricyclic agent such as desipramine, which has a very favorable side-effect profile. If this is unsuccessful, trying other TCAs is warranted. If this also is unsuccessful, trying the alternative agents is recommended (see Chapter 4 for dosing for these agents). In conclusion, we believe that although the stimulants are felt to be somewhat more effective in the treatment of ADHD than desipramine and other antidepressants, and have a very favorable side-effect profile in nonabusing adolescent patients (particularly methylphenidate and dextroamphetamine), the risks of abuse for the patient, and often the family, contraindicates their use in this population, especially since there are other nonaddictive agents that are known to be effective in the treatment of ADHD.

Case History

A 13-year-old boy was referred for a psychiatric evaluation after being discharged from a rehabilitation center for drug and alcohol abuse. He had begun smoking cigarettes at the age of 9 and now smoked a pack and a half to two packs a day. When he was 12, some friends with whom he often smoked cigarettes cajoled him into skipping school with them and getting "stoned." Subsequently, he began to play truant from school and go off with friends to use drugs and alcohol. His pattern of abuse continued to escalate, so that at the time of detoxification and inpatient rehabilitation admittance, he had been drinking a fifth of whiskey per day and "more" on weekends. He was also smoking several joints a day and had experimented with cocaine, acid (LSD), and quaaludes "a few times." Alarmingly, he had begun to indulge his drug and alcohol use even when alone and now felt that he needed "a fix."

The boy had done well in rehabilitation and had responded favorably to psychosocial interventions, including a 12-step approach. After 14 days of being drug-free and having completed the rehabilitation program, it was noted that the patient continued to have problems with inattention, distractibility, and fidgetiness, and great difficulty in waiting his turn in group situations. He was impulsive and described as "chronically hyper." He was also noted to suffer chronic low self-esteem.

Psychiatric evaluation revealed a boy who had a long history of disruptive behaviors. His mother recalled that he was "wild even in my womb." She reported that he had always been more "hyper" than her three other children. He often took unnecessary risks, such as running into the street without looking and jumping off roofs. Moreover, she said that he had chronic difficulty in school and that teachers had commented on his inability to stay in his seat ever since nursery school. Reports of inattentiveness and easy distractibility with difficulty staying focused were abundant. His mother also reported that he had suffered from low self-esteem ever since she and his father had divorced five years earlier. Both she and her son denied other neurovegetative symptoms of depression. Suicidal ideation was also denied. There was no evidence of an oppositional or conduct disorder, nor was there a history of manic depression.

The family history was significant in that the patient's mother reported that all her and her ex-husband's male relatives were "on the wild side." They had never undergone psychiatric evaluation, but they had had problems at home and in school, with high levels of motoric activity, distractibility, difficulty paying attention, and impulsivity. Both the mother and father had significant histories of substance abuse. The patient's mother admitted IV drug use and abuse. She said that she was trying to quit, but that her ex-husband, with whom her son still had regular contact, continued to use and sell drugs. There was no history of mood disorder in the family.

The patient was diagnosed with ADHD, rule out dysthymia, and polysubstance abuse in remission since rehabilitation. In view of his significant history of substance abuse and the positive family history of current drug and alcohol use, the treating psychiatrist was reluctant to prescribe psychostimulant medication (i.e., dextroamphetamine, methylphenidate). Instead, a behavioral modification program was put into place and a desipramine trial was initiated to target the patient's ADHD symptoms. Implementation of a comprehensive behavioral management program combined with an ultimate desipramine dose of 50 mg t.id. (plasma level 106 ng/ml) resulted in marked improvement in the patient's ADHD symptoms. The patient suffered no adverse side effects from the medication.

Other Substance Abuse Concerns in Adolescents

Anabolic Steroids

The use of anabolic-androgenic steroids (AS) has received a lot of public and media attention secondary to that focused on athletes, who have been using them to enhance their performance.[162] Investigation thus far has mostly concentrated on the effects and health risks of AS use in adults.[163–167] While most of the effects in adults may be reversible, adolescents may be at risk of suffering permanent effects from AS use,[168–170] primarily premature skeletal maturation, spermatogenesis, and an increased risk of skeletal muscle injury. It must be emphasized that the evidence regarding steroid-induced complications in adolescents is largely anecdotal and limited to case reports. In addition, these side effects seldom, if ever, appear with steroids such as the glucocorticoids, or mineralcorticords (which are commonly employed to treat medical problems in adolescents) when used in recommended doses. Unlike AS, these agents are *not* considered to be drugs of abuse.

Anabolic steroid use is believed to be increasing since first reported among athletes in the 1950s, although very few studies have appeared assessing its incidence and prevalence, and those that have been conducted have been restricted mostly to the athletic population.[171,172] A study by Buckley and colleagues[174] to identify AS use among males in the general adolescent population focused on 3403 12th-grade teenage boys in 46 private and public schools across the country. The researchers found that 6.6% of these students currently used or had used AS, and that over two-thirds of the user group started such use when they were 16 years old or younger. This is significant since 27% of adolescents achieve Tanner Stage V after 16 years of age, placing them at permanent risk for permanent effects of AS use.[167–170] Of greater concern was the finding that 21% of the users reported that a health professional was their primary source of AS. Another study, by the Hazelton Foundation in Minneapolis, found that in 1986 the rate of current or previous AS use was reported as 3% for all the students polled in grades 8, 10, and 12.[175] Among the 12th graders, 5% of the males and 1% of the females used or had used steroids. At one of the high schools, 8% of the senior males admitted to having used AS. This emphasizes the need for educational intervention strategies that should begin in elementary school, and should be directed toward the entire student body rather than just the athletes.[175] Nonetheless, it needs to be emphasized that the data thus far are not definitive and remain controversial. Indeed, a look at AS use nationally as opposed to that in selected areas shows that less than 2% of U.S. high school student have used AS.

Steroids have been reported to cause mood alterations in adults, including depression, mania, psychosis, and delirium. Very little has been written about the psychopharmacologic treatment of steroid-induced destabilization of mood in children and adolescents, and the psychiatric sequelae of AS for these patients have not been well documented. Reports of increased aggressiveness have surfaced, but depression, suicide, and psychosis appear to be unusual. Clinical experience indicates that treatment strategies are similar to those used for adults.

Reducing the steroid dose to the lowest possible effective dose is the first intervention. Sometimes, this intervention alone will result in amelioration of the psychiatric symptoms. If it is not possible to reduce the steroid dose because of a life-threatening medical condition, and/or if the dose reduction is not effective in eliminating the psychiatric symptoms, the use of adjunctive medication to target the patient's psychiatric symptoms is indicated. Steroid use does not contraindicate antipsychotic, antidepressant, or lithium use. Actually, lithium may have both a prophylactic and stabilizing effect in some steroid-induced manic states.[178] This is an area that deserves further investigation and evaluation in the child and adolescent population.

It is important to point out that when Moss and associates[194] recently assessed the relationship between the use of AS and specific personality dimensions in 50 male bodybuilders who were current or past users as compared with a sample of 25 age-matched, "natural" bodybuilders who never used AS, they failed to confirm prior (largely anecdotal) reports of AS use being associated with significant psychopathology. Surprisingly, the authors found no personality differences between the groups. When they looked specifically at the relationship between current AS use and the presence of variations in mood state, hostility, and psychiatric symptomatology, they found that current AS users scored higher than nonusers *only* on psychometric scales measuring hostility, aggression, and somatization.[194]

Perry and colleagues[195] conducted a controlled retrospective study to characterize psychiatric symptom patterns and mental status changes precipitated by AS abuse in which they compared 20 male weight lifters who were currently using AS with 20 male weight lifters who had never used AS. The AS users had significantly more somatic, depressed, anxious, hostile, and paranoid complaints when using AS than they did when they were not using the drugs. But while AS users complained much more frequently of depression, anxiety, and hostility during cycles of AS use than did weight lifter controls, no differences in the occurrence of major mental disorders were found between the two groups.[195] The authors concluded that the organic mood changes associated with AS abuse most often present as a subsyndromal depression not severe enough to be characterized as a psychiatric disorder. Further controlled study is necessary before definitive conclusions can be drawn.

Prenatal Exposure to Drugs and Alcohol

Drug and alcohol abuse in pregnancy can result in a wide spectrum of abnormalities in the developing fetus and child, including the fetal alcohol syndrome and behavior and learning difficulties.[179–181] This has important implications for the adolescent population in view of the current epidemic of teenage pregnancies in this country. Many of the pregnant teenage girls are in the very-high-risk group; they often are high school dropouts or are not doing well in school and are of a lower socioeconomic status. Many of them have been abused, and, as noted, substance abuse is significantly more common in abused adolescents. These girls may not get appropriate prenatal care, especially considering their major risk factors. As there is a direct relationship between the use of alcohol and/or drugs and the absence of prenatal care, clinicians must consider the possibility of pregnancy in any adolescent female. In addition, substance abuse often results in decreased inhibitions and impulsive acts, including unprotected sex. Screening for this is thus mandated so that the young mother-to-be and her unborn child can receive appropriate medical care. The risk to the adolescent female of acquiring a sexually transmitted disease such as AIDS or hepatitis B, and the consequences for both mother and child, is a major concern in this population.

The care of infants born to drug-abusing and addicted mothers is largely supportive, including fluid management and nutritional supplementation as necessary. Psychopharmacologic intervention is not utilized in this population, and it has not been found necessary to withdraw infants born to drug- and alcohol-addicted mothers.

Alternative Treatment Options

The major controversy regarding the psychopharmacologic management of substance abuse disorders has centered on whether such an approach is indicated at all for these patients. Uncontrolled studies have shown that otherwise healthy patients in drug or alcohol withdrawal can be treated safely and successfully without using psychotropic medications.[174,176,177] As we have also mentioned, there are front-line nonphysician clinicians who are often adamantly opposed to the use of psychotropic medications for patients who have preexisting substance abuse disorders, recommending instead that such patients seek nonchemical solutions to their problems.

Because of the effectiveness and proliferation of self-help groups and psychosocial interventions, pharmaceutical companies have shown limited interest in searching for effective pharmacologic agents for the management of substance abuse disorders. Disulfiram, for instance, is the only medication in the United States that is indicated for alcohol dependence, and this agent was first introduced in Europe in 1948. Moreover, as mentioned, it is not likely to be useful for the adolescent alcohol-abusing patient.

Despite the fact that there is no convincing evidence supporting the claim by front-line nonphysician clinicians that all psychoactive drugs are dangerous for patients with substance abuse problems, the drug-free approach has continued to reign for 40 years. Now, however, recent advances in the pharmacology of alcohol, cocaine, and other drugs of abuse, and recent studies of the biological and genetic basis of inherited forms of substance abuse disorders, have heightened interest in potential psychopharmacologic interventions directed toward these disorders.[6] We believe that, in view of the significant morbidity and mortality caused by substance abuse, the search for effective and safe psychopharmacologic interventions to be used in conjunction with psychosocial interventions must continue. This supports what we are discovering in general psychiatry as well—that a multimodal combined psychosocial and psychopharmacologic approach will prove to be the most efficacious for many psychiatric conditions.

References

1. Bass, J., Gallagher, S., Mehta, K. (1985). Unintentional injuries among adolescents and younger adults. *Pediatr Clin North Am, 32*, 31–39.

2. Morrison, M.A. (1991). Overview—kids and drugs. *Psychiatr Ann, 21(2)*, 72–73.

3. MacDonald, D.I. (1984). Drugs, drinking, and adolescence. *Am J Dis Child, 138*, 117–125.

4. Mensch, B.S., Kandel, D.B. (1988). Underreporting of substance use in a national longitudinal youth cohort: Individual and interviewer effects. *Public Opinion, 52*, 100–124.

5. Bailey, G.W. (1991). Substance use and abuse. In J.M. Wiener (Ed.), *Textbook of Child and Adolescent Psychiatry* (pp. 439–452). Washington, D.C.: American Psychiatric Press.

6. Moss, H.B. (1991). Pharmacotherapy. In A.S. Bellack, M. Hersen (Eds.), *Handbook of Comparative Treatment for Adult Disorders* (pp. 506–520). New York: Wiley.

7. Stowell, R.J.A. (1991). Dual diagnosis issues. *Psychiatr Ann, 21(2)*, 98–104.

8. Levy, J.C., Deykin, E.Y. (1989). Suicidality, depression, and substance abuse in adolescents. *Am J Psychiatry, 146*, 1462–1467.

9. Deykin, E.Y., Levy, J.C., Wells, V. (1986). Adolescent depression, alcohol and drug abuse. *Am J Public Health, 76*, 178–182.

10. Singer, M.I., Petchers, M.K. (1989). The relationship between sexual abuse and substance abuse, among psychiatrically hospitalized adolescents. *Child Abuse Neglect, 13*, 319–325.

11. Cohen, F.S., Densen-Gerber, J. (1982). A study of the relationship between child abuse and drug addiction in 178 patients: Preliminary results. *Child Abuse Neglect, 6*, 383–387.

12. Rohsenow, D.J., Corbett, R., Devine, D. (1988). Molested children: A hidden contribution to substance abuse? *J Substance Abuse Treat, 5*, 13–18.

13. Christie, K.A., Burke, J.D., Regier, D.A., et al. (1988). Epidemiologic evidence for early onset of mental disorders and higher risk of drug abuse in young adults. *Am J Psychiatry, 145,* 971–975.

14. Wood, D., Wender, P.H., Reimherr, F.W. (1983). The prevalence of attention deficit disorder, residual type, or minimal brain dysfunction, in a population of male alcoholic patients. *Am J Psychiatry, 140,* 95–98.

15. Smith, D.E., Ehrlich, P., Seymour, R.B. (1992). Current trends in adolescent drug use. *Psychiatr Ann, 21(2),* 74–79.

16. Schwartz, R.H. (1991). Heavy marijuana use and recent memory impairment. *Psychiatr Ann, 21(2),* 80–82.

17. Tinklenberg, J.R., Melges, F.T., Hollister, L.E., et al. (1970). Marijuana and immediate memory. *Nature, 226,* 1171–1172.

18. Melges, F.T., Tinklenberg, J.R., Hollister, L.E., et al. (1970). Marijuana and temporal disintegration. *Science, 168,* 1118–1120.

19. Abel, E.L. (1970). Marijuana and memory. *Nature, 227,* 1151–1152.

20. Abel, E.L. (1971). Marijuana and memory: Acquisition or retrieval? *Science, 173,* 1038–1040.

21. Dornbrush, R.L., Fink, M., Freedman, A.M. (1971). Marijuana, memory, and perception. *Am J Psychiatry, 128,* 194–197.

22. Darley, C.F., Tinklenberg, J.R., Hollister, L.E., et al. (1973). Influence of marijuana on storage and retrieval processes in memory. *Memory Cognition, 1,* 196–200.

23. Seymour, R.B., Smith, D.E., Inaba, D., et al. (1989). *The New Drugs: Look Alikes, Drugs of Deception and Designer Drugs.* Center City, Minn.: Hazelden.

24. Robbins, L.N., Helzer, J.E., Weissman, M.M., et al. (1984). Lifetime prevalence of specific psychiatric disorders in three sites. *Arch Gen Psychiatry, 41,* 949–958.

25. U.S. Department of Health and Human Services (1987). *Sixth Special Report to Congress on Alcohol and Health from the Secretary of Health and Human Services.* Rockville, Md.: U.S. Department of Health and Human Services.

26. Rogers, P., Silling, S.M., Adams, L.R. (1991). Adolescent chemical dependence: A diagnosable disease. *Psychiatr Ann, 21(2),* 91–97.

27. Kandel, D., Faust, R. (1975). Sequence and stages in patterns of adolescent drug use. *Arch Gen Psychiatry, 32,* 923–932.

28. Kandel, D., Logan, J. (1984). Periods of drug use from adolescence to young adulthood: 1. Periods of risk for initiation, continued use, and discontinuation. *Am J Public Health, 74*, 660–666.

29. Single, E., Kandel, D., Faust, R. (1985). Patterns of multiple drug use in high school. *J Health Soc Behav, 32*, 344–357.

30. Harwood, H.J., Napolitano, D.M., Kristiansen, P.L., et al. (1984). *Economic costs to Society of Alcohol and Drug Abuse and Mental Illness.* Research Triangle Park, N.C.: Research Triangle Institute.

31. Newcomb, M., Maddahian, E., Bentler, P. (1986). Risk factors for drug use among adolescents: Concurrent and longitudinal analyses. *Am J Public Health, 76*, 525–531.

32. Forney, M., Forney, P., Ripley, W. (1989). Predictor variables of adolescent drinking. *Adv Alcohol Substance Use, 8*, 97–117.

33. Mezzich, A., Tarter, R., Hsieh, T., et al. (1992). Substance use severity in female adolescents: Association between age of menarche and chronological age. *Am J Addictions, 1*, 217–221.

34. Mezzich, A., Moss, H., Tarter, R. (1991). Psychiatry comorbidity and drug abuse patterns in alcohol abusing female adolescents. Paper presented at the meeting of the Research Society on Alcoholism, Marco Island, Fl.

35. Rogers, P.D., Harris, J., Jarmuskewicz, J. (1987). Alcohol and adolescence. *Pediatr Clin North Am, 34*, 289–303.

36. Kalant, H., LeBlanc, A.E., Gibbins, R.J. (1971). Tolerance to and dependence on some non-opiate psychotropic drugs. *Pharmacol Rev, 23*, 135–191.

37. Tabakoff, B., Melchior, C.L., Hoffman, P. (1984). Factors in ethanol tolerance. *Science, 224*, 523–524.

38. American Psychiatric Association. (1987). *Diagnostic and Statistical Manual of Mental Disorders (3rd ed., rev.).* Washington, D.C.: American Psychiatric Association.

39. American Psychiatric Association (1980). *Diagnostic and Statistical Manual of Mental Disorders (3rd ed.).* Washington, D.C.: American Psychiatric Association.

40. Vingelis, E., Smart, R.G. (1981). Physical dependence on alcohol in youth. In Y. Israel, F.B. Glaser, H. Kalaut, et al. (Eds.), *Research Advances in Alcohol and Drug Problems.* New York: Plenum Press.

41. Nichols, J.R., Headlee, C.P., Coppock, H.W. (1956). Drug addiction: I. Addiction by escape training. *J Am Pharm Assoc, 45*, 788–791.

42. Fischman, W.M., Schuster, G.R. (1982). Cocaine self-administration in humans. *Fed Proc, 41*, 241–246.

43. Henningfield, J.E., Griffiths, R.R. (1980). Effects of ventilated cigarette holders on cigarette smoking by humans. *Psychopharmacology, 68*, 115–119.

44. Wikler, A. (1952). A psychodynamic study of a patient during self-regulation readdiction to morphine. *Psychiatr Q, 26*, 270–293.

45. Mello, N. K., Mendelson, J.H. (1978). Behavioral pharmacology of human alcohol, heroin, and marijuana use. In J. Fishman (Ed.), *The Bases of Addiction*. Berlin: Dahlem Konferenzen.

46. Mello, N.K., Mendelson, J.H. (1980). Buprenorphine suppresses heroin use by heroin addicts. *Science, 207*, 657–659.

47. Mendelson, J.H., Mello, N.K. (1966). Experimental analyses of drinking behavior of chronic alcoholics. *Ann NY Acad Sci, 133*, 828.

48. Leonard, K.E., Bromet, E.J., Parkinson, D.K., et al. (1984). Agreement among Feigner, RDC, and DSM-III criteria for alcoholism. *Addict Behav, 9*, 319–322.

49. Tarter, R.E., Arria, A.M., Moss, H., et al. (1987). DSM-III criteria for alcohol abuse: Associations with alcohol consumption behavior. *Clin Exp Res, 11*, 541–543.

50. Selzer, M. (1971). The Michigan Alcoholism Screening Test (MAST): The quest for a new diagnostic instrument. *Am J Psychiatry, 127*, 1653–1658.

51. Valliant, G. (1983). *The Natural History of Alcoholism*. Cambridge, Mass.: Harvard University Press.

52. Mirin, S.M., Weiss, R.D., Michael, J., et al. (1988). Psychopathology and substance abusers: Diagnosis and treatment. *Am J Drug Alcohol Abuse, 14*, 139–157.

53. Bukstein, O.E., Brent, D.A., Kaminer, Y. (1989). Comorbidity of substance abuse and other psychiatric disorders in adolescents. *Am J Psychiatry, 146*, 1131–1141.

54. Demilio, L. (1989). Psychiatric syndromes in adolescent substance abusers. *Am J Psychiatry, 146*, 1212–1214.

55. Nace, E.P. (1989). Substance use disorders and personality disorder: Comorbidity. *Psychiatr Hosp, 20*, 65–69.

56. Estroff, T.W., Schwartz, R.H., Hoffman, N.G. (1989). Adolescent cocaine abuse: Addictive potential, behavioral and psychiatric effects among adolescent substance abusers. *Clin Pediatr, 28*, 550–555.

57. McLellan, A.T. (1986). Psychiatric severity as a predictor in outcome from substance abuse treatments. In R. Meyer (Ed.), *Psychopathology and Addictive Disorders* (pp. 97–139). New York: Guilford Press.

58. Schuckit, M.A. (1985). The clinical implications of primary diagnostic groups among alcoholics. *Arch Gen Psychiatry, 42*, 1043–1049.

59. Rounsaville, B.J., Dolinski, Z.S., Babor, T.F., et al. (1987). Psychopathology as a predictor of treatment outcome in alcoholics. *Arch Gen Psychiatry, 44*, 505–513.

60. Kofoed, L., Kania, J., Walsh, T., et al. (1986). Outpatient treatment of patients with substance abuse and coexisting psychiatric disorders. *Am J Psychiatry, 143*, 867–872.

61. Gfeerer, J. (1987). Correlation between drug use by teenagers and drug use in older family members. *Am J Drug Alcohol Abuse, 13*, 95–108.

62. Hughes, S.O., Power, T.G., Francis, D.J. (1992). Defining patterns of drinking in adolescence: A cluster analytic approach. *J Stud Alcohol, 53*, 40–47.

63. Marden, P., Zylamn, R., Filmore, K.M., et al. (1976). Comment on "A national study of adolescent drinking behavior, attitudes, and correlates." *J Stud Alcohol, 37*, 1346, 1358.

64. Moberg, D. (1983). Identifying adolescents with alcohol problems: A field test of the Adolescent Alcohol Involvement Scale. *J Stud Alcohol, 44*, 701–721.

65. White, H.R. (1987). Longitudinal stability and dimensional structure of problem drinking in adolescence. *J Stud Alcohol, 48*, 541–550.

66. White, R., Labouvie, E.W. (1989). Towards the assessment of adolescent problem drinking. *J Stud Alcohol, 50*, 30–37.

67. Thompson, W.L., Johnson, A.D., Maddrey, W.L. (1975). Diazepam and paraldehyde for treatment of severe delirium tremors. *Ann Intern Med, 82*, 175–180.

68. Rankin, H., Hodgson, R., Stockwell, T. (1979). The concept of craving and its measurement. *Behav Res Ther, 17*, 389–396.

69. Meyer, R.E. (1986). Anxiolytics and the alcoholic parent. *J Stud Alcohol, 47*, 269–273.

70. Williams, H.L., Rundell, D.H. (1981). Altered sleep physiology in chronic alcoholics: Reversal with abstinence. *Alcoholism: Clin Exp Res, 5*, 318–325.

71. Khan, A., Ciravlo, D.A., Nelson, W.H., et al. (1984). Dexamethasone suppression test in recently detoxified alcoholics: Clinical implications. *J Clin Psychopharmacol, 4*, 94–97.

72. Hughes, J.R., Hatsukami, D.K., Krahn, R.W., et al. (1984). Effect of nicotine on the tobacco withdrawal syndrome. *Psychopharmacology* (Berlin), *83*, 82–87.

73. Kissin, B. (1975). The use of psychoactive drugs in the long-term treatment of chronic alcoholics. *Ann N Y Acad Sci, 252*, 385–395.

74. Dackis, C.A., Gold, M.S. (1985). Pharmacological approaches to cocaine addiction. *J Substance Abuse Treat, 2*, 139–145.

75. Kleber, H., Gawin, F. (1986). Psychopharmacological trials in cocaine abuse treatment. *Am J Drug Alcohol Abuse, 12*, 235–246.

76. Borg, V. (1983) Bromocriptin in the prevention of alcohol abuse. *Acta Psychiatr Scand, 68*, 100–110.

77. Jaffe, J.H. (1980). Drug addiction and drug abuse. In L.S. Goodman, A. Gilman (Eds.), *The Pharmacological Basis of Therapeutics* (pp. 535–584). New York: Macmillan.

78. Jaffe, J.H. (1987). Pharmacologic agents in treatment of drug dependence. In H.Y. Meltzer (Ed.), *Psychopharmacology: The Third Generation of Progress* (pp. 1605–1616). New York: Raven Press.

79. Jaffe, J.H., Martin, W.R. (1987). Opioid analgesics and antagonists. In H.Y. Meltzer (Ed.), *Psychopharmacology: The Third Generation of Progress* (pp. 494–534). New York: Raven Press.

80. Gold, M.E., Redmond, D.C., Kleber, H.D. (1978). Clonidine blocks acute opiate-withdrawal symptoms. *Lancet, 2*, 599–602.

81. Charney, D.S., Sternberg, D.E., Kleber, H.D., et al. (1981). The clinical use of clonidine in abrupt withdrawal from methadone. *Arch Gen Psychiatry, 38*, 1227–1273.

82. Charney, D.S., Heninger, G.R., Kleber, H.D. (1986). The combined use of clonidine and naltrexone as a rapid, safe, and effective treatment of abrupt withdrawal from methadone. *Am J Psychiatry, 143*, 831–837.

83. Isbell, H., Fraser, H.F., Wikler, A. (1955). An experimental study of the etiology of "rum fits" and delirium tremors. *Q J Stud Alcohol, 16*, 1–13.

84. Kaim, S.C., Klett, C.J., Rothchild, B. (1969). Treatment of the acute alcohol withdrawal state: A comparison of four drugs. *Am J Psychiatry, 125*, 1640–1646.

85. Sampliner, R., Iber, F.L. (1974). Diphenylhydantoin control of alcohol withdrawal seizures. *JAMA, 230,* 1430–1437.

86. Runion, H.I., Fowler, A. (1978). A double-blind study of chlordiazepoxide and hydroxyzine HCI therapy in acute alcohol withdrawal. *Proc West Pharmacol Soc, 21,* 303–309.

87. Wegner, M.E., Fink, D.W. (1965). Chlordiazepoxide compared to meprobamate and promazine for the withdrawal symptoms of acute alcoholism. *Wis Med J, 64,* 436–440.

88. Baskin, S.I., Easdale, A. (1982). Is chlordiazepoxide the rational choice among benzodiazepines? *Pharmacotherapy, 2,* 110–119.

89. Sellers, E.M., Naranjo, C.A., Harrison, B., et al. (1983). Diazepam loading: Simplified treatment of alcohol withdrawal. *Clin Pharmacol Ther, 34,* 822–826.

90. Caille, G., Lacasse, Y., Vezina, M., et al. (1980). A novel route for benzodiazepine administration: A sublingual formulation of lorazepam. In L. Manzo (Ed.), *Advances in Neurotoxicity* (pp. 375–389). New York: Pergamon.

91. Spencer, J. (1980). Use of injectable lorazepam in alcohol withdrawal. *Med J Aus, 2,* 211–212.

92. Wilkins, A.J., Jenkins, W.J., Steiner, J.A. (1983). Efficacy of clonidine in the treatment of alcohol withdrawal state. *Psychopharmacology, 81,* 78–80.

93. Baumgartner, G.R., Rowen, R.C. (1987). Clonidine vs. chlordiazepoxide in the management of acute alcohol withdrawal. *Arch Intern Med, 147,* 1223–1226.

94. Van Rossum, J.M., Hurkman, J.A. (1964). Mechanism of action of psychomotor stimulant drugs: Significance of dopamine in locomotor stimulant action. *Int J Neuropharmacol, 3,* 227–238.

95. Ross, S.B., Renyi, A.L. (1966). Uptake of some tritrated sympathomimetic amines by mouse brain cortex in vitro. *Acta Pharmacol Toxicol, 24,* 297–309.

96. Taylor, D., Ho, B.T. (1977). Neurochemical effects of cocaine following acute and repeated injection. *J Neurosci Res, 3,* 95–101.

97. Taylor, D.L., Ho, B.T., Fagan, J.D. (1979). Increased dopamine receptor binding in rat brain by repeated cocaine injections. *Commun in Psychopharmacol, 3,* 137–142.

98. Tennant, F.S. (1985). Effect of cocaine dependence on plasma phylalenine and tyrosine levels and on urinary MHPG excretion. *Am J Psychiatry, 142,* 1200–1201.

99. Banerjee, S.P., Sharma, V.K., Kung-Cheung, L.S., et al. (1979). Cocaine and d-amphetamine induces changes in central beta-adrenoceptor sensitivity: Effects of acute and chronic drug treatment. *Brain Res, 175*, 119–130.

100. Charney, D.S., Menkes, D.B., Heninger, G.R. (1981). Receptor sensitivity and the mechanisms of action of antidepressant treatment. *Arch Gen Psychiatry, 38*, 1227–1273.

101. Koide, T., Matsushita, H. (1981). An enhanced sensitivity of muscarinic cholinergic receptors associated with dopaminergic receptor sub-sensitivity after chronic antidepressant treatment. *Life Sci, 28*, 1139.

102. Flemenbaum, A. (1974). Does lithium block the effects of amphetamine? *Am J Psychiatry, 131*, 7.

103. Van Kammen, D.P., Murphy, D.L. (1975). Attenuation of the euphoriant and activating effects of d- and l-amphetamine by lithium carbonate treatment. *Psychopharmacologia* (Berlin), *44*, 215–224.

104. Cronson, A.J., Flemenbaum, A. (1978). Antagonism of cocaine highs by lithium. *Am J Psychiatry, 135*, 856–857.

105. Huey, L., Janowsky, D., Lewis, J., et al. (1981). Effects of lithium carbonate on methylphenidate induced mood, behavior, and cognitive processes. *Psychopharmacology, 73*, 161–164.

106. Angrist, B., Gershon, S. (1979). Variable attenuation of amphetamine effects by lithium. *Am J Psychiatry, 136*, 806–810.

107. Gawin, F.H., Kleber, H.D. (1984). Cocaine abuse treatment: An open pilot trial with lithium and desipramine. *Arch Gen Psychiatry, 41*, 903–910.

108. Kline, N.S., Wren, J.C., Cooper, T.B., et al. (1974). Evaluation of lithium therapy in chronic and periodic alcoholism. *Am J Med Sci, 268*, 15–22.

109. Merry, J., Reynolds, C.M., Bailey, J., et al. (1976). Prophylactic treatment of alcoholism by lithium carbonate: A controlled study. *Lancet, 2*, 481–482.

110. Judd, L.L., Hubbard, R.B., Huey, L.Y. (1977). Lithium carbonate and ethanol induced "highs" in normal subjects. *Arch Gen Psychiatry, 34*, 463–467.

111. Linnoila, M., Saario, I., Maki, M. (1974). Effect of treatment with diazepam or lithium and alcohol on psychomotor skills related to driving. *Eur J Clin Pharmacol, 7*, 337–342.

112. Judd, L.L., Huey, L.Y. (1984). Lithium antagonizes ethanol intoxication in alcoholics. *Am J Psychiatry, 141*, 1517–1521.

113. Fawcett, J., Clark, D.C., Aagesen, C.A., et al. (1984). A double-blind, placebo-controlled trial of lithium carbonate therapy for alcoholism. *Arch Gen Psychiatry, 44*, 248–256.

114. Dole, U.P., Nyswander, M. (1965). A medical treatment for diacetylmorphine (heroin) addiction: A clinical trial with methadone hydrochloride. *JAMA, 193*, 646–650.

115. McLellan, A.T., Lubrosky, L., O'Brien, C.P. (1982). Is substance abuse treatment effective? Five different perspectives. *JAMA, 247*, 1423–1427.

116. Ginzburg, H.M.. Naltrexone: Its clinical utility. In B. Stimmel (Ed.), *Advances in Alcohol and Substance Abuse* (pp. 83–101). New York: Haworth.

117. Resnik, R.B., Schuyten-Resnik, E., Washton, A.M. (1980). Assessment of narcotic antagonists in the treatment of opioid dependence. *Ann Rev Pharmacol Toxicol, 20*, 463–474.

118. Hald, J., Jacobson, E. (1948). A drug sensitizing the organism to ethyl alcohol. *Lancet, 255*, 1001–1004.

119. Fuller, R.K., Williford, W.O. (1980). Life-table analysis of abstinence in a study evaluating the efficacy of disulfiram. *Alcoholism: Clin Exp Res, 4*, 298–301.

120. Fuller, R.K., Branchley, L., Brightivell, D.R., et al. (1986). Disulfiram treatment of alcoholism: A Veteran's Administration cooperative study. *JAMA, 256*, 1449–1455.

121. Goyer, P.F., Major, L.F. (1979). Hepatoxicity in disulfiram-treated patients. *J Stud Alcohol, 40*, 133–137.

122. Rainey, J.M. (1977). Disulfiram toxicity and carbon disulfide poisoning. *Am J Psychiatry, 134*, 371–378.

123. Bennet, A., McKeeve, L., Turk, H. (1951). Psychotic reactions during tetraethylthiuram disulfide (antabuse) therapy. *JAMA, 145*, 483.

124. Knee, S.T., Razani, J. (1974). Acute organic brain syndrome: A complication of disulfiram therapy. *Am J Psychiatry, 131*, 1281–1282.

125. Major, L.F., Lerner, P., Ballenger, J.C., et al. (1979). Dopamine-beta-hydroxylase in the cerebrospinal fluid: Relationship to disulfiram-induced psychosis. *Biol Psychiatry, 14*, 1423–1427.

126. Heath, R.G., Neeselhof, W., Bishop, M.P., et al. (1965). Behavioral and metabolic changes associated with the administration of tetraethylthiuram disulfide (Antabuse). *Dis Nerv Sys, 26*, 99–105.

127. Brent, D.A., Perper, J.A., Goldstein, C.E., et al. (1988). Risk factors for

adolescent suicide: A comparison of adolescent suicide victims with suicidal inpatients. *Arch Gen Psychiatry, 45*, 581–588.

128. Brent, D.A. (1987). Correlates of the medical lethality of suicide attempts in children and adolescents. *J Am Acad Child Psychiatry, 26*, 87–89.

129. Garfinkel, B., Froese, A., Hood, J. (1982). Suicide attempts in children and adolescents. *Am J Psychiatry, 139*, 1257–1261.

130. Asarnow, J.R., Carlson, G.A., Guthrie, D. (1987). Coping strategies, self-prescriptions, hopelessness and perceived family environments in depressed and suicidal children. *J Contemp Clin Psychol, 55*, 361–366.

131. Brent, D.A., Kalas, R., Edelbrock, C., et al. (1986.) Psychopathology and its relationship to suicidal ideation in childhood and adolescents. *J Am Acad Child Psychiatry, 25*, 666–673.

132. Kazdin, A.E., French, N.H.Y., Unis, A.S., et al. (1983). Hopelessness, depression, and suicidal intent among psychiatrically disturbed inpatient children. *J Contemp Psychol, 51*, 504–510.

133. Shafii, M., Carrigen, S., Whittinghill, J.R., et al. (1985). Psychological autopsy of completed suicide in children and adolescents. *Am J Psychiatry, 142*, 1061–1063.

134. Mello, N.K., Mendelson, J.H., Bree, M.P., et al. (1989). Buprenorphine suppresses cocaine self-administration by rhesus monkeys. *Science, 245*, 859–862.

135. Dorus, W., Ostrow, D.G., Anton, R., et al. (1989). Lithium treatment of depressed and nondepressed alcoholics. *JAMA, 262*, 1646–1652.

136. Ciraulo, D.A., Barnhill, J.G., Ciraulo, A.M., et al. (1989). Parental alcoholism as a risk factor in benzodiazepine abuse: A pilot study. *Am J Psychiatry, 146*, 1333–1335.

137. Ciraulo, D.A., Sands, B.F., Shader, R.I. (1988). Critical review of liability for benzodiazepine abuse among alcoholics. *Am J Psychiatry, 145*, 1501–1506.

138. Kissin, B. (1975). The use of psychoactive drugs in the long-term treatment of chronic alcoholics. *Ann NY Acad Sci, 252*, 385–395.

139. Christensen, J.K., Ronstead, P., Vaag, U.H. (1984). Side effects after disulfiram. *Acta Psychiatr Scand, 69*, 265–273.

140. Branchey, L., Davis, W., Lee, K.K., et al. (1984). Psychiatric complications in disulfiram treatment. *Am J Psychiatry, 144*, 1310–1312.

141. Naranjo, C.A., Sellers, E.M., Raoch, C.A., et al. (1984). Zimelidine-in-

duced variations in alcohol intake by nondepressed heavy drinkers. *Clin Pharmacol Ther, 35*, 374–381.

142. Naranjo, C.A., Sellers, E.M., Lawrin, M.O. (1985). Moderation of ethanol intake by serotonin uptake inhibitors. In C. Shagass (Ed.), *Biological Psychiatry* (pp. 708–710). Amsterdam: Elsevier Science.

143. Naranjo, C.A., Cappel, H., Sellers, E.M. (1981). Pharmacological control of alcohol consumption: Tactics for identification and testing of new drugs. *Addict Behav, 6*, 261–269.

144. Tennant, F.S., Rawson, R.A. (1982). Cocaine and amphetamine dependence treated with desipramine. In *Problems of Drug Dependence*. Washington, D.C.: National Institute of Drug Abuse.

145. Kosten, T.R., Rounsaville, B.J., Kleber, H.D., et al. (1987). A 2.5 year follow-up of cocaine use among treated opioid addicts. Have our treatments helped? *Arch Gen Psychiatry, 44*, 281–284.

146. Milby, J.R., Gurwitch, R.H., Wiebe, D.J., et al. (1986). Prevalence and diagnostic reliability of methadone maintenance detoxification fear. *Am J Psychiatry, 143*, 739–743.

147. Meyer, R.E. (1986). Anxiolytics and the alcoholic parent. *J Stud Alcohol, 47*, 269–273.

148. Jensen, S.B., Christofferson, C.B., Noerregaard, A. (1977). Apomorphine outpatient treatment of alcohol intoxication and abstinence: A double-blind study. *Br J Addict, 72*, 325–330.

149. Wadstein, J., Ohlin, H., Sternberg, P. (1978). Effects of apomorphine and apomorphine-L-dopa carbidopa on alcohol postintoxication symptoms. *Drug Alcohol Dependence, 3*, 281–287.

150. Kline, N.S., Wren, J.C., Cooper, T.B., et al. (1974). Evaluation of lithium therapy in chronic and periodic alcoholism. *Am J Med Sci, 268*, 15–22.

151. Ditman, K.S. (1966). Review and evaluation of current drug therapies in alcoholism. *Psychosom Med, 28*, 248–258.

152. Ciraulo, D.A., Jaffe, J.H. (1981). Tricyclic antidepressants in the treatment of depression associated with alcoholism. *J Clin Psychopharmacol, 1*, 146–150.

153. Ciraulo, D.A., Alderson, L.M., Chapron, D.J., et al. (1982). Imipramine disposition in alcoholics. *J Clin Psychopharmacol, 2*, 2–7.

154. Roy, A., Linnoila, M. (1988). Suicidal behavior, impulsiveness and serotonin. *Acta Psychiatr Scand, 78*, 529–535.

155. Asberg, M., Nordstrom, P., Traskman-Benz, L. (1986). Biological factors in suicide. In A. Roy (Ed.), *Suicide* (pp. 47–71). Baltimore, Md.: Williams & Wilkins.

156. Pool, D., Bloom, W., Mielke, D.H., et al. (1976). A controlled evaluation of loxitane in 75 adolescent, schizophrenic patients. *Curr Ther Res, 19,* 99–104.

157. Geller, B. (1988). Pharmacotherapy of concomitant psychiatric disorders in adolescent substance abusers. *NIDA Research Monographs, 77,* 94–112. DHHS Publication (ADM)88-1523. Rockville, Md.: Department of Health and Human Services.

158. Alcoholics Anonymous. (1984). The AA member—medications and other drugs: A report from a group of physicians in AA. New York: Alcoholics Anonymous World Services.

159. Meyer, R.E. (1978). Behavioral pharmacology of marijuana. In A. DiMascio, K.F. Killam (Eds.), *Psychopharmacology: A Generation of Progress* (pp. 1639–1652). New York: Raven Press.

160. Glassman, A.H. (1984). The newer antidepressant drugs and their cardiovascular effects. *Psychopharmacol Bull, 20,* 272–279.

161. Hillard, J.R., Vieweg, W.V.R. (1983). Marked sinus tachycardia resulting from the synergistic effects of marijuana and nortriptyline. *Am J Psychiatry, 140,* 626–627.

162. Cowart, V. (1987). Steroids in sports: After four decades, time to return these genies to bottle? *JAMA, 257,* 421–427.

163. Lamb, D.R. (1984). Anabolic steroids in athletes: How well do they work and how dangerous are they? *Am J Sports Med, 12,* 31–38.

164. Wright, J.E. (1978). *Anabolic Steroids in Sports.* Natick, Moss, Sports Science Consultants.

165. Haupt, H.A., Rovere, G.D. (1984). Anabolic steroids: A review of the literature. *Am J Sports Med, 12,* 469–484.

166. Strauss, R.H., Wright, J.E., Finerman, G.A.M., et al. (1983). Side effects of anabolic steroids in weight-trained men. *Phys Sports Med, 11,* 87–96.

167. Shephard, R.J., Killinger, D., Fred, T. (1977). Response on sustained use of anabolic steroid. *Br J Sports Med, 11,* 170–173.

168. Rosenfeld, R.G., Northcraft, G.B., Hentz, R.L. (1982). A prospective, randomized study of testosterone treatment of constitutional delay of growth and development in male adolescents. *Pediatrics, 68,* 681–687.

169. Strauss, R.H. (1987). Anabolic steroids. In R.H. Strauss (Ed.), *Drugs and Performance in Sports* (pp. 59–67). Philadelphia: W.B. Saunders.

170. Blether, S.L., Gaines, S., Weldon, V. (1984). Comparison of predicted and adult heights in short boys: Effect of androgen therapy. *Pediatr Res, 18,* 467–469.

171. Wilson, D.M., Kei, J., Hintz, R.L., et al. (1988). Effects of testosterone therapy for pubertal delay. *Am J Dis Child, 142,* 96–99.

172. Anderson, W., McKeag, D. (1986). *The Substance Use and Abuse Habits of College Student Athletes.* Mission, Kansas: National Collegiate Athletic Association.

173. Yesalis, C., Herrick, R., Buckley, W.E., et al. (in press) Self-reported use of anabolic-and rogenic steroids by elite power lifters. *Phys Sports Med.*

174. Buckley, W.E., Yesalis, C.E., Friedl, K.E., et al. (1988). Estimated prevalence of anabolic steroid use among male high school seniors. *JAMA, 260,* 3441–3445.

175. Newman, M. (1986). *Michigan Consortium of Schools Student Survey.* Minneapolis: Hazelton Research Services.

176. Shaw, J.M., Kolesar, G.S., Sellers, E.M., et al. (1981). Development of optimal treatment tactics for alcohol withdrawal: I. Assessment and effectiveness of supportive care. *J Clin Psychopharmacol, 1,* 382–389.

177. Whitfield, E.L., Thompson, G., Lamb, A., et al. (1978). Detoxification of 1,024 alcoholic patients without psychoactive drugs. *JAMA, 293,* 1409–1410.

178. Stoudemire, G.A., Levenson, J.L. (1991). Psychiatric consultation to internal medicine. In A. Tasman, S.M. Goldfinger, C.A. Kaufmann (Eds.), *Review of Psychiatry (volume 9)* (pp. 360–381). Washington, D.C.: American Psychiatric Press.

179. Miller, J.C., Friedhoff, A.J. (1980). The effect of prenatal exposure to ethanol or opiates on brain catecholamine activity. In H. Parvez, S. Parvez (Eds.), *Biogenic Amines in Development* (pp. 709–723). Amsterdam: Elsevier/ North Holland Biomedical Press.

180. Barrison, I.G., Waterson, E.J., Murray-Lyon, I.M. (1985). Adverse effects of alcohol in pregnancy. *Br J Addict, 80,* 11–22.

181. Shaywitz, S.E., Cohen, D.J., Shaywitz, B.A. (1980). Behavior and learning difficulties in children of normal intelligence born to alcoholic mothers. *Pediatrics, 96(6),* 978–982.

182. Johnston, L.D., O'Malley, P.M., Bachman, J.G. (1991). *U.S. Department of Health and Human Services: Drug Use Among American High School Se-*

niors, College Students and Young Adults, 1975–1990. Vol. 1 NIDA. DHHS Publication No. (ADM)91-1813.

183. Marks, I., Lader, M. (1973). Anxiety states (anxiety neurosis): A review. *J Nerv Ment Dis, 156,* 3.

184. Centers for Disease Control (1985). *Suicide Surveillance 1970–1980.* Atlanta: U.S. Department of Health and Human Services, Public Health Service, Violent Epidemiology Branch, Center for Health Promotion and Education.

185. Shaffer, D., Fisher, P. (1981) The epidemiology of suicide in children and young adolescents. *J Am Acad Child Psychiatry, 20,* 545–565.

186. Brent, D.A., Perper, J.A., Allman, C. (1987). Alcohol, firearms and suicide among youth: Temporal trends in Allegheny County, PA, 1960–1983. *JAMA, 257,* 3369–3372.

187. Klerman, G.L., Lavori, P.W., Rice, J., et al. (1985). Birth cohort trends in rates for major depressive disorder among relatives of patients with affective disorder. *Arch Gen Psychiatry, 42,* 689–695.

188. Friedman, I.M. (1985). Alcohol and unnatural deaths in San Francisco youths. *Pediatrics, 76,* 191–193.

189. Myer, R.E. (1986). Anxiolytics and the alcoholic patient. *J Stud Alcohol, 47,* 269–273.

190. Volpicelli, J.R., Alterman, A.I., Hayashida, M., et al. (1992). Naltrexone in the treatment of alcohol dependence. *Arch Gen Psychiatry, 49,* 876–880.

191. O'Malley, S.S., Jaffe, A.J., Chang, G., et al. (1992). Naltrexone and coping skills therapy for alcohol dependence. *Arch Gen Psychiatry, 49,* 881–887.

192. Arndt, I.O., Dorozynsky, L., Woody, G.E., et al. (1992). Desipramine treatment of cocaine dependence in methadone-maintained patients. *Arch Gen Psychiatry, 49,* 888–893.

193. Kosten, T.R., Morgan, C.M., Falcione, J., et al. (1992). Pharmacotherapy for cocaine-abusing methadone-maintained patients using amantadine or desipramine. *Arch Gen Psychiatry, 49,* 894–898.

194. Moss, H.B., Panzack, G.L., Tarter, R.E. (1992). Personality, mood, and psychiatric symptoms among anabolic steroid users. *Am J Addictions, 1(4),* 315–325.

195. Perry, P.J., Yates, W.R., Andersone, K.H. (1990). Psychiatric symptoms associated with anabolic steroids: A controlled, retrospective study. *Ann Clin Psychiatry, 2,* 11–17.

Appendix

This appendix provides the reader with easy access to major places in the book that discuss the diagnoses in childhood and adolescence for which pharmacologic intervention may be therapeutically indicated. This appendix does not refer to every citation; that purpose is served by the index. We wish to emphasize that the indications and dosages of all drugs in this book have been recommended in the medical literature and conform to practices in the general medical community. The medications prescribed do not necessarily have specific FDA approval for use for the diseases and in the dosages recommended. The package insert for each drug should be consulted for use and dosage as approved by the FDA. Because standards for usage change, it is advisable to keep abreast of revised recommendations, particularly those concerning new drugs.

Acute Psychoses:
antipsychotics; benzodiazepines (anxiolytics)

Akathisia:
anticholinergics; antipsychotics; beta-adrenergic blockers; benzodiazepines (anxiolytics); clonidine

Alcohol Abuse (Chapter 14—Substance Abuse):
antidepressants; benzodiazepines (anxiolytics); disulfiram; lithium

Alcohol Withdrawal (Chapter 14—Substance Abuse):
benzodiazepines (anxiolytics); beta-adrenergic blockers; carbamazepine; clonidine

Anxiety:

> **Overanxious Disorder/Separation Anxiety Disorder:** antidepressants; benzodiazepines (anxiolytics); beta-adrenergic blockers; buspirone; clonidine; diphenhydramine

> **Performance Anxiety:** benzodiazepines (anxiolytics); beta-adrenergic blockers

Situational Anxiety: benzodiazepines, buspirone (anxiolytics)

Phobias: antidepressants; benzodiazepines (anxiolytics); beta-adrenergic blockers

Attention-Deficit Hyperactivity Disorder:
stimulants; antidepressants; clonidine; MAOIs; antipsychotics; lithium

Atypical Psychoses—Schizoaffective and Schizophreniform Disorders:
lithium; carbamazepine; antipsychotics

Bipolar Disorder:

Acute Mania: lithium; antipsychotics; carbamazepine; valproic acid; benzodiazepines (anxiolytics); clonidine

Bipolar Depression: lithium; antidepressants; MAOIs

Bipolar Prophylaxis: lithium; carbamazepine; antipsychotics; valproic acid; clonazepam

Rapid Cycling: lithium; carbamazepine, valproic acid, clonazepam

Bulimia:
antidepressants; lithium; MAOIs; antipsychotics

Conduct Disorder:
antipsychotics; lithium; beta-adrenergic blockers; stimulants

Cyclothymia:
lithium

Delirium and Organic Psychoses:
antipsychotics; benzodiazepines (anxiolytics)

Dyscontrol Syndromes:
antipsychotics; lithium; beta-adrenergic blockers; carbamazepine; valproic acid

Functional Encopresis:
lithium

Functional Enuresis:
antidepressants; benzodiazepines (anxiolytics); carbamazepine

Insomnia:
benzodiazepines (anxiolytics); antidepressants; diphenhydramine; hydroxyzine

Lithium-Induced Tremor:
beta-adrenergic blockers

Major Depression:
antidepressants; lithium; MAOIs

Mental Retardation:
antipsychotics; lithium; fluoxetine; propranolol; naltrexone; stimulants

Narcolepsy:
stimulants; antidepressants; MAOIs

Nicotine Withdrawal (Chapter 14—Substance Abuse):
nicotine transdermal system; nicotine polacrilex chewing gum; clonidine; propranolol

Obesity (Chapter 13—Consultation–Liaison Psychiatry):
psychostimulants; fluoxetine; sertraline

Obsessive-Compulsive Disorder:
antidepressants; benzodiazepines (anxiolytics)

Opioid Withdrawal (Chapter 14–Substance Abuse):
clonidine; methadone; naltrexone

Organic Psychoses (Chapter 13—Consultation–Liaison Psychiatry):
antipsychotics; carbamazepine; valproic acid

Pain (Chapter 13—Consultation–Liaison Psychiatry):
antidepressants; carbamazepine; stimulants

Pervasive Developmental Disorder:
antipsychotics; fluoxetine; fenfluramine; naltrexone; stimulants

Panic Disorder:
benzodiazepines (anxiolytics); antidepressants; beta-adrenergic blockers; clonidine

Parkinsonian Symptoms:
anticholinergics; antipsychotics

Personality Disorders:
antidepressants; antipsychotics; carbamazepine; clonidine; beta-adrenergic blockers; carbamazepine

Posttraumatic Stress Disorder:
antidepressants; beta-adrenergic blockers; clonidine; benzodiazepines (anxiolytics)

Schizophrenia:
antipsychotics; benzodiazepines (anxiolytics); clonidine; lithium

Sleep–Wake Schedule Disorder:
benzodiazepines (anxiolytics); diphenhydramine; hydroxyzine

Sleep Terror Disorder:

benzodiazepines (anxiolytics); carbamazepine

Sleepwalking Disorder:

benzodiazepines (anxiolytics)

Tourette's Disorder:

antipsychotics; stimulants; clonidine; clonazepam

Name Index

Subject Index

About the Authors

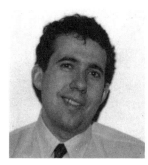

David R. Rosenberg, M.D., is Assistant Professor of Psychiatry, Division of Child and Adolescent Psychiatry, Western Psychiatric Institute and Clinic, University of Pittsburgh, Pittsburgh, PA.

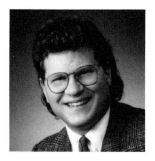

John Holttum, M.D., is Attending Psychiatrist, Children's Psychiatric Treatment Center, Mayview State Hospital, Bridgeville, PA. He has 12 years' experience in basic pharmacological research and studies of childhood behavioral disorders. His most recent work explores the neuroanatomic correlates of autism, for which he was recognized with a Charter Fellowship from the AACAP and the Pittsburgh Clinical Neuroscience Award.

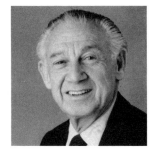

Samuel Gershon, M.D., is Associate Vice Chancellor for Research, Health Sciences; Vice President for Research; and Professor of Psychiatry, University of Pittsburgh Medical Center, Pittsburgh, PA.